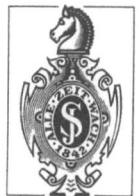

LASER
Optoelectronics in Medicine

Proceedings of the 7th Congress
International Society for Laser Surgery and Medicine
in Connection with Laser 87 Optoelectronics

Edited by Wilhelm and Raphaela Waidelich

With 382 Figures

Springer-Verlag Berlin Heidelberg GmbH 1988

Dr. rer. nat. Wilhelm Waidelich
Professor, Head, Institute for Medical Optics, University of Munich

Raphaela Waidelich
Physician, Munich

ISBN 978-3-540-18130-9   ISBN 978-3-642-72870-9 (eBook)
DOI 10.1007/978-3-642-72870-9

This work is subject to copyright. All rights are reserved, whether the whole or part of the material is concerned, specifically the rights of translation, reprinting, re-use of illustrations, recitation, broadcasting, reproduction on microfilms or in other ways, and storage in data banks. Duplication of this publication or parts thereof is only permitted under the provisions of the German Copyright Law of September 9, 1965, in its version of June 24, 1985, and a copyright fee must always be paid. Violations fall under the prosecution act of the German Copyright Law.

© Springer-Verlag Berlin Heidelberg 1988
Originally published by Springer-Verlag Berlin Heidelberg New York in 1988

The use of registered names, trademarks, etc. in this publication does not imply, even in the absence of a specific statement, that such names are exempt from the relevant protective laws and regulations and therefore free for general use.

2362/3020-543210

Introductory Remarks

Since the 7th Congress of the International Society for Laser Surgery and Medicine is being organized by one of our founding members, Prof. Wilhelm Waidelich, whose experience in organising congresses is indisputable, we can look forward with confidence to a meeting both stimulating and informative whereas Mrs. Raphaela Waidelich will, I am sure, see to it that it will also be most enjoyable.

All this in spite of the fact that, speaking from experience, Murphy's Law seems to apply as much to the organisation of congresses such as this, as to technical equipment.

Judging from the program, many new applications of different lasers will be presented so that one feels justified in repeating what one has said so often even at the risk of appearing to preach: When introducing a laser into one's armamentarium, one must bear in mind the physical properties of the particular wavelength of the laser under consideration in the light of the purpose for which it is to be acquired. This one can avoid a relatively large capital investment the justification of which may result in an attempt to do things with it for which it was never designed.

This will inevitably lead to discrediting an otherwise invaluable piece of equipment, while at the same time undermining one of the main purposes of our society which is to "spread the gospel".

In conclusion, one would like to take the opportunity of wishing the organisers every success on behalf of Masha and myself. I am sure that this meeting will leave us fond memories for many years to come.

					Isaac Kaplan

Preface

With the development of lasers, human intellect has created a source of radiation, for which nature offers no model. The coherence of laser radiation opens up exciting new opportunities.

The most evident and direct advantages of laser technology can be found in the field of medicine. The spontaneous research activities of individual scientists - in accordance with the principles of laser - were stimulated by the founding of the International Society for Laser Surgery and Medicine. The international congresses, which have been held every two years since 1975, act as forums, where experiences can be exchanged.

In the summer of 1987, the 7th International Congress was held in Munich in connection with the 8th International Congress ans Trade Fair "Laser Optoelectronics Microwaves" (organized by MMG). Munich, the capital of Bavaria, is an excellent location for undertaking research into new radiation sources. It was here that Röntgen discovered X-rays, and a basis for medical laser research was established here at an early date.

The 7th congress comprised the entire spectrum of laser medicine. In addition to the classic subjects (surgery, neurosurgery, gastroenterology, gynaecology, urology, dermatology, ophthalmology, ENT), the contributions focussed on basic science, endoscopy, lithotripsy, PDT, cardiovascular, biostimulation.

This book includes the contributions to the congress, providing a "first-hand" survey of the state-of-the-art in laser medicine and showing the future development trends.

We would like to thank all those who participated in the congress, especially the authors and the Springer publishing house, for their collaboration.

May the cooperation between physicians, physicists and engineers lend wings to the further development of laser medicine:
"Lasers for the good of man!"

Munich, March 1988   Wilhelm and Raphaela Waidelich

Contents

Contributors XXIII

BASIC SCIENCE

LASER HOSPITAL -- IT'S CLINICAL AND ENGINEERING RESULTS --
K. Atsumi, N. Nimsakul, A. Ihara, Y. Shiokawa, H. Koyama, N. Suenaga/J 3

REMOTIZED LASER BEAM DISTRIBUTION SYSTEM FOR SURGICAL APPLICATIONS
P. Spinelli, M. Dal Fante, M. Pascucci, N. Ridi/I 7

DIFFUSELY REFLECTING SURFACES FOR LASER SURGICAL INSTRUMENTS
W.-G. Wrobel, U. Fink, M. Reindl, E. Unsöld/D 11

EXCIMER LASER FOR MEDICINE - PROSPECTS FOR COMPUTER GUIDED SURGERY
K. Hohla, H.-W. Henke, J. Pfaff, W. Würth/D 15

A NEW ARGON LASER SYSTEM WITH KALEIDOSCANNER AND ITS CLINICAL APPLICATIONS
T. Morita, R. Tanino, M. Miyasaka, M. Nishimura, M. Osada, K. Iwasaki, S. Shimizu/J 19

THE CLINICAL POTENTIAL OF THE HOLMIUM LASER
I. Kaplan, D. Aravot, S. Giler, Y. Gat, D. Sagie, J. Kagan/Il 23

MEDICAL APPLICATIONS OF KrF EXCIMER LASER
U. Kubo, K. Okada/J 27

COMPARATIVE STUDY ON EXCIMER, CO_2 AND ND:YAG LASER FOR BIOLOGICAL TISSUE CUTTING
T. Yonezawa, T. Onomura, K. Motomura, Y. Abe, K. Mabuchi, T. Chinzei, T. Imachi, K. Atsumi/J 31

NEODYMIUM-YAG LASER AT 1064 AND 1320 NM: LASER-TISSUE INTERACTION AT VARYING IRRADIATION PARAMETERS AND APPLICATION TECHNIQUES
J. Hochberger, Ch. Ell/D 35

PHOTOABLATION THRESHOLD OF HUMAN AORTA AS A FUNCTION
OF WAVELENGTH
G. Müller, H.-P. Berlien, B. Biamino, K. Dörschel, H. Kar/D 38

FIRST EXPERIENCES WITH DISPOSABLE FIBRE DELIVERY SYSTEMS
FOR THE NEODYM:YAG LASER
T. Müller-Schwefe, M. Siemon, M. Thermann/D 42

INFRARED PLASTIC WAVEGUIDES FOR SURGICAL APPLICATIONS
J. Dror, D. Mendlovic, E. Goldenberg, N. Croitoru/Il 45

HOLLOW LIGHT GUIDE FOR MEDICAL CO_2 LASER
U. Kubo, Y. Hashiahin/J 49

MEDICAL APPLICATIONS OF SILVER HALIDE OPTICAL FIBERS
D. Gal, A. Katzir/Il 53

DETECTION AND ANALYSIS OF THE ULTRA-WEAK PHOTON
EMISSION FROM VARIOUS BIOLOGICAL MATERIALS
B. Yoda, Y. Goto, Y. Taguchi, T. Miyazawa, A. Saeki, H. Inaba/J 57

MINIATURIZED OPTOELECTRONIC TRANSCEIVER FOR
APPLICATION AND PICK-UP OF BIOLOGICAL SIGNALS
V. Annovazzi-Lodi, S. Donati/I 61

APPLICATIONS OF OPTICAL PHASE CONJUGATION IN MEDICINE
B.W. Stewart/USA 67

POTENTIAL APPLICATIONS OF LASERS IN DIAGNOSIS AND
PREOPERATIVE ASSESSMENT OF LESIONS USING THREE
DIMENSIONAL IMAGING
R.A.S. Blackie, J. Drinkwater, S. Hart/GB 71

NEUROSURGERY

HOMO FABER AMPLIFICUS LUCIS - STATE OF THE ART
F. Heppner/A 77

LASERS IN NEUROSURGERY - STATE OF THE ART
P.W. Ascher/A 87

THE USE OF CONTACT LASER IN NEUROSURGERY
V.A. Fasano, R.M. Ponzio/I 92

A REVIEW OF 500 CASES OF BRAIN TUMORS OPERATED
WITH MULTIPLE LASER SOURCES IN COMPARISON WITH
CONVENTIONAL TOOLS
G.F. Lombard, G. Mazzotta, E. Gallo Lassere/I 98

LASER-ASSISTED NERVE ANASTOMOSES USING A 1,3 µM ND:YAG
LASER WITH LONG-TERM OBSERVATIONS
F. Ulrich, T. Sander, R. Schober, W.J. Bock/D 101

TIME COURSE OF THE BLOOD-BRAIN BARRIER DEFECT
FOLLOWING LASER IRRADIATION AND OTHER INJURIES
OF THE RAT FOREBRAIN
H.R. Eggert, J. May, M. Hornyak, V. Kallmeyer/D 104

EFFECT OF ND:YAG LASER AT 1.44 µM ON RABBIT BRAIN
R. Martiniuk, J.D.S. McKean, J. Tulip, B. W. Mielke, J. Bauer/Can 108

USE OF THE ND:YAG LASER IN MICROSURGERY OF INTRACRANIAL
TUMORS
H. R. Eggert, J. May/D 113

SURGERY AND PLASTIC SURGERY

THE CO_2-LASER IN CLINICAL SURGERY
PAST, PRESENT AND FUTURE - STATE OF THE ART
I. Kaplan/Il 119

OPERATIVE TREATMENT OF HEMORRHOIDS WITH CO_2-LASER
AND NEODYM:YAG LASER RESPECTIVELY
Ch. Armbruster, K. Dinstl, H. Greiner, A. Tuchmann/A 127

ENDOBRONCHIAL LASER THERAPY IN PNEUMOLOGICAL
EMERGENCY
H.D. Becker/D 130

SURGERY OF BREAST CANCER WITH THE CO_2-LASER -
REPORT ON 449 OPERATIONS
K. Dinstl, St. Kriwanek, G. Platthy, A. Tuchmann/A 133

THE COMBINED 1,06 µm AND 1,32 µm ND:YAG LASER IN SURGERY
L. Horak, J. Fanta, J. Kabat, J. Marek/CS 136

CLINICAL EXPERIENCES IN LASER RESECTION OF LIVER,
SPLEEN AND KIDNEY IN CHILDREN - INDICATIONS AND
MORPHOLOGICAL RESULTS
H. Meier, K.H. Dietl, J. Morcate, E. Unsöld, G.H. Willital/D 138

POSTOPERATIVE ANALGESIA AND ND:YAG LASER SURGERY
K.C. Moore, A. Steger, N. Hira/GB 142

APPLICATION OF THE LASER SPECKLE METHOD FOR THE BLOOD
FLOW DETERMINATION AT PATIENTS WITH ARTERIAL
OCCLUSIVE DISEASE
B. Ruth, D. Abendroth, L. Sunder-Plassmann, W. Waidelich/D 144

TWO STEP EMERGENCY TREATMENT OF MALIGNANT TRACHEAL
STENOSES
H. Seibold, O. Sigg, D. Bunjes/D 148

MORPHOLOGICAL PECULIARITIES IN LASER WOUNDS HEALING
V.I. Yeliseenko, V.E. Normansky/UDSSR 153

COMPARATIVE ASSESSMENT OF CONVENTIONAL AND LASER
TREATMENT FOR SUPPURATIVE WOUNDS
O.K. Skobelkin, P.I. Tolstykh, V.I. Ryabov, V.A. Derbenev/UDSSR 154

12-YEAR EXPERIENCE OF CO_2-LASER APPLICATION IN
SURGERIES ON HOLLOW ORGANS OF GASTRO-INTESTINAL TRACT
O.K. Skobelkin, E.I. Brekhov, G.D. Litvin, M.V. Smoljaninov,
V.I. Ryabov/UDSSR 156

MORPHOLOGIC ASPECTS OF ND:YAG LASER APPLICATION ON
LUNG TISSUE
A. Rolle, E. Unsöld, L. Ruprecht, W. Permanetter, F. Frank/D 159

INDICATION AND TECHNIQUE OF LASERAPPLICATION IN PANCREAS-
RESECTION IN CHILDREN - FIRST RESULTS
G.H. Willital, H. Meier, M. Maragakis, G. Stöhr/D 164

ULTRASONOGRAPHIC GUIDED LASERTHERAPY FOR LIVER
CANCERS - EXPERIMENTAL TEMPERATURE MEASUREMENTS
AND CLINICAL APPLICATION
D. Hashimoto, K. Yabe, Y. Uedera, S. Yumoto, Y. Idezuki/J 168

APPLICATION OF THE CO_2-LASER IN THORACIC SURGERY
H.R. Herrera, J.R. Hinshaw, R.J. Lanzafame/USA 172

USE OF CARBON DIOXIDE LASER IN GENITAL SYSTEM
CORRECTIVE OR RECONSTRUCTIVE SURGERY
R. Pariente/I 176

LASER SCALPEL IN PANCREATIC SURGERY
E.I. Brekhov, G.D. Litvin, A.G. Kirpitchov, V.V. Kalinnikov,
A.N. Severtsev/UDSSR 177

EXPERIENCE WITH THE USE OF CO_2 LASER AND INFRA-
RED LOW ENERGY LASER IN AESTHETIC PLASTIC
SURGERY OF THE FACE
R.E. Amar/F 180

HEMORRHOIDECTOMY AND FISTULECTOMY WITH Nd:YAG LASER
S. Zhao, Y. Chen/PRC 182

THE EFFECTS OF LASER SMOKE ON THE LUNGS OF RATS
M.S. Baggish, M. Elbakry/USA 183

ORTHOPEDY

CO_2 LASER IN ORTHOPAEDIC SURGERY
P. Balasubramaniam/FRCS 187

LASER AS AN OPERATIVE TOOL IN ENDOSCOPIC
OPERATIONS IN ORTHOPAEDIC SURGERY
W.E. Siebert, D. Kohn, S. Breitner, H.J. Refior/D 191

GASTROENTEROLOGY

ENDOSCOPIC LASER TREATMENT IN THE GASTROINTESTINAL
TRACT - STATE OF THE ART
P. Kiefhaber, K. Kiefhaber, G. Nath/D 199

ENDOSCOPIC Nd:YAG LASERTHERMIA: EXPERIMENTAL STUDY
ON CARCINOMA-BEARING BDF_1 MICE
N. Kanemaki, H. Tsunekawa, C. Brünger, M. Nishida, H. Nishikawa,
H. Kato, K. Hattori, N. Daikuzono/J 200

ENDOSCOPIC Nd:YAG LASERTHERMIA IN DEPRESSED EARLY
GASTRIC CARCINOMA
C. Brünger, H. Tsunekawa, N. Kanemaki, M. Nishida, H. Nishikawa,
H. Kato, K. Hattori, N. Daikuzono/J 204

PSYCHOLOGICAL AND QUALITY OF LIFE ANALYSIS OF THE
PALLIATIVE TREATMENT OF OESOPHAGEAL CANCER
H. Barr, N. Krasner/GB 208

Nd:YAG LASER TREATMENT OF MALIGNANT GASTRO-
INTESTINAL TUMORS
K. Dittrich, Ch. Armbruster, K. Dinstl, H. Günter/A 211

CLINIC EXPERIENCE IN ENDOSCOPIC YAG-LASER THERAPY
FOR LARGE INTESTINAL POLYPS
Wang Rui-zhong, Wang Zhen-he, Wang Shu-shen, Bai Yu-gang/PRC 215

NEW VASCULAR OCCLUSION METHOD WITH LATERAL LASER
AIMING PROBE
D. Hashimoto, H. Koyama, K. Yabe, Y. Uedera, S. Yumoto, Y. Idezuki/J . . 218

Nd:YAG LASER IN THE MANAGEMENT OF GASTROINTESTINAL
BLEEDING IN RELATION TO INTENSITY
B. Jereb, R. Pulanić, V. Salamon, M. Rosandić-Pilaš, B. Vucelić,
N. Hadžić, S. Knežević, V. Borčić, F. Golem/Y 222

LASERS IN RECTOSIGMOID TUMORS
J.M. Brunetaud, V. Maunoury, J.P. Ancelin, D. Cochelard,
A. Cortot, J.C. Paris/F 226

ENDOSCOPIC ELECTRIC SURGERY AND Nd:YAG LASER THERAPY
FOR GASTROINTESTINAL CANCERS
K.L. Wu, T.C. Cheng/ROC 230

BLEEDING ULCERS - RESULTS WITH Nd-YAG LASER
COAGULATION
H. Schönekäs/D 233

Nd:YAG LASER TREATMENT IN EARLY GASTRIC CANCER IN
OUR INSTITUTION
H. Fujimura, I. Tanabe, T. Otani, T. Aibe, T. Noguchi, Y. Okazaki,
T. Takemoto, S. Kawamura, S. Ariyama, T. Sasayama, M. Tanabe,
H. Kawano/J 237

Nd:YAG LASER WITH WATER JET STREAM - A NEW TRANSMISSION
SYSTEM WITH A WATER-GUIDED LASER BEAM
R. Sander, H. Poesl, F. Frank, P. Meister, M. Strobel, A. Spuhler,
E. Unsöld/D 241

LASER TREATMENT OF COLORECTAL TUMORS - INITIAL
RESULTS OF CLINICAL STUDIES WITH THE Nd:YAG LASER,
WAVELENGTH 1318 NM
R. Sander, H. Poesl, A. Spuhler, M. Strobel, E. Unsöld/D 245

LASER TREATMENT OF A STENOSIS AFTER CONTINUITY
RESECTION OF THE COLON
T. Müller-Schwefe, P. Dreverhoff/D 249

GYNECOLOGY

LASER DIAGNOSTIC CYLINDRICAL EXCISION VERSUS COLD KNIFE
CONIZATION - A CLINICAL EXPERIENCE OF 60 CASES
A. C. Wang, T.Z. Chang, S. Hsueh, M.C. Kao/ROC 253

CO_2 LASER-APPLICATION IN THE LOWER FEMALE GENITALTRACT
FOR TREATMENT OF CERVICAL INTRAEPITHELIAL NEOPLASIA,
BARTHOLIN DUCT CYSTS AND CONDYLOMATA ACUMINATA
U. Heckmann/D. 255

NEW METHODS IN TREATMENT OF THE PORTIO DYSPLASIAS BY
CARBON DIOXIDE LASER
L. Kovacs, A. Bartsch, P. Unk/H 257

IMMEDIATE, SHORT AND LONG-TERM EFFECTS OF CO_2 LASER
THERAPY ON CERVICAL EPITHELIUM
G.H. Faktor, E. Avram/Il 262

TREATMENT OF CONDYLOMATA ACUMINATA BY MEANS OF
CO_2 LASER
A. Bartsch, L. Kovacs/H 265

THE USE OF CONTACT LASER PROBE IN GYNECOLOGICAL
ENDOSCOPY
J. Keckstein, A.S. Wolf, R. Steiner/D 269

THE Nd:YAG LASER-SAPPHIRE TIP IN REPRODUCTIVE SURGERY -
A PRELIMINARY REPORT
D. Wallwiener, A. Morawski, D. Pollmann, G. Bastert/D 273

SAPPHIRE TIP IN TREATMENT OF RECURRENCE OF BREAST
CANCER OF THE VULVA AND TUMOR REDUCTION
A. Morawski, D. Wallwiener, G. Bastert/D 276

Nd:YAG LASER-SAPPHIRE TIP IN OPERATIVE HYSTEROSCOPY -
A PRELIMINARY REPORT
A. Morawski, D. Wallwiener, G. Bastert/D 279

HISTOLOGICAL DIFFERENCES IN THE TISSUE-EFFECT; AS WELL AS
THE HEALING PROCESS AFTER THE UTEROTOMY PERFORMED ON
RATS WITH THE USE OF CO_2 LASER (SHARPLAN 1060) -
SUPER-PULSED WAVE VERSUS CONTINUOUS WAVE
D. Wallwiener, A. Morawski, R. Damböck, G. Bastert/D 282

COMPLEMENTARY LASER APPLICATION IN GYNAECOLOGY
U. Herrmann/DDR. 285

CLINICAL EXPERIENCE ON CO_2 LASER-TREATMENT OF VAGINAL
AND VULVAL DISEASES
W. Albrich, A. Götz, H. Hepp, K. Richter, W. Waidelich/D 291

LASER TECHNIQUE FOR NON-SURGICAL FEMALE STERILIZATION
AND REVERSAL OF STERILIZATION BY TISSUE WELDING
E. Lachman, A. Shulman, C. Bahari, D. Aravot, S. Giler,
I. Kaplan, D. Sagie, J. Kagan, Y. Kalisky/Il 297

UROLOGY

LASERS IN UROLOGY - STATE OF THE ART
A. Hofstetter/D 303

LASER ASSISTED URETHROTOMIA INTERNA
A. Schilling, A. Friesen, R. Böwering/D 309

CONTACT Nd:YAG LASER SURGERY IN UROLOGY
E.J. Sacknoff/USA 313

VALUE OF THE NEODYMIUM:YAG LASER IN THE THERAPY OF
PENILE CARCINOMA
K.H. Rothenberger/D 317

INDURATIO PENIS PLASTICA: LASER-CHEMO-THERAPEUTIC
TREATMENT
M. D'Ovidio, G. Leonelli/I 322

TRANSURETHRAL LASER SURGERY FOR BLADDER TUMOR.
WITH REFERENCE TO TUMOR RECURRENCE
K. Okada, S. Kiyotaki, H. Asaoka, A. Nakano/J 323

ARGONLASER-URETHROTOMY IN MALE: RESULTS AND
PROBLEMS
H.D. Nöske, J. Kraushaar, M. Wolf, C.F. Rothauge/D 327

ENDOSCOPIC YAG-LASER THERAPY FOR LOCALISED CARCINOMA
OF THE PROSTATE
T.A. Mc Nicholas, C. Charig, S.St.C. Carter, J.E.A. Wickham,
E.P.N. O'Donoghue/GB 329

CARCINOMA OF THE PENIS TREATED WITH THE NEODYMIUM:YAG LASER
R. Malloy, A.J. Wein, V.L. Carpiniello/USA 332

ULTRASOUND GUIDED LASERTREATMENT OF UROTHELIAL
TUMORS
A. Baumüller, R. Vannahme/D 336

HISTOPATHOLOGICAL FINDINGS OF BIOPSIES GAINED FROM
UROTHELIAL TUMORS FOLLOWING LASER THERAPY
G.E. Schubert, A. Baumüller, R. Sonnenberg/D 338

LASER APPLICATION IN PEDIATRIC UROLOGY
H.-P. Berlien, W. Biewald, J. Waldschmidt, G. Müller/D 341

COMPARATIVE STUDY OF MICROVASCULAR ANASTOMOSIS
USING A CO_2 LASER, A NEODYMIUM:YAG LASER AND
CONVENTIONAL SUTURE TECHNIQUES
R.A. Bürger, C.-D. Gerharz, P. Küppers, U. Engelmann,
R. Hohenfellner/D 345

LASER SURGERY OF THE BLADDER NECK AND PROSTATE
R.S. Warner, M.S. Cohen/USA 349

LASER NEONYDIUM YAG IN UROLOGY
R.A. Olmedo, P.M. Minuzzi, P.G. Minuzzi, F.G. Minuzzi,
S.I. Minuzzi, J.A. Saenz/Arg 355

LITHOTRIPSY

LASER-INDUCED SHOCK WAVE LITHOTRIPSY (LISL)-BIOLOGIC
EFFECTS AND FIRST CLINICAL APPLICATION
R. Hofmann, R. Hartung, H. Schmidt-Kloiber, E. Reichel/D 361

LASER LITHOTRIPSY: MEASUREMENT OF PRESSURE AND
SHOCK-WAVES IN STONES
Th. Meier, E. Keckeis, R. Steiner/D 365

LASER INDUCED SHOCKWAVES FOR MEDICAL APPLICATIONS
E. Steiger, W. Uebelacker/D 369

PHYSICAL FOUNDATIONS OF THE LASER-INDUCED SHOCKWAVE
LITHOTRIPSY (LISL)
E. Reichel, H. Schmidt-Kloiber, H. Schöffmann, G. Dohr,
R. Hofmann, R. Hartung/A 375

LASER FRAGMENTATION OF URINARY CALCULI:
IN VITRO STUDIES
R. Friedrichs, R. Poprawe, R. Kohnemann, W. Schäfer, H. Rübben/D . . . 380

LASER-INDUCED SHOCK WAVE LITHOTRIPSY (LISL)
N. Schmeller, A. Hofstetter, J. Pensel, F. Frank, F. Wondrazek/D . . . 384

LASER LITHOTRIPSY OF GALLSTONES BY MEANS OF PULSED
Nd:YAG LASERS
Ch. Ell, J. Hochberger, D. Müller, G. Lux, L. Demling/D 386

GALLSTONE - LITHOTRIPSY BY PULSED Nd:YAG LASER
H. Wenk, V. Lange, K.O. Möller, F.W. Schildberg, A. Hofstetter/D 389

ENT

LASER SURGERY - ENT (UPPER AERO-DIGESTIVE TRACT) -
STATE OF THE ART
W. Steiner/D 395

ENDOSCOPIC THERAPY OF LARYNGEAL CARCINOMAS WITH
THE CO_2 LASER
H. Rudert/D 398

VAPORIZATION OF ORO-PHARYNGEAL LYMPHOID TISSUES -
INDICATIONS, TECHNIQUES AND RESULTS IN 40 CASES
M. Remacle, M. Hamoir, P. Van Heule, Y. Fredericks, B. Bertrand/B . . . 401

BENEFIT AND RISKS OF LASER SURGERY IN CARCINOMAS
OF THE LARYNX AND PHARYNX
T. Lenarz, J. Haels/D 404

LASER TURBINECTOMY
R.A. Kirschner/USA 407

CO_2 LASER MICROSURGERY IN CHOANAL ATRESIA -
HOW TO PROTECT THE ALAR SKIN FROM BURNING
B. Bertrand, Ph. Eloy, M. Remacle/B 410

USE OF A MICROSPOT MICROMANIPULATOR FOR CO_2 LASER
SURGERY IN OTOLARYNGOLOGY
S.M. Shapshay, R. Wallace, J.F. Kveton, R. Hybels, R.K. Bohigian,
S. Setzer/USA 411

ROLE OF LASER SURGERY IN THE MANAGEMENT OF
RECURRENT MALIGNANCIES AT THE BASE OF SKULL
N. Kunaratnam/FRCS 412

REFORM OF TRADITIONAL TREATMENT OF NASAL POLYPS BY
USING LASER
De Min Liu, Hong Deng, Pei Zhong Wang/PRC 413

ORAL SURGERY

PROGRESS REPORT ON LASER THERAPY IN ORAL AND
MAXILLO-FACIL SURGERY
H.-H. Horch, M. Herzog/D 417

THE CARBON DIOXIDE LASER IN ORAL SURGERY
S. Barak, I. Kaplan, I. Rosenblum/Il 422

SOCIO-ECONOMIC APPRAISAL OF DENTAL TREATMENT
USING CO_2 LASER
F. Melcer, J. Melcer, J.Dejardin/F 428

THE ADVANTAGES OF THE CO_2 LASER BEAM IN INTENTIONAL
REPLANTATION, IMPLANTATION
J. Melcer, F. Melcer, Ph. Tardieu, J.-P. Brun/F 430

CONVENTIONAL AND Nd:YAG LASER HYPERTHERMIA
(LASERTHERMIA): EFFECTS ON RABBIT TONGUE TISSUE
Y. Watanabe, H. Tsunekawa, K. Takeuchi, H. Okumura, K. Fujitsuka,
S. Kitayama, T. Toyoda, Y. Kameyama, K. Hiranuma, C. Brünger/J 433

NEODYNIUM:YAG LASER IN ORAL CANCER
REPORT OF 200 CASES - MINIMUM FOLLOW UP OF ONE YEAR
D.D. Patel/In 437

THERMAL COMBINATION OF DENTAL ALLOYS WITH A
COMMERCIAL Nd:GLASS COMPACT-LASER
T. Kasenbacher, E. Dielert/D 440

CARDIOLOGY / ANGIOLOGY

APPLICABILITY OF 10 WATT ARGON-LASER TO RECANALISATION
OF OBLITERATED ARTERIAL SEGMENTS
C. Norden, F. Dähne, St. Müller, H. Heine, W. Ebert/DDR 445

CARDIOVASCULAR STABILITY DURING CONTACT Nd:YAG LASER
SURGERY IN THE ABDOMINAL CAVITY
K.C. Moore, A. Steger, N. Hira/GB 448

FUNDAMENTAL RESEARCH IN LASER ANGIOPLASTY(1):
EFFECTS OF Nd:YAG, ARGON-ION AND EXCIMER LASERS ON
HUMAN AORTIC WALL WITH OR WITHOUT ATHEROMATOUS PLAQUE
M. Iwasaki, K. Kamiya, A. Ueno/J 451

MORPHOLOGICAL BASIS FOR LASER ISOLATION OF THE ECTOPIC
FOCI IN ATRIA
V.A. Obelienius, A.J. Knepa, E.J. Burneckis/UDSSR 455

ENERGY THRESHOLD FOR ARGON LASER ABLATION OF
ARTERIAL PLAQUE
R.W. Gammon, K.R. Fox, A.A. Coster/USA 459

AN EVALUATION OF PROSTAGLANDIN ACTIVITY AND
PATHOLOGIC CHANGES FOLLOWING CARBON DIOXIDE
LASER ENDARTERECTOMY
F.W. Gamache, B. Weksler, D. Alonso/USA 463

LASER APPLICATION IN THE FIELDS OF CARDIOVASCULAR
SURGERY; EXPERIMENTAL AND CLINICAL STUDIES
M. Okada, Y. Tsuji, M. Yoshida, K. Shimizu, H. Ikuta, H. Horii, K. Nakamura/J . 466

LASER ANGIOPLASTY BY MEANS OF SAPPHIRE CONTACT PROBE
J. Lammer, E. Pilger, H. Shreyer, P.W. Ascher/A 477

OPHTHALMOLOGY

THE USE OF Nd:YAG LASER IN THE TREATMENT OF
HYPERPLASTIC PERSISTENT PUPILLARY MEMBRANE
C.L. Lin, J.K. Wu, J.H. Liu/ROC 485

INTRAOCULAR MICROSURGERY BY SHORTPULSED Nd:YAG
LASER EFFECTS, CLINICAL APPLICATION AND ITS
MICROSURGICAL ALTERNATIVES
V.-P. Gabel, R. Birngruber/D 489

INFRARED VERSUS VISIBLE LASER PHOTOCOAGULATION
IN THE TREATMENT OF SPECIFIC EYE DISEASES
B. Lorenz, R. Birngruber/D 493

THE ROLE OF HEAT DISSIPATION IN LIVING TISSUE DURING
AND AFTER LASER EXPOSURE
R. Birngruber, V.-P. Gabel, B. Lorenz/D 497

OUR CLINICAL EXPERIENCE WITH THE NEW SCANNING LASER
OPHTHALMOSCOPE - A PRELIMINARY REPORT
M. Mertz, E. Fabian, Chr. Foos/D 500

INTERACTION OF Q-SWITCHED AND MODE-LOCKED Nd:YAG LASER
PULSED WITH OCULAR MEDIA: AN EXPERIMENTAL ANALYSIS
C.A. Sacchi, F. Docchio/I 505

INTRAOCULAR PRESSURE CHANGES AFTER Nd:YAG LASER
CAPSULOTOMY
K.S. Wang, L. Wang/PRC 506

CORNEAL LASER TRAUMA
E. Fabian/D 507

DERMATOLOGY

LASER DERMATOLOGY - STATE OF THE ART
T. Ohshiro, R.G. Calderhead/J 513

ARGON LASER TREATMENT OF PORTWINE STAIN,
ITS APPLICATION AND LIMITATIONS
T. Matsumoto, T. Ohura/J 522

LASER TREATMENT OF CUTAN AND DEEP VESSEL ANOMALIES
H.-P. Berlien, J. Waldschmidt, G. Müller/D 526

ARGON LASER PHOTODERMOABRATION FOR CICATRICAL ACNE
SEQUELLA TREATMENT
M.A. Trelles, M. Martinez-Morillo, E. Mayayo, J. Rigau, I. Sánchez,
P. Sala-Francino/E 529

POSSIBILITIES FOR THE INCREASE OF THE COAGULATION DEPTH
IN SKIN WITH THE ARGONLASER
D. Haina, M. Landthaler, W. Waidelich/D 539

IMPROVEMENT OF THERAPY RESULTS IN TREATMENT OF PORT
WINE STAINS WITH THE ARGONLASER
D. Haina, W. Seipp, M. Landthaler, W. Waidelich/D 543

NEW LIGHT GUIDE WITH A SAPPHIRE TIP FOR THE ARGON LASER
M. Landthaler, D. Haina, E. Weimel, W. Waidelich, O. Braun-Falco/D ... 547

A COMPARATIVE STUDY OF THE WAVELENGTH DEPENDENT EFFECT
OF THE ARGON, Nd:YAG AND CO_2 LASERS IN ddY MOUSE SKIN
T. Ohshiro/J 550

EFFECTS OF LASERLIGHT OF LOW POWER DENSITY ON SEBACEOUS
GLANDS
M. Landthaler, D. Haina, C. Ohngemach, W. Waidelich, O. Braun-Falco/D .. 555

LARGE SCALE TREATMENT OF DERMATOSES USING HeNe AND
IR LASER RADIATION
S. Chlebarov/D 558

TUNABLE LASERS IN DERMATOLOGY: DETERMINATION OF ACTION
SPECTRA
A. Anders, M. Knälmann, E.-G. Niemann, H. Tronnier/D 563

MORPHOLOGIC EFFECTS OF SHORT ARGON AND DYE LASER PULSES
K. Klepzig, M. Landthaler, D. Haina, W. Waidelich, O. Braun-Falco/D ... 566

CO_2 LASER MICROSURGERY FOR SKIN LESIONS
G. Bandieramonte, O. Santoro, P. Lepera, G. Fava, G. de Palo/I 571

CO_2 LASER AND CAVERNOUS HAEMANGIOMAS
F. Laffitte, J.P. Chavoin, D. Rouge, H. Costagliola/F 574

DERMABRASION VERSUS CO_2 LASER IN THE REMOVAL OF TATTOOS -
A COMPARATIVE STUDY
U. Hohenleutner, M. Landthaler, D. Haina, W. Waidelich, O. Braun-Falco/D . 576

Nd:YAG LASER ABLATION OF SUPERFICIAL VARICES
R.A. Kirschner/USA 578

POSSIBILITY OF TREATING HYPERPIGMENTED SKIN LESIONS
USING THE Nd:YAG LASER
K. Iwasaki, S. Shimizu, M. Osada, R. Tanino, M. Miyasaka/J 582

Nd:YAG LASER TREATMENT OF TATTOOS
R.A. Kirschner/USA 586

THE PERCUTANEOUS AND SUBCUTANEOUS APPLICATION OF THE
Nd:YAG LASER FOR ANIMAL EXPERIMENTS
D. Katalinic/D 590

NEW DIODE LASER FOR IMMEDIATE PAIN ATTENUATION
FOLLOWING SNOWY DRY ICE TREATMENT FOR NAEVUS OF OHTA
T. Ohshiro, J. Kubota, K. Iwahira, I. Tanaka/J 597

ABNORMAL SKIN MICROCIRCULATORY REFLEX IN DIABETIC
PATIENTS WITH AUTONOMIC NEUROPATHY DETECTED BY THE
USE OF LASER DOPPLER FLOWMETER
L.T. Ho, K.T. Tang, J.T. Wang, H.C. Lam, S.H. Li, L.C. Hsiao,
J.C. Perng, Y.F. Liu/ROC 602

PDT

PDT - STATE OF THE ART
P. Spinelli, M. Dal Fante/I 609

ENDOSCOPIC Nd:YAG LASER PHOTOCOAGULATION IN ONCOLOGY:
A 5 YEAR EXPERIENCE
P. Spinelli, M. Dal Fante/I 618

THE EFFECTS OF PHOTORADIATION THERAPY AND
HYPERTHERMIA ON MICE BEARING SUBCUTANEOUS TUMOR
D.M. Hau, H. Chang, M.C. Kao, H.Y. Hsu/ROC 624

LASER INACTIVATION OF BLAST LYMPHOCYTES BY
PHOTODYNAMIC EFFECT WITH HEMATOPORPHYRIN SPECIES
S. Satomi, Y. Taguchi, H. Inaba, S. Mashiko, S. Sato/J 628

TWO-PHOTON EXCITED VISIBLE FLUORESCENCE AND
PHOTODYNAMICAL EFFECT OF PHEOPHORBIDE A ON
CULTURED TUMOR CELLS USING A Nd:YAG LASER
S. Mashiko, H. Inaba, S. Sato, Y. Taguchi, S. Kimura/J 633

INTRACELLULAR AND IN VIVO COMPOSITION OF HEMATO-
PORPHYRIN DERIVATIVE BY VARIOUS FLUORESCENT COMPONENTS
H. Schneckenburger, M. Frenz, J. Feyh, A. Götz/D 637

DYNAMICAL PROCESSES ASSOCIATED WITH SINGLET OXYGEN
GENERATIONS IN PORPHYRIN SOLUTIONS
I. Tanabe, H. Fujimura, Y. Okazaki, T. Takemoto, Y. Kanemitsu, Y. Tanaka,
H. Kuroda/J 641

AN IN VITRO COMPARISON OF LASER PARAMETERS FOR
PHOTODYNAMIC THERAPY
B.W. Stewart, M. La Plant, S. B. Kim, C. Distler/USA 645

HISTOLOGICAL ANALYSIS OF COTTONTAIL RABBIT PAPILLOMA
VIRUS-INDUCED PAPILLOMAS TREATED WITH HEMATOPORPHYRIN
PHOTODYNAMIC THERAPY
M.J. Shikowitz, B.M. Steinberg, R.L. Galli, A.L. Abramson/USA 650

BIODISTRIBUTION OF INDIUM-III DIHEMATOPORPHYRIN ETHER
IN PAPILLOMAS AND BODY TISSUES AND ITS RELEVANCE TO
PHOTODYNAMIC THERAPY
M.J. Shikowitz, R. Galli, D. Bandyopadhyay, S. Hoory/USA 653

PHOTODYNAMIC THERAPY (PDT) OF SUPERFICIAL BLADDER TUMOR
H.D. Nöske, J. Kraushaar, C. F. Rothauge/D 656

HPD MEDIATED PHOTOCHEMOTHERAPY FOR SELECTIVE
TREATMENT OF LEUKEMIC CELLS VS NORMAL CELLS
T. Patrice, M.T. Foultier, V. Praloran, D. Cloarec, L.Le Bodic/F 660

INDIRECT APPRECIATION OF THE PDT EFFECT ON THE TUMOR
VASCULATURE
T. Patrice, M.T. Foultier, M.F. Le Bodic, L. Le Bodic/F 662

"ROSETTE" ARGON LASER PHOTOTHERAPY WITH RHODAMINE 123:
A NEW METHOD FOR ERADICATION OF MELANOMA TUMORS
IN NUDE MICE
D. J. Castro, R.E. Saxton, H.R. Fetterman, P.H. Ward/USA 663

PHOTODYNAMIC THERAPY OF ORAL CANCER IN HAMSTERS
M. Herzog, H.-H. Horch, Th. Meyer, S. Enders/D 664

LOW POWER LASER/BIOSTIMULATION

LOW POWER LASER IN MEDICINE AND SURGERY -
STATE OF THE ART
K. Atsumi/J 673

EFFECTS OF LOW DOSE LASER RADIATION ON BACTERIAL GROWTH
M. Džinić, N. Nanušević, O. Nanušević/Y 681

PRELIMINARY OBSERVATION AND APPROACH OF THE LASER
BIOLOGICAL EFFECT OF THE IMMUNE LIVER RNA IN THE
ACTION OF MALIGNANT TUMOR
Fu-Shou Yang, Da-Wen Xu/PRC. 685

LOW POWER CO_2 LASER TREATMENT OF THE FACIAL NEOPLASM -
3,000 PATIENTS
Fu-Shou Yang/PRC. 691

STUDIES OF LASER-INDUCED CELL GROWTH WITH YEAST IN
CONTINUOUS CULTURE
A. Gfrörer, J. Spahn, W.-D. Wagner, W. Waidelich/D 695

THE CONCEPT OF "BIOLOGON" AND THE INFLUENCE OF LASER
LIGHT ON VITAL ACTIVITIES
P. Greguss/H 699

LOW ENERGY LASER IRRADIATION PREVENTS THE EARLY
MORPHOLOGICAL AND ELECTROPHYSIOLOGICAL EFFECTS OF
OPTIC NERVE INJURY
M. Rosner, M. Belkin, M. Erlich, J. Friedman, M. Schwartz/Il 703

APPLICATION OF THE CO_2 LASER IN THE RHEUMATOID HAND
H.R. Herrera, J.R. Hinshaw, R.J. Lanzafame/USA 706

Na^+-K^+ TRANSPORT, COTRANSPORT AND CELL VOLUME OF RATS
ERYTHROCYTES SUBMITTED TO HELIUM-NEON LASER RADIATION
H. Juri, J. Palma, F. Frank, R. Lapin, J. Lillo, S. Yung/Arg 707

BIOLOGICAL EFFECTS OF LOW LASER IRRADIATION ON
CULTIVATED RAT BRAIN CELLS
M.C. Kao, Jui-Chang Tsai, Teh-Cheng Jou/ROC 713

IMMUNOLOGICAL ASPECTS OF LASER THERAPY
H. Klima, L. Schindl, D. Adamiker/A 717

LOW POWER LASER RADIATION ACTS ON MAST CELLS
DEGRANULATION
E. Mayayo, M.A. Trelles, L. Miro, J. Rigau, G. Baudin/E 724

DATA FOR LASER BIOSTIMULATION IN WOUND-HEALING
A. Mester, A.F. Mester/USA 731

CLINICAL EXPERIENCE ON MIX HeNe AND I.R. LOW ENERGY
LASER - A REVIEW OF 404 CASES
P. Hasan, A. Rijadi, S. Purnomo, H. Kainama/In 736

LASER TREATMENT OF BACKPAIN AND ENTHESIOPATHY IN
ANKYLOSING SPONDYLARTHRITIS
C. Gärtner, A. Becker/D 742

A DOUBLE BLIND STUDY OF LOW POWER HeNe LASER THERAPY
IN RHEUMATOID ARTHRITIS
Y. Oyamada, R. Satodate, J. Nishida, S. Izu, Y. Aoki/J 747

POSTOPERATIVE HELIUM-NEON-LASER IRRADIATION IN THE
FACE AND NECK REGION
H. Porteder, E. Rausch, U. Jaskulka. K. Vinzenz, P. Schenk/A 751

LASER STIMULATION THERAPY USING A DIODE LASER
C. Shiroto, K. Ono, T. Ohshiro/J 755

TREATMENT OF PERIPHERAL AND CENTRAL NERVOUS SYSTEMS
AFTER INJURY USING LOW ENERGY LASER IRRADIATION:
EXPERIMENTAL RESULTS
S. Rochkind, M. Nissan, L. Barr-Nea, R. Lubart, N. Brusovalnic,
N. Razon, Y.D. Heilbronn, A. Bartal/Il 760

INVESTIGATIONS ON DIFFERENT LASER WAVELENGTHS AND
POWER IN PERIPHERAL AND CENTRAL NERVOUS SYSTEM
R. Lubart, S. Rochkind, M. Nissan, L. Barr-Nea/Il 763

EFFECT OF LOW POWER LASER RADIATION ON EXPERIMENTAL
BURNS AND THEIR APPLICATION IN CLINICS
M.A. Trelles, E. Mayayo, F. Dalmases, C. Romero/E 766

EFFECT OF LASER RADIATION OVER ZUSANLI POINT ON EGG
OF THE AGED
Peng Yue, Gao Hui He, Zhang Dong/PRC 779

PRELIMINARY STUDY ON THE BIOSTIMULATION OF LOW POWER
LASER THERAPY
K. Kamikawa/J. 781

HISTOLOGICAL EVALUATION OF EFFECT OF LOW POWER LASER ON THE
SYNOVIAL MEMBRANE OF RHEUMATIC ARTHRITIS
J. Nishida, T. Iwasaki, R. Satodate, M. Abe, Y. Oyamada/J 784

CONT. WAVE INFRARED LOW POWER APPLICATION
SIGNIFICANTLY ACCELERATES CHRONIC PAIN RELIEF REHABILITATION
OF PROFESSIONAL ATHLETES. A DOUBLE BLIND STUDY
C. Diamantopoulos, O. Emmanouilidis/Gr 788

Contributors

Abe, Y. 31
Abe, M. 784
Abendroth, D. 144
Abramson, A.L. 650
Adamiker, D. 717
Aibe, T. 237
Albrich, W. 291
Alonso, D. 463
Amar, R.E. 180
Ancelin, J.P. 226
Anders, A. 563
Annovazzi-Lodi, V. 61
Aoki, Y. 747
Aravot, D. 23, 297
Ariyama, S. 237
Armbruster, Ch. 127, 211
Asaoka, H. 323
Ascher, P.W. 87, 477
Atsumi, K. 3, 31, 673
Avram, E. 262

Baggish, M.S. 183
Bahari, C. 297
Bai Yu-gang, 215
Balasubramaniam, P. 187
Bandieramonte, G. 571
Bandyopadhyay, D. 653
Barak, S. 422
Barr, H. 208
Barr-Nea, L. 763, 760
Bartal, A. 760
Bartsch, A. 257, 265

Bastert, G. 273, 276, 279, 282
Baudin, G. 724
Bauer, J. 108
Baumüller, A. 336, 338
Becker, A. 742
Becker, H.D. 130
Belkin, M. 703
Berlien, H.-P. 38, 341, 526
Bertrand, B. 401, 410
Biamino, B. 38
Biewald, W. 341
Birngruber, R. 489, 493, 497
Blackie, R.A.S. 71
Bock, W.J. 101
Böwering, R. 309
Bohigian, R.K.
Borčić, V. 222
Braun-Falco, O. 547, 555, 566, 576
Breitner, S. 191
Brekhov, E.I. 156, 177
Brünger, C. 200, 204, 433
Brun, J.-P. 430
Brunetaud, J.M. 226
Brusovalnic, N. 760
Bürger, R.A. 345
Bunjes, D. 148
Burneckis, E.J. 455

Calderhead, R.G. 513
Carpiniello, V.L. 332
Carter, S.St.C. 329

Castro, D.J. 663
Chang, H. 624
Chang, T.Z. 253
Charig, C. 329
Chavoin, J.P. 574
Chen, Y. 182
Cheng, T.C. 230
Chinzei, T. 31
Chlebarov, S. 558
Cloarec, D. 660
Cochelard, D. 226
Cohen, M.S. 349
Cortot, A. 226
Costagliola, H. 574
Coster, A.A. 459
Croitoru, N. 45

D'Ovidio, M. 322
Dähne, F. 445
Daikuzono, N. 200, 204
Dal Fante, M. 7, 609, 618
Dalmases, F. 766
Damböck, R. 282
de Palo, G. 571
De Min Liu 413
Dejardin, J. 428
Demling, L. 386
Deng, Hong 413
Derbenev, V.A. 154
Diamantopoulos, C. 788
Dielert, E. 440
Dietl, K.H. 138

Dinstl, K. 127, 133, 211
Distler, C. 645
Dittrich, K. 211
Docchio, F. 505
Dörschel, K. 38
Dohr, G. 375
Donati, S. 61
Dong, Zhang 779
Dreverhoff, P. 249
Drinkwater, J. 71
Dror, J. 45
Džinić, M. 681

Ebert, W. 445
Eggert, H.R. 104, 113
Elbakry, M. 183
Ell, Ch. 35, 386
Eloy, Ph. 410
Emmanouilidis, O. 788
Enders, S. 664
Engelmann, U. 345
Erlich, M. 703

Fabian, E. 500, 507
Faktor, G.H. 262
Fanta, J. 136
Fasano, V.A. 92
Fava, G. 571
Fetterman, H.R. 663
Feyh, J. 637
Fink, U. 11
Foos, Chr. 500
Foultier, M.T. 660, 662
Fox, K.R. 459
Frank, F. 159, 241, 384, 459, 707
Fredericks, Y. 401
Frenz, M. 637
Friedman, J. 703
Friedrichs, R. 380

Friesen, A. 309
Fujimura, H. 237, 641
Fujitsuka, K. 433

Gabel, V.-P. 489, 497
Gärtner, C. 742
Gal, D. 49
Galli, R.L. 650, 653
Gallo Lassere, E. 98
Gamache, F.W. 463
Gammon, R.W. 459
Gat, Y. 23
Gerharz, C.-D. 345
Gfrörer, A. 695
Giler, S. 23. 297
Götz, A. 291, 637
Goldenberg, E. 45
Golem, F. 222
Goto, Y. 57
Greguss, P. 699
Greiner, H. 127
Günter, H. 211

Hadžić, N. 222
Haels, J. 404
Haina, D. 539, 543, 547, 555, 566, 576
Hamoir, M. 401
Hart, S. 71
Hartung, R. 361, 375
Hasan, P. 736
Hashiahin, Y. 49
Hashimoto D. 168, 218
Hattori, K. 200, 204
Hau, D.M. 624
He, Gao-Hui 779
Heckmann, U. 255
Heilbronn, Y.D. 760
Heine, H. 445
Henke, H.-W. 15

Hepp, H. 291
Heppner, F. 77
Herrera, H.R. 172, 706
Herrmann, U. 285
Herzog, M. 417, 664
Hinshaw, J.R. 172, 706
Hira, N. 142, 448
Hiranuma, K. 433
Ho, L.T. 602
Hochberger, J. 35, 386
Hofmann, R. 361, 375
Hofstetter, A. 303, 384, 389
Hohenfellner, R. 345
Hohenleutner, U. 576
Hohla, K. 15
Hoory, S. 653
Horak, L. 136
Horch, H.-H. 417, 664
Horii, H. 466
Hornyak, M. 104
Hsiao, L.C. 602
Hsu, H.Y. 624
Hsueh, S. 253
Hybels, R. 411

Idezuki, Y. 168, 218
Ihara, A. 3
Ikuta, H. 466
Imachi, T. 31
Inaba, H. 57, 628, 633
Iwahira, K. 597
Iwasaki, K. 19, 582
Iwasaki, M. 451
Iwasaki, T. 784
Izu, S. 747

Jaskulka. U. 751
Jereb, B. 222
Jou, Teh-Cheng 713
Juri, H. 707

Kabat, J. 136
Kagan, J. 23, 297
Kainama, H. 736
Kalinnikov, V.V. 177
Kalisky, Y. 297
Kallmeyer, V. 104
Kameyama, Y. 433
Kamikawa, K. 781
Kamiya, K. 45
Kanemaki, N. 200, 204
Kanemitsu, Y. 641
Kao, M.C. 253, 624, 713
Kaplan, I. 23, 119, 297, 422
Kar, H. 38
Kasenbacher, T. 440
Katalinic, D. 590
Kato, H. 200, 204
Katzir, A. 53
Kawamura, S. 237
Kawano, H. 237
Keckeis, E. 365
Keckstein, J. 269
Kiefhaber, K. 199
Kiefhaber, P. 199
Kim, S.B. 645
Kimura, S. 633
Kirpitchov, A.G. 177
Kirschner, R.A. 407, 578, 586
Kitayama, S. 433
Kiyotaki, S. 323
Klepzig, K. 566
Klima, H. 717
Knälmann, M. 563
Knepa, A.J. 455
Knežević, S. 222
Kohn, D. 191
Kohnemann, R. 380
Kovacs, L. 257, 265
Koyama, H. 3, 218
Krasner, N. 208

Kraushaar, J. 327, 656
Kriwanek, St. 133
Kubo, U. 27, 49
Kubota, J. 597
Küppers, P. 345
Kunaratnam, N. 412
Kuroda, H. 641
Kveton, J.F. 411

La Plant, M. 645
Lachman, E. 297
Laffitte, F. 574
Lam, H.C. 602
Lammer, J. 477
Landthaler, M. 539, 543, 547, 555, 566, 576
Lange, V. 389
Lanzafame, R.J. 172, 706
Lapin, R. 707
Le Bodic, L. 660, 662
Le Bodic, M.F. 662
Lenarz, T. 404
Leonelli, G. 322
Lepera, P. 571
Li, S.H. 602
Lillo, J. 707
Lin, C.L. 485
Litvin, G.D. 156, 177
Liu, J.H. 485
Liu, Y.F. 602
Lombard, G.F. 98
Lorenz, B. 493, 497
Lubart, R. 760, 763
Lux, G. 386

Mabuchi, K. 31
Malloy, R. 332
Maragakis, M. 164
Marek, J. 136
Martinez-Morillo, M. 529

Martiniuk, R. 108
Mashiko, S. 628, 633
Matsumoto, T. 522
Maunoury, V. 226
May, J. 104, 113
Mayayo, E. 529, 724, 766
Mazzotta, G. 98
Mc Nicholas, T.A. 329
McKean, J.D.S. 108
Meier, H. 138, 164
Meier, Th. 365
Meister, P. 241
Melcer, F. 428, 430
Melcer, J. 428, 430
Mendlovic, D. 45
Mertz, M. 500
Mester, A. 731
Mester, A.F. 731
Meyer, Th. 664
Mielke, B.W. 108
Minuzzi, F.G. 355
Minuzzi, P.G. 355
Minuzzi, P.M. 355
Minuzzi, S.I. 355
Miro, L. 724
Miyasaka, M. 19, 582
Miyazawa, T. 57
Möller, K.O. 389
Moore, K.C. 142, 448
Morawski, A. 273, 276, 279, 282
Morcate, J. 138
Morita, T. 19
Motomura, K. 31
Müller, D, 386
Müller, G. 38, 341, 526
Müller, St. 445
Müller-Schwefe, T. 42, 249

Nakamura, K. 466

Nakano, A. 323
Nanušević, O. 681
Nanušević, N. 681
Nath, G. 199
Niemann, E.-G. 563
Nimsakul, N. 3
Nishida, J. 747, 784
Nishida, M. 200, 204
Nishikawa, H. 200, 204
Nishimura, M. 19
Nissan, M. 760. 763
Nöske, H.D. 327, 656
Noguchi, T. 237
Norden, C. 445
Normansky, V.E. 153

O'Donoghue, E.P.N. 329
Obelienius, V.A. 455
Ohngemach, C. 555
Ohshiro, T. 513, 550, 597, 755
Ohura, T. 522
Okada, K. 27, 323
Okada, M. 466
Okazaki, Y. 237, 641
Okumura, H. 433
Olmedo, R.A. 355
Ono, K. 755
Onomura, T. 31
Osada, M. 19, 582
Otani, T. 237
Oyamada, Y. 747, 784

Palma, J. 707
Pariente, R. 176
Paris, J.C. 226
Pascucci, M. 7
Patel, D.D. 437
Patrice, T. 660, 662
Pensel, J. 384
Permanetter, W. 159

Perng, J.C. 602
Pfaff, J. 15
Pilger, E. 477
Platthy, G. 133
Poesl, H. 241, 245
Pollmann, D. 273
Ponzio, R.M. 92
Poprawe, R. 380
Porteder, H. 751
Praloran, V. 660
Pulanić, R. 222
Purnomo, S. 736

Rausch, E. 751
Razon, N. 760
Refior, H.J. 191
Reichel, E. 361, 375
Reindl, M. 11
Remacle, M. 410, 404
Richter, K. 291
Ridi, N. 7
Rigau, J. 529, 724
Rijadi, A. 736
Rochkind, S. 760, 763
Rolle, A. 159
Romero, C. 766
Rosandić-Pilaš, M. 222
Rosenblum, I. 422
Rosner, M. 703
Rothauge, C.F. 327, 656
Rothenberger, K.H. 317
Rouge, D. 574
Rübben, H. 380
Rudert, H. 398
Ruprecht, L. 159
Ruth, B. 144
Ryabov, V.I. 154, 156

Sacchi, C.A. 505
Sacknoff, E.J. 313

Saeki, A. 57
Saenz, J.A. 355
Sagie, D. 23, 297
Sala-Francino, P. 529
Salamon, V. 222
Sánchez, I. 529
Sander, R. 241, 245
Sander, T. 101
Santoro, O. 571
Sasayama, T. 237
Sato, S. 628, 633
Satodate, R. 747, 784
Satomi, S. 628
Saxton, R.E. 663
Schäfer, W. 380
Schenk, P. 751
Schildberg, F.W. 389
Schilling, A. 309
Schindl, L. 717
Schmeller, N. 384
Schmidt-Kloiber, H. 361, 375
Schneckenburger, H. 637
Schober, R. 101
Schöffmann, H. 375
Schönekäs, H. 233
Schubert, G.E. 338
Schwartz, M. 703
Seibold, H. 148
Seipp, W. 543
Setzer, S. 411
Severtsev, A.N. 177
Shapshay, S.M. 411
Shikowitz, M.J. 650, 653
Shimizu, K. 466
Shimizu, S. 19, 582
Shiokawa, Y. 3
Shiroto, C. 755
Shreyer, H. 477
Shulman, A. 297
Siebert, W.E. 191

Siemon, M. 42
Sigg, O. 148
Skobelkin, O.K. 154, 156
Smoljaninov, M.V. 156
Sonnenberg, R. 338
Spahn, J. 695
Spinelli, P. 7, 609, 618
Spuhler, A. 241, 245
Steger, A. 142, 448
Steiger, E. 369
Steinberg, B.M. 650
Steiner, R. 269, 365
Steiner, W. 395
Stewart, B.W. 67, 645
Stöhr, G. 164
Strobel, M. 241, 645
Suenaga, N. 3
Sunder-Plassmann, L. 144

Taguchi, Y. 57, 628, 633
Takemoto, T. 237, 641
Takeuchi, K. 433
Tanabe, I. 237, 641
Tanabe, M. 237
Tanaka, I. 597
Tanaka, Y. 641
Tang, K.T. 602
Tanino, R. 19, 582
Tardieu, Ph. 430
Thermann, M. 42
Tolstykh, P.I. 154
Toyoda, T. 433
Trelles, M.A. 529, 724, 766

Tronnier, H. 563
Tsai, Jui-Chang 713
Tsuji, Y. 466
Tsunekawa, H. 200, 204, 433
Tuchmann, A. 127, 133
Tulip, J. 108

Uebelacker, W. 369
Uedera, Y. 168, 218
Ueno, A. 451
Ulrich, F. 101
Unk, P. 257
Unsöld, E. 11, 138, 159, 241, 245

Van P. Heule, 401
Vannahme, R. 336
Vinzenz, K. 751
Vucelić, B. 222

Wagner, W.-D. 695
Waidelich, W. 144, 291, 539, 543, 547, 555, 566, 576, 69
Waldschmidt, J. 341, 526
Wallace, R. 411
Wallwiener, D. 273, 276, 279, 282
Wang, A.C. 253
Wang, J.T. 602
Wang, K.S. 506
Wang, L. 506
Wang, Pei Zhong 413
Wang Rui-zhong, 215

Wang Shu-shen, 215
Wang Zhen-he, 215
Ward, P.H. 663
Warner, R.S. 349
Watanabe, Y. 433
Weimel, E. 547
Wein, A.J. 332
Weksler, B. 463
Wenk, H. 389
Wickham, J.E.A. 329
Willital, G.H. 138, 164
Wolf, A.S. 269
Wolf, M. 327
Wondrazek, F. 384
Wrobel, W.-G. 11
Wu, J.K. 485
Wu, K.L. 230
Würth, W. 15

Xu, Da-Wen 685

Yabe, K. 168, 218
Yang, Fu-Shou 685, 691
Yeliseenko, V.I. 153
Yoda, B. 57
Yonezawa, T. 31
Yoshida, M. 466
Yue, Peng 779
Yumoto, S. 168, 218
Yung, S. 707

Zhao, S. 182

Basic Science

Laser Hospital – It's Clinical and Engineering Results

Kazuhiko Atsumi, Narong Nimsakul*, Akio Ihara*, Yuichi Shiokawa*,
Hiroshi Koyama* and Norihiro Suenaga**
Institute of Medical Electronics, Faculty of Medicine,
University of Tokyo, 7-3-1 Hongo, Bunkyo-ku, Tokyo, 113, Japan
*Nahtmec Nanasato Hospital, **NIIC

Introduction

In order to use the multiple lasers simultaneously for better treatment, to save the staff and space more effectively, to perform more reliable safety program, to educate and train laser surgeons, physicians, nurses, and para-medical personnels, the laser hospital was planned in 1983.

The challenge to apply high laser technology has been performed in cooperation with the Japanese industries, and the hospital was finally opened in Japan, in September, 1985.

The hospital has been operating well without a major trouble until now, and over three hundred patients have been treated by this system during the last 18 months.

The laser hospital -- Nanasato High-Tech Medical Center -- located at Nanasato, Omiya City, 20 miles north of Tokyo.

In 1985, the first stage of the hospital was started with 300 beds for laser surgery, neurosurgery and cardiac surgery.

1) The Hardware and Software on the Laser System

Two Nd-YAG laser units of 100 watts output, one Argon laser unit of 7.5 watts, and one Argon-dye laser unit of 1.5 watts, are installed in the central supply room in the second floor of the hospital. (Photo(1))

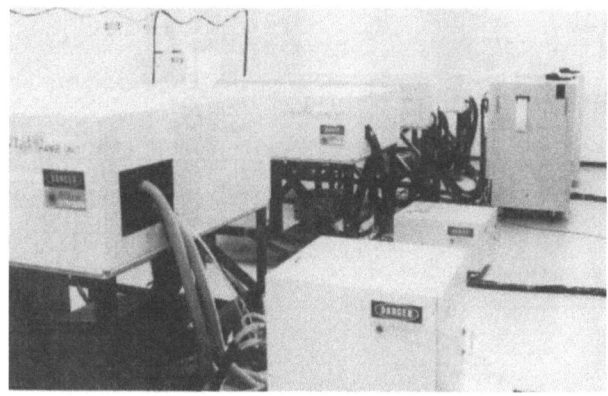

Photo(1)
The two Nd-YAG laser, an argon laser and an argon-dye laser units are installed in the central supply room

The laser units are connected with optical fibers to two operating rooms, and seven outpatient treatment rooms -- ophthalmology, otolaryngology, endoscopy, plastic surgery, urology, gynecology and general surgery -- as shown in the Figure(1). The maximal length of the optical fiber is 100 m in length.

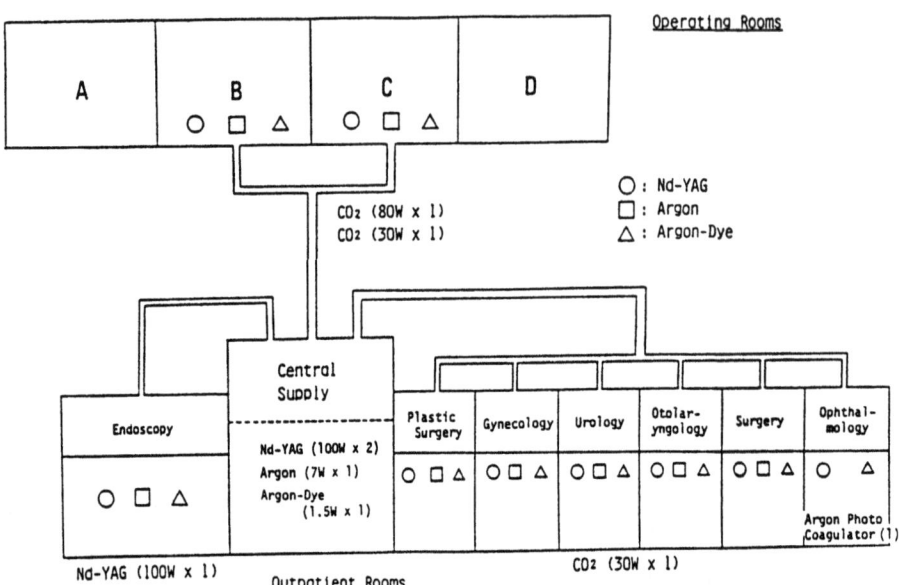

Fig.(1) Arrangement of Medical Laser System in Nanasato High-Tech. Medical Center

Each laser unit can deliver laser beam into the nine terminal rooms by the mechanical switching interfaces, which are controlled by the central computer.

Surgeons can control the laser selection, the output, duration, and scheduling, etc., through the terminals which are connected with the central computer. (Photo(2))

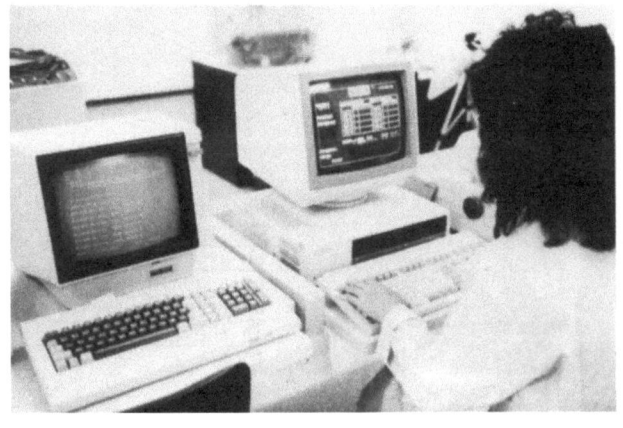

Photo(2)
The doctor and nurse can input their orders and requirements into the computer by the terminals

When the laser unit is occupied by the requirement from a surgeon, the other surgeon can not use the same laser unit, because one unit is to be used only by one line.

However, only with Nd-YAG laser, the surgeon's requirement can be complemented by the other unit.

The back-up system which is essential, when the centralized system is in the trouble. For this purpose, two mobile Nd-YAG laser units of 100 watts, and two CO_2 laser units of 80 and 30 watts are installed for emergency use.

Furthermore, low energy laser units of three diode lasers(30 mW and 60 mW), two He-Ne lasers(15mW) and Nd-YAG laser(300 mW) are used in the pain clinic and in the other application.

In future, gold-vapor laser and excimer laser will be installed for photodynamic therapy and laser-angioplasty.

2) Clinical Application

Up to May 10, 1986, 366 cases have been treated by the central laser supply system, with most of the cases in plastic surgery (147 cases) and general surgery (130 cases). (Photo(3), (4))

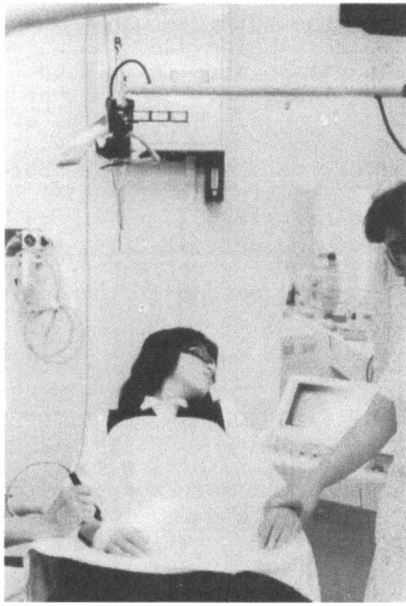

Photo(3)
Outpatient room for plastic surgery.
A patient treated by argon laser which is delivered through optical fiber from the central supply system

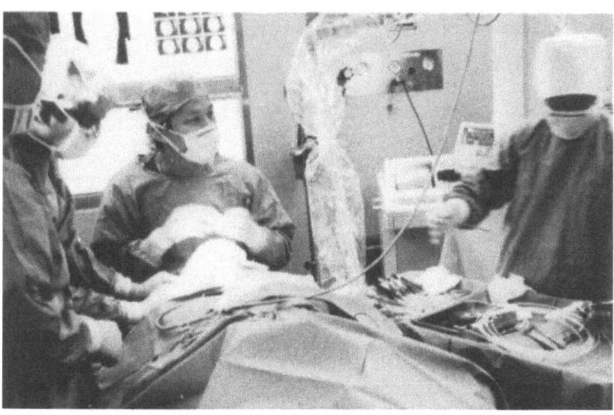

Photo(4)
Surgical operation room.
Nd-YAG, argon, argon-dye and CO_2 lasers can be used simultaneously

Discussion

The central supply system has many advantage as follows.
1. Laser technician staffs can be saved by the central supply system. In actual operation, two full time technicians and one part time engineer can operate the whole system.
2. Installation of the hugh laser units, including cooling system and accessories, can be avoided in the operating room and outpatient treatment room.
   At the laser operation, only the sterilized optical fibers are necessary to be provided.
3. The terminal control unit to input the required data can be operated easily by a surgeon or nursing staff.
4. The safety in the treatment room is reliable, because the room is separated from the laser units.

However, there still be some of the problems as listed below, needed further improvement.
1. At the present, even though the total terminal output of the YAG is 100 watt, and 30 watt is being used somewhere, the remaining laser energy can not be parallelly used.
   If the laser energy of each laser unit can be shared and be delivered simultaneously to the laser-rooms, the efficiency of the laser utility will be improved significantly.
2. Even though the optical fiber for CO_2 laser has been developed technically, but there still remain the financial and safety problems before it can be centralized.
3. The durability and safety of the optical fiber system was approved for one and a half years' experiments. The regular check of the fiber's safety will be one of the most important problem.

Summary

The laser hospital was constructed and opened in September of 1985 in Japan. The central supply system utilizing optical fibers and computer control have been operating well without a major trouble.

At the present time, the experience has been too primitive to evaluate the usefulness, safety, economy, etc..

However, the trial can be appreciated as a mile-stone for the future application of laser surgery and medicine.

Remotized Laser Beam Distribution System for Surgical Applications

P.Spinelli, M. Dal Fante, Divisione Endo-
scopia, Istituto Nazionale Tumori (INT),
Milan/I and
M.Pascucci, N. Ridi, Direzione Ricerca e
Sviluppo, Società Cavi Pirelli, Milan/I

Introduction

The laser technique is continuously spreading among the medical community, but many institutions are discouraged by the cost of a medical laser, evaluable in about 150.000 US$. Furthermore, during a normal operation, the sum of the durations of the laser shots may be up to a few minutes, because of the "dead times" needed to prepare each patients, to aim the lesion with the endoscope and later to disengage the room. Of course, could the system be shared by several specialists in different rooms, these dead times could be cross-linked so not to interfere with each other, and the equipment could therefore be used much more intensely. The solution of a portable laser has a major drawback in the unavoidable misalignment of the cavity resulting from the vibrations and pushes involved in the moving. Our system consists of a commercial Nd:YAG laser, originally portable and now kept fixed, provided with a fiber distribution system of the laser beam to 6 different rooms of the Endoscopy Department of the INT, Milan. In each room it is possible to control via software the functioning of the laser in each detail.

Materials and methods

A commercial Nd:YAG laser, 100 W output, was modified in both the coupling to the fiber and the controls. The coupling device to one fiber is constituted by a special couple of lenses, allowing a maximum loss of less than 1 dB at peak power (about 100 W). Six connectors of this kind are set on a computer driven rotator, and each bears a fiber conveying radiation in a different surgery room. The radiation conveyed is actually made up of two collinear beams, the infrared one from the Nd:YAG and the red one from the He-Ne, the latter necessary as an aiming beam. Into each operating room the fiber terminates into a fiber-to-fiber connector. The distal end of the latter bears a length of disposable fiber and a connection to gas and/or liquid manometers. The fiber is sheated into a thin tube which enters the endoscope: one of the uses of the tube is that of protecting the soft inside of the endoscope from the sharp edges of the fiber and the other is that of conveying the fluids necessary to keep cool and clean the tip of the fiber. The disposable connector is also provided with a sensor revealing the actual presence of both the infrared beam and the red He-Ne beam: should some technical failure occur for which the laser was conveyed in the wrong room, the sensor would warn the system which would immediately turn the laser off. Under normal conditions the presence of the red guiding light (He-Ne) or the availability of the YAG laser is signalled by pulsing lights (LEDs) and the actual arriving of the beam by the usual buzzer.

A computerized system (mP) serves for the remote control of the laser and for the reservations any surgeon may make up to thirty days ahead of the intervention. A terminal placed in each room allows to communicate with the mP and make or change the above mentioned reservations. The surgeon must impost his identification and a priority code for the intervention he is scheduling, plus general information about the nature of the intervention and the identification of the patient. He then imposts data about the room he intends to occupy, the time of the data at which the operation is scheduled, and possibly some data about the indicative quality of the beam to be used (power and lenght of the laser pulses). Whenever two or more surgeons reserve the laser for the same day, the mP proceeds to an authomatic optimization of the schedule, taking into account the "priority" data in the case the schedule presented any overlap of use.

On each day, as soon as turned on from the central terminal, the mP reads the schedule of the day, identificates the room in which the first intervention must take place, and positions the right connector in front of the laser. This is then turned on with the appointed parameters, and then waits for the surgeon to operate the usual foot-switch, which raises the metal shutter blocking the beam from the remote room. The surgeon may of course change any of the required parameters of the beam any times, and does so by means of a small conseole fastened to the bed. On this a couple of kays is provided to increase or decrease power, pulse length, and frequency and the set up values are numerically displayed. Keys are also provided to open or close the electrovalves of the fluids and to stop the laser (a first-level security). On the console several LED's signal the presence or the availability of the beam and the presence of the fluids in the sheath. In case of an emergency, from a terminal placed in each room it is also possible to call for the laser if not already present or to ask for an extended use of the same. This shifts the schedule of the whole day and each room is warned of the situation on its own terminal. In each room is also placed a red button for a hard reset of the whole system should any technical emergency take place. These turn off the power from the laser, and the system does not allow the laser to be turned on again until the several appointed check-ups have been made. At the end of each day a printer documents all that has been done in each room and the same information is also stored on hard disk for future reference.

Results

The prototype system installed serves 6 room 50 to 15 meters away. The energy transfer ahead of the disposable part has an efficiency of at least 80% at peak power. The disposable connection is still under development and these first units cut 30 to 40% of the incident power. The fiber used for both the remotization of the beam and for the disposable length is a 400 micron core PCS fiber (area 0.12 square mm) against the normal 600 micron core (0.28 square mm): the rigidity of the fiber is therefore reduced by a factor two. This fact is a great help in specialties like flexible endoscopy in which a tight curve of the tip is often necessary.

Discussion

In comparison with a portable laser, a system like the one described allows a better utilization of the available spaces, being it possible, for example, to place the laser and the mP in some room unsuitable as an operating room, and leave them there without the necessity of moving anything from one room to another. In terms of technical reliability this brings a certain improvement as explained in the introduction. Leaving the machine still allows therefore for a reduced need for assistance and an increased life of the cavity itself. It is furthermore possible to place more than one laser in the same room (for example, an argon or a dye laser besides the Nd:YAG) connected to a parallel distribution system to the same or to other rooms, creating this way a source room serving the whole department through a network of optical fibers. The next improvement may come from the use of an industrial or scientific laser instead of a medical one: the technical characteristics of the former (power available vs. beam diameter and divergence, and their stability) satisfy much higher standards, and the cost of the machine is inferior. The addition of all the options necessary to dedicate them to medical functions plus the whole distribution system (hardware plus software) turns the cost into about the double of the price of a medical dedicated laser. Such an expense provides the medical institution with an equivalent of six (or more) lasers.

Diffusely Reflecting Surfaces for Laser Surgical Instruments

W.-G. Wrobel, U. Fink, M. Reindl
Aesculap-Werke AG, D-7200 Tuttlingen

E. Unsöld
Zentrales Laserlabor, Gesellschaft
für Strahlen- und Umweltforschung mbH
D-8042 Neuherberg

Introduction

Makers of surgical instruments are proud of the bright stainless steel surfaces of their products. However used in conjunction with a laser such surfaces are a dangerous source of inadvertently reflected light.

As an obvious solution, instruments with a blackened rough finish are commercially available. When these instruments are hit by a laser beam the instrument is heated up rapidly, and not only does thermal contact become dangerous, but also delicate instruments may glow and melt quickly. The ideal instrument surface therefore should not absorb light: it should reflect and disperse it.

For a long time, laser researchers have known that surfaces which appear dull to the eye may still be quite good reflectors at the 20 times longer wavelength of CO_2 lasers.

In conclusion, the ideal surface for CO_2 laser instruments should be much rougher than is required for visible light, and it should be coated with a highly reflecting material, gold (R > 95 % at 10.6 µm) being the best.

Measurement of specular reflectivity

The specularly reflected radiation is superimposed on a diffusely reflected component, the magnitude of which depends on the solid angle of the detector. In order to separate the two correctly, and to measure the specularly reflected radiation only, an aperture was placed in front of the detector a Scientech calorimeter 361 (Fig. 1). The 3 W laser beam (Edinburgh Instruments waveguide laser WL-4)

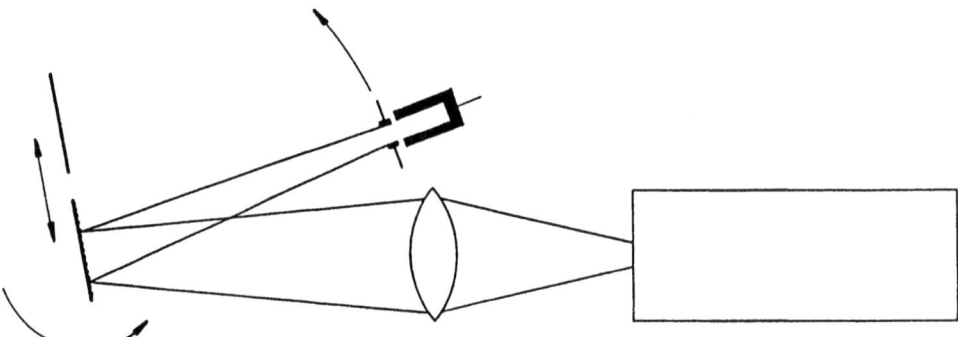

Fig. 1. Experimental set-up for measuring the specular reflectivity only

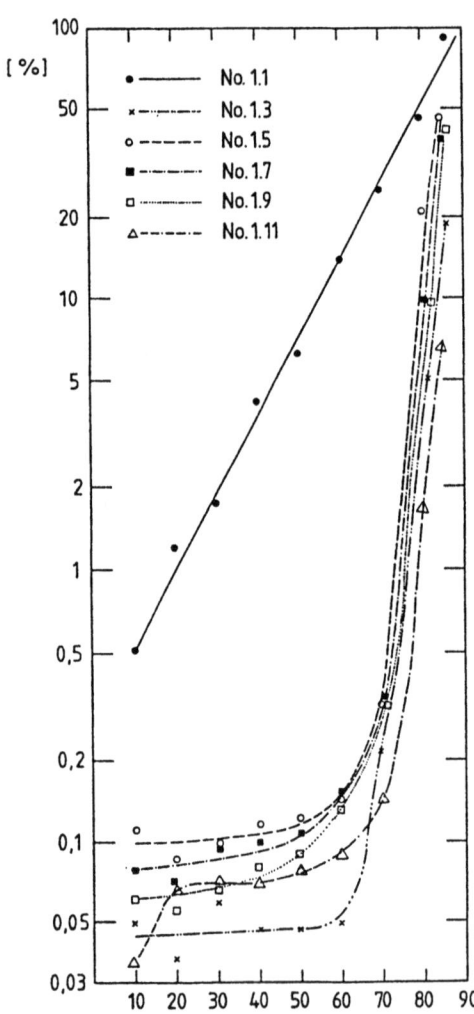

Fig. 2. Specular reflectivity measurements for different samples as a function of the angle of incidence

was focused by a f = 300 mm NaCl lens onto the aperture, with the sample positioned between lens and aperture. In this way, the contribution of the diffusely reflected radiation could be minimized. Both sample and calorimeter head were rotated independently. The minimum angle of incidence was 10°. A gold mirror (R = 95 ... 99 %) was used as a reference for all the measurements.

For the samples, plane stainless steel plates were roughened in different ways and coated with gold (sample 1.3 - 1.11). For comparison, sample 1.1 is the black spatula mentioned previously.

For the gold-coated samples, the reflectivity at near normal incidence was 0.04 % to 0.1 % (Fig. 2), with the surface 1.3 being the optimum. These values are approximately constant up to 60° and then increase sharply because the surface starts to appear "smooth". The black spatula (sample 1.1) has a minimum reflectivity of 0.5 %. Reflectance increases monotonically with the angle of incidence, since the oxide layer acts as a dielectric interface.

In conclusion, rough gold surfaces can reduce the risk of perforation by up to two orders of magnitude for a wide angular range.

Scattered profile measurements

Fig. 3 shows the intensity of the diffusely reflected light as a function of the angular deviation from the specular direction for different sample surfaces.

Sample 1.1 reflects light almost specularly into a narrow cone of a 2° apex angle. The total amount of light scattered in this cone is 6 %, whereas 94 % of the radiation is absorbed.

Sample 1.7 reflects into a cone with a 60° apex angle. In this geometry the specular part of the scattered light is observed as a small peak in the center only.

Sample 1.3 performs even better and approximates a perfectly diffusing Lambertian surface.

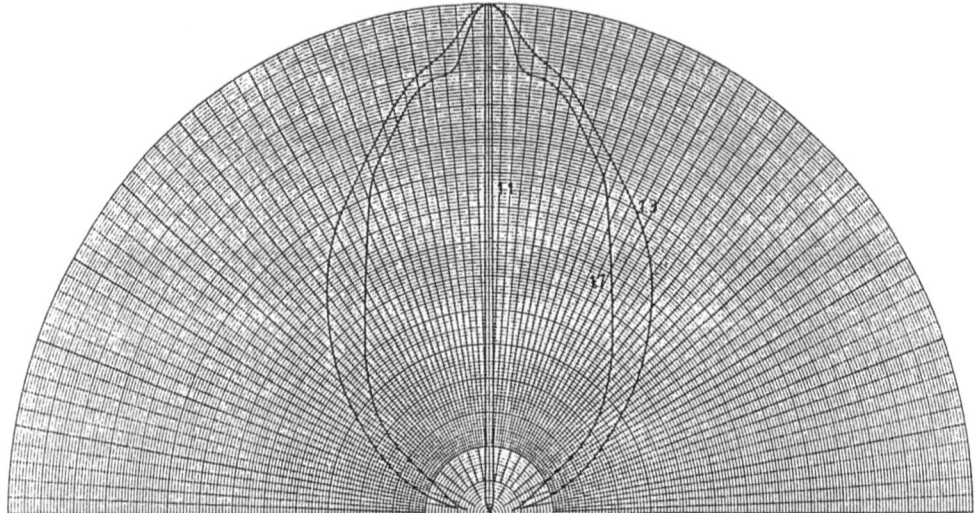

Fig. 3. Distribution of the diffusely reflected radiation for different sample surfaces

Thermal damage

Instruments have a complicated thermal response. We therefore tested some representative Aesculap® instruments with different coatings. A 30 W laser beam was directed on a point near the distal tip of the instruments and the temperature on the rear side was measured. Black instruments started to glow red after a few seconds only and began to melt, whereas gold coated instruments were not damaged in any way.

Possible use with other lasers

We did not measure the properties of these surfaces for 1.06 μm Nd-YAG radiation. It is obvious that they are also useful for Nd-YAG lasers since the 10-times shorter wavelength reduces the roughness requirements, and the reflectivity of gold at 1.06 μm is still quoted at 98 %. However, even diffusely scattered Nd-YAG radiation is extremely dangerous for the eyes. For Argon lasers, gold surfaces are not advisable (R ~ 40 % at 0.5 μm).

Conclusions

We have investigated CO_2 laser light reflection from rough gold coated surfaces. Surgical instruments with these surfaces offer more safety for both, the patient and the surgeon. In addition, the thermal effects of the laser beam do not damage them.

Excimer Laser for Medicine – Prospects for Computer Guided Surgery

K. Hohla, H.-W. Henke, J. Pfaff, W. Würth
TECHNOLAS Laser Technik GmbH
Lochhamer Schlag 19, 8032 Gräfelfing, BRD

A) INTRODUCTION

In contrast to the cutting effect by heat transfer from Argon, Nd:Yag and CO_2 laser beams the excimer laser can remove organic tissue without almost any heat transfer to adjacent material. This ablative effect depends strongly on the intensity of the laser beam at the target: The ablation rate is in the μm range per laser shot, therefore many pulses are required to ablate tissue layers.

Lasers have been studied with a view, not only to their application for removing material, but also to their suitability for identifying tissue material by flourescence spectroscopy. It has been demonstrated that the pattern of the fluorescence is closely related to the chemical properties of the organic tissue. These experiments have been performed with N_2, Argon and Dye lasers at low intensities.

We have used excimer lasers at high intensities for the identification of tissue. It could be demonstrated that the fluorescence light can also act as a fingerprint of the ablated material. It is possible to simultaneously identify and ablate the tissue and to control the laser by the identifying pattern.

B) EXCIMER LASER BASICS

In excimer lasers gases are used as the laser medium. The gas is composed of a mixture of rare gases and halogene gases in which the laser action is initiated by a fast electrical discharge. During the discharge the rare gases are excited in such a way that they start to react with the halogene molecules to form rare gas halide molecules. These molecules excist only in the excited state, that is why they are called excimers.

Depending on the gas mixture within the discharge tube different molecules (excimer molecules) are formed which emit light at different wavelengths. Using Argon and Fluorine with a large amount of Helium or Neon results in the emission of 193 nm. Similarly Krypton and Fluorine gives the Krypton-Fluorid laser emitting at 248 nm and Xenon and Chlorine the Xenon-Chloride laser at 308 nm. Even so other combinations of halogenes and rare gases can also be excited to lase, they play a minor role in the practise. The total pressure required to get the laser action is in the order of 2 to 3 bars.

Excimer lasers are repetitively pulsed to emit up to 1000 pulses per sec (pulse energy of 10 to 300 mJ). The gas within the discharge chamber is degraded by the sputtering of the electrodes during the discharge and by chemical reactions of the halogenes with the wall material. For this reason the laser gas has to be replaced after a certain period of time or after a certain number of shots (which depends on the gas in use).

The optical quality of excimer laser radiation is very poor in terms of "normal" laser radiation. The divergence of the radiation is pretty big because thousands of modes are emitting. The beam cross-section is rectangular with dimensions of about 6x20 mm².

Table 1 comprises the characteristic features of normally used excimer lasers. For special applications in industry or science excimer lasers with higher energies per pulse or other pulse durations have been developed but they are of no concern in the medical field up to now.

Table 1: typical values for excimer lasers

	wavelength	gas pressure	pulse duration	pulse energy	rep. rates
ArF	193 nm	2-3 bar	10-20 ns	50-200 mJ	20-200 Hz
KrF	248 nm	"	"	"	"
XeCl	308 nm	"	"	"	"

C) MEDICAL EFFECT OF EXCIMER LASER RADIATION

Excimer laser show qhite a different cutting mechanism than the Argon, Nd:Yag and CO_2 laser beams which relay on heat transfer. The wavelengths of nearly all the excimer lasers are so short, the energies per quantum are so high that molecules are dissociated by direct bond breaking yielding volatile fragments. As a consequence only directly irradiated molecules are disrupted, the adjacent tissue layers remain uneffected and cold. The ablative effect depends strongly on the intensity of the laser beam at the target and varies between 0.5 and 20 µm per laser shot. The threshold for the intensity corresponds to 0.1 and 3 J/cm² for 20 ns long laser pulses. The threshold depends also on the wavelength with 193 nm laser radiation yielding the smallest heat effect.

D) TISSUE IDENTIFICATION WITH EXCIMER LASER

Lasers have been studied not only to remove material but also to identify tissue material by fluorescence spectroscopy. It has been demonstrated that the pattern of the fluorescence is closely related to the chemical properties of the organic tissue. These experiments have been performed with N_2, Argon and Dye laser at low intensities.

We have investigated the fluorescence properties of various tissue samples under the influence of excimer laser radiation. The purpose of this investigation was to combine the diagnostic properties of excimer laser irradiation with the ablative (therapeutic) effect. In this way the fluorescence analyses of the tissue could control the laser beam intensity and the cutting depth.

The experimental setup to investigate the fluorescence of the human tissue is depicted in Fig. 1.

We use for the experiment the excimer laser MAX-10 from Technolas. The laser emitted up to 400 mJ KrF radiation (248 nm), with a pulse length of 16 ns. This gives a maximum

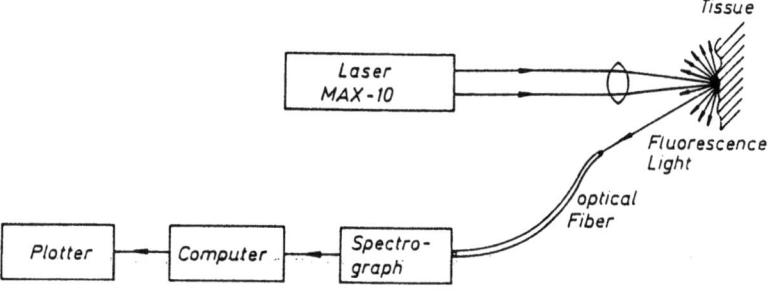

Fig. 1. Experimental setup for the investigation of the fluorescence of human tissue under the irradiation of excimer laser beam.

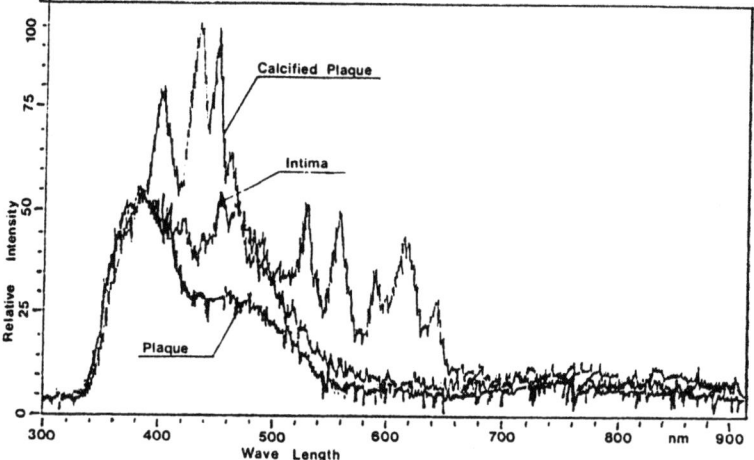

Fig. 2. Time integrated fluorescence spectrum of the inner layer of an artery (intima), of plaque and of calcified human artery tissue.

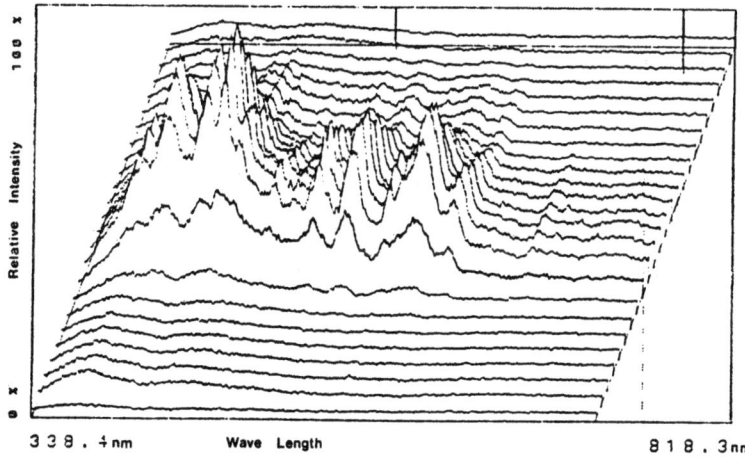

Fig. 3. Three-dimensional presentation of the spectra of the various layers of human artery during the ablation with excimer laser radiation. Each of the curves represent the spectrum of a removed layer of approximately 10 μm thickness.

laser power of 10(7) Watt. The laser pulse energy was monitored and kept constant during the experiment by microprocessor control. The focusing length of the lense to concentrate the laser beam amount to be 30 cm. The laser pulse energy was reduced in order not to exceed 5 J/cm². In this way we assured that the fluence on the target did lay well above threshold for the ablation effect of the tissue. The experiments were performed at repetition rates of 5 shots per sec. The targets were placed in air and no gas stream was applied to the target to remove the degradation products.

To monitor the fluorescence from the irradiated target we used an OSMA multichannel analyzer system (Spectroscopy Instruments). The fluorescence spectrum was analyzed by a 30 cm spectrograph with a resolution of 1 nm. The light was guided by an optical fiber from the target to the spectrograph. The spectra were displayed on a screen and/or written by a plotter. We observed one spectrum per laser shot. Fresh samples of human arteries obtained during autopsies served as targets for the laser beam.

E) RESULTS AND DISCUSSIONS

Artery tissue samples without any pathological changes were given single laser shots, each of which produced a fluence of 5 Joule/cm². A typical fluorescence spectrum of the inner layer of the artery (intima) is shown in Fig. 2. Single shot irradiation of artherosclerotic plaques (without calcium deposition) resulted in a different pattern of the spectrum (Fig.2). Calcified plaques presented quite a different behavior. Strong line emission was observed throughout the visible wavelength regime as demonstrated in Fig. 2. The distinction between calcified and non-calcified material was quite obvious.

In an additional experiment we penetrated the artery with a sequence of laser shots from the inner to the outer layer (Fig. 3). We selected an obviously severely pathological part of the artery wall. Each of the laser pulses removed a 10-20 μm layer of the tissue and simultaneously produced a fluorescence spectrum. The spectra of the various laser shots were recorded and superimposed in a three dimensional representation. As tissue ablation proceeded we observed the various spectral patterns obtained in the single shot experiments. Each of the spectra identified the ablated tissue layer.

The combination of tissue diagnosis and ablation is a unique capability of excimer laser irradiation. The tissue can be removed μm by μm while analyses is done simultaneously. This provides information about the character of tissue to be removed with the next shot. Setups which use the tissue identification can controle the cutting. All this can be done by a computer which automatically compares the observed spectrum with a spectral library. In this way the excimer laser may be the best tool to realize computer guided surgery (CGS).

A New Argon Laser System with Kaleidoscanner and its Clinical Applications

T.Morita,R.Tanino,M.Miyasaka,M.Nishimura
M.Osada,K.Iwasaki*,S.Shimizu**
Dept.of Plast.Surg.,Tokai Univ.,Kanagawa,Japan
*Toshiba Corporation,Tokyo,Japan
**Toshiba Medical Engineering Co.,Ltd.,Tokyo,Japan

Introduction

   The argon laser has become a well-accepted modality for physicians interested in treating superficial vascular cutaneous lesions. It has become well-established and is the most commonly and successfully used treatment. However, conventional practical argon laser therapy for port wine stains is extremely difficult and often results in uneven and excessive local dosage during the treatment and operator fatigue is common, due to small laser beam size and uneven power distribution curve. We have developed the "Kaleidoscope"(a glass light-guiding rod) to obtain a uniform power distribution over the irradiated area and then applied it to the handpiece for a ruby laser system for treatment of hyperpigmented skin lesions On the basis of our kaleidoscope system we have developed a new argon laser system incorporating a kaleidoscanner for treatment of vascular cutaneous lesions.
   The following is a report on our new argon laser system with kaleidoscanner and its clinical applications.

Principle of the "Kaleidoscope"

   A laser beam cross section through a optical fiber is normally circular and has a uneven curve power distribution. This nature often makes it unsuitable for treatment of vascular cutaneous lesions and hyperpigmented skin lesions. To obtain a square, sharply defined power distribution, a "Kaleidoscope"(a glass light-guiding rod) was developed. Fig.1 shows the principle of the "Kaleidoscope". The laser beam is focused by a lens and the divergent beam enters a square quartz rod. The laser beam propagates through the rod, reflecting off the quartz walls several times and emerging with a uniform intensity distribution over the beam

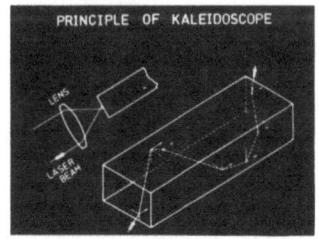

Fig.1. Principle of kaleidoscope

cross section at the end of the rod. Fig.2 shows the beam profiles of both the conventional method and that of the "Kaleidoscope". The uniform square intensity distribution pattern is better realized in the "Kaleidoscope" method. Fig.3 shows the configuration of the new argon laser system with kaleidoscanner.

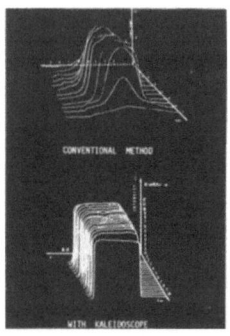

Fig.2. Beam profiles of both the conventional method and that of the kaleidoscope.

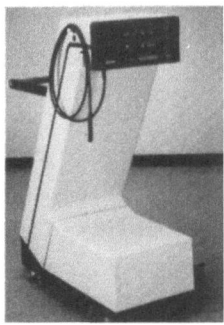

Fig.3. New argon laser system with kaleidoscanner

Kaleidoscanner

Using the kaleidoscope(a glass light-guiding rod), we are able to obtain a uniform power distribution over the irradiated area. The hand held apparatus houses 16 small kaleidoscopes (2x2mm each) in 4 rows, each row arranged 1mm apart in order to treat port wine stains in a striped pattern. An optical fiber is attached to the back of each kaleidoscope. A laser beam is introduced sequentially and automatically into each rod through the optical fibers and we are able to obtain an 8x11mm homogeneous irradiated area by a single scanning. (Fig.4,5)

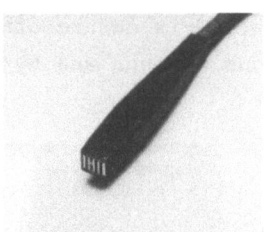

Fig.4. Handpiece of kaleidoscanner

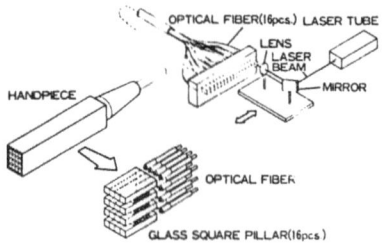

Fig.5. Configuration of "Kaleidoscanner"

Fig.6 shows the actual measured values of output from each rod, which are 4.5W maximum and 4.0W minimum with dispersion within ±5%. Four types of interchangeable handpiece are included in this system:

kaleidoscanner type, kaleidoscope type using a glass rod, two conventional lens types.

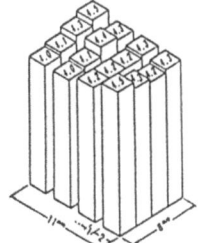

Fig.6. Actual measured values of output from each pillar of kaleidoscanner

Technique

Practical argon laser therapy for port wine stains using the kaleidoscanner is described below. After local anesthesia by 1% xylocaine without epinephrine(general anesthesia in small children), the handpiece of the kaleidoscanner incorporates a template which is applied to the irradiated area and when the foot switch is depressed, the laser irradiation begins to scan automatically. (Fig.7) The handpiece is then moved according to the template and next irradiation is started. We always use a pulse duration of 0.2sec. and output power of 2.0-3.0W.

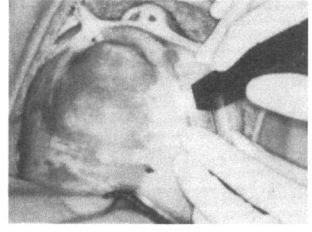

Fig.7. Practical argon laser therapy for port wine stain using the kaleidoscanner

Clinical application

From 1985 to 1987, we have treated 65 patients with vascular cutaneous lesions using our new argon laser system. Fifty-seven patients had port wine stains. Eight patients had strawberry marks and vascular spiders. Thirty of the port wine stain patients were treated by kaleidoscanner. Some representative port wine cases using the kaleidoscanner are shown in Figures 8 and 9.

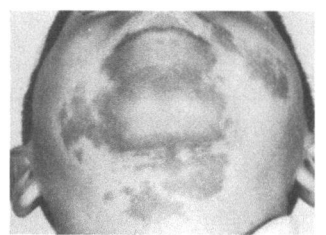 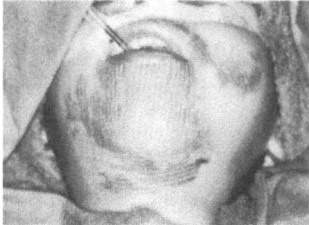

Fig.8. Port wine stain case using kaleidoscanner
(left) A condition after test irradiation
(right) Immediately after irradiation

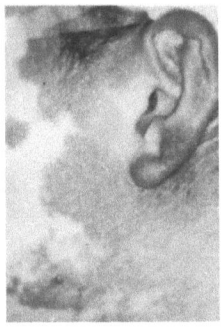 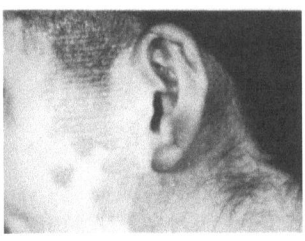

Fig.9. Port wine stain case
(left) Preoperative condition
(right) Condition at 4 months
      after irradiation

Discussion

   Because of the small laser beam size, the conventional practical argon
laser therapy for port wine stains is extremely difficult resulting in
uneven and excessive local dosage in the treatment and operator fatigue
is common. Thus the conventional practical argon laser sometimes results
with hypertrophic scarring and the efficiency is not good. To overcome
these problems, we have developed a new argon laser system which uses
many small kaleidoscopes and an automatic scanning system. This laser
scanning system is called "Kaleidoscanner".
   In our clinical experience, the advantages of this system are:
1. Less complication of hypertrophic scarring through more homogeneous
   irradiation with the kaleidoscope (a glass light-guiding rod).
2. Greater efficiency and less operator fatigue through automatic scanning of a wider area.

Conclusion

   Sixty-five patients presenting a variety of superficial vascular lesions were treated by our new argon laser system with kaleidoscanner.
Thirty port wine stain patients were treated by kaleidoscanner. We have
concluded that the kaleidoscanner method facilitated uniform irradiation
through automatic scanning of a wider area. As a next step, we would
like to collect more basic experimental data and make them available for
clinical application.

References

M.Miyasaka,T.Morita,M.Nishimura,et al: EXPERIENCE OF LASER IRRADIATION
ON THE HYPERPIGMENTED SKIN SESION. Lasers Surg.Med. 7:97, 1987.
K.Iwasaki,S.Shimuzu,R.Tanino,et al: Argon Laser System with "Kaleido-
scanner". J.Japan Soc. Laser Med. 6:339-342, 1986.
Apfelberg D B,Smith T,Maser MR,et al: Dot or Pointillistic Method for
Improvement in Results of Hypertrophic Scarring in the Argon Laser
Treatment of Portwine Hemangiomas. Lasers Surg.Med. 6:552-558, 1987.

The Clinical Potential of the Holmium Laser

I. Kaplan, D. Aravot, S. Giler, Y. Gat, D. Sagie, Y. Kagan
Chilewich Chair of Plastic Surgery, Tel Aviv University
Ramat-Aviv, 69978 Tel-Aviv, Israel

The Holmium Laser has a wavelength of 2.1 microns. This falls between the NdYag (1.06) and the CO_2 (10.6) both of which are established as lasers which have a clinical application.
Theoretically, therefore, the Holmium Laser should prove to be a better photo-coagulator than the CO_2 laser and a better "light knife" than the NdYag.

In addition, the ability to transmit the beam through an optical fibre may well render this laser the one of choice for various endoscopic procedures.

Accordingly a multidisciplinary team was recruited in order to investigate the possible clinical application of this laser which was provided by Rotem Industries Ltd. of Israel.

We would like here to report our experience to date in relation to some of the investigations undertaken in the framework of the above program viz the application of the Holmium laser in tissue fusion and intravascular coagulation.

All experiments were performed on dogs.

The following procedures were undertaken in connection with tissue fusion:

1) Welding of a longitudinal incision in the femoral artery.
   After exposure of the artery, blood flow was occluded with the aid of clamps. Two holding sutures were placed through the arterial wall and a longitudinal incision of 1 cm. made.
   The incision was then welded with 750 milliwatts using the holding sutures to prevent damage to the intact wall by maintaining tension.
   After welding was completed the clamps were removed and the vessel found to be patent without leaking.

2) A similar procedure was performed on the femoral vein with success.

3) End to end anastomosis of the femoral artery was performed again using 750 milliwatts. Approximation of the cut end was achieved by inserting a hypodermic needle through the wall on one side out of the lumen of the same side, into the lumen of the opposite side and out through the wall. The two ends were then approximated by sliding them together on the needle. The ends were then welded and the needle withdrawn.
The anastomosis was found to be patent and the sutures were removed.

4) End to side anastomosis of saphenous vein to the femoral artery, in order to create an arterio-venous fistula.
This was found to be patent.

5) Interpositional graft of femoral vein into the femoral artery.
Thus creating another arterio-venous shunt.
This was also found to be patent.

6) Welding of stab wound of the left ventrical.
An incision 1 cm. in length was made transmurally in the left ventrical within a purse-string suture.
The suture was tightened and the incision welded.
On removing the suture the incision was found to be sealed and the cardiac function maintained.

7) The bile duct was opened with a longitudinal incision 0.5 cm. in length and the opening welded by means of the laser at 1 watt output. No leak of bile was observed.

8) A cube of tissue was taken from the spleen, transplanted into a defect of the same size made in the liver and the capsule welded with the laser at an output of 2 watts.

9) The uterine horn in a pregnant bitch was opened at 2 sites of foetuses, and sealed by welding. At one site the foetus was left and at the other removed.

10) End to end anastomosis of small bowel was easily accomplished at an output of 750 milliwatts.

So far we are able to state with confidence that the Holmium laser is easy to handle and that tissue fusion can be performed with it with confidence. It might well prove to be the laser of choice for this purpose.

THE HOLMIUM LASER IN INTRA VASCULAR COAGULATION

During our various experiments with the Holmium laser in dogs, we were impressed with the ability to perform photocoagulation even in the presence of blood. This led us to embark on a project designed to test the ability to seal blood vessels through a suitable catheter thus avoiding the necessity to expose and tie such vessels. This was with a view to performing non-invasive procedures in order to treat such conditions as aneurisms, patent ducts, varicose veins, varicoceles, cavernous haemangiomas, etc.

The following experiments were performed with the above object in view:

1) The blood flow in the saphenous vein was arrested by inserting the optical fibre through a venous canula and firing a pulse at low power.

2) The femoral artery was occluded by inserting a catheter according to the Seldinger technique, the optical fibre being inserted into the artery through the catheter.
   A pulse of two watts succeeded in occluding the artery both during blood flow and cessation of blood flow.
   Perforation was avoided by the catheter maintaining centralisation of the optical fibre.

3) A shunt was created by end to end anastomosis of the femoral artery to the femoral vein by the laser at 750 milliwatts. This was then occluded by passing the optical fibre through the iliac artery to the site of the shunt.

   It is worthy of mention that the Hene guide light transilluminates and enables one to position the fibre aaccurately.

4) A model of a berry aneurysm was created by anastomosing a segment of the femoral vein to the femoral artery through the stump of which a No 8 Foley catheter was inserted, inflated and tied in position.

One week later the catheter was removed and the free end of the venous stump tied, leaving an aneurysm into which a cardiac catheter was inserted and the laser fired at 1.5 watts. This resulted in obliteration of the aneurysm, the artery remaining patent.

5) A model of patent ductus arteriosis was created by implanting a segment of femoral artery between the aorta and the pulmonary artery.

A cardiac catheter was introduced via the femoral artery into the "patent duct" under direct vision, and the optica fibre inserted through the catheter.

The "patent duct" was occluded with a pulse at 2 watts leaving the two arteries patent without leaks.

The results of the above auger well for the eventual clinical application of the Holmium laser in intra-vascular procedures, where to date, no satisfactory solution has been forthcoming, apart from major invasive surgery.

Medical Applications of KrF Excimer Laser

U. Kubo, K. Okada
Kinki University, Dept. of Electrical Enginerring
Kowakae, Higashiosaka, Osaka 577, Japan

In the laser technology, as new laser it is put great emphasis on development of short wavelength lasers. It is one of the ultraviolet lasers, that is excimer laser, being noticed much lately[1,2]. We will introduce some example of excimer laser and tissue interactions.

Medium	KrF
Wavelength	0.248 μm
Pulse Duration	23 nsec
Repetition Rate	2~200 Hz
Average Power	45 W (Max)
Peak Power	14 MW
Beam Cross Section	7x22 mm

Fig.1. Characteristics of KrF excimer laser

Figure 1 shows the characteristic of KrF excimer laser[3]. The laser medium is Krypton and Fluoride mixing gas, wavelength is 248nm. The laser is repeat pulse oscillation, pulse width is ca. 23ns. The repeat frequency is under 200 pulses per second. The mean power is ca. 45W maximum, the pulse peak power is ca. 14MW, the beam cross section pattern is 7 x 22mm rectangular.

The irradiation beam was focused to line shape by the cylindrical lens.

Figure 2 shows the comparison of cutting surface of the beef with the KrF excimer laser and the cotinuous CO_2 laser. In the case of KrF excimer laser irradiation, not carbonization on cutting surface, it can very sharp cut. This is true of not only the beef but also a bone. It is possible to cut clearly, even a cartilage as shown in Fig.3.

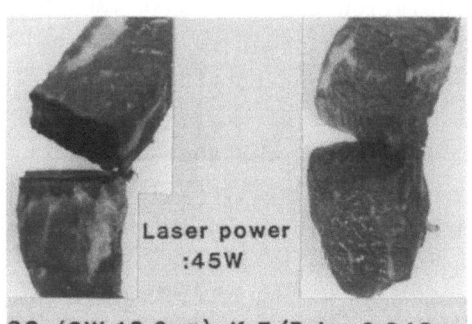

Fig.2. Comparison of cutting surface of the beef with KrF and cw-CO_2 lasers

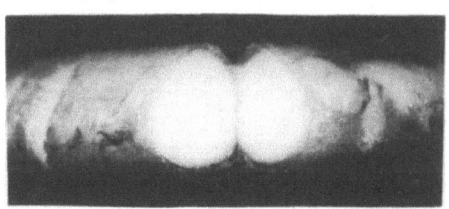

Fig.3. Cutting surface of cow's bone with KrF laser

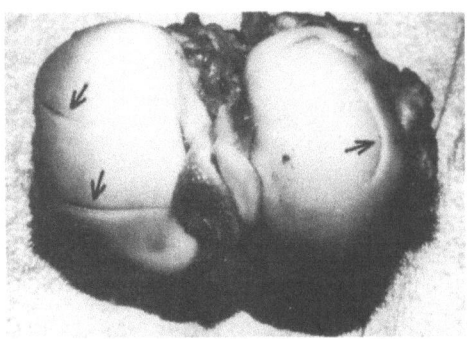 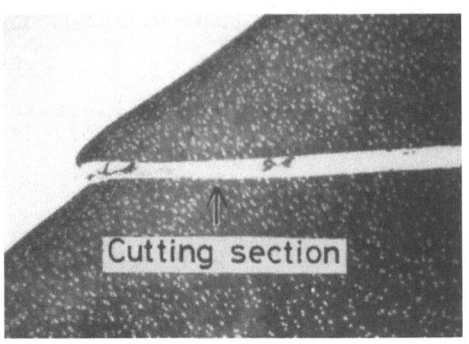

Fig.4. Photograph of pig's articulatio genus used as cutting sample

Fig.5. Microphotograph of cutting part cross section of the sample with KrF laser beam

Figure 4 shows the photograph of pig's articulatio genus as cutting sample. Figure 5 shows the microphotograph of cutting part cross section of pig's articulatio genus with KrF excimer laser irradiation. We found that it was possible to cut it without disorder of bone's cell at around of cutting part.

However, KrF excimer laser dose not have an effect of stopping bleeding. Figure 6 shows the bleeding from living mouse with KrF excimer laser irradiation. Namely, KrF excimer laser is hardly thermal coagulation, so that it is neccessary to find out some applications to use excimer laser effectively.

Main deferent points of both lasers(KrF, CO_2) is absorption by water. As is well known, CO_2 laser is very strong absorbed by water and that resultant water was eliminated by the vaporization. In the case of KrF excimer laser, the absorption by water is very weak, therefore, we have cosidered that the cooling effect of irradiated tissue by water.

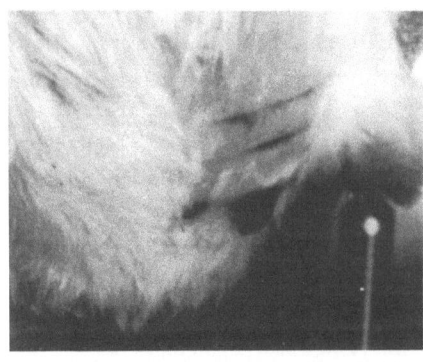

Fig.6. Bleeding from cutting part of living mouse with KrF laser irradiations

On the other hand, the interval of irradiation pulse is most important condition in order to prevent of carbonize about cutting tissue. The intervals of irradiation pulse are above 20ms for the water rich tissue(for example:beef) and above 50ms for dry tissue(for example:bone) respectively. Namely, the interval of irradiation pulse is closely connected with the thermal effect. If shorten the interval of irradiation pulse, a carbonization appea-

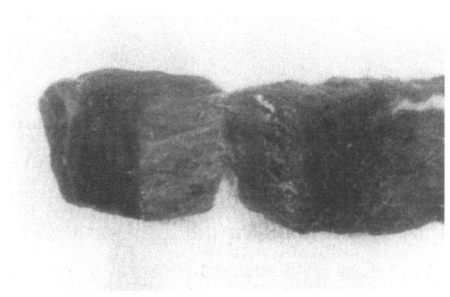
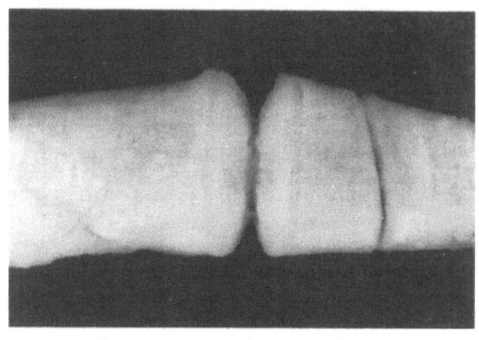

Fig. 7. Cutting surface of the beef with TEA CO_2 laser irradiation

Fig. 8. Cutting surface of the cow's bone with TEA CO_2 laser irradiation

red on the irradiated tissue surface.

An expected finding was made during the very latest experiments. It is the fact that also slow repeat higher pulse CO_2 laser have sharp cut ability to tissue without the carbonization as KrF excimer laser. We have used CO_2 laser that called TEA CO_2 laser[4], the TEA CO_2 laser is repeat pulse oscillation(TEA:Transversely Excited Atmospheric pressure). The maximum repeat pulse frequency is 10 pulses per second, wave length is 10.6um, the pulse width is ca.80ns, the mean power is ca.25W maximum, the pulse peak power is ca.30MW, the beam cross section pattern is 20 x 15mm rectangular. These characteristics is similar to KrF excimer laser expect pulse width.

Figure 7 shows the photograph of clear sharp cutting part of the beef with the TEA CO_2 laser. The irradiation repeat pulse interval is ca.200ms(5Hz). This is true of not only the beef but also a bone, it exactly similar to the case of KrF excimer laser. Figure 8 shows the the cutting part of the cow's bone with the pulse CO_2 laser irradiation. The cutting surface is not carbonized, it can very sharp cut. Figure 9 shows the photograph of TEA CO_2 laser apparatus.

From the present experiments, fact that of following items were clarified. (1)The sharp cut laser is not only excimer laser. (2)The higher peak power

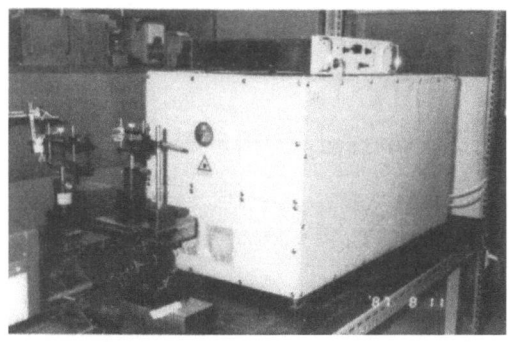

Fig. 9. Appearance of TEA CO_2 laser device (repeat pulse laser)

and short width pulse laser will have the ability of non carbonized cutting. In the details of the laser-tissue interactions by defference of the wavelength is still being studied.

We have obtained the following items as conclusions.

(a) KrF excimer laser(repeat pulse) have sharp cutting ability to tissue.
(b) Repeat pulse CO_2 laser(TEA type) have also sharp cut ability, comparison with KrF excimer laser somewhat inferior cutting ability.
(c) In the present experimental results, both lasers about same ability to the cutting tissue is stand point from the macroscopic view. The microscopic details unknown, this problem will be clarify in the near future(effects of different wavelength, UV and middle infrared).
(d) The medical applications of higher peak power and short width repeat pulse lasers will be become very important in the near future(application of quick photoablation effect).
(e) Developments of UV optical fibers.

There is a close connection between human's tissue and light. Therefore, laser of miracle light gives us new therapy. We belive as stand point of laser physicist, medical application is most important of all. Because it gets most close relation between human and high technology which is the lasers.

The authors would like to thank Mr.S.Yoshikawa, Mr.Y.Kyusho and Mr.A.Wakaiki. This work was supported by Laser Device Division, NEC Corporation and MIKASA SHOJI Company.

References

1) S.P.Kern: SPIE, vol.712, Lasers in Medicine, p.86, 1986.
2) R.G.caro, D.F.Muller: SPIE, vol.712, Lasers in Medicine, p.95, 1986.
3) U.Kubo: Medical Applications of Lasers, OHMSHA(Tokyo), p.59, 1985(in Lapanese).
4) M.J.Beesley: Lasers and their applications, Taylor & Francis(London), p.124, 1976.

Comparative Study on Excimer, CO_2 and Nd: YAG Laser for Biological Tissue Cutting

* T.Yonezawa, * T.Onomura, K.Motomura, Y.Abe, K.Mabuchi, T.Chinzei, K.Imachi, K.Atsumi.

* Department of Orthopedics, Osaka Medical College
Inst. of Med. Electr., Faculty of Med., University of Tokyo

INTRODUCTION

The mechanism of biological tissue cutting was investigated using excimer laser compared with CO2 and ND-YAG lasers. Tissue cutting by excimer laser is different from others. Tissues are cut sharply, and bleeding from tissue can not be coagurated by using excimer laser. No or a minimal thermal effect can be observed from the postoperative tissues. Many hypotheses have been published the mechanism of tissue cutting by excimer laser; thermal effect, photochemical effect, photon effect, plasma effect and others. From thermographic analysis and histological studies, we confirmed that biological tissues are destroyed by cutting organelle, especially mitochondria. Cells and tissue blow out following to the organelle explosion. It is true that the generation of heat causes and sometimes makes carbonated layer. But the generation of heat is the result following to tissue explosion. The energy balance, between generated and lost heat, makes defferences of tissue effect.

MATERIALS AND METHODS

The irradiation was carried with Lambda Physix pulsed excimer laser equipped for Xe-CL opelation at 308nm. Before irradiating biological tissues, wood and the white of an egg had been used for thermographic anaiysis. And wister rat and rabbit were used for this study. Postoperative tissues (skin, musle and bone) were used for light and electro microscopic study. The specimens for light microscope were stained with hematoxylin-eosin and for electoromicroscope were fixed with glutalaldehyde.

RESULT

Wood was irradiated at 1Hz and 20Hz, a point focus of 0.2mm square. Irradiating at 1Hz, the temperature of the irradiated point rised up only 34 degrees C, and subtraction thermograph showed that the irradiated surface was equal balance between generated and lost heat. The surface cuold not be accepted carbonated layer. Irradiating at 20Hz, the temperature rised up to above 50 degrees C and carbonated layer was recognized.

The white of an egg was irradiated at 1Hz, 5Hz, 10Hz, 30Hz and 60Hz. Irradiating at 1Hz, the irradiated point had no remarkable change in spite of ablation of the white of an egg. The temperature rised up to 27.6 degrees C and subtruction thermogram shows the same significance as wood irradiated at 1Hz. And the generation of heat partialy diffused surrounding tissue. The result of irradiating at 5Hz was almost same besides the temperature rised up to 43 degrees C. Irradiating over 10Hz, the temperature rised above 50 degrees C and heat degeneration was caused obviously.

Rat's subcutaneouos muscle and rabit's muscle were irradiated in a physical saline solution. A liner laser beam was used for light micrscope and defocused beam for SEM and TEM. The muscle change irradiating without carbonated layer (100 - 130 Hz) was that; Tissue fragments were ablated away. Nucleuses were also ablated but not in peaces. The ends of muscle fibers was observed as like as teared off strings. At the bottom of the irradiated parts, muscle fibers made irregular wave formation. These findings were also confirmed by SEM. The muscles for TEM study were irradiated at 5Hz and 10Hz, by defocused beam (7J/mm2). The results irradiated at 5Hz followed; Many mitchondrias were destroyed their structures and swollen. In the intersttial tissue around the vessel, Many mitochondrias, which had been emmitted from cells,were seen.(Fig.1) Myofibril and sarcoplasmic reticurum were normal and mitochondria's changes were same as Fig.1.(Fig.2) From these changes, it may be considered that there is no thermal effect in the mechanism of tissue cutting and selective organelle distruction is a characteristic histological change.

The results irradiated at 10Hz were as follows; Chlomatin of the nucleus was coagurated, which meant the death of cell.(Fig.3) Myofilaments especially Z and M-bands were degenerated in addition to the findings of specimen which was irradiated at 5Hz.(Fig.4)
This degeneration of tissue protein would be caused by thermal effect.

MUSCLE (RABIT), TEM.

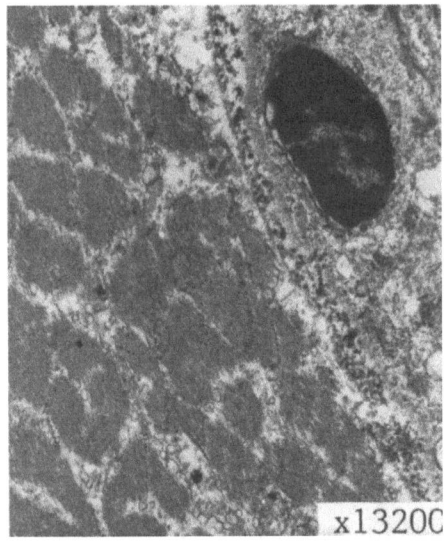

Fig.1. Many mitchondrias were destroyed

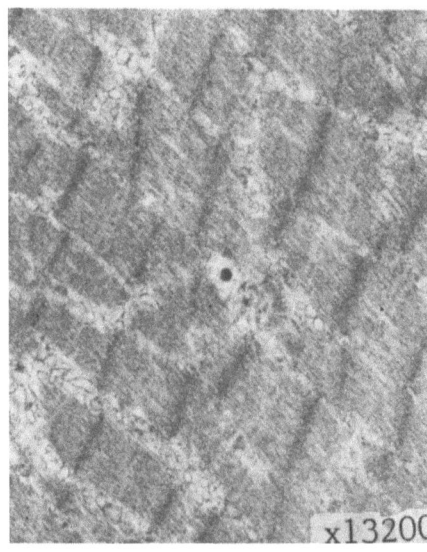

Fig.2. Myofibril and sarcoplasmic reticurum were normal

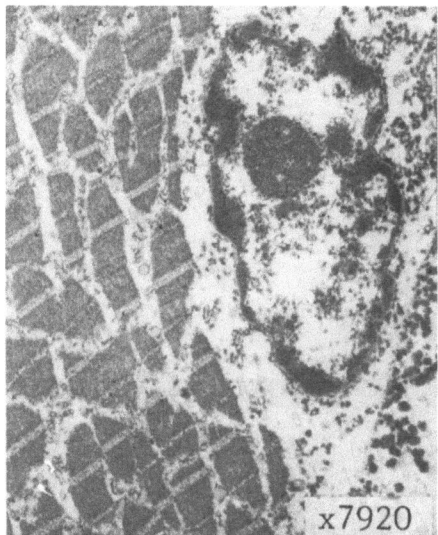 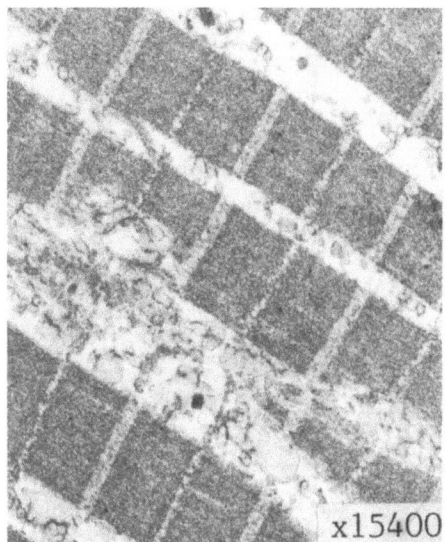

Fig.3. Chlomatin of the nucleus was coagurated

Fig.4. Myofilaments especially Z and M-bands were degenerated

DISCUSSION

From the results, we guessed the mechanism of tissue cutting as follows;
When excimer laser irradiates to the biological tissue, selective organelle distruction causes. Mitchondria and others blow out.
Following this, cells and tissue blow out. Tissue fragments ablate away from tissue. So the tissue is cut sharply. At the same time, organelle and cell's explotion causes the generation of heat secondary and ablation causes jet cooling. Including the environment and the heat which diffuse to surrounding tissue, the energy balance between generated and lost heat, makes difference of tissue cutting. If the heat generate too much, combined tissue cutting, namely, non-thermal and thermal effect, occurs.(Fig.5)

CONCLUSIONS

1. Thermographic analysis shows that even below 50 degrees C, excimer laser operates for tissue cutting.
2. Histological findings indicates that selective organelle distruction is the starting point of tissue cutting.
3. The generation of heat is the secondary phenomenon.
4. When excimer laser irradiate, conbined tissue cutting occurs.

Now we are studying the reason why selective organelle distruction is occured.

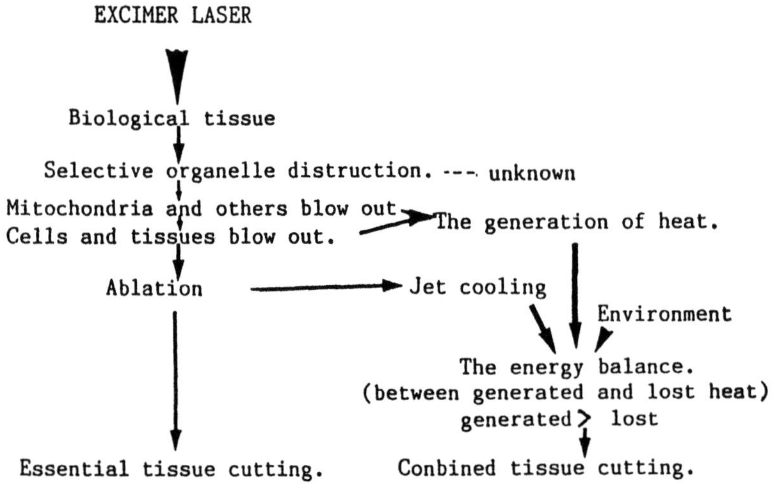

```
EXCIMER LASER
      ▼
   Biological tissue
      ↓
   Selective organelle distruction. --- unknown
      ↓
   Mitochondria and others blow out
   Cells and tissues blow out.        →  The generation of heat.
      ↓                                        ↑
   Ablation    ─────────→  Jet cooling          │
                                   ↘    ↓   ↗ Environment
                                  The energy balance.
                              (between generated and lost heat)
                                     generated > lost
      ↓                                     ↓
   Essential tissue cutting.      Conbined tissue cutting.
```

Fig.5 The mechanism of biological tissue cutting

Neodymium-YAG Laser at 1064 and 1320 NM: Laser Tissue Interaction at Varying Irradiation Parameters and Application Techniques

J. Hochberger, Ch. Ell
Medizinische Universitätsklinik Erlangen
Krankenhausstraße 12, D - 8520 Erlangen, W-Germany

It was the aim of this study to compare the tissue effects of the 1,318 µm with the ones of the 1,064 µm Nd-YAG laser in in vitro tests and in the acute animal experiment under conditions oriented on the gastroenterological endoscopic practice before applying the method in man.

Material and method: We used two continuous wave Nd-YAG lasers made by MBB, Ottobrunn, West Germany, with a wave length of 1,064 µm (mediLas 2) and a power output of 100 W as well as a prototype laser with a wave-length of 1,318 µm and a maximum power of 40 W. The energy was transmitted via a flexible endoscopic transmission system with a quartz fibre of 600 µm in diameter and a low hydroxide (OH^-) content.

As practice related irradiation parameters we chose in the non-contact method a constant light guide - tissue distance of 5 mm. This means with a beam opening angle of 10° a beam diameter of 1,5 mm on the tissue surface and a irradiation area of 1.7 mm².

In the non-contact method serial tests were carried out with a constant application time and varying power settings in 1,064 µm (power density 1169-5260 W/cm²) and in 1,318 µm (power density 468-2104 W/cm²). Then we examined the tissue effects after application of a constant amount of total energy (irradiation dose: 1,064 µm: 14600 J/cm²; 1,318 µm: 5850 J/cm²) using varying laser power. Orientating tests with the contact method were carried out with a constant irradiation time (3 sec) and varying laser power (4-18 W) in both the 1,064 µm and the 1,318 µm laser.

Results: For the 1,064 µm laser with a constant irradiation time of 3 seconds and within the whole range of 20-90 W we stated tissue lesions in the form of a central vaporisation defect with a surrounding coagulation zone changing with increasing laser power to sugar-cone form reaching into the depth of the tissue. With the augmentation of the laser power not only the depth and the diameter of the central vaporisation defect increased continuously but also the width of the surrounding coagulation zone increased continuously.

As in 1.064 µm in 1.318 µm a central vaporisation defect could be achieved in the whole range from 8-36 W. In the range above 8 W, this defect reached into the tissue in the form of a cylinder, but increased only slightly in its width. The coagulation zone was always wider in 1,318 µm than in 1,064 µm and homogeneously surrounded the central vaporisation defect in constant thickness almost irrespective of the power used . When the irradiation energy was constant and the laser power varied the resulting tissue defects varied considerably in 1,064 µm (250 J) regarding their form, vaporisation/coagulation ratio and extension. In the low power range (20-40 W) there was a long, acute-angled, narrow vaporisation channel going deep into the tissue with a small surrounding coagulation seam, while in high laser power and short exposition time there was a V-shaped vaporisation defect which was wide on the surface, but not very deep with a broad surrounding coagulation zone. In 1,318 µm this highly power dependent variation of the tissue defect could not be observed. The lesions were always of about the same size independent of the chosen laser energy, usually showing the shape of a U with an almost constant size of the vaporisation and coagulation zone. In the first tests concerning the contact method the differences between the two wave lengths observed in the non-contact method could be stated in basically the same way.

In order to achieve an identical vaporisation volume in a constant time, the 1,318 µm laser in the contact method required the lowest energy the 1,064 µm laser in the non-contact method the highest energy. Equivalent vaporisation volumes at a constant irradiation time (3 sec) could be achieved with: 12 W - 1,318 µm contact, 16 W-1,064 µm contact, 32 W - 1,318 µm non-contact, 5u W - 1,064 µm non-contact, corresponding roughly to a ratio of 0,75 : 1 : 2 : 3 - for Laser power needed. At these power settings leading to an equivalent vaporisation volume, the relationship of the totally denatured amount of tissue (vaporisation plus coagulation) was about 1 : 1, 1 : 1, 3 : 3 for 1064 µm C: 1.318 µm C: 1064 µm NC: 1.318 µm NC. The results found in the in vitro tests could be confirmed in the acute animal experiments. In contrast to the in vitro tests, however, the coagulation zone was always greater at the expense of the vaporisation zone in both wave lengths.

Summing up the results concerning the clinical use for the removal of tumours in the gastro-intestinal tract, both the 1,064 µm and the 1,318 µm Nd-YAG laser are suitable. The laser of the wave length 1.318 µm needs for vaporisation as well as for coagulation significantly less energy than the 1.064 µm laser in the contact as well as in the non-contact method. Since vaporisation in 1.318 µm is always accompanied with a higher coagulation effect compared to 1.64 µm the risk of complications in palliative tumour therapy with the late necroses and resulting perforation is increased. Thus the 1.318 µm laser appers to offer no advantages for endoscopic tumour treatment compared to the 1.064 µm laser.

Photoablation Threshold of Human Aorta as a Function of Wavelength

G. Müller, H.-P. Berlien, B. Biamino, K. Dörschel, H. Kar

Laser-Medizin-Zentrum GmbH, Berlin, Krahmerstr. 6-10, D 1000 Berlin 45

In Fig. 1 an artist's view of laser angioplasty is shown. The goal is to transport energy from short pulsed lasers through fibers via a catheter system, probably a balloon-dilatation catheter, to photoablate plaques in coronary and peripheral arteries.

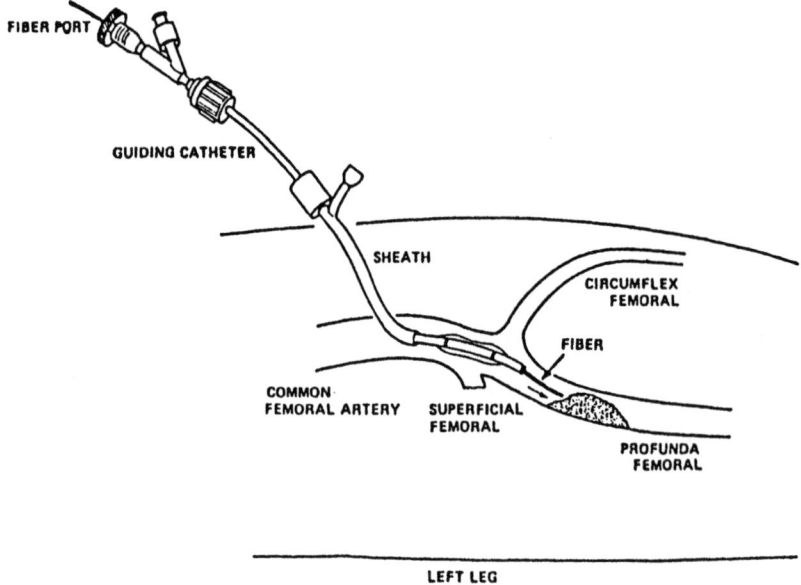

Fig. 1. Laser angioplasty

Photoablation (Fig. 2) is a non-thermal process of removing tissue. No removal of tissue occurs using short pulsed laser irradiation with low energy density (Fig. 3). But removal of tissue started suddenly at a critical energy density and then the ablation rate, i.e. the removal depth of tissue for one laser shot per unit area, rises steeply and then saturates. The reason for saturation is the formation of a plasma above the tissue surface, which functions as an optical shield.

All Excimer wavelengths were investigated as well as, the wavelength of the Nd:YAG laser and its harmonics, and the CO_2 laser at the wavelengths 9.6 µm and 10.6 µm.

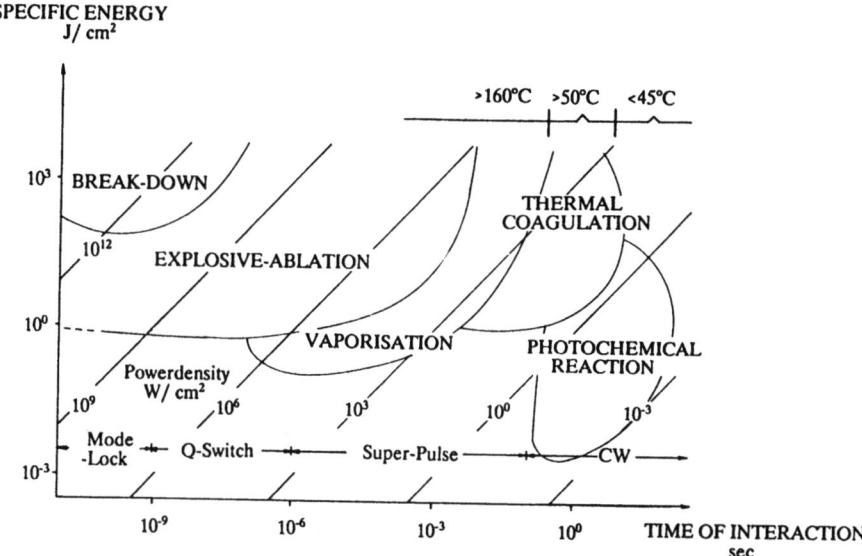

Fig. 2. Distribution of the different laser interactions on tissue in an interaction time-energy density diagram

In the experimental set up, the intima of a human aorta was irradiated at normal incidence through a pinhole, and the laser pulses needed to perforate the vessel wall were counted. Then the ablation rate was calculated by taking the thickness of the aorta and the number of laser pulses required for perforation. The results are shown in Fig. 4-6.

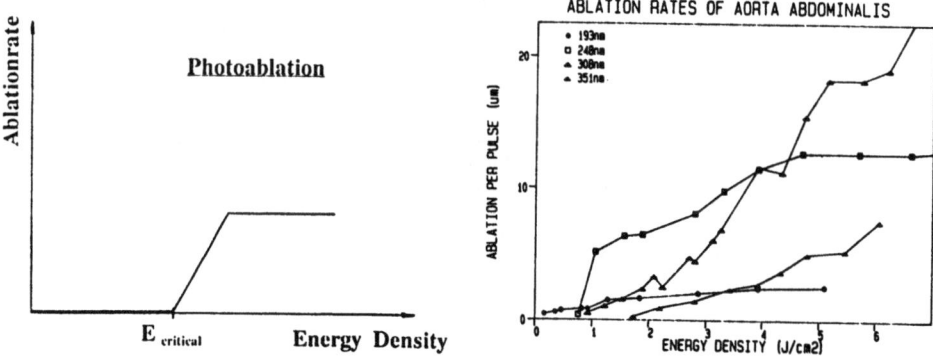

Fig. 3. Principle behaviour of the photoablation rate as a function of energy density

Fig. 4. Experimental ablation rate of aorta at the Excimer laser wavelengths

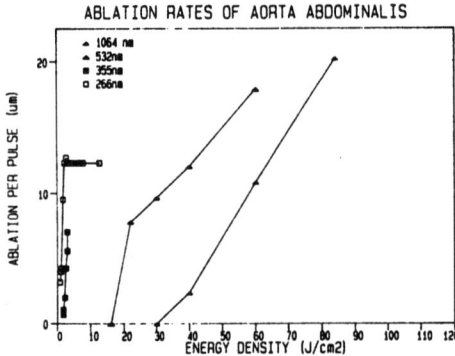 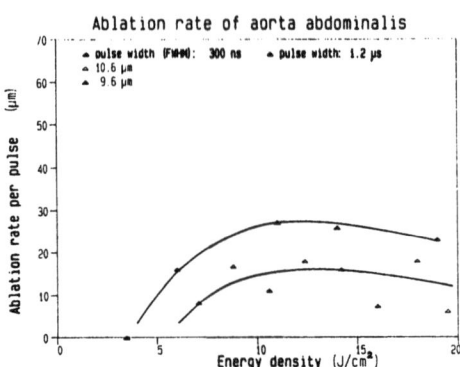

Fig. 5. Experimental ablation rate of aorta for the Nd:YAG laser wavelength and its harmonics

Fig. 6. Experimental ablation rate of aorta using the CO_2 laser at wavelengths 9.6 µm and 10.6 µm

To get an insight into the photoablation process, the threshold energy was plotted versus wavelength (Fig. 7). The data at 2 µm and 3 µm are calculations taken from literature [1] [2]. This diagram also shows the absorption coefficient of water [3]. It can be seen clearly that the threshold energy density forms a mirror-like pattern of the absorption coefficient of water and this leads to the assumption that the linear absorption coefficient might play a major role.

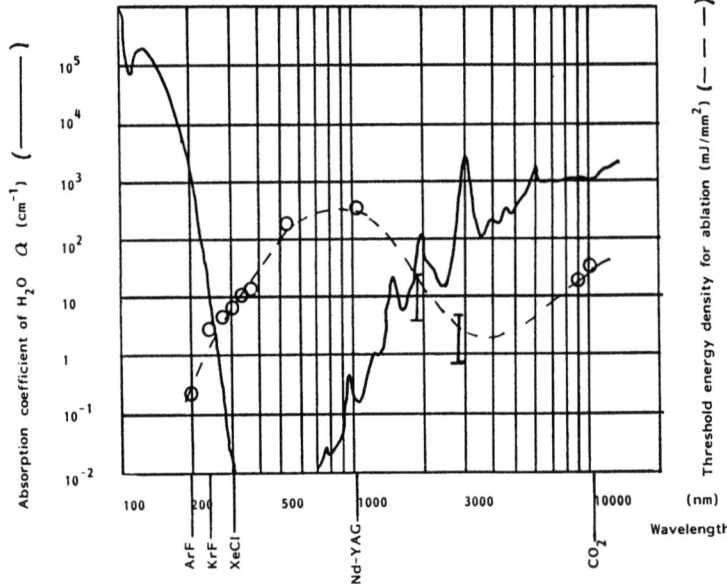

Fig. 7. Energy-densities at threshold as a function of wavelength (- o - this paper, - I - calculated from the literature [1] [2]). The absorption of water [3] (solid line) resembles a mirror image of the threshold data.

As a proof an aorta segment was stained with Doxycyclin, an antibiotic, which has an absorption maximum at about 350 nm (Fig. 8a). The results with stained and unstained aorta obtained with the same experimental procedure as above are shown in Fig. 8b.

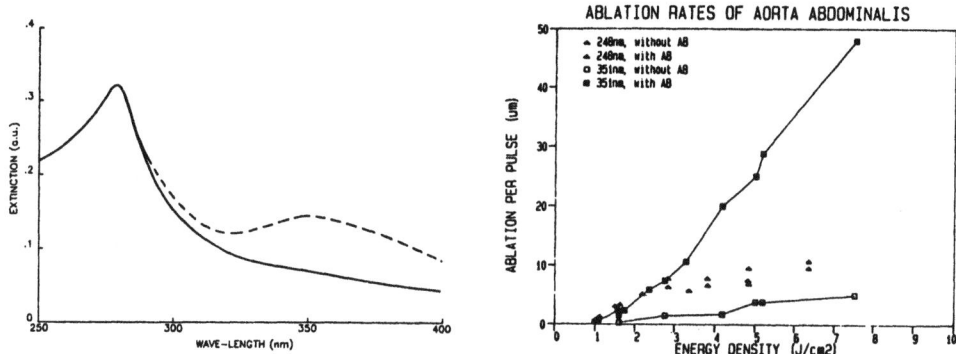

Fig. 8a/b. a: Absorption of aorta unstained (———) and stained (- - - -) with Doxycycline.
b: Experimental ablation rate for unstained and stained aorta. The ablation rate is about ten times higher at 351 nm. At 248 nm the absorption and hence the ablation rate is unchanged.

For the stained aorta at 351 nm the ablation rate increased dramatically and the threshold energy density decreased. At 248 nm no change was effected by staining either in the absorption coefficient or in the ablation rate. This supports the hypothesis, that for photoablation the linear absorption coefficient and the linear penetration depths is of major importance.

All samples were examined histologically and it was found that at none of the wavelengths tested there is any thermal damage larger than about 5 times the ablation rate when the threshold is surpassed. There is only some mechanical damage increasing with the linear absorption depths of the radiation, but this mechanical damage heals "in vivo" within hours.

One can conclude that non-thermal photoablation could be performed at any wavelength.

Literature

1. M. L. Wolbarsht et al.
   VII. Meeting of the American Society for Laser Medicine and Surgery
   San Francisco, USA, 1987

2. T. Seiler et al.
   Lasers in Ophthalmology, Vol. 1, 1986, pp 49-60

3. Boulnois, J.-L.
   Photophysical Processes in Recent Medical Laser Development:
   a review
   Laser in Medical Science, Vol. 1, No. 1, Jan. 1986, pp 47-66

First Experiences with Disposable Fibre Delivery Systems for the Neodym-YAG-Laser

T.Müller-Schwefe, M.Siemon, M.Thermann
Städtische Krankenanstalten Bielefeld-Mitte
Ölmühlenstraße 26, 4800 Bielefeld/Germany

For a few month sterile packed, for single use designed laserprobes of the british Pilkington company are available.
Aim of our abstract is to present first expiriences in the handling of these fibres as well as to draw conclusions for medical and economical indications of their application.
As essential for a sensefull application we consider
- Easiness of handling
- Versatilenes
- Medical profit
- Economocal profit

Comparing the application of the disposable fibres with that of conventional repairable fibres, so first of all we perceive, that as far as we know, disposable fibres are only available for the non-touch-techniuqe. This means, that their employment is mostly limited to the endoscopical field.
The second point is: The fibres are conditioned by construction not repairable.
The technical dates of disposable fibres are, as can be seen, identical with those of normal repairable fibres.
Only the maximal flow of cooling gas is limited for the 1.8mm fibre to 26 ml/sec and for the 2.1mm fibre to 33 ml/sec.
To connect the disposable fibre with the laser, it is merely necessary to insert an adapter into the laser aperture and fix it.
The silica fibre of the disposable probe is at the distal tip so prcisely manufactured and is compared with the self repaired tips of superior quality, as far as the laser users do not send the damaged laser probes for repairs to the makers, which takes quite a long time and can be expensive.
About the application of disposable fibres the following general statements can be made:
- Application is limited to non-touch-tech.
- Technically easyly exchangeable with re-

                            pairable fibres
                        - Available in two diameters for G-I-endoscopy
                        - Precisely worked tips and length of fibres
                          allways sufficent.

In using the fibres in 27 cases no problems during application occured.
Time for exchanging the fibres were short and we had no repair times.
The technical applyability given, the main question has to be concerning the medical use of disposable fibres.
In endoscopy today it is in general use and normal, to clean the endoscopes after every exploration thoroughly and if necessary to disinfect the equipment and sterilize it.
In laserprobes a similar proceeding has not been observed so far.
Although the contamination of laserprobes is only possible at the distal part, the gasflow of cooling gas can not avoid the entry of liquids as blood and small tissue particles in rinse liquid through capillary force into the metal tip and the outer canula.
Because of the dimensions and the method of construction thorough mechanical cleaning is hardly possible so that a certain hygienic risk of transmission of infections must be calculated.
Several bacterial probes taken from the laserfibres after endoscopical lasertreatments of patients with infections of the upper gastro-intestinal tract showed pathological bacterial contamination even after cleaning the fibres.

Especally for patients with a week immunological system as we find it in tumorpatients, an infection transferred by the physician is a unbearable risk.
So with patients with infectious diseases as hepatitis or AIDS out of medical indications it is recommended to use disposable fibres as a protection for the following patients.

Economically the disposable fibre with an average price of 100.-DM is in comparison to the repairable fibre with an price of 1500.-DM in some fields an true alternative. In case of damage and shortage of normal repairable laserprobes the disposable probes, some of which we used several times without any problem, can be taken as an transitional solution and hereby render superfluous stockpiling of repairable fbres, which one normaly needs in two diameters.
Last but not least, time for repairs and cleaning of damaged or dirty distal tips as well as the price of the relarively expensive distal metal tips have to be calculated.

In case of technical difficult laserapplication, when damage of probes is likely, the employment of disposable fibres is sometimes advisable.

To sum up, in our opinion the application of disposable fibres

        is necessary   for patients with known serious infective diseases as hepatitis or AIDS as well as in suspected cases of AIDS

        is recommendable for patients with immundeficency in some cases of endobronchial treatment

        usefull   as a substitute and reserve in case of damage of repairable fibres or tips

        useless   for the daily routine

because the repairable fibre is a more economical alternative without any medical disatvantage.

Infrared Plastic Waveguides for Surgical Applications

J. Dror, D. Mendlovic, E. Goldenberg and N. Croitoru
Dept. of Electron Devices, Faculty of Engineering,
Tel-Aviv University, Ramat Aviv 69978, Israel

Introduction

For successful use of the IR lasers in medicine a good type of waveguide is essential to be devised. The known IR transparent materials, from which fibers might be drawn (1-3) have several disadvantages such as: sensitivity to light, chemicals and humidity, or high toxicity and limited flexibility. In this paper we present a new type of hollow fiber made of plastic tubes which were covered, on the inside walls, with metallic or metallic and dielectric films. The metallic and dielectric films were obtained by depositing successively a metal film followed by a dielectric one. These hollow plastic waveguides are good waveguides and do not suffer from the above shown disadvantages.

Theoretical and Experimental Results

The theoretical calculations for energy transmission in waveguides (4-7) consider the bending of the fiber as a small perturbation. The main difficulties of such an approach are: (a) Difficult mathematical procedure, (b) Inability to compute the attenuation in a practical situation when the laser gaussian beam is coupled into the waveguide with a lens.

In our previous papers (8,9) these difficulties were avoided by using a 3-D ray model, where the gaussian distribution of the laser beam, which is coupled to the hollow fiber through a lens, is represented as a bundle of 200 rays. The waveguide is represented as a thoroid, and the path of every ray was traced through a series of reflections from the walls of the waveguide. By totalling all the intensities of the rays, at the output and, comparing them with the intensity at the input, the transmission yield was calculated.

Several types of plastic tubes made of polythylene, polystyrene, fluoropolymers, nylon and polyuretanes were internally coated with Silver or other metals. Silver was deposited by using electroless methods with special techniques to get uniform deposition on the inner wall of the small diameter plastic tubes. Energy transmission measurements were done with CO_2 laser ($\lambda = 10.6$ μm).

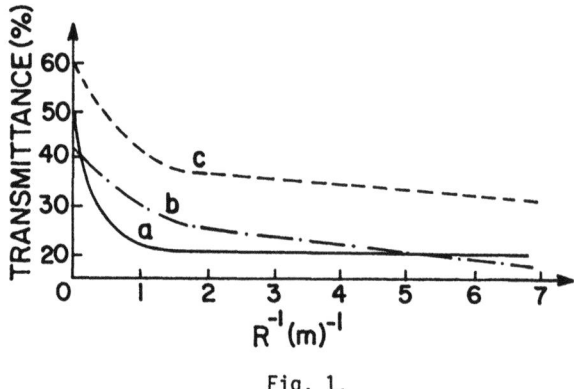

Fig. 1.

Energy transmission vs. curvature (R^{-1}) of a plastic waveguide (length - 500 mm, internal diameter - 3 mm) a. Theoretical calculation for silver coated inner walls. b. Experimental results for silver coated inner walls. c. Experimental results for silver and dielectric (AgI) coated inner walls

As can be seen from Fig. 1 there exists a satisfactory agreement between the results predicted by the theoretical calculations (8,9), Fig. 1a, and the experimental data, Fig. 1b. By depositing dielectric film (AgI) over the metallic film (Ag) of the waveguide, higher energy transmissions were achieved, Fig. 1c. The energy transmissions in bent hollow fibers was investigated as a function of the following parameters: (a) Curvature (R^{-1}, where R is the radius of the curvature), (b) Internal diameter, (c) Coupling mode. From Fig. 2 and 3 it can be seen that when the curvature (R^{-1}) increases (the bends get sharper) the transmitted energy decreases but, it does not decrease proportionally with the bending. By increasing the curvature, a sharp decrease in energy transmission appears at the subtle bends, and for further increases in curvature the transmitted energy remains practically constant. The variations of the internal diameter between 3 and 4 mm (Fig. 2a and 3a respectively) have very small influence on the energy transmission. The internal diameter might be decreased to a value comparable with the diameter of the incident laser beam.

The coupling mode does have an influence on the transmitted energy. This can be seen by comparing data shown in Fig. 2a with 2b and 3a with 3b. Fig. 2a and 3a were achieved by using a coupling done by directing the laser beam through a positive ZnSe lens with f = 110 mm, towards the center of the tube. Data in Fig. 2b and 3b was obtained by measuring the beam directed towards the

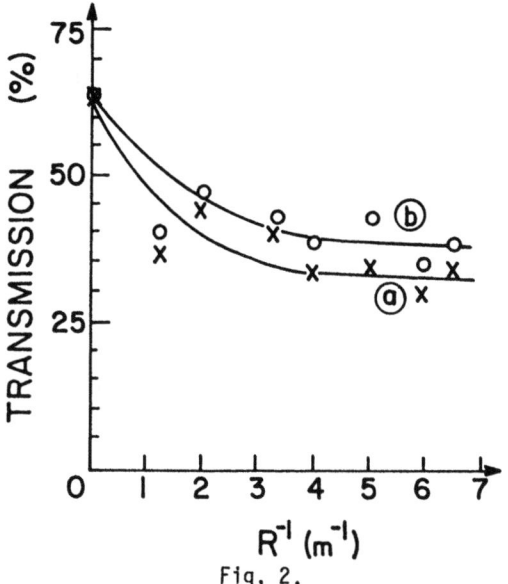

Fig. 2.
Experimental results of energy transmission vs. R^{-1} of the same waveguide as in Fig. 1. a. Silver coated inner walls with coupling to the center. b. Same as a but coupling to the wall

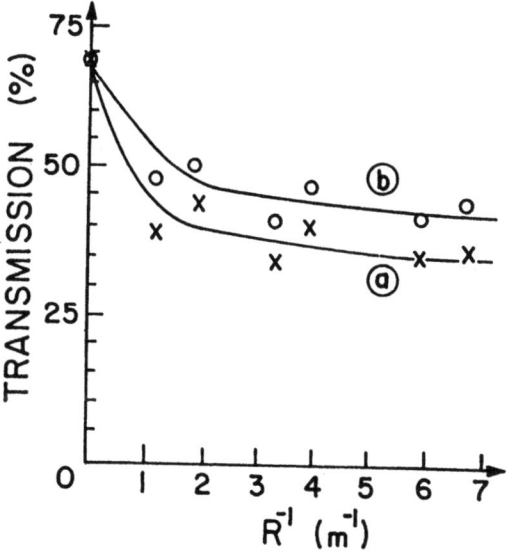

Fig. 3.
Experimental results of energy transmission vs. R^{-1} of the same waveguide as in Fig. 1 but internal diameter 4 mm. a. Silver coated inner walls with coupling to the center. b. Same as a but coupling to the wall

metal wall of the hollow fiber. This gives a higher transmission but such a coupling is very unstable, when small vibrations and distortions apppear. Conversely, the centrally focused coupling mode is very stable and might simulate the practical situation when the laser coupled to a fiber will be used in medical applications. Energies of about 11 watts were obtained at the output of a straight fiber, for a few minutes. For radius of curvature between 350 mm and 155 mm, the energy at the output decreased to about 6-4 watts respectively.

Further research is carried out in order to increase the thermal resistance of the plastic tube, to decrease the diameter of the tube and to improve the input and output coupling by using non-imaging optics. Investigations of such hollow guides on animals have begun in cooperation with physicians.

References

1. A. Bornstein, N. Croitoru and E. Marom, J. Non-crystal Solids (1985) 74 57.

2. A. L. Gentile, Optical Properties of Highly Transparent Solids. eds. S.S. Mitra and B. Bendow. Plenum, New York, p. 105, (1975).

3. D.A. Pinnow, Applied Phys. Lett. (1978) 33 28.

4. E.A.J. Marcatili and R.A. Schmeltzer, Bell Sys. Tech. J. (1964) 43, 1783.

5. M. Miyagi and S. Kawakami, IEEE J. Lightwave Technol. (1984) LT3 , 116.

6. M. Miyagi, K. Harda and S. Kawakami, J. Microwave Theory and Technol. (1984) MTT32, 513.

7. M.E. Marhic. Proc. SPIE, Advances in Infrared Fibers (1982), 320 II, 79.

8. N. Croitoru, D. Mendlovic, J. Dror, S. Ruschin and E. Goldenberg. Lase '86, Sept. 1986, Cambridge, M.A., U.S.A. Proc. of SPIE, Laser in Medicine, (1986) 713 in press.

9. N. Croitoru, J. Dror, E. Goldenberg, D. Mendlovic and S. Ruschin. Fourth International Symposium on Optical and Optoelectronic Applied Science and Engineering, 30 March - 3 April, 1987, Haag, Holland. Proc. SPIE, New Materials for Optical Waveguides, (1986), 799 in press.

Hollow Light Guide for Medical CO_2 Laser

U.Kubo, Y.Hashiahin
Kinki University,Dept.of Electrical Enginerring
Kowakae,Higashiosaka,Osaka 577,Japan

We have developed a flexible CO_2 laser beam guide with metal and polymer compound hollow tube.[1] These previous experimental results reported in the 6th congress at Ilsarem.[2] In this paper,we will be report improvement experimental results of since the year before last congress.

It was concentrated the research as following two points:
(1)We have forward tyial product small size guide tube.[3] (2)The high power pulse CO2 laser beam transmission. These guide tube formed by three compornents materials. The mirror finished aluminum foils were used as light beam reflector,and thin teflons were used as spacer between aluminum foils. These elements were formed rectangularly with soft polymer coat.

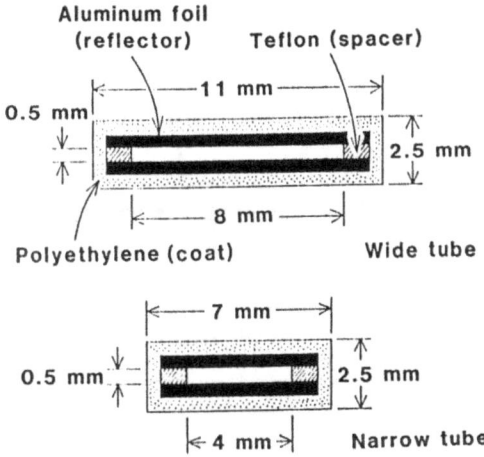

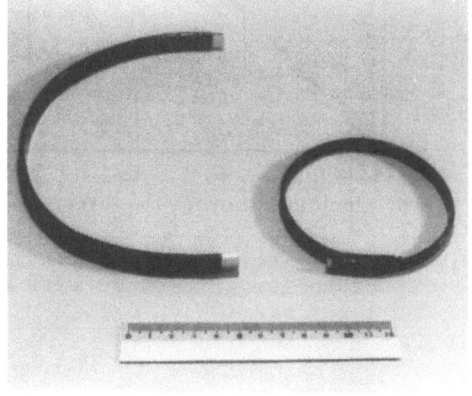

Fig.1. Cross section of hollow guide tubes

Fig.2. Appearance of guide tubes

Figure 1 shows the cross section of guide tube. In this experiments, two kind size tubes were used, cross section of beam transmission space were 8 x 0.5mm and 4 x 0.5mm rectangular space. The outside size are 11 x 2.5mm(wide tube) and 7 x 2.5mm(narrow tube) rectangular cross

section tube. The appearance of guide tubes is shown in Fig.2.
The aluminum foil surface is mirror finished, reflectance is ca.99.5%
for CO_2 laser beam. The characteristics of incident power versus emitted power, at straight shape guide tube as shown in Fig.3, the transmission length is 30cm. The incident laser beam is contenuous wave
and power range from 0 to 20W. The emission power increased lineally
by increasing incident power. The slope represents the transmittance
of guide tube. In this case, transmittance is ca.93% both tubes. In
the results, the transmittance of both tubes were same characteristics.

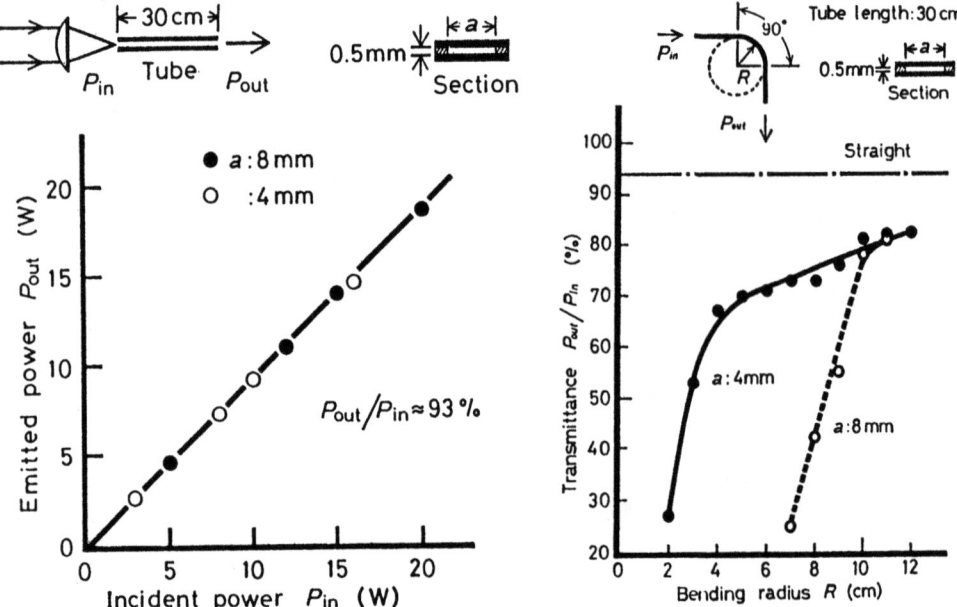

Fig.3. Transmission characteristics of hollow guide tube with CO_2 laser beam(CW)

Fig.4. Comparison of CO_2 laser beam transmittance change by bending radius with two kind aperture size

Figure 4 shows the comparison of transmittance change by bending
radius with both tubes. The effective bending radius of narrow is
reduced to 4cm. It is transmittance is ca.70%. In the wide tube,
effective bending radius is 10cm, transmittance is 77%. The flexibility
was improved as compared with wide tube.

We are having also experiments of higher pulse power CO_2 laser beam
transmission. The characteristics of incident beam is 500kW peak pulse

power, 80ns pulse width and 5Hz repeat pulse. One pulse energy is ca. 40mJ. The experiment was transmittance one meter wide type tube. From the experimental results, the pulse beam transmittance was obtained ca.90% at straight shape tube. The emitted pulse was 450kW peak power, 36mJ per pulse. The pulse width was not change as shown in Fig.5.

Figure 6 shows the bending dependence on emission power and pulse shape, bending radius ca.15cm. In this case, transmittance is ca.80%, pulse shape is not change almost.

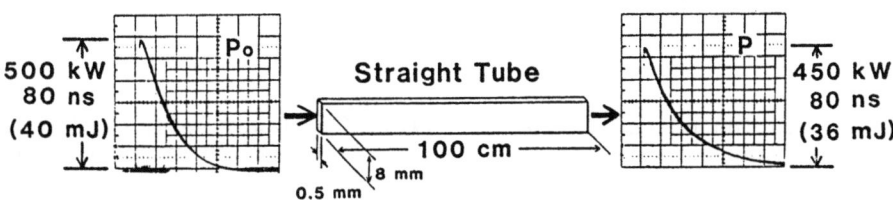

Fig.5. Transmission characteristics of hollow guide tube with higher peak power, short pulse width CO_2 laser beam

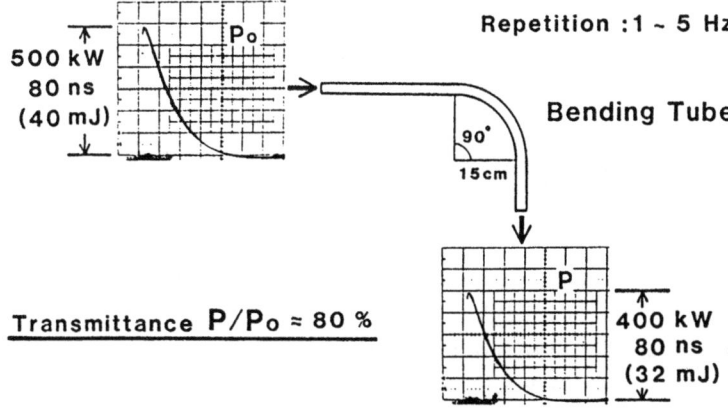

Fig.6. Transmission characteristics of bent tube with pulse CO_2 laser beam

We have made the CO_2 laser scalpel as a trial according to the system adopted the wide type hollow guide tube. Figure 7 shows the perforation of cow's thigh bone by the horizontal system. It is more practically that the laser oscillator is placed above the operator, and light

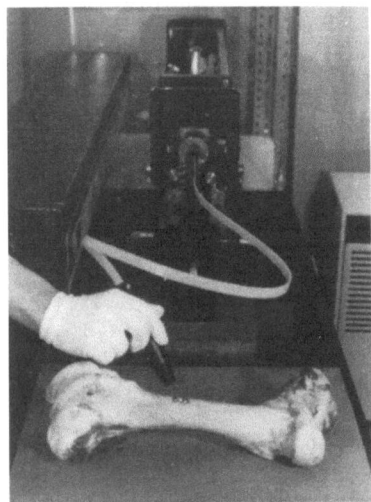 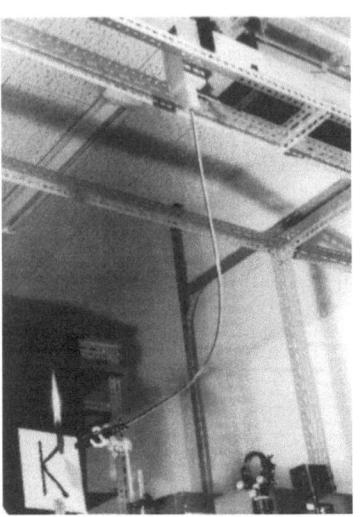

Fig.7. Perforation of cow's bone by CO_2 laser using the horizontal beam guide system

Fig.8. CO_2 laser device using the vertical beam guide system

guide is hung down from high place. Figure 8 shows the trial apparatus was made according to the vertical system. The laser oscillator is movable on the rail structure.

In the near future, if moreover the guide tube improved, CO_2 laser scalpel using the hollow tube beam guide system will be become to compactly.

We have obtained the following items as coclusions. (a)The small size hollow guide tube was made that the width of aperture was reduced from 8mm to 4mm width. In this result, flexibility improved as compared with 8mm width tube. (b)The hollow beam guide tube is also useful flexible guide tube for higher pulse power CO_2 laser beam transmission.

The authors would like to thank Mr.S.Yoshikawa, Mr.Y.Kyusho and Mr. A.Wakaiki. This work was supported by Laser Device Division, NEC Corporation and MIKASA SHOJI Company.

References

1) E.Garmire et al.;Appl.Phys.Lett.,vol.29,p.254,1976.
2) U.Kubo et al.;SPIE,vol.494,Novel Optical Fiber Techniques for Medical Applications, p.79,1984.
3) U.Kubo et al.;SPIE,vol.713,Optical Fibers in Medicine II,p.17,1986.

Medical Applications of Silver Halide Optical Fibers

Dov Gal[a] and Abraham Katzir[b]

School of Physics and Astronomy, Tel Aviv University, Tel Aviv, Israel

(a) Present Address: Box 70, New England Medical Center, 171 Harrison Street, Boston, Mass. 02111, U.S.A.
(b) Present Address: M.I.T. Bldg. 20A-108, Cambridge, Mass. 02139, and Boston University, School of Medicine, Boston, Mass. 02215, U.S.A.

Since the early eighties, when lasers were first used in cardiology, intensive investigation has been carried on to develop a system consisting of a laser and an optical fiber for percutaneous transluminal laser angioplasty. Argon and Nd:YAG lasers were first used, since quartz fibers capable of transmitting visible light were commercially available (1). A persistent high rate of arterial wall perforation has jeopardized _in vivo_ experiments with these two lasers. This arterial wall perforation has been attributed to the thermal mechanism by which the tissue was ablated (2). In the last two years it has been demonstrated that lasers such as dye, excimer, CO_2 TEA and Er:YAG -emitting ultrashort, energetic pulses of light, which are strongly absorbed by tissue - should be selected to obtain tissue ablation with minimal thermal damage (3-5). Yet excimer laser pulses shorter than 300 nanometer are poorly transmitted through fused silica optical fibers, while good optical fibers for the transmission of the Er:YAG light at 2.43 micrometer are not yet commercially available. The CO_2 laser was also considered a good candidate for cardiovascular applications. As a system, the CO_2 laser is extremely well developed, featuring continuous (CW), chopped and pulse modes of energy delivery and almost an unlimited variety of energy profiles in the pulsed mode including ultrashort high energy pulses. The lasers are small, efficient, reliable, easy to operate and thus do not require high technical skills. Nevertheless, this laser was not considered a good candidate for endoscopic applications because of the problems involved with transmission of infrared (IR) light through optical fibers. It was our goal, at Tel Aviv University, to develop suitable fibers and to demonstrate that a system based on CO_2 laser and an IR optical fiber is potentially an excellent candidate for endoscopic surgery.

We have developed and fabricated, since 1981, silver halide optical fibers which transmit the 10.6 micrometer wavelength. Silver halide crystals can be extruded to form optical fibers which are nontoxic, water insoluble and fairly flexible. They can transmit CO_2 laser radiation with power densities greater than 3×10^4 W/cm^2 in the CW mode or short pulses with power densities on the order of 5×10^6 W/cm^2. The losses at 10 micrometer are lower than 0.3 dB/m, and a 0.9 mm diameter fiber can transmit continuously more than 20 watts. The total transmission of 1 meter of fiber is about 70% and it remains invariable with bending down to a radius r = 5 cm. The far field pattern of the beam is Gaussian, having a full width at half maximum (FWHM) of about 20 degrees (5). All these properties make these fibers good candidates for endoscopic laser surgery.

One of the major problems in endoscopic surgery is the propagation of the light from the distal end of the fiber, through the fluid medium to the target tissue. The efficiency of ablation of lasers such as argon, excimer, Er:YAG and CO_2 in a flowing blood field was believed to be compromised since their radiation is at wavelengths which are strongly absorbed by blood. While flushing away the blood with saline solution of perfluorochemical was beneficial in the case of the argon, it was useless for wavelengths shorter than 300 nanometers (deep UV) and longer than 2 micrometers (far infrared). Recently, a successful transmission of excimer laser light through a saline-tissue interface has been reported (6). We have demonstrated that pulsed CO_2 laser radiation may be transmitted through "opaque" liquids by a cavitation effect (7). This effect occurred when the following requirements were met:

(i) strong absorption of the laser beam in the liquid.
(ii) sufficiently high energy (E) per pulse.
(iii) sufficiently high repetition rate (f).

A simple theoretical model describing the relation between h, f and E was studied, and the conditions for keeping an open cavity were found. As an example, a beam with energy of 30 mJ/pulse at repetition rate of 500 Hz penetrated 2 mm of water! Therefore pulsed CO_2 laser radiation can propagate from the distal face of a silver halide fiber, onto tissue even through saline or blood interface.

Since 1982 we have been using the CO_2 laser and the silver halide fibers to perform several *in vitro* and *in vivo* experiments most of them in cardiology (8). Some of the important experiments will be described below:

In one of these *in vivo* experiments five segments of human femoral atherosclerotic arteries, harvested during amputation surgery or shortly thereafter, were transplanted, each in the right carotid artery of a mongrel dog. After 10 to 18 days, the CO_2 laser catheter was inserted into the exposed carotid artery and angioplasty was performed using pulsed CO_2 laser energy. Radiation parameters measured from the distal face of the fiber were as follows: CW delivery of 1.0 to 3.5 joules and pulsed delivery of 20 to 40 mJ per pulse, for a total of 60 to 231 joules delivered over a time span of several minutes. Two of the dogs were sacrificed immediately after the laser procedure, and the other three were followed-up from 10 to 21 days. Three of the totally occluded xenografts were successfully recanalized using the pulsed mode; the CW mode, which was used only once, failed to recanalize the occluded xenograft. In one dog, while lasing, three small carbonized spots (size of a pin hole) appeared on the xenograft wall, one of which was microscopically identified as a thermal perforation.

In a second *in vivo* experiment we studied the feasibility of a percutaneous atrial laser septostomy in five mongrel dogs. The laser catheter was introduced via a cut-down of the femoral vein, it was advanced and its tip was positioned, under fluoroscopic guidance, against the interatrial septum. Laser light was then delivered in the pulsed mode with energy levels of 20 to 40 mJ per pulse. In four of the dogs, the interatrial septum was performed by the laser beam, creating holes of about 2 mm diameter each. Pre and post-lasing blood counts and coagulation parameters were assessed in one dog and were found to be similar.

In a third experiment we explored the feasibility of using the CO_2 laser radiation to coagulate bleeding gastric ulcers in vivo, using a CO_2 laser endoscope. Ulcers were made, using a mechanical disruption, in three mongrel dogs. The dogs were divided into acute and chronic groups. In the acute group the coagulative properties of the CO_2 laser radiation were studied. The chronic group was made to study the long-term effects of the laser light on the healing process by comparing treated and non-treated control ulcers. A silver halide fiber 180 cm long and 0.9 mm in diameter, clad with a loose Teflon tube, was inserted in the irrigation channel of a 12 mm flexible gastroscope (Stortz model 13211). Energy was delivered either in the CW or the pulsed mode. The results indicated that the use of CW mode was more effective in coagulating moderately bleeding ulcers than the use of pulsed mode. Results from the chronic study indicated that histologically there were not significant differences between the healing process of the treated and non-treated ulcers. After thirty days, both the treated and non-treated ulcers looked almost identical macroscopically.

Infrared fibers, and especially silver halide ones, have a wide range of applications in medicine. These fibers would serve as waveguides for the transmission of IR laser radiation (eg. CO_2) for surgical applications. They would also be a part of diagnostic systems, such as the fiber-optic radiometers used for non-contact surface temperature measurements. With the development of good cladding, an ordered bundle of such fibers may even be used for endoscopic thermal imaging inside the body. Our in vivo experiments, which were briefly discussed in this paper, have demonstrated the feasibility of cardiovascular and gastrointenstinal application of the CO_2 laser catheter. We are convinced that a system composed of a laser and a silver halide fiber will enable physicians to easily perform safe percutaneous and endoscopic procedures.

ACKNOWLEDGEMENT

The development of silver halide fibers, and their applications, involved many researchers. The authors wish to thank all members of the Applied Physics Group at Tel Aviv University, Ramat Aviv, Israel.

REFERENCES

1) G. S. Abela, S. Normann, D. Cohen, R. L. Feldman, E. A. Geiser, C. R. Conti, "Effects of CO_2, Nd:YAG and argon laser radiation on coronary atheromatous plaques", Am. J. Cardiol., Vol. 50, pp. 1199-1205, 1984.

2) G. Lee, D. Seckinger, M. C. Chan, A. Embi, D. Stobbe, R. V. Thomson, N. A. Sanchez, R. M. Ikeda, R. L. Reis, D. T. Mason, "Potential complications of coronary laser angioplasty", Am. Heart J., Vol. 108, pp. 1577, 1984.

3) W. S. Grundfest, F. Litvack, J. S. Forrester, T. Goldenberg, H. J. C. Swan, L. Morgenstern, M. Fishbein, I. S. Mcdermid, D. M. Rider, T. J. Pacala, J. B. Laudenslager, "Laser ablation of human atherosclerotic plaque without adjacent tissue injury", J. Am. Coll. Cardiol., Vol. 5, pp. 929-933, 1985.

4) R. F. Bonner, P. D. Smith, M. Leon, L. Esterowitz, M. Storm, K. Levin and D. Tran, "Quantification of tissue effects due to a pulsed Er:YAG laser at 2.9μm with beam delivery in a wet field via zirconium fluoride fibers", SPIE Proc., Vol. 713, pp. 2-5, 1986.

5) A. Saar, F. Moser, S. Akselrod and A. Katzir, "Infrared optical properties of polycrystalline silver halide fibers", Appl. Phys. Lett., Vol. 49, pp. 305-307, 1986.

6) J. M. Isner, R. H. Clarke, A. Katzir, D. Gal, S. T. Dejesus, K. R. Halaburka, "Transmission characteristics of individual wavelengths in blood do not predict ability to accomplish laser ablation in a blood field: inferential evidence for the "Moses Effect", Circulation, Vol. 74, II, p. 361, 1986.

7) A. Saar, D. Gal, R. Wallach, S. Akselrod and A. Katzir, "Transmission of pulsed laser beam through "opaque" liquids by a cavitation effect", Appl. Phys. Lett., Vol. 50, pp. 1556-1558, 1987.

8) D. Gal and A. Katzir, "Silver halide optical fibers for medical applications", IEEE J. Quant. Elect., Vol. QE-23, pp. 1827-1835, 1987.

Detection and Analysis of the Ultra-Weak Photon Emission from Various Biological Materials

B. YODA[1,2], Y. GOTO[2], Y. TAGUCHI[1,3]
T. MIYAZAWA[4], A. SAEKI[6] and H. INABA[1,5]

[1]Research Development Corporation of Japan (JRDC), [2]Department of Medicine and [3]Department of Surgery, School of Medicine, [4]Department of Food Chemistry, Faculty of Agriculture and [5]Research Institute of Electrical Communication, Tohoku University, and [6]Tohoku Institute of Technology, Sendai, JAPAN

This paper describes an unique phenomenon of the spontaneous chemiluminescence of human blood samples. An extremely sensitive single photon counter was developed using a carefully selected, highly effective photomultiplier and the very weak light emissions from various biological samples including human blood specimens were measured. As the most representative results obtained, ultra-weak chemiluminescence of human blood plasma samples taken from subjects under certain living conditions and disease states are presented. The intensities of very weak light emission of smokers' plasma samples reached substantially higher levels than those of nonsmokers'. Chemiluminescence of smokers' and nonsmokers' urine samples, cigarette smoke itself, cigarette smoke absorbed into organic solvents were also examined. Effects of cigarette smoke on organ chemiluminescence were experimentally tested in an animal model. Ultra-weak chemiluminescence of blood plasma samples of certain liver diseases also showed higher chemiluminescence levels than those of healthy subjects. Oxygen requirement was generally observed for these light emissions. It is interesting to speculate that this higher chemiluminescent property of the plasma samples might be somehow related to health disorders.

METHODS AND MATERIALS

Human studies: A group of healthy male volunteers were used for cigarette smokers' experiment. These subjects were divided into smokers and nonsmokers. In this study the nonsmokers included ex-smokers and never smokers. The amount of cigarettes smoked by these subjects and the duration of smoking were based on the statements made by the subjects. The types of cigarettes and the inhalation habit of each smoker were not considered. Patients with various health disorders were also studied. Informed consents were obtained from all subjects.

Animal study: A group of male rats were used as the animal model of cigarette smoking. The animals were placed in an inhalation chamber for smoking experiment.

Experimental samples: In human studies blood samples were collected by venous punctures from the cubital veins in the morning. A small amount of heparin was used to prevent coagulation. Blood samples were then span at 3,000 rpm for 10 min at 4°C and resulting plasma portions were used for chemiluminescence assay. Urine samples were collected around at 10.00 a.m. without restriction on eating and drinking. In an animal study blood and other organ samples were taken from the experimental animals and the chemiluminescence was measured. Cigarette smoke was passed through organic solvents in a rubber topped flask to absorb cigarette smoke components.

Measurement of ultra-weak chemiluminescence: A single photon counter of high performance (Chemiluminescence Analyzer OX-7, Tohoku Electronic Industrial Co., Ltd., Sendai, Japan) was used to assess extremely weak chemiluminescence of blood plasma and other experimental materials. The equipment was carefully tuned up to achieve high sensitivity and low electrical noise. A specially selected photomultiplier was used for this purpose. Aliquots of plasma and other samples were placed in a stain less steel dish-type counting cell of 5 cm diameter and the single photoelectron pulses were counted at 37°C with a continuous air flow. In some experiments samples were put in a closed type counting cell and atmosphere was replaced with oxygen or nitrogen. Results were arbitrarily expressed as the number of observed photons per 10 sec.

RESULTS

Chemiluminescence intensities of smokers' and nonsmokers' plasma and urine: Chemiluminescence intensities of smokers' and nonsmokers' blood plasma were plotted against their age. Though the distribution of the chemiluminescence intensities of both smokers' and nonsmokers' plasma samples had no direct correlation with their age, smokers' plasma showed an approximately twice higher averaged chemiluminescence level than nonsmokers' plasma (1). An arbitrarily set line at a level of the chemiluminescence intensity of about 90 counts per 10 sec almost clearly separated the distribution of smokers' and nonsmokers' plasma chemiluminescence. The intensities of smokers' plasma chemiluminescence possessed a weak positive correlation with the number of cigarettes consumed per day by these smokers. Duration of smoking had no correlation with the chemiluminescence levels of smokers' plasma. Smokers' urine samples showed a tendency to have higher chemiluminescence levels than those of nonsmokers'. Atmospheric conditions influenced the chemiluminescence levels of smokers' and nonsmokers' plasma samples. Both smokers' and nonsmokers' plasma showed decreased chemiluminescence levels under nitrogen flow than air flow. Oxygen caused some increases in the chemiluminescence levels of both smokers' and nonsmokers' plasma. Situations were almost similar in case of urine samples. These results suggested that the chemiluminescence of smokers' and nonsmokers' plasma and urine might involve oxidative mechanism.

Chemiluminescence of cigarette smoke and smoke absorbed into solvents: Cigarette smoke itself was directly passed into a closed type measuring cell and the chemiluminescence was measured. Cigarette smoke gave relatively higher chemiluminescence levels and the chemiluminescence levels decreased quickly. The same phenomenon was observed in cigarette smoke absorbed into organic solvents. These chemiluminescence levels were far higher than those of smokers' plasma and urine. Oxygen augmented these chemiluminescence intensities and nitrogen suppressed them.

Animal model experiment: A group of rats were exposed to cigarette smoke in a closed glass chamber for approximately 5 min. The animals were killed and the organ chemiluminescence was analyzed (Table 1). The organs including blood plasma from cigarette smoke exposed rats showed elevated levels of chemiluminescence than those of control rats.

Table 1. ORGAN CHEMILUMINESCENCE OF CIGARETTE SMOKE EXPOSED RATS

Animals	Chemiluminescence (counts/10sec)		
	Lung	Liver	Plasma
Smoke exposed	457	59	597
Control	25	51	49

This experimental result may well coincide with and support the observed findings of elevated chemiluminescence in smokers' plasma.

Patients' blood plasma chemiluminescence: Liver diseases tended to show higher plasma chemiluminescence. Plasma from patients with obstructive jaundice typically showed higher levels of chemiluminescence (Table 2). The intensities of the plasma chemiluminescence of patients with obstructive jaundice increased with time during assay, while the chemiluminescence levels of control plasma from healthy subjects remained constant. Atmospheric conditions also influenced these chemiluminescence intensities of patents' plasma as of smokers' plasma.

Table 2. PLASMA CHEMILUMINESCENCE OF PATIENTS WITH OBSTRUCTIVE JAUNDICE

Time in assay (min)	Chemiluminescence (counts/10sec)		
	Control	Patient A	Patient B
0	---	425	823
15	55	902	1,250
30	---	1,230	1,878

DISCUSSION

Participation of free radicals and active oxygens in the aging process, carcinogenesis, and other physical disorders are a present matter of interest (2-6).

In the early latter half of the 20th century Vassilev already indicated that a weak chemiluminescence observed in certain chemical reactions was attributable to the oxidative reaction involving molecular oxygen and free radicals (7). Singlet oxygen molecules, one of active oxygens and electronically exited states of oxygen molecules, emit light in visible and near infrared regions as shown by Kahn and Kasha in chemical reactions (8).

The biological significance of the present findings and the exact mechanisms of the increased light emitting properties of plasma and other organs are not yet clear. It may be worthy enough to speculate that the observed phenomena of chemiluminescence of these biological materials are somehow related to certain health disorders including carcinogenesis through the generations of free radicals and active oxygens.

REFERENCES

1) Yoda, B., Goto, Y., Sato, K., Saeki, A. and Inaba, H.: Arch. Environ. Health: 40, 148-150 (1985)
2) Nagata, C., Kodama, M., Ioki, Y. and Kimura, T: in Free Radicals and Cancer (Floyd, R.A. ed) pp 1-62 (Dekker, New York, 1982)
3) Demopoulos, H.B.: Fed. Proc., 32, 1859-1861 (1973)
4) Halliwell, B.: in Age Pigments (Sohal, R.S. ed) pp 1-62 (Amsterdam Elsevier, 1981)
5) Harman, D.: J. Gerontol., 11, 298-300 (1956)
6) Totter, J.R.: Proc. Natl. Acad. Sci. (USA), 77, 1763-1767 (1980)
7) Vassilev, R.F. and Vichutinskii, A.A.: Nature, 194, 1276-1277 (1962)
8) Kahn, A.U. and Kasha, M.: Am. Chem. Soc., 92, 3293-3000 (1970)

Miniaturized Optoelectronic Transceiver for Application and Pick-Up of Biological Signals

Valerio Annovazzi-Lodi, Silvano Donati, Dipartimento di Elettronica, Università di Pavia, Pavia, Italy

Summary

We present a two-way optoelectronic transmission system for telemetry between a main instrument and a satellite mobile unit to be mounted on a laboratory animal. The link employs a pair of LED/photodiode transmitters and receivers operating in regime of diffused infrared radiation from laboratory walls and ceiling.

The system offers an accuracy of 0.5% in amplitude and a signal bandwidth of 1KHz with a high degree of immunity to electromagnetic noise and ambient illumination.

The small size of the mobile unit implemented in surface mount technology (SMT) and the low-voltage, low-power design, make it well-suited for an indoor telemetry link with a freely moving animal of small size. This transceiver system has been routinely utilized for polarographic in-vivo determination of brain metabolites (DOPAC, 5-HIAA) in rats.

1. Introduction

Transmission via diffused radiation is a well-known technique [1,2] which allows indoor operation over short range distances (several meters) and medium range bandwidth (up to 1MHz), exploiting the diffusion of the transmitted light or infrared radiation over walls and ceiling towards a receiver.

This technique is characterized by a high degree of immunity to electromagnetic interference; it implements a mobile link without the requirement of tracking; moreover, a very compact design is possible as well as low power consumption, thus allowing battery operation. These features make the technique attractive for transmission of biological signals because it avoids wiring-induced disturbances and also greatly reduces perturbations of the animal behaviour, a major problem, e.g., in neurological experiences.

2. Analysis of the diffused channel

The diffuse radiation channel is schematized in Fig. 1 where a LED on the transmitter emits, over an angle θ_{FOI}, an optical power P_t a part of which (P_r)

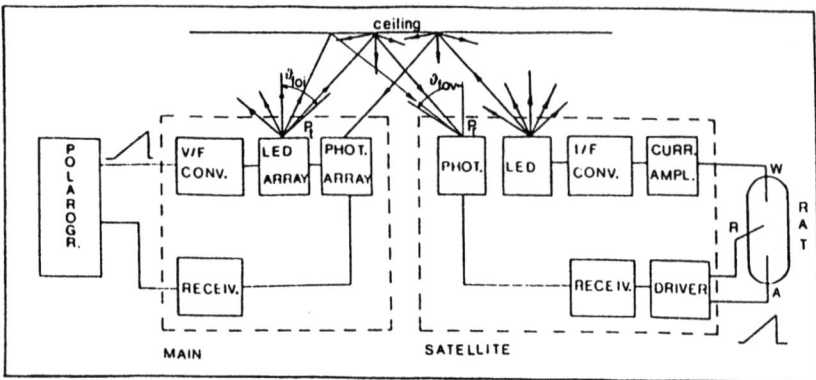

Fig. 1. Diffused radiation channel geometry and block scheme of the two-way transceiver as connected for polarographic experiences

is collected after diffusion by the receiver photodiode whose angle of aperture is θ_{FOV}. The channel has been characterized in terms of attenuation, bandwidth, S/N ratio and the most important results of this analysis [2] are summarized in the following.

2.1 Attenuation

In the case of moderate fied of illumination ($\theta_{FOI} < 1$ sr) and neglecting the contributions of multiple path diffusion, the channel attenuation P_r/P_t amounts to

$$P_r/P_t = (\delta/\pi) A_r / (H^2(1+d^2/H^2)) \qquad (1)$$

where δ is the ceiling diffusivity, A_r the detector area and a complete overlap of the field of view (f.o.v.) over the field of illumination (f.o.i.) is assumed. The attenuation diagram is reported in Fig. 2 for different values of the ceiling height H

2.2 Bandwidth

An intrinsic limitation for the diffused channel bandwidth B arises from the multipath propagation, i.e., the multiplicity of lightpaths connecting the transmitter to the receiver, each with a different delay. This delay spreading depends on the device parameters θ_{FOI}, θ_{FOV} as well as on the room height H and the relative distance d. Though a more general analysis can be performed [2], here we limit ourselves to report an approximate result, valid for $\theta_{FOV} \leq 1$, $d/H \ll 1$. These hypotheses allow to obtain the solution in a compact form, i.e.:

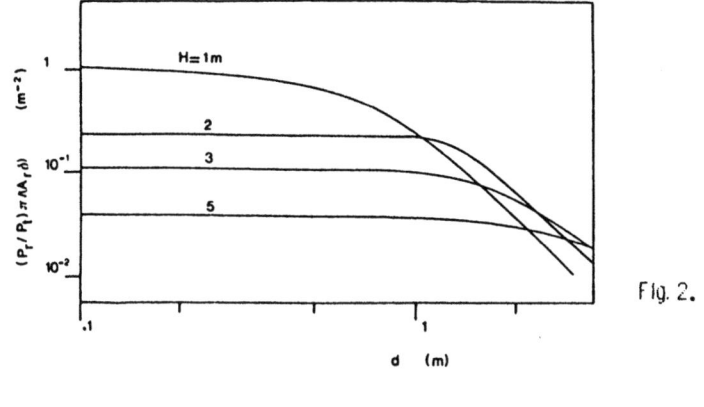

Fig. 2. Attenuation diagram

$$B = 0.22 \, (c/H)(\cos \theta_{FOI}/(1-\cos \theta_{FOI})) \qquad (2)$$

From eq (2) it follows that the channel can be characterized in terms of a distance-bandwidth product BH, once θ_{FOI} has been fixed. As an example, for $\theta_{FOI} = \pi/6$, we get BH = 427 MHz m. Thus, a bandwidth of at least a few hundred MHz is in principle available in all practical cases. In Fig. 3 we report the plot of the distance-bandwidth product as a function of the angle of illumination θ_{FOI}, $\theta_{FOI} \leq \theta_{FOV}$.

2.3 Signal to noise ratio

The signal to noise ratio is defined as $S/N = I_s/I_n$. In most applications, where at least a moderate level of background illumination is present, the shot noise due to the stray light photogenerated current I_L, i.e.:

$$I_N = (2q \, I_L B)^{1/2} = (2q\sigma^* A_r E B)^{1/2} \qquad (3)$$

is the main contribution to noise [2]. In eq.(3), σ^* is the luminous sensitivity (A/lm), E the illumination (lux), B the front-end bandwidth.

On the other hand, the photogenerated signal current on the photodiode can be expressed as

$$I_S = \sigma P_r = \sigma A_r K P_t \qquad (4)$$

where σ is the radiant sensitivity (A/W) and

$$K = (\delta/\pi) \quad L = H^2(1 + d^2/H^2)^2 \qquad (5)$$

as can be found using eq.(1)

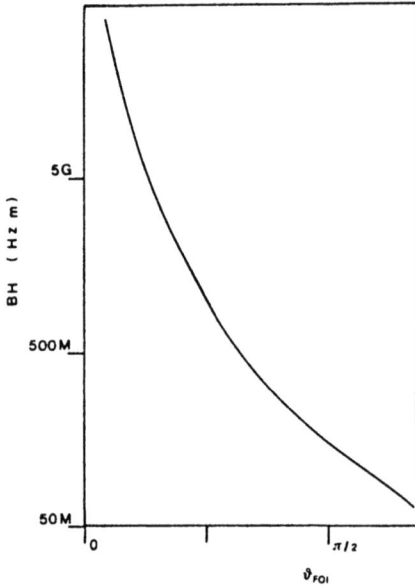

Fig. 3. Distance-bandwidth product as a function of the angle of illumination θ_{FOI}

3 The optoelectronic transceiver

In Fig 1 we report the block scheme of the two-way transceiver as connected for an experience of three-electrode pulse polarography [3]. The main unit transmits the slow voltage ramp generated by the polarograph to the mobile unit on the rat. On the receiver, after demodulation, the ramp is applied to the electrodes implanted in the rat brain. The response current is amplified and the signal is sent back, via the return channel, to the polarograph, where the information about the metabolite concentration is extracted. Square wave voltage to frequency conversion has been used as the modulation scheme and electrical multiplexing allows to separate channels, whose subcarries are located at 8KHz (first channel) and 80 KHz (return channel). The optical carrier is at $\lambda = 950$ nm for both channels. This choice allows to maximize the LED efficiency ($\simeq 10\%$) and LED/photodiode matching.

An electronic feedback loop has been implemented around the front-end amplifiers, where the well-known cold resistance scheme is employed, as detailed in Fig. 4. A current generator sinks the photogenerated current in a frequency range from d.c. to about 500 Hz, so as the effect of sun and lamps is cancelled, at the expense of a 3 dB deterioration of the S/N ratio. This scheme prevents the front-end from saturation allowing to operate in presence of relatively high levels of ambient illumination.

To achieve a higher level of EMI immunity a dummy wiring has been made in close proximity to each photodiode using high value (6 MΩ) resistors connected to the non-inverting input of the operational amplifier [4]. Since the dummy

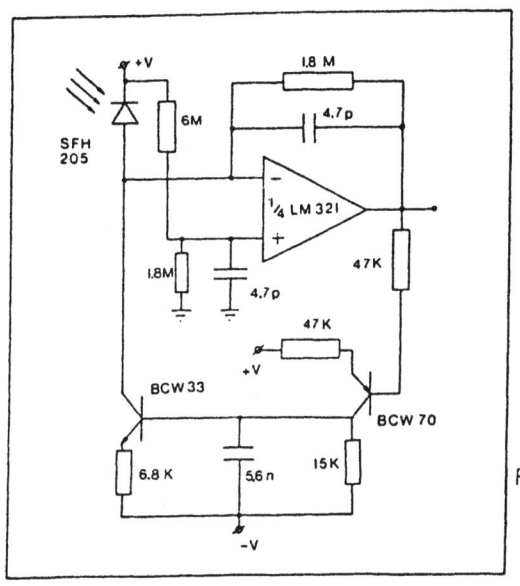

Fig.4. Front-end amplifier with EMI reduction network and stray light cancellation feedback (satellite unit)

wires collect nearly exactly the same electrical interference as the photodiode, the two contribution cancel each other at the output. In tipical operating conditions, the S/N ratio can be improved of about 30 dB.

The main tranceiver includes an array of 6 LEDs and 6 photodiodes while single components are used on the satellite, which has been designed for low voltage, low drain supply (it requires two thin Li-batteries for a few hour operation). The circuit has been made compact (35 x 35x 5 mm) by SMT technology implementation and using miniaturized components. As shown in Fig. 5, it consists of two double face printed circuit boards, with components on one side only to be cemented back to back.

The transmission system allows to implement a link in the range of a few meters with a good S/N ratio. As an illustration of the performances in typical operating conditions, the S/N ratio has been calculated from eqs.(3),(4) for E = 300 lux, L= 5 m, thus obtaining S/N=60 dB for the first channel and S/N= 30dB for the return channel.

The tranceiver offers a maximum bandwidth of about 1KHz, a dynamic range of ± 1 V and a linearity error less than 1%. The baseline drift is less than 20 mV over the whole battery life.

In Fig. 6 we report a polarogram relative to a determination of DOPAC in the accumbens of a rat using the optoelectronic transceiver. After injection of Haloperidol (0.5 mg/Kg I.P.) a 300% increase in metabolite concentration is found, as expected. Though this brain area is quite sensitive to stress, the recorded peaks are regular in shape and the measurement is not sensibly effected by environmental disturbances. Fig.7 outlines the experimental arrangement showing the implantation, the electrode holder/positioner and the satellite transceiver.

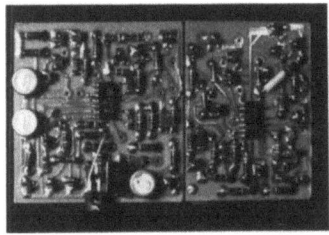

Fig.5. Satellite circuit implemented in SMT. The two boards are to be cemented back to back

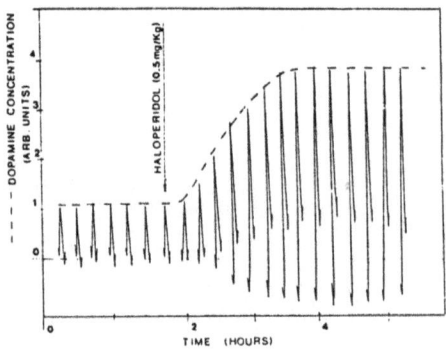

Fig. 6. Polarographic determination of DOPAC in a rat using the optoelectronic transceiver (see text)

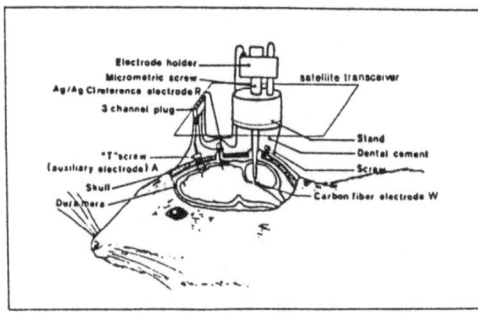

Fig.7. Schematics of the experimental arrangement for in vivo three--electrode polarography using the optoelectronic transceiver

References

1. F.R. Gfeller, U. Bapst, Proc. IEEE, 67(11) (1979), 1474-85.
2. V. Annovazzi-Lodi, S. Donati, to be published.
3. L.L. Iversen, S.D. Iversen, S.H. Snyder: "New Techniques in Psychopharmacology", Plenum Press, New York, (1977).
4. S. Donati, G. Martini, Proc. Laser 81, Springer Verlag, Berlin, (1982), 434-9

Applications of Optical Phase Conjugation in Medicine

B.W. Stewart, Ph.D.
Dept. of Mechanical and Industrial Engineering
University of Cincinnati
Cincinnati, Ohio 45221
USA

Abstract

In this paper we introduce optical phase conjugation to the laser-medical community as well as to speculate on several possible applications of this phenomenon.

I. Introduction

Optical phase conjugation (opc) has been explored by the physicist since 1972. In the last fifteen years, however, little effort has been made toward application of this phenomenon to medicine. In fact, it appears that those possible applications described by physicists (Refs. 1,2) have not been realized as of yet in the laboratory. It is believed that this phenomenon has great potential in diagnostic medicine. At the very least opc theoretically has the potential to eliminate scattering effects in non-ionizing radiography (Ref. 2) and to eliminate modal dispersion in single optical fibers thus making a single fiber imaging endoscope possible (Ref. 1). Many other medical applications may be developed in the near future.

The remainder of this paper is organized as follows. We begin with an introduction to opc. It will not be an in-depth examination of the physical mechanisms behind opc but will serve to illustrate some of the possible uses of opc in medical diagnostics. Following will be a section describing one such possible application.

II. Optical Phase Conjugation

Zel'dovich and collaborators first observed the phenomenon in 1972. By passing the beam of light from a pulsed ruby laser through a frosted glass plate, they intentionally distorted it. The distorted beam was then directed on a tube containing high-

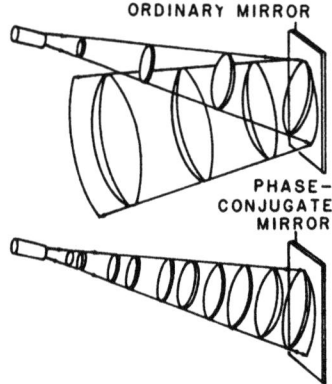
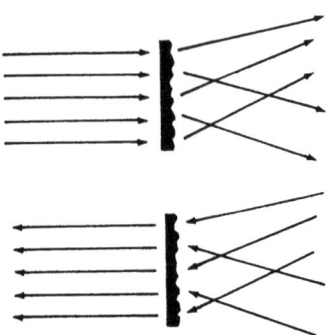

Figure 1. Properties of a phase conjugate mirror as compared with those of an ordinary mirror. The phase-conjugate mirror redirects the diverging beam so that a converging beam is formed independent of the angle of incidence.

Figure 2. A plane wave is scattered and degraded when transmitted through a nonuniform glass plate. The beam is restored when the rays are reversed (through opc) and transmitted back the same glass plate.

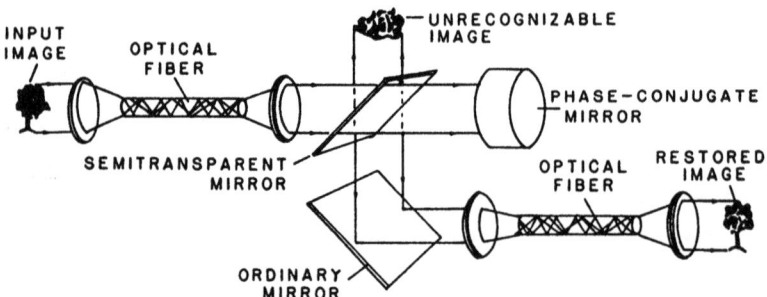

Figure 3. Distortions due to optical fibers can be removed by a phase conjugate mirror. The distortions arise due to modal dispersion (see text). After opc, all modes transverse the same paths, in reverse, and the image is restored.

pressure methane gas. Through stimulated Brillouin scattering the beam was reflected backward. Thus the gas acted as a mirror (a "phase conjugate" mirror). After the reflected beam passed back through the frosted plate, the investigators were surprised to find that it emerged nearly undistorted. The distortion inflicted by the first passage through the plate was reversed by the second passage. If the gas were replaced by an ordinary mirror, the distortion would have been increased by the second passage.

Additionally, phase conjugation devices have been used to eliminate distortion effects in the transmission of information in single fiber optics (Ref. 3). One of the problems involved here arises from modal dispersion in the fiber. This distortion is present anytime the object one desires to image (a tumor, lesion, etc.) is large compared to the fiber diameter. Each point on the object is a source of light. The rays emanating from the object then enter the fiber at different angles. After the light enters the fiber it is reflected many times before reaching the exit. This multiple reflection effectively scrambles the image; the spatial relationship between rays originating from nearby points has undergone considerable change during the propagation through the fiber. The resulting image pattern bears little resemblance to the object producing it. Optical phase conjugation can be used to reverse the scrambling as described below.

III. Dual Fiber Endoscope

Although recent advances in fiber optic technology have made possible the development of submillimeter diameter optical fibers, current imaging endoscopes are limited somewhat due to the fact that many (500-1000) such fibers (a "fiber bundle") are needed to provide distortion-free imaging. In addition to the effect this number of fibers has on the size (diameter) of the endoscope, the flexibility is also adversely affected. Since in certain potential applications both size restrictions and flexibility requirements are important, the fiber bundle-based imaging endoscope cannot be employed. If distortion-free, dual fiber endoscopes (one fiber for illumination/treatment and one for imaging) could be developed, endoscopic size and flexibility would not limit their application as severely.

The dual fiber endoscope described here would use opc in order to eliminate the distortion present in a single optical fiber imaging system. In the application presented here, we make use of two imaging fibers, one in the endoscope itself (i.e., inside the body) and an "identical" fiber which remains outside the body. The phase conjugate mirror should be of the four wave mixing variety (Ref 1). The intensity of the image is then not of concern in relation to the activation of the phase conjugating process. The use of the "identical" fiber mimics the correction mechanism achieved by allowing the image to exactly retrace its path. The real problem is the development of fibers with "identical" modal-scrambling properties. This needs to be investigated experimentally.

IV. Conclusions

The dual fiber endoscope described above is capable, in principal, of illumination, imaging, and treatment. Endoscope flexibility is increased and the endoscope size requirements are reduced, possibly opening up many areas of the body for endoscopy that are currently inaccessible.

References

1. Pepper, D.M., Sci. Am <u>254</u>, 74 (1986).
2. Stewart, B.W., "Conceptual Application of Phase-Conjugation in Tumor Detection", Proceedings of LASERS '86 (SOQUE, in press).
3. Yariv, A., IEEE J. Quant. Elect. <u>QE14</u>, 650 (1978).

An excellent review of the concepts of phase conjugation can be found in:

Zel'dovich, B.Ya., Pilipetsky, N.F., and Shkunov, V.V., <u>Principles of Phase Conjugation</u>. Springer-Verlag, 1985.

Potential Applications of Lasers in Diagnosis and Preoperative Assessment of Lesions Using Three Dimensional Imaging

R. A. S. Blackie, J. Drinkwater[*], S. Hart[*].

Dept. of Histopathology, Charing Cross and Westminster Medical School, Fulham Palace Road, London W6 8RF, U.K.
[*] Dept. of Physics, Imperial College, London SW7, U.K.

INTRODUCTION

The investigation of disease in a living patient employs many techniques. In diagnostic pathology, one of those most frequently used is the microscopic examination of thin slices of the diseased tissue.

The examination of thin cross sections, however, reduce bulky organs such as the brain or liver which have their own three dimensional organisation, to what are, in effect, flat or two dimensional slices. A considerable amount of information about the internal structure of an organ can be gained by this means. Though it is possible to assemble a mental picture of the arrangement of the whole organ from a series of these thin sections, it is probable that important interrelationships are not appreciated because of the limitations imposed by the use of only two dimensions.(Blackie, 1986)

Two dimensional cross sectional images of tissues can be produced not only by physical means but can also be generated by computer. Recently, radiologists have begun studying cross-sectional images of the body by means of computerised axial tomographic (CAT) scans. CAT scans can be made of any part of he body but they are particularly useful as a non-invasive means of demonstrating lesions behind the abdominal cavity and within the skull.

Holography is a technique in which three dimensional images can be produced. In these images the three dimensional characteristics of the original object, such as parallax, are preserved so that the image can be examined, within limits, from different points of view.

The purpose of our project was to investigate whether the three dimensional nature of organs, and lesions within them, could be recreated and more easily studied using this technique.

HOLOGRAPHY

In holography, a beam of laser light is split. One beam, the reference beam, shines directly onto a photographic plate. The other beam, the object beam, is first reflected off the object onto the same photographic plate. When the two beams of light meet, they interact with each other like ripples on a pond. Where the light waves are in phase, with the crests of one light wave coinciding with the crests of the other beam of light, they produce a larger, brighter point of light. Conversely, if the crest of one light wave coincides with the trough of another, the two beams of light cancel each other out and the result in an area of darkness. The overall result is the formation of a complex interference pattern which can be recorded on photographic film.

This interference pattern of which a hologram is composed is a form of optical code in which information is preserved about not only the amplitude of the light from the subject but also its phase difference.

When a beam of light is subsequently directed at the hologram, it is diffracted by the complex interference pattern and the optical effect is the creation of a three dimensional image. This process is called reconstruction.

One of the properties of holography is that it one can superimpose several exposures onto a single photographic plate. It is this property which we have exploited in our aim to reconstruct composite three dimensional pictures from a series of two dimensional sections.

A series of cross sections are accurately aligned with one another. Each cross section in turn is then exposed by the object beam. Between each exposure, the same photographic plate is moved along the axis of the object beam a distance proportional to the thickness of the cross sections. The resultant hologram is called a multiplex hologram and consists of several images "stacked" one on top of another. When it is reconstructed, a composite three dimensional image is created. This original hologram can be used to make a transfer hologram in which can be optically manipulated to produce a brighter and clearer image which can be seen in ordinary light.(Drinkwater, 1987)

HOLOGRAPHIC RECONSTRUCTION OF MULTIPLE CAT AND NMR SCANS

Radiology is the study of images created by beams of X-rays. Formerly, all radiographs were records of the X-ray shadows created behind radio-opaque tissues. The recent development of CAT scans, however, has enabled the shape of organs, and lesions within them, to be demonstrated in cross section. This development has overcome the problem encountered in which important lesions may be obscured because they are situated in the shadow of a denser structure.(Hounsfield, 1973)

A CAT scanner consists of an X-ray source and an array of detectors are mounted on a scanning gantry which moves around the patient. The detectors record the number of X-ray photons emerging from the patient as the gantry rotates. The information recorded by the detectors is processed in a computer and the reconstructed image is displayed as a series of cross sectional images. The depth of these cross sections may be selected, the chosen range commonly lying between a few millimetres and several centimetres depending on the organ involved and the size of the lesion.

A permanent record of a series of these multiple, computer processed cross sectional images can be made, usually in the form of photographic negatives. By either aligning these negatives or by manipulating the data from the computer directly, a multiplexed hologram can be made from them to form a single, composite, three dimensional image.

We show examples of holograms produced in this manner. Because properties such as parallax are preserved, it will allow a radiologist or a surgeon to "look around" the lesion and to see it from different perspectives so that they may be more easily able to visualise and to appreciate preoperatively the size and extent of the lesion, its distorting effects, and its relationship to anatomical landmarks and important adjacent structures such as blood vessels.

Three dimensional reconstructions of other computer generated images have also been made. These include Nuclear Magnetic Resonance (NMR) scans, which, by using the magnetic properties of atomic nuclei to report on the amount and environment of these nuclei in complex chemical mixtures, can be used as a non-invasive means of examining the metabolism of living tissues.

HOLOGRAPHIC RECONSTRUCTION OF HISTOPATHOLOGICAL SECTIONS

Pathology is the scientific study of disease. It attempts to reconstruct the development of the disease process from its inception to its termination. The treatment of the patient may depend on the histopathological diagnosis.

One of the techniques most frequently used in the histopathological investigation and diagnosis of disease within the the body include the microscopic examination of slices of the tissue involved. Representative samples of the tissues are first chemically processed, and thin sections of the tissue are appropriately mounted for examination by light or electron microscopy and are stained to demonstrate structures of interest.

The tissue slices, or sections, are cut as thin as is feasible to allow both the transmission of light through the stained specimen into the optical system of the microscope and to minimise the number of times that other structures overlap and obscure features of importance or interest. Sections prepared for light microscopic examination are commonly 2 - 5µ thick, but electron microscopic section may be 80 nm. thick.

To investigate the feasibility of reconstructing these microscopic sections, we selected a morphologically simple cell, the lymphocyte. It is a small cell which measures 6µ in diameter. It has a round nucleus and few organelles in the surrounding narrow rim of relatively featureless cytoplasm.

Lymphocytes can be readily obtained from a sample of peripheral blood. An enriched suspension of peripheral blood lymphocytes were prepared and examined under the electron microscope. A suitable lymphocyte was selected and serially sectioned to form multiple 80nm. slices. These sections were stained with the electron dense chemicals, uranyl acetate and lead citrate. In an electron microscope, structures coated with these chemicals cast a shadow in the electron beam and this is recorded on a black-and-white photographic plate. A selection of these electron microscopic images were photographed on transparencies and were approximately aligned. A multiplexed hologram was made from them as described previously.

On viewing the hologram, parallax between the sections was clearly visible. Regions within the nucleus of electron dense material which represent deposits of inactivated, condensed nucleoprotein apparently move relative to one another on varying one's viewing angle. It provided a primitive example of a three dimensional image of the nucleus of the lymphocyte as seen from its centre.

We have also found that holographic reconstruction can complement other techniques such as immunofluorescent microscopy.

DISCUSSION

Our investigations into the use of multiplex holography as a means of displaying and aiding the interpretation of three dimensional information have shown that it works. In many cases, the information could previously only be studied as a series of two dimensional slices. The technique is at an early stage of development and we are now attempting to refine the technique and to improve its results.

One of the major difficulties in using holograms in general is that of viewing them, requiring, as they do, special lighting conditions and positioning of the holograms and observers. The first of these problems has, in part, been overcome by the production of holograms which can be viewed in white light. This has obviated the need for laser illumination which would have probably rendered the routine use of holography impractical. The viewing box based on dispersion compensation developed by Bazargan (1985) has provided a means by which small groups can easily see the three dimensional transmission holographic image in ordinary ambient lighting conditions. For large audience viewing, the use of television and video technology has been required to provide the best means of illustrating holograms.

The production of holograms of solid objects can be simple: the production of multiplex holograms is more complex. One of the major problems inherent in this technique is the problem of alignment of the individual sections.

Sections of pathological material are discrete physical objects which are often mounted by hand onto individual glass microscope slides. At present, photographic transparencies of the enlarged microscopic images have to be aligned by eye. The imprecision of this method results in a reduction in the quality of the final holographic image. It also, at present, prevents detailed measurements being made directly from the hologram. If this problem can be overcome by, for instance, superimposing a hologram of a three dimensional grid of known dimensions, the value of holography will be increased.

In holography it is important to be selective and to display the most appropriate information. Though a hologram is capable of recording a lot of information in a compact form, the visual interpretation of a complex biological structure may suffer if it is obscured by a mass of irrelevant detail. A two stage procedure is needed in which unimportant information is deleted.

These two important aspects, alignment and selectivity of detail, are more easily dealt with in images from a CAT scanner and, as a result, the formation of multiplexed holograms of CAT scans has progressed further than the other applications and show that the stage has been reached where its value in clinical practice can be demonstrated. In the CAT scanner, the individual images are aligned by the computer and transparencies of these images can be aligned accurately using a pin-registered camera. The computer in the CAT scanner can be programmed to select or highlight only the important features and to ignore unimportant detail so that the final hologram is clearer and appears less cluttered.

Holography, in its many forms, may have widespread potential applications in medicine. Computer images are easier to manipulate but require considerable computing power and sophisticated software. However, as holograms can be made from computer generated data, these two fields of endeavour may be complementary. Though the difficulties exist, holography is sure to prove to be an aid in the diagnosis of a lesion and in assessing the optimal therapeutic approach. In addition, the comparison of two relevant holograms of a lesion may allow its response to chemotherapy to be more clearly demonstrated and assessed.

Holography does not give any information other than that already available, but it can present that information in a form that is easier to visualise and interpret.

REFERENCES

Bazargan, K.(1985) A Practical Portable System for White Light Display of Transmission Holograms using Dispersion Compensation. Proc. SPIE, 524,24.
Blackie, R.A.S. et al. (1986) Reconstruction of Three Dimensional Images of Tissues using Holography. J. Path. 149, 220-221A.
Drinkwater J. and Hart S. (1987) Multiplex Holography for Display of Three Dimensional Information Fourth International Symposium on Optical and Optoelectronic Applied Science and Engineering. The Hague, Netherlands (in press)
Hounsfield G.N. (1973) Computerised Transverse Axial Scanning. Part 1. Description of System. Brit. J. Radiol. 46, 1016-1022.

Neurosurgery

Homo Faber Amplificus Lucis – State of the Art

F. Heppner
Department of Neurosurgery, University of Graz, A-8036 Graz

Surgery with lasers constitutes without any doubt one of the most outstanding achievements of civilization in the age of technology. The scientific investigation of brain functions which forms its base and is still being carried on by this discipline has been a consequence of keen observation of nature, which had already started in antiquity, and ingenious nature studies, as manifested by clinical research in the 19th and electrobiology in the 20th centuries. Modern technology has enriched the arsenal of our diagnostic tools by neuroimaging, which permits visualization of nerve structures with a degree of accuracy as achieved by any anatomical atlas, while evoked potentials and their monitoring in vivo safeguard maximum precision in the scanning of neural paths and centers. Neurosurgery thus represents the apex of the application of up-to-date technological tools and highly sophisticated surgical methods, including lasers of varying wavelength, to the human brain. From times immemorial, generations of thinkers and researchers have contributed with industry and tenacity to the exponential development of new means and ways for saving human lives or making them again worth living, thus gradually opening up new perspectives to the knowledge of mankind. They all have been guided by a law of nature demanding of man not only survival and preservation of his species but also urging him on to progress from the old to the new.

Tracking the phylogenetic development of Homo sapiens from the first lines of his evolution, Ramapithecus in the Miocene, up to the Paleolithic age, we can see the first decisive transition at the moment when he changed from living as an arboreal animal in the dense jungles to life in the open steppe, based on the apparently mad decision to give up the so far reliable mode of locomotion on four feet and to walk upright therefrom - a crazy idea indeed, which, however, was a step towards new possibilities. As a further consequence, these entailed the development of language, a system of communication based on the formation and utterance of words, and thus also a further enlargement of his intellectual capacity. This presupposed most probably the separation of the ego from the non-ego in man's consciousness, and therefore also the development of the distance to his environment necessary for mastering it in a rational way. It also implied a farewell to the paradise of his childlike innocence and entailed the recognition of his own mortality. The gaining of this consciousness and knowledge constitutes the main difference between man and animal, and this is also what Nestroy meant to convey by his phrase: "An ape, if he knew that he were an ape, would be a human being."

This early development enabled primitive man to produce weapons and implements and to make fire serve his purpose. This feat of his inventive mind dates back some 400,000 years, as proved by finds in the cave of Chou-Kou-Tien near Peking, where skulls and skull fragments of Sinanthropus pekinensis were found beside ashes and bone particles scorched by fire. The harnessing of fire entailed immense progress, as it enabled man to change from raw to cooked food and to keep away the cold in winter.

There have been frequent contemplations as to whether man invented the wedge, the lever, the roll and finally the wheel in a playful way or by a conscious effort of his mind. In the former case, the invention is said to have been due to Homo ludens, in the latter, to Homo faber. I am convinced that in reality there has been no such alternative, since each and every invention must have been due to a stroke of genius of an individual, as is still true of all great works of art and feats of technology - two fields which are derived from one and the same matrix and therefore cannot be strictly separated. There is a well-known saying that genius consists only of 10 % inspiration but 90 % perspiration. Both the inventor and the artist are urged on to create something novel by a mysterious extrapersonal force, but real creativity also requires immense assiduity, dedication and even self-denial on their side - just remember, for example, Michelangelo, Kepler, Lavoisier, Beethoven and many others.

Hand in hand with early technological progress, characterized by the settling down of man and the sensational venture of not simply living on the fruits offered to him by nature but growing them himself according to his needs, there came the formation of communities and societies. Previously, in the thick of wilderness, the individual had to utter shouts in order to find his or her partner for mating, and the mother had to guide her child by her voice lest he or she got

lost in the dusk. Now the family started to flourish, hordes
joined to form clans and tribes on the basis of a primitive kind of
social contract, still far from establishing a veritable state. The
purpose of these forms of association was to help and protect each
other, which meant, however, to sacrifice more and more of the freedom
that once had seemed boundless to mutual consideration and respect.
Many a youngster in the steppe had to unwillingly recognize that
freedom and safety are not identical but complementary: the growing
demand for greater safety is accompanied by growing pressure to integrate into the social structure offering safety. This fact is an
undeniable reality, giving rise to many problems up to the present
day, making youth unruly and rebellious and causing many to "drop out".
The most boundless of all forms of freedom is the freedom of the
outlaw, a state in which the individual finds himself completely outside society, in a situation where everybody tries to get hold of him
so that he is forced to develop the alertness of a wary animal. But
even this state of outlawry, with its manifold tests of one's moral
and physical stamina, may be a gratifying sensation, as the author
knows from his own experience gained in 1946.

This constraint to conform exerted on archaic society resulted in
many practical inventions such as the substitution of fur clothing
by textile garments, but it also forced man to develop new phychological traits such as leadership, voluntary subordination, obedience,
loyalty, and it also domesticated the concepts of property and love.
The raising of the brood and their training for life presupposed
strong family ties, the willingness to learn on the side of the younger generation, and a sense of responsibility on that of the parents.
This process has been extremely laborious and is far from being complete. The elemental power of love, for instance, has not yet been
really domesticated so far. Konrad Lorenz characterizes this stage on
the way from cerebration to humanization when he says: "The transition
from ape to man - that's us.".

The origin of science, as we understand it, dates back to the 6th
century B.C. On the eastern and western fringes of the land inhibited
by the ancient Greeks, in Asia Minor and in Sicily, there appeared men
who did not content themselves with merely looking at nature - they
were eager to look into it. Thales of Miletus considered water to be
the source of life. Anaximander, his disciple, theorized that the beginning of all life was to be found in the sea. Anaximenes, on the

other hand, believed to recognize the principle of life in pneuma, the air, thus formulating a concept that was to remain active until the 18th century. Heraclitus assumed that fire, i.e. processes of combustion, was at the base of all phenomena of life. Democritus developed an atomistic theory which already anticipated essential elements of modern nuclear physics. Aristarchus of Samos described the heliocentric system with its planets fifteen centuries before Copernicus, and Empedocles was the first philosopher to formulate a near-Darwinist theory of the origin of species. One of his contemporaries was Hippocrates, with his first methodical description of neurological phenomena such as the crossing of nerve pathways; he also recognized that epilepsy did not have supranatural but pathophysiological causes. Of no lesser importance for the future fate of mankind was Socrates, as it was he who discovered human conscience. This discovery doomed him to death, because he who replaces the verdict of the Delphic Oracle by the voice of man's conscience within himself urging him to do good will destroy the ingenuousness which so far had been characteristic of the view of life of ancient Greece. He who removes the highest authority from Olympus, placing it into the heart of man, will burden him with a hitherto unknown load of responsibility.

This enormous revolution, seizing all fields that man had conquered so far and to which he had given the names of physics and philosophy, tore down the ancient heaven of gods and created a vacuum to be filled by the teachings of the Man from Bethlehem. He directed the aspirations of mankind away from life in this world, promising fulfillment in the other world. This withdrawal put an end to all scientific research for almost a thousand years; it also stopped social development for the same span of time, as the medieval state was regarded as a divine institution and any criticism of or rebellion against its hierarchic structure was considered to be sinful.

After around 800 A.D. learned clerics in the occident, starting out from philosophy, began to ponder upon the origin of all kinds of phenomena, thus laying the foundations for a new approach, not merely looking at nature, as the ancient Greeks did, but asking questions about it. They were righteous and pious men, not beset by theological doubts: Erigena, Duns Scotus, Bacon of Verulam, Nicholas Cusanus, and, above all, Albertus Magnus, archbishop of Cologne. It was the latter who finally implemented this questioning of nature by devising the

experimental approach. Surgery, however, was still excluded from this
new start, as the Council of Rouen in 1038 stated: "Ecclesia abhorret
a sanguine." It thus transferred surgery from the hands of monks into
those of barbers and tonsors.

During the age of European Renaissance, which followed this period of
newly aroused scientific interest, reason, with its insatiable longing
for knowledge and recognition, began to take the place of faith. Already at that time - long before Lenin - Machiavelli, in his "Principe",
stated that religion was opium for the people. The Church, however,
still the keeper of all knowledge, was fully aware of the dangers
that might arise to the existing and so far successful system if it
were to permit philosophical and/or scientific questioning beyond the
barriers of traditional dogma. It should, however, be considered that
the Holy Office sitting in judgment upon Galilee consisted of educated
and learned men who probably within their hearts sympathized and
agreed with the accused but nevertheless indicted and condemned him
on the charge that his teachings were godless. It was not knowledge
as such that was dangerous; it was the radical change of the existing
order that was considered to be sinful.

Galilee is also said to have formulated the phrase that everything
measurable should be measured and everything that could not be
measured should be made measurable. One might argue that it was only
by meeting this requirement that all the achievements contained in
the modern physical conception of the world have become possible.
Recent developments, however, seem to show that research and the
application of its results are now going far beyond Galilee, aiming
at an even farther goal: that everything makeable should be made and
that everything that cannot be made should be made makeable. In this
connection, one is reminded of the history of creation in the book
of Genesis, where we read: "So he drove out the man; and he placed
at the east of the garden of Eden cherubim, and a flaming sword
which turned every way, to keep the way of the tree of life."
Faced with the destruction of the natural environment, uncheckable
so far, and perhaps also in view of the perspectives opened up by
genetic engineering, one might ask whether man, in his endeavor to
make everything makeable, is already on his way to the tree of
life with its forbidden and unattainable fruit. Who knows: Was it
perhaps already the cherub's flaming sword that flashed over
Hiroshima and Nagasaki ? The atomic bomb constitutes not only an

entirely novel achievement in arms technology; it also marks a biological incision of which Arthur Koestler justly remarked: "In human consciousness, death always meant the end of the life of the individual. But the day of Hiroshima has reduced our entire species to the state of mortality."

The employment of nuclear energy for peaceful and military purposes occurs at an advanced stage in the development of mankind where mechanically operated systems spare man a large amount of physical labor while computerized systems also save him a great deal of intellectual effort. Biologically speaking this means a leveling of natural differences in muscular strength and intelligence; sociologically speaking it means the loss of social positions which had been based on these differences. This leveling in the production process has not only led to the disappearance of traditional professional and vocational categories such as certain trades and crafts and their guilds; it has already questioned the esteem and reputation of all traditional estates, and it now goes about questioning the sense of human labor as such. In primitive society, labor was synonymous with the struggle for survival, but during the further development of humanity it acquired its own meaning and dignity so that it filled man's life with sense and satisfaction. His soul beamed with pride when he looked at the work of his hands; a cultivated field, a fine garment, a work of art, or a service rendered to the community. Just as a mountaineer will experience true happiness on a peak which he has conquered after a strenuous climb, the worker will only be proud of his work when it has cost him great effort.

The call to do one's job is duty; the potential of effort exerted is diligence; the reward obtained is satisfaction. These ethical concepts combine with the desire to acquire additional property and increase one's health. This sense of individual property is innate in man: its origins go back to the instinct of older vertebrae to build nests, holes, dens and lairs. Just as a fox will only feel safe in his earth, man needs a home where he and she will be comfortable and cosy, where they can relax and raise a family: "My home is my castle", and thus the paragon of privite property.

Like so many new sociological phenomena which we owe to the Second Industrial Revolution, the commune is an interesting experiment which, however, - as far as we can tell - has not yet found its final solution. Social experiments have a particular fascination, especially for young people. It is certainly true that every younger generation has felt the desire to try, test and even change the world into which it had been born without being asked. This is quite understandable, as I myself would't feel fine either in a flat where I'm not even allowed to rehang the pictures on the walls. From this aspect, this test of strength between sons and fathers, between young citizens and the authorities, is not something perverse but a physiological phenomenon. A society unable to stand this test would be ripe for reforms, or even in for a revolution. Constructive lack of respect is a prerequisite for progress and a new quality of life; it is not a sign of decay but a behavioral pattern serving to overcome obsolete taboos and to keep society healthy and active.

Modern technocracy, the unbridled rule of the machine over man, has taken hold of this desire and imparted to it some new and rather menacing features. When Herbert Marcuse, for instance, recommends to blow up the state like a prison, without having something better to offer in its place, this is no real alternative to the many vexations by which the state keeps annoying us. Despite of its untoward features the modern state is an elaborate structure, the result of many thousand years of human effort. The trouble it must have taken to develop and build it occasionally becomes visible in our days where such well-designed political structures are lacking, e.g. in certain parts of the Third World.

In the 20th century, the concept of democracy also has undergone very strange interpretations which neither the forefathers of Enlightenment nor the patriarchs of Socialism would ever have dreamt of. The call for equal chances at the starting line has been perverted into the claim for an equal prize at the finishing post, which favors the lazy and discriminates against the hardworking who now has to toil for both. The state, originally conceived as an agency for protecting safety and promoting the free development of its citizens, has now assumed the role of being a guardian for all; in many places it has turned into an end in itself, into a power mechanism in the hands of a resolute minority which controls all means of production and directs the masses, to its own very material advantage, by giving them panem et circenses or by exerting psychic pressure.

In the train of the machine which Homo faber had construed to his own relief and which, as we have seen, leveled out so many differences between individuals, the missionaries of new teachings approach young people in an attempt to discredit traditional ethical values such as diligence, responsibility, faith, work morale, patriotism, trying to replace them by idleness, submersion into anonymity and moral unrestraint. They decry work as something sickening, at the same time pursuing the objective of destroying young people's attachment to the place where they live and to their inner sense of belonging, which also includes the elevating power of art. Pleasure gain and risklessness on one's entire path through life rank supreme in their scale of values. This also includes that authority as exercised by a superior or father is equated with repression, that a girl's virtue is ridiculed, and that wives and mothers are continuously deceived by telling them that the work done by them is not gainful and therefore despicable. The call for equal rights for women is in reality a call for equal duties for women which they can only follow when they give up their original destination as core and focus of the family. The real meaning of the slogan of equal rights for women became clear to me when I was a prisoner in that Eastern country where women were made to quarry stones and carry bricks but decried the sad fate of their poor sisters in Switzerland who at that time did not have the right to vote.

Two other sociological endeavors now under way seem to me to be in close correspondence with an erroneous understanding or conscious misinterpretation of the concept of democracy: They consist, on the one hand, in an effort to turn people against each other by stirring up envy and jealousy among them, and, on the other, in wrapping them up in deceitful care in the disguise of social welfare, which, however, only aims at their intellectual incapacitation. The obvious objective of these endeavors is, of course, to come to or cling to power by securing a sufficient number of votes: The "Brave New World" is built on the backs of submissive and uncritical subjects.

In practice this is achieved by imposing sanctions against heritage and talent, setting different social groups at variance and bringing them down on each other: pupils on their teachers, children on their parents, students on their professors, apprentices on their masters, subalterns on their superiors, soldiers on their officers, farmhands on their farmers, and even wives on their husbands. Under the slogan of equal rights harmony is replaced by repression. Once authority has been equated with oppression it can easily be undermined by calling for a full share in all decisions - without any share in corresponding responsibility, as a matter of fact.

A primitive behavioral pattern innate in man (which may be permissible in the tropics but has already been overcome in more temperate climates) is being artificially reactivated: Its most characteristic traits are arrogant idleness, a disinclination to learn and to work, distance for any achievement and aversion to assume any responsibility, the unrestrained wish to dawdle and play around; its declared ideals are enjoyment of all pleasures and satisfaction of all desires - without any responsibility whatsoever, but with full claims to care and maintenance. This is exactly the situation of a kindergarten child: As innocent victims of a far too permissive education the younger generations have never learnt how to establish and keep order; nobody stops them when they are noisy and start destroying things, but like children unrestricted by any forbiddance they turn angry and become violent. While they abuse democratic principles and wrongly advocate socialist goals, neglect, noise and filth are spreading over the globe like a rash. The world as a kindergarten gone wild: this is something Engels, Marx, Kautsky, Bebel, Lassalle, Liebknecht or Plechanov would never have dreamt of.

The outcome of hedonistic seduction, however, is not lust and pleasure but weariness, unfulfillment and boredom, of which both fiction and the theater are replete since the days of "Bonjour Tristesse", "La Noia" and "Magic Afternoon". The past is either detracted or seen in nostalgic transfiguration so that many of those who are disenchanted with the present just drop out or seek refuge with one or the other sect. But he who, fully conscious of the biological development of man, praises those traits to which man owes the present high level of his civilization, will be condemned as a representative of social Darwinism, on the assertion that man, being exempted from any order ruling in the animal kingdom, occupies a privileged position in nature. This assumption is erroneous. As the only living creature on this planet man has won for himself the liberty of cutting off his own roots, but if he really makes use of this freedom this will be the end of him: There can be no existence contrary to the laws of life. The laws of nature govern not only man's physiology but also his psyche. There are many illustrations of this fact, apart from love which, as already mentioned, does not always conform to "law and order". And in its essence the protest of the young against law and order is nothing but the rebellion of good old Tarzan, who does not want to be lulled by welfare and safety but wishes to prove his worth. In former days, wars constituted such a challenge to test one's strength to the very bounds of one's existence. Nowadays the machine makes war appear obsolete even in its function as an instrument of biological selection so that it is very difficult indeed for the young to prove to themselves and others what they are capable of doing and achieving. Competitive sports, military missions for peaceful purposes, extreme accomplishments above and under water, exploits on mountains over 20.000 feet, protest actions including participation in terrorist commando raids - all these practicable for the few. The majority, however, will find other opportunities to prove their moral and physical stamina, e.g. in a profession that demands extreme efforts and offers extreme rewards.

Both things apply to laser surgery - to an extent not attained by any other discipline. The day-to-day confrontation with the extreme frontiers of human existence, with the struggle between the patient's ego and his metaphysical forces, the resolute decision to save lives and the consequent efforts to this end by day and night, whether on duty or off duty, regardless of material reward - all this, and additionally the handling of this exciting new tool that promises much and fulfils even more - all this constitutes the unmatched burden and unparalleled fascination of surgical work by means of lasers.

Lasers in Neurosurgery: State of the Art

P. W. Ascher
Department of Neurosurgery, University of Graz, A-8036 Graz

Abstract

When we were first confronted with the laser, in 1975, it was not considered useful for neurosurgery (1,2,3). We were nonetheless fascinated by the potential of a non-touch instrument and attempted to demonstrate its applicability. After theoretical considerations and animal experiments, we performed the first laser operation on a patient on July 28, 1976. Since then we have performed over 1,100 procedures with the CO_2 and Nd:YAG lasers (4-8). Our early hopes for the laser have been realized and new indications added.

Not long after Maiman, Patel, and Polanyi (3) constructed the first lasers, these were evaluated and accepted by a number of medical fields (Goldman). Neurosurgical experiments with a ruby laser on mice produced catastrophic results and led to the false impression that the laser, any laser, was much too powerful and uncontrollable to be used in the central nervous system (1,2). Stellar used an early commercial CO_2 laser (that was meant for general surgery) in a small number of neurosurgical patients. While recognizing the CO_2 laser's potential, Stellar used the wrong type of instrument for the wrong indications and came to the same conclusions as his predecessors. Our own analysis of Stellar's results led us to conclude that lasers designed for general surgery were not necessarily ideal for neurosurgical operations (just as other instruments from that field are not always useful in ours).

Novelty is not enough. New methods and instruments must provide additional benefit to be justified. The CO_2 laser allows non-touch technique, does not clutter the narrow neurosurgical operating field, and maximizes precision, thus allowing surgery of previously inaccessible tumors. Only an instrument under visual control, such as the CO_2 laser - and certainly not a high-power laser - can be used safely in the nervous tissue.

Experience has confirmed these virtues but the CO_2 laser did not meet our expectations in the coagulation of bleeding vessels. While both the argon and the Nd:YAG lasers are used for coagulation elsewhere, only the latter is applicable in neurosurgery (9-12).

It is essential to define exactly the indications for use of either the CO_2 or Nd:YAG laser. The CO_2 laser is used to cut and vaporize tissue and, in combination with the operating microscope, in microsurgery; it is not suitable for protein denaturation by radiation. In contrast, the Nd:YAG laser is well suited to the coagulation of both venous and arterial vessels and to protein denaturation. Developed in conjunction with optic fibers, this laser was soon used endoscopically. Microadaptors now permit its use in microsurgery.

Physical Characteristics

It is not up to us to teach physics - we aim only to clarify abstruse concepts for the surgeon. The principle underlying all surgical lasers is the absorption of light energy and its conversion to heat by tissue. Schalow permitted me, for physicians, to use the following simplified formula:

Laser light + nervous tissue = heat by absorption.

The absorption of light depends on its wavelength. The CO_2 laser, which has a wavelength of 10.6 um, is absorbed in water almost completely, and therefore also at the surface of human tissue. Used in focus, this laser penetrates the tissue and permits sharp cutting (especially in the super-pulsed mode). Depending on the energy density, a defocused beam can vaporize thin sheets of tissue at the surface.

The Nd:YAG laser has a shorter wavelength (1.06 um) and thus penetrates into tissue. The scattering effect and delayed absorption of a defocused beam result in slow heating and denaturation of protein. A focused Nd:YAG, especially at high energy output, not only vaporizes surface tissue but also causes denaturation in the depths that is difficult to estimate and control. The now available 1.32-um Nd:YAG laser is better for cutting than the original device but still not comparable to the CO_2 laser.

These concepts, while simplified, have suffuced to explain the lasers' effects to physicians. The introduction of tumor dyes and new instruments, such as the ultraviolet laser (Excimer), will soon make new explanations necessary. We are studying photosensibilization and other photochemical reactions.

Clinical Experience

In the last 11 years, we have operated on over 1,100 patients with the laser (Table 1). Absolute indications for the laser were uncommon - only 0.8% to 1.0% of all our patients. However, these select patients were otherwise inoperable. In contrast, 10% of our total patients presented with relative indications, meaning that advantages to the patient and/or surgeon were to be expected by using the laser. Advantages include less postoperative cerebral edema, less postoperative pain, better scarring, and shorter hospitilisation for the patient and less bleeding, better visibility, less stress, and more elegant technique for the surgeon.

Table 1. Laser operations performed at the Universitätsklinik für Neurochirurgie in Graz, Austria; July 28, 1976 - June 15, 1987. The Table shows the total number of procedures (1,107) with the different lasers.

```
Glioblastomas.............................................. 247
Astrocytomas............................................... 188
Meningiomas................................................ 143
Metastases................................................. 117
Other...................................................... 125

    Tumors of the pineal gland....... 10
    Adenomas of the pituitary gland.. 12
    Plexus papillomas................  5
    Medulloblastomas................. 17
    Craniopharyngeomas...............  6
    Acoustic nerve tumors............ 10
    Angiomas and AVMs................ 27
    Ependymomas...................... 33
    Tumors of the corpus callosum....  5

Other (unclassified tumors)................................  26

Other intracranial lesions.................................  49

    Hemorrhagic cysts................ 18
    Arachnoidal cysts................  8
    Abscesses........................  8
    Tuberculomas.....................  1
    Procedures on epileptics......... 13

Operations on the spinal cord..............................  77

    Extramedullary tumors............ 38
    Intramedullary tumors............ 18
    Functional surgery...............  7
    Nucleus pulposus vaporization.... 14

Operations on peripheral nerves............................  33
Sympaticus surgery.........................................   2
Craniostenosis.............................................   7
Operations on vessels......................................  37
Miscellaneous..............................................  56
```

The laser is not indicated when conventional techniques produce the same or better results or when its purpose is the satisfaction of the surgeon's curiosity. The Nd:YAG laser is contraindicated in critical areas such as the brainstem and spinal cord and when the surgeon is inexperienced.

Table 2. Laser operations on and in the brainstem (1976 - 1987)

Astrocytoma	27
Ependymoma	17
Medulloblastoma	12
Meningioma	13
Pineal tumors	6
Angiomatous lesions	11
Spongioblastoma	3
Cholesteatoma	1
Papilloma	3
Lipoma	1
Epidermoid cyst	1
Sarcoma	1
Glioblastoma	1
Neurinoma	1
Unclassified	3
Metastases	4
Total	105

Table 3. Laser surgery in or close to the lower brainstem (1976-1987). The Table lists lesions in or close to the pons (P), rhombencephalon (R), cerebellum-pons (CP), and cerebellum-rhombencephalon (CR).

	P	R	CP	CR	T
Medulloblastoma	1	5	-	7	13
Astrocytoma	1	3	1	1	6
Spongioblastoma	1	-	-	1	2
Ependymoma	1	7	1	2	11
Papilloma	1	1	-	-	2
Sarcoma	1	-	-	-	1
Angioma	4	1	1	-	6
Metastases	-	-	2	1	3
Unclassified	-	1	1	1	3
Total	10	18	6	13	47

Postoperative mortality (3 weeks) was 8%, an excellent result considering the poor prognosis of these mostly histologically benign but nonetheless deadly lesions.

Future Considerations

With the laser, we have developed completely new neurosurgical techniques such as non-touch cutting and vaporization. Coagulation without tissue sticking to metal instruments certainly makes surgery easier. Denaturation of malignant cells allows treatment of previously inaccessible tumors. Also, the lasers in use today permit the bonding of tissue.

Fiber optics are revolutionizing endoscopic neurosurgery. We are studying the intravascular endoscopic application of the laser to atherosclerotic disease of the carotid artery. Sapphire-tipped Nd:YAG lasers have shown the feasibility of this procedure. A further clinical study will evaluate the vaporization of the nucleus pulposus of the intervertebral disc as an outpatient procedure for selected patients with disc disease.

Experimentally, tumor dyes and corresponding lasers may be able to elicit photochemical reactions that selectively destroy malignant cells. A further aspect is the introduction of interstitial thermotherapy of central tumors with the 1.06-um Nd:YAG laser. The laser is applied stereotactically under CT control; the procedure and the denaturation of the tumor can be followed by realtime NMR imaging. Thus the heat application can be limited to the lesion. This treatment is being planned at our hospital; the difficulties are mainly logistic. The probes are being designed and made of plastics and carbon fiber so as to avoid interference with the magnetic field. This is a potential breakthrough in the treatment of the malignant gliomas, the greatest challenge to modern neurosurgery.

References

1. Fox JL et al. The effects of laser radiation on intracranial structures. In: Abstract book: 1st Ann Biomed Laser Conf. Boston 1965.
2. Rosomoff HL. Effect of ruby laser on brain and neoplasm. In: Abstract book: 1st Ann Biomed Laser Conf. Boston 1965.
3. Stellar S et al. Lasers in surgery. In: Laser appl in medicine and biology, p 241. New York 1972.
4. Ascher PW. Der CO_2 Laser in der Neurochirurgie. Monographie. Molden Vlg, Wien 1977.
5. Ascher PW. CO_2 laser in neurosurgery. Neurosurg Rev 7; 1984.
6. Heppner F, Ascher PW. Über den Einsatz des Laserstrahls in der Neurochirurgie. Medizinalmarkt 12, p 424. 1976.
7. Ascher PW, Cerullo L. Chapter 9:Laser use in neurosurgery. In: Surgical Appl of Lasers. Year Book Med Publ, Chicago, pp 163-74 1983
8. Heppner F, Ascher PW. The CO_2 laser in neurosurgery. In: Int Adv in Surg Oncology, Vol 5. Alan R Liss, New York, pp385-96.1982.
9. Ascher PW. Different lasers in neurosurgery: a comparison of Nd:YAG and CO_2. In Neodymium:YAG laser in med and surg. Elsevier. pp 119-125. 1983.
10. Ascher PW, Heppner F. Clinical applications of lasers in neurosurgery. In: Lasers in medicine. John Wiley & Sons, New York, pp 1-14. 1980.
11. Ascher PW. Chapter 23: Neurosurgery. In: Microscopic and endoscopic surgery with the CO_2 laser. pp 298-314. John Wright, Boston 1982
12. Ascher PW et al. Surgery of tumors in the midline. Eur Soc for Pediatric Neurosurgery, 8th Congr, Abstracts p 24, Rennes 1982.
13. Lammer J et al. Transfemorale Katheter-Laser-Thrombendarteriektomie der Arteria carotis. DMW 16, pp 607-10. 1986.

The Use of Contact Laser in Neurosurgery

V.A.Fasano,R.M.Ponzio
Institute of Neurosurgery.University of Torino
Via Cherasco, 15 - 10126 Torino Italy

Introduction

Recent technological improvement consents to deliver a laser beam directly in contact with the tissue and to restore that tactile feed-back the operator had lost with usual laser instruments.
The artificial $AL2O3$ sapphire experimented by Daikuzono and Joffe in 1985,is able to deliver more than 90% of laser light causing no tissular adhesion phenomena(1).From the chemical poin of view,this is a neutral crystal with a hardness and a mechanical resistence,strenght enough to prevent the possibility of breaking the tip;these contact probes reduce the depth of tissue damage and allows for much lower power of laser energy to be used.Moreover the efficiency of the system is proportionately increased by the absence of backscattering effect,which is responsible,during conventional irradiation,for a waste of energy of 30-40%.
Experimental data on the Nd:YAG contact laser exclude the possibility of a direct thermic effect.As a matter of fact,when tissue adhesion is avoided,thermal delivery averages 1/1000 of the total power(3).Furthermore,it has been shown that as far as contact lasers are concerned(0.6 mm sapphire's tip diameter),the 80% of delivered power is emitted in a 90° cone shaped beam and that the power density at the tip corresponds to 2500 watt/cm2 for a delivered laser power of 6.5 watt.In the conventional non-contact systems,the 80% of energy is however focused in a 12° cone and the power density at the end of the fibre is about 400 watt/cm2 for a delivered power of 13 watt(3).This accounts for the vaste energy at the target and instantaneous tissue evaporation produced by Nd:YAG contact irradiation.
Owing to the great width of the emission cone,in contact systems,the power density reduces itself to 40 watt/cm2 at a distance of 2 mm from the tip,while with non-contact laser at a distance of several cm from the end of the fibre power density still corresponds to 400watt/cm2.This is responsible for the less extent of tissue damage in depth after contact irradiation(2).
Experimental studies show moreover that in contact laser systems,the thermic diffusion and consequently the damage of surrounding tissues are reduced(3).
The table(Fig.1)shows as the extension in mm of thermic diffusion,calculated for 42°C temperatures(thresold of cellular damage),60°C(thermal coagulation),100°C(permanent cellular damage),is drastically reduced as far as conventional laser systems are concerned in case that equivalent emission powers from a surgical point of view are considered(3).
Histological studies made on different tissues after incision with contact Nd:YAG show the absence of carbonization whereas the area of coagulative necrosis spreads for 15-40 micron only into extracranial tissue(temporal muscle) and for 100-200 micron into cerebral tissue(2).
The ultrastructural study of the effects on adjacent tissues(evidence of tissular lesions 1.5-3 mm away from the centre of the lesion),shows different pictures

	T	42° C	60° C	100° C
CONTACT LASER	25	14.6 (9.9)	10.0 (5.3)	5.9 (1.2)
	28	15.2 (10.4)	10.6 (5.8)	6.4 (1.7)
	31	15.6 (10.9)	11.0 (6.3)	6.9 (2.2)
NONCONTACT LASER	15	11.0 (6.3)	6.4 (1.7)	2.3 (-)
	18	11.8 (7.1)	7.3 (2.5)	3.2 (-)
	21	12.6 (7.9)	8.0 (3.3)	3.9 (-)

Fig.1.Thermal effect in the cerebral tissue

after Nd:YAG and Argon irradiation.
The latter causes slight modifications like erythrocytes,endothelial cells and neurons vacuolization,along with a total preservation of vessel perviety and tissue structure(Fig.2a-2b).
Nd:YAG laser instead causes clear damage as far as microcirculation and tissue are concerned:astrocyte pedicles and endothelial cells shows always nuclear and cytoplasmic lesions(Fig.3a-3b),while in some samples erytrocytes are aggregated.

Surgical technique

Contact laser systems can be fit to different non-contact laser units on the market.However,it is to be stressed that in some of these the instability of low power energy delivery causes the maneuver to be discontinuous and can easily induce melting of the sapphire tip.This is easily visible in power surgical lasers.
The sapphire connection with the optic fibre is easily performable simply confronting the two surfaces.A cooling system avoids the tip overheating assuring in the same time the removal of smokes and gases produced by tissue burning.
Contact cutting probes combine the coagulating properties of the Nd:YAG laser with cutting capabilities previously only seen with the carbon dioxide laser.
Sapphire of the following kinds are available:
sapphires with a 0.2 up to 1.2 mm diameter and with 19 up to 9 mm lenght,these last ones being employed for dissection maneuvers into cavities;
a sapphire with a 0.05 mm diameter employed for microsurgical purposes;
a frosty surface sapphire by means of which there is a delivery coming both from the tip and from lateral faces,very useful where the cutting of highly vascularized tissues(cerebral cortex,tumoral vascularized tissue) is required.
Contact laser is to be employed like a usual scalpel and can be combined with

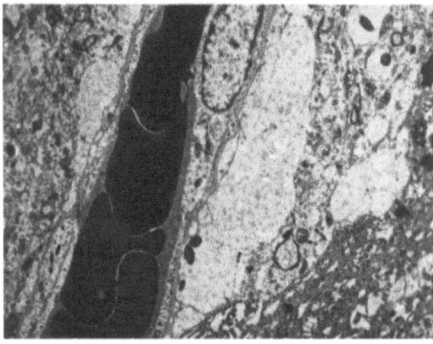 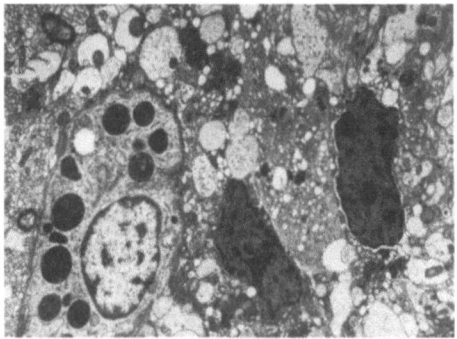

Fig.2:
Argon laser:This source produces minimal tissutal changes,consisting in appearance of vesicles into endotelial cells and basement membrane.
Fig.2a shows a cerebral capillary with the endothelial cells,basement membrane and erytrocytes into the lumen.Only vesicles into basement membrane are evident.
Fig.2b shows normal cerebral tissue:nuclei,granules of pigment,astrocyte pedicles and myelinic sheats are evident.The laser-induced damage is limited to the apnearance of several intracytoplasmic vesicles.

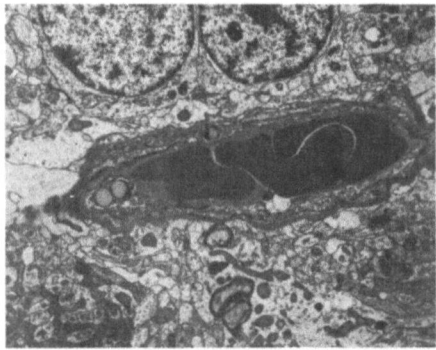 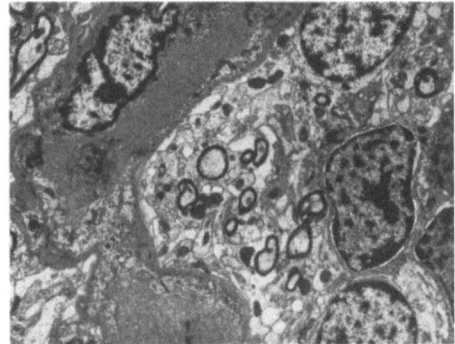

Fig.3:
Nd:YAG laser:This source produces marked histological changes,consisting in swelling of cells and basement membrane and in appearance of intracytoplasmic vesicles.
Fig.3a shows a cerebral capillary.The structure is preserved.Swelling of the endothelial cells and vesicles into the basement membrane are observed.
Fig.3b shows the cerebral tissue.The tissue architecture with nuclei,granules of pigments and myelinic sheats are observed.Astrocyte pedicles are swelled and several intracytoplasmic vesicles are detectable.

operation miccroscope employing the 0.05 mm tip with no visual encoumber.Contact is obtained with a minimal trauma simply grazing the tissue.Energy delivery must be stopped when the contact with the tissue is interrupted thus preserving the sapphire's tip melting.
A possible tissue adhesion to the tip requires the sapphire substitution.A direct,continuous control of the cutting surface is compulsory to make a hemostatic cut.
For the hemostasis,some sapphire tips with a medium diameter(0.6-1mm) whose tip and portion of the lateral surface are frosty,are being used,and a low power(1-4 watts) is delivered when touching the external vessel wall with the tip.
Once the hemostasis is performed in this way,the cutting of the tissue will be done increasing the power values.
The section of the much less vascularized white matter is performed with normal tips of a smaller diameter(0.2-0.8mm) with a power of 10-20 watt.
As far as the tumoral surface incision is concerned,variables sapphires and powers are employed according to the tissue hardness.The sapphire is included between 0.8-1.2 mm in case of hard tissues,with a power ranging from 12 to 18 watts.The peeling of tumor from the surrounding healthy tissue is performed with 0.2 up to 0.6 sapphire tips.

Results and indications

Contact laser offers some remarkable advantages in cutting and dissection maneuvers if compared both to traditional and to non-contact laser systems.
The section made with bipolar forceps is more traumatic,irregular and wider;moreover the coagulation of tille vessels often causes a remarkable extension of tissular damage.
The cut with CO2 laser has a wider diameter.Tumoral lesions always show indented edges and irregular growth as far as surrounding tissues are concerned,requiring and indented cutting.With CO2 laser,dissection is much less precise and the risk of a beam deviation on adjacent tissues is greater.The procedure is slower,the hemostasis less complete and the control of incision depth is less direct.
Other advantages of the contact laser are represented by the absence of smoke in the operative space and the possibility to use lower energies thus limiting the thermic diffusion.This last characteristic will make possible the employ of generators reduced in size.
The main indications for contact laser are represented by incision in depth and dissection of fibrous-connective structures adjacent to the tumor.The cutting maneuver is less efficacious in case of hard or calcifying tissues.The hemostasis is limited to the non bleeding vessels,not superior to 1 mm in diameter.
Our experiences concerns 154 cases affected from super and subtentorial intra-axial and extra-axial neoplasia.The showed tables illustrate the surgical results and the series of cases(Fig.4-5).
Contact and non-contact irradiation techniques can be associated.
Non-contact irradiation is indicated for surface irradiation,contact laser for deeper penetration and dissection.

CONTACT LASER	
Incision of cortex and white matter	Reduced width of cut (0.05 mm) Complete hemostasis
Peeling of residual tumors from the adjacent tissues and dissociation of nervous-vascular structures	Reduced width of cut (0.05 mm), reduced lateral thermal diffusion, reduced side effects and mechanical trauma
Contact hemostasis of arteries up to 1 mm and veins up to 3 mm	Low power required for vessel closure Use of bipolar forceps limited to bleeding vessels and larger arteries
Resection of tumor emplant	Rapid and bloodless resection of dural and fibrous structures (falx and tentorium)
Fig.4.MANEUVERS PERFORMABLE WITH	ADVANTAGES

PATHOLOGY	N° OF CASES
Cortico-subcortical gliomas	45
Deep-seated gliomas	15
Convexity endotheliomas	15
Parasagittal meningiomas	14
Falx and tentorial meningiomas	10
Sphenoid wing meningiomas	6
Posterior fossa meningiomas	5
Ependimomas	5
Cerebellar hemangioblastomas	1
Cerebellar Spongioblastomas	15
Metastases	13
Abscesses	7
Radionecrosis	3

Fig.5.SERIES OF CASES:154

References

1. Daikuzono N, Joffe SN: Sapphire probe for contact photocoagulation and tissue vaporization with the Nd:YAG laser. Medical Instrumentation :173-178,1985.

2. Diaz FG, Dujovny et al: Use of the contact Nd:YAG laser scalpel in neurosurgery. Proceedings of the 4th general and scientific Meeting of the LANSI(Laser Association of Neurological Surgeons International),Venice,1986. In press.

3. Fasano VA, Ponzio R.M. et al: The use of contact laser(Nd:YAG-Argon)in Neurosurgery. Clinical and experimental data. Proceedings of the 4th general and scientific Meeting of the LANSI,Venice,1986. In press.

A Review of 500 Cases of Brain Tumors Operated with Multiple Laser Sources in Comparison with Conventional Tools

Lombard G.F., Mazzotta G., Gallo Lassere E.
Institute of Neurosurgery ,Director Prof.V.A.Fasano
University of Turin,Italy

In this review we have considered the surgical results of the treatment of cerebral gliomas and meningiomas with multiple laser sources,microscope,CUSA and intraoperative echography in comparison with conventional tools. The laser (1,2,3,4,5) is utilized for cutting,vaporization,hemostasis. There are different laser sources with peculiar characteristics. CO_2 laser is utilized for dissection and vaporization in restricted and hardly approachable areas. It has a limited thermic and hemostatic effect. Nd;YAG laser presents considerable depth of penetration and a better hemostatic effect in comparison with CO_2 laser. Recently Nd:YAG laser has been utilized as contact laser coupled with a sapphire tip. (6,7,8,9,10,11,12)
CUSA (Ultrasonic aspirator)(12,14) presents three different functions: fragmentationn,irrigation and aspiration of the pathologic tissue.
Microscope is utilized when a high precision of surgical manouvres is required.
Intraoperative echography(15,16,17) is usually utilized both in A-mode and B-mode. It is very useful to improve the radicality of the operation.
Cerebral gliomas.
We have examinated 250 cases of gliomas treated with modern technologies and 100 cases operated with conventional tools. Then for each group we have separeted high malignancy gliomas from low malignancy gliomas. We have taken account of postoperative morbidity,time and quality of survival. We used Karnofsky scale(18) to evaluate the neurologic and general condition of the patients.
Postoperative morbidity.
The patients with high malignancy gliomas treated with laser surgery presented a preop. Karnofsky score of 84,5, a postop. score of 85,5 and a score at the discharging of 85,8.
The patients with high malignancy gliomas treated with traditional tools presented respectively these scores:80;59;68,6.
The patients with low malignancy gliomas treated with laser surgery presented a preop. Karnofsky score of 91,2, a postop. score of 78,2 and a score at discharging of 85,9.
The patients with low malignancy gliomas treated with conventional tools presented respectively these scores: 91; 72,8; 83,8.
Time of survival.
The patients with high malignancy gliomas operated with conventional tools and radiotherapy present an average time of survival of 17,7 months. The patients treated with laser surgery and radiotherapy present an average time of survival of 17,4 months.
The time of survival in low malignancy gliomas are respectively of

38,4 and 39 months.

Quality of survival.
We have considered only the patients with a Karnofsky score ranging 80-100 at discharging.
After 6 months the 81,3% of patients with high malignancy gliomas treated with laser surgery have a score over 80, after 12 months 50%, after 24 months 40,6%. The patients treated with traditional surgery present respectively these percentages: 71,4%, 42,8% and 35,7%.
In the patients with low malignancy gliomas treated with laser surgery the 91,7% have a score ranging 80-100 after 12 months, 83,3% after 24 months, 70,8% after 36 months.
In the patients with low malignancy gliomas operated with conventional tools the percentages are respectively of 75%; 56,2% and 43,8%.

Meningiomas.
We have considered 70 cases of meningiomas treated with traditional tools and 80 cases treated with laser surgery.
We controlled the postoperative morbidity and the percentage of recurrences.
The postop. morbidity is reduced in the cases operated with laser surgery. The patients operated with laser presented a Karnofsky score over 80 in 92,2% of the cases in comparison with the 71,7% of the patients treated with conventional tools.
To evaluate the recurrences of meningiomas we have previously classified the exereses in accord to the classification of Simpson(19).
In the exereses grade I the recurrences after laser surgery have been of 7%; after traditional surgery of 7,3%.
In the exereses grade II the percentages have been respectively of 7,8% and 10%; in the exereses grade III the percentages have been respectively of 9,8% and 10,2%.

Discussion.
The use of laser shows an evident improvement of the postoperative morbidity both in the high malignancy gliomas and in low malignancy gliomas. The laser should be able to reduce the collateral effects and mainly the postop. edema.
The time of survival seems to be not influenced by the use of modern or conventional techniques.
The quality of survival has improved in the patients treated with laser and other modern technologies.
The laser surgery confirms also in the treatment of meningiomas the improvement of postop. morbidity and quality of life.
No differences have been noticed in the recurrences?

Conclusions.
We may conclude that laser surgery offers some important advantages in comparison with traditional surgery(1,3,4,5,8,9,20,21):
a) an improvement of the radicality of the operation, in relation also to the use of intraoperarive echography;
b) reduction of bleeding and of postop. edema with shortening of hospitalitation;
c) duration of operation no longer than traditional surgery;
d) reduction of postoperative morbidity;

e) improvement of quality of life.

References
1) Edwards M.S.B.: The laser in neurological surgery, J.Neurosurg.59, 555-566,1983.
2) Fasano V.A.: Principles of laser surgery. In: Advanced intraoperative technologies in neurosurgery,97-102,Springer-Verlag,Wien,1986.
3) Hara M.: Evaluation of brain laser surgery. In:Laser surgery III; part one,158-165;Tel-Aviv:OT-PAZ;1979.
4) Takizawa T.: Laser surgery of brain tumors which were difficult to extirpate with conventional modalities.Laser surgery III,part one 133-144,Tel-Aviv:OT-PAZ;1979.
5) Takizawa T.:Laser surgery of brain tumors. No Shinkeigeka 9,743, 1978.
6) Beck O.J.: The use of Nd:YAG and CO2 laser in neurosuregery.Neurosurg.Rev.3,261-266,1980.
7) Inaba Y.: CO2 laser microsurgery for brain tumor. In:Laser Surgery III,part one,119-127;Tel-AVIV: OT-PAZ,1979.
8) Mattos Pimenta L.H.: Evaluation of diddicult placed meningiomas operated with CO2 laser. In: Laser Surgery III,145-146.Tel-Aviv:OT-PAZ,1979.
9) Perria C.: The value and limitations of the CO2 laser in neurosurgery.Neurochirurgia 26,6-11,1983.
10) Burke L.P.: Nd:YAG laser in neurosurgery. In:Nd:YAG laser in Medicine and Surgery;141-148. New York- amsterdam-Owford:Elsevier,1983.
11) FasanoV.A.:Prime osservazioni preliminari sull'uso del laser scalpel ad Argon ed Nd:YAG in neurochirurgia. In: Proceedings of the International Congress on laser in meddicine and surgery.Bologna, June 26-28,1985.
12) Fasano V.A.: Preliminary experiences with contact Nd:YAG and Argon laser in neurosurgery.Experimental data. 4th Annual and Scientific Meeting of the LANSI.Venice,March 19-22,1986.
13) Brock M.: Ultrasonic aspirator in neurosurgery.Neurosurg.Rev.7,173-177,1984.
14) FasanoV.A.: Ultrasonic aspirator in the surgical treatment of intracranial tumors.J.Neurosurg.Sci.25, 35-40,1981.
15) Fasano V.A.:Preliminary experience with real-time intraoperative ultrasonography associated to the CUSA in neurosurg. Surg.Neurol. 19,318-323,1983.
16) Fasano V.A.: Intraoperative A-mode echoencephalography in neurosurgery.In:Advanced intraoperative technologies in neurosurgery,20-26. Wien-New York:Springer Verlag,1986.
17) Chandler W.F.: Intraoperative use of real-time ultrasonography in neurosurgery. J.Neurosurg.57,157-163,1982.
18) Karnofsky D.A.: The clinical evaluation of chemoterapeutic agents in cancer. In: Evaluation of chemotherapeutic agents. New York, Columbia University press, 192-205,1949.
19) Simpson D.:The recurrence of intracranial meningiomas. J.Neurosurg. Psych.,20:22-39,1957.
20) Kelly P.J.:Computer-assisted stereotaxic laser resection ot intraaxial brain neoplasms.J.Neurosurg. 64,427-439,1986.
21) Heppner F.:CO2 laser surgery of the spinal cord.In:Laser surgery III,part one,57-59, Tel-Aviv:OT-PAZ,1979.

Laser-Assisted Nerve Anastomoses Using a 1,3 µm Nd: YAG Laser with Long-Term Observations

F. Ulrich, T. Sander, R. Schober*, W. J. Bock
Department of Neurosurgery and Department of Neuropathology*
University of Düsseldorf, FRG

Summary

Laser-assisted nerve anastomoses (LANA) of the left sciatic nerve of 30 adult albino rats were carried out with the 1,318 µm Nd:YAG laser in the following way: The nerves are cut through with microscissors. The proximal and the distal nerve stumps are adapted by two lateral epineural sutures. The epineurium, adapted by means of tweezers, is welded together on the upper side and the lower side by a few laser fusion points (12,5 W; 0,1 sec; 0,2 mm diameter) and then the epineural tube is closed.
After being removed following several weeks 28 laser-assisted nerve anastomoses showed perfect continuity.

Introduction

Although use of the laser in nerve anastomosis produced results similar to the traditional suture technique, the potential for its use in nerve repair is promising. Because the power density, length of exposure, and optical attenuation play a role in laser beam tissue response.
Sciatic nerves of rats were severed with steel scalpel blades and subsequently anastomosed with epineurial sutures and laser-aided techniques. Morphometric analysis of myelinated nerve fibers proximal and distal to the anastomosed region revealed that the laser had no deleterious effects on the degree of retrograde axonal degeneration or regeneration potential as compared to the traditional suture technique (1). By changing the walvelength and by conversion of the beam geometry, using 2 (10:0) stay sutures, we have performed rat sciatic nerve microepineurial anastomoses with the modified 1,318 um Nd:YAG laser.

Materials

30 Operations on the left sciatic nerve of adult rats, 20 nerve anastomosis and 10 nerve transplantions, were carried out with the modified Nd:YAG laser in the following way: The nerve was cut through. The proximal and the distal nerve stumps are adapted by two lateral epineural sutures. The epineurium, adapted by means of tweezers, is welded together on the upper side and the lower side by laser fusion points with 0,2 mm diameter, 12,5 watt/0,1 sec and thus the epineural tube is closed. For the nerve transplantations no sutures are necessarey.

Results

Of 30 laser-assisted anastomoses, 28 were optimally functional after being removed following several weeks.
All remaining 28 laser-assisted nerve anastomoses showed perfect continuity without sacculation and could be identified only on the basis of the sutures left behind.
Histological findings will be presented in detail elswhere, but it has to be pointed out that reactive changes were minimal and foreign body granulomas were exclusively observed around the silk sutures. In this respect, the 1.319 μm Nd:YAG laser seems distinctly advantageous to other laser types that induce carbonaceous deposits potentially give rise to scarring detrimental to nerve repair and even to adverse immunologic reactions (2).

Conclusions

The 1.319 μm Nd:YAG laser seems to be particularly useful as an auxilary instrument in peripheral nerve microsurgery. Its welding property alteration of intrinsic supportive tissue structures without induction of a foreign reaction may render it advantageous in other fields as well (2).

Besides the shortening of the operation time of laser-assisted vascular anastomoses, an improvement of integrity could be achieved compared to the conventional technique.
But long-term evaluation by electrophysiological methods are required before safe clinical application.

Literature

1. Beggs, J.L., Fischer D.W., Shetter, A.G.:
   Comparative study of rat sciatic nerve microepineural anastomoses made with Carbon Dioxide Laser and sutures techniques: Part 2
   Neurosurgery, Vol 18, No 3, 266-269, 1986

2. Schober, R., Ulrich F., Dürselen, R., Sander, Th.:
   Laser-induced alteration of collagen substructure enables microsurgical tissue welding.
   Science, Vol 232, 1421-1422, 1986

Time Course of the Blood-Brain Barrier Defect Following Laser Irradiation and Other Injuries of the Rat Forebrain

H.R.Eggert, J.May, M.Hornyak, V.Kallmeyer
Neurochirurgische Universitätsklinik, D-7800 Freiburg,FRG

Laser irradiation of the brain surface of an experimental animal results in a lesion consisting of 3 to 6 discernible zones (1). The outermost zone of the lesion is usually an edematous zone, due to the break down of the blood-brain barrier (4). Similar vasogenic brain edema may be produced by focal freezing of the brain cortex (3) and by local laceration (5). In order to evaluate the time needed for restoration of blood-brain barrier function impaired by the trauma, blood-brain barrier function was investigated at different times after Nd-YAG- and CO_2-laser irradiation, cold injury and focal laceration of the rat forebrain using Evansblue as an indicator.

MATERIALS AND METHODS

Male Wistar rats (200-250 g) were used as experimental animals. Operations and final perfusion were perfomed using neurolept analgesia (Thalamonal$^{(R)}$ 2 ml/kg bw). In order to avoid artifacts caused by the trepanation, a left sided parietal osteoplastic trepanation was performed 48 hours before trauma. For traumatization the skull was reopened and the dura was left intact except from the animals with a laceration trauma. In 56 animals, the exposed brain surface was irradiated by the focussed beam of a Nd-YAG-laser (medilas I, MBB-AT,München) using a focussing handpiece (focal length 3 cm). Output power was 30 W, irradiation time 1 s, energy density 462 J/cm^2. In 18 animals a carbondioxide laser (medilaser-S,MEL-444-S, Mochida Pharmaceutical Co.,Ltd.,Tokyo,Japan) was used for irradiation in connection with an adapter to the operating microscope. In order to produce a lesion similar in shape and size to that of the Nd-YAG laser group, a slightly divergent defocussed beam was used. Output power was 30 W, irradiation time 0.3 s. In 41 animals, a freezing lesion was produced by putting a stainless steel rod of 2.9 mm in diameter previously cooled in liquid nitrogen on the exposed dura for 60 seconds. In 42 animals the cortex was lacerated by dipping a ball-shaped drill of 3.9 mm in diameter running with approximately 5000 rpm into the brain surface.

The animals were allowed to survive for 0.5, 2, 4, 12, 24 and 48 hours. Thirty minutes before the end of the survival time, 0.5 ml of Evansblue 2 % was administered via a femoral vein. At the end of the survival time perfusion fixation was performed as described earlier (2). Following dissection of the fixated brains, coronal sections through the centre of the lesion were documented photographically. In these photographs 3 zones were evaluated planimetrically (MOP-AMO, Contron, Zürich). The "entire lesion" included a central necrosis and a perifocal area stained by Evansblue. The "edema"-zone consisted of the area outside the central necrosis stained by Evansblue. Since Evansblue was injected only 30 min before perfusion, this "edema"-zone does not correspond to the zone of brain edema in histological preparations. But it may serve as a measure for the amount of blood-brain barrier dysfunction. The "center" of the lesion consisted of the unstained central coagulation necrosis in Nd-YAG laser irradiated animals. In CO_2-laser irradiated animals the "center" included the central defect due to vaporization. After cold injury the "center" corresponded to a central deeply blue stained area in contrast to a less stained perifocal area. After laceration trauma, the "center" included the area of disrupted brain tissue or a cortical defect. Additionally to the planimetrical evaluation, in 72 of the Nd-YAG laser irradiated, the cold lesioned and the mechanically lacerated animals the amount of extravasated Evansblue of the traumatized hemisphere was measured photometrically after extraction by chloracetic acid (6).

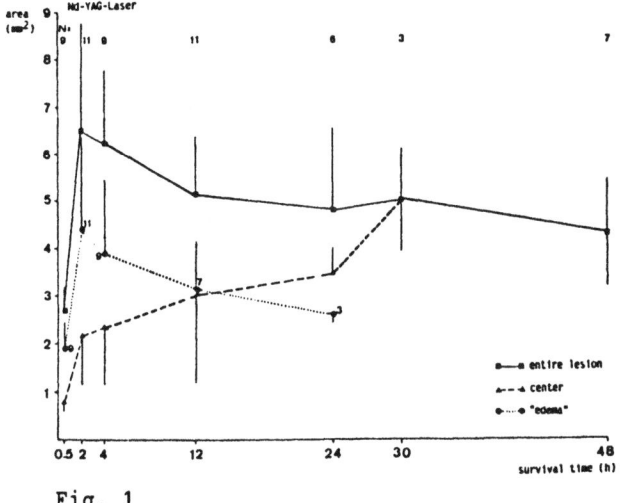

Fig. 1.

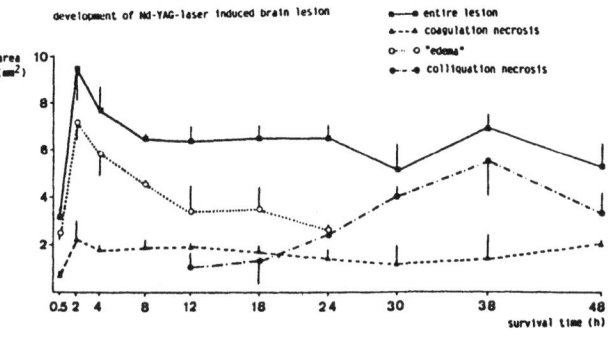

Fig. 2.

RESULTS

Following Nd-YAG laser irradiation, the entire lesion increased significantly within 2 hours and decreased gradually up to 48 hours. The initial increase was mainly due to an enlargement of the stained "edema"-zone which decreased in size up to 24 hours survival time. At longer survival times, staining of the tissue outside the central necrosis was not observed (Fig.1). Primarily, the central necrosis consisted only of a coagulation necrosis. At 12 hours survival time, a surrounding colliquation necrosis appeared which increased gradually (Fig.2). By this mechanism, the size of the entire necrosis was nearly four times larger at 48 hours compared to 30 minutes

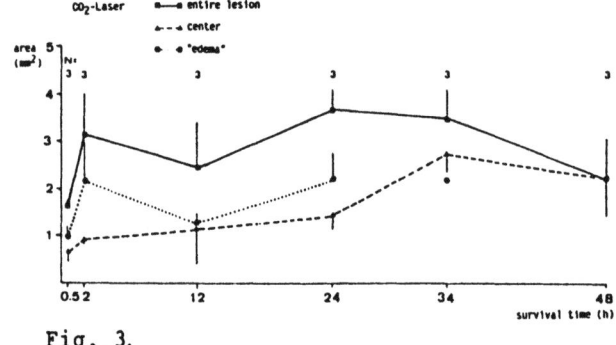

Fig. 3.

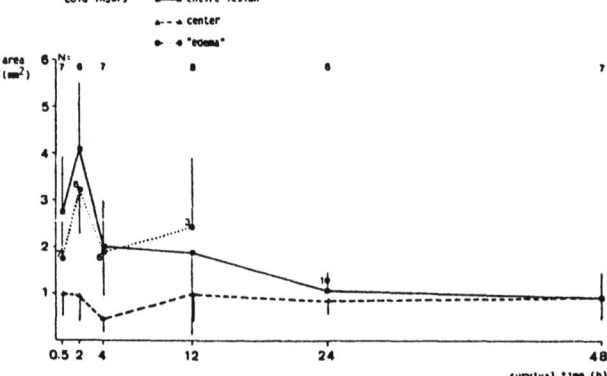

Fig. 4.

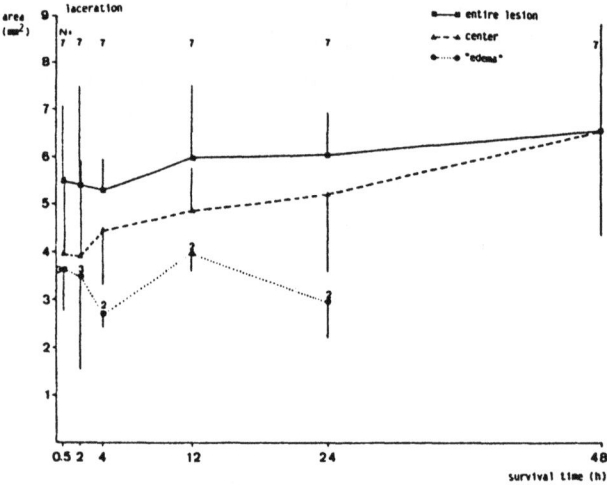

Fig. 5.

after irradiation.

After CO_2-laser irradiation, the size of the entire lesion increased also within 2 hours after irradiation due to a perifocal edematous zone. Again, perifocal staining was observed up to 24 hours. But the extension of the stained zone was much smaller than following Nd-YAG-laser irradiation (Fig.3). Nevertheless, the size of the central necrotic area at 48 hours was double as large as at 30 minutes after irradiation.

After cold injury perifocal staining was more transient than after laser irradiation. Even 12 hours after trauma in only 3 out of 8 animals perifocal staining could be observed (Fig.4). The size of the necrotic area did not increase up to 48 hours.

Mechanical laceration of the cortex produced only in a few animals visible perifocal staining, which did not last longer than 24 hours after trauma. The size of the necrotic lesion increased littel but not significantly within 48 hours after the trauma (Fig.5).

Corresponding to the size of the "edema"-zone, the extravasation of Evansblue increased after Nd-YAG laser irradiation. After cold injury it decreased

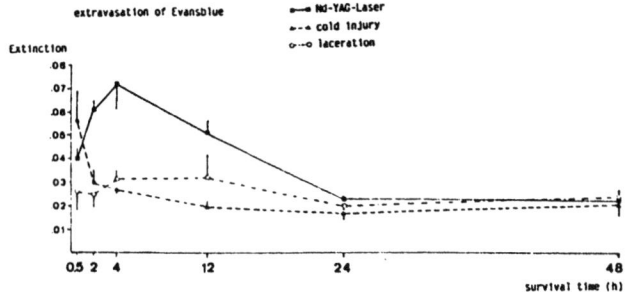

Fig. 6.

steeply. After mechanical laceration only a small amount of extravasated Evansblue could be measured (Fig.6).

Conclusions

1. Blood-brain barrier disruption is more pronounced and is later restored after laser irradiation than after cold injury or mechanical laceration.

2. In contrast to cold injury and to mechanical laceration, the size of the necrotic lesion increases after laser irradiation of the rat forebrain up to 48 hours.

3. Blood-brain barrier disruption as well as secondary increase of the necrotic lesion are more pronounced after Nd-YAG- than after CO_2-laser irradiation.

References
1. BOGGAN JE, EDWARDS MSB, DAVIS RL et al.; Neurosurgery 11, 609-616, 1982
2. EGGERT HR, KIESSLING M, KLEIHUES P; Neurosurgery 16, 443-448, 1985
3. KLATZO I; J.Neuropath.Exp.Neurol. 26, 1-14, 1967
4. LAMPERT PW, FOX JL, EARLE KM; J.Neuropath.Exp.Neurol. 25, 531-541, 1966
5. PERSSON LI, ROSENGREN LE, HANSSON HA; Acta Neurol.Scand. 57, 405-417, 1978
6. RÖSSNER W, TEMPEL K; Med.Pharmacol.Exp. 14, 169-182, 1966

Effect of Nd:YAG Laser at 1.44 μm on Rabbit Brain

R. Martiniuk, J.D.S. McKean, J. Tulip, B.W. Mielke, J. Bauer

Departments of Surgery and Electrical Engineering

University of Alberta, Edmonton, Canada

Laser vaporization of tissue is highly dependent upon the wavelength of the applied radiation. In the near infrared, absorption is dominated by the water content of tissue. There is a large variance of the absorption spectrum of water over a relatively small range of radiation wavelength (Fig. 1). Consequently, a small change in the operating wavelength of an infrared laser will dramatically influence tissue response. Several laser emission wavelengths and their corresponding absorption coefficients in water are shown in Fig. 2. The absorption coefficient increases from approximately 2 cm^{-1} at the Nd:YAG wavelength of 1.32 μm to 30 cm^{-1} at 1.44 μm. This study was undertaken to quantify some of the differences in laser interaction with brain tissue at 1.06 μm and 1.44 μm.

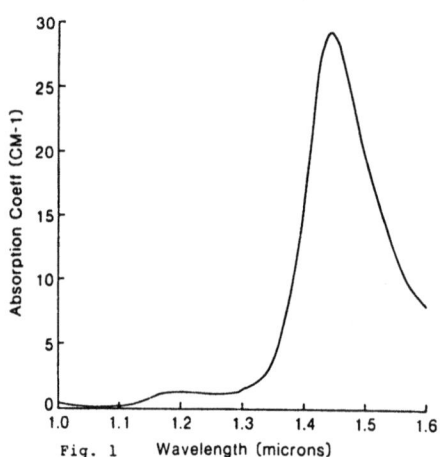

Fig. 1

ABSORPTION COEFFICIENT OF WATER FOR VARIOUS LASER WAVELENGTHS

LASER	λ (micron)	α (cm^{-1})
Nd:YAG	1.06	0.174
Nd:YAG	1.32	2.01
Nd:YAG	1.44	29.7
CO_2	10.6	800

Fig. 2

Method

Laser radiation close to the water absorption peak at 1.44 μm was generated by a Nd:YAG laser developed at the University of Alberta. This laser would also generate radiation at the conventional Nd:YAG wavelength of 1.06 μm. The power available at the target site was set at 5, 10, and 20 Watts as measured by a Coherent® 201 power meter. This energy was delivered, multimode, to the target area via a mirror-lens assembly. This assembly was configured to produce consistent spot sizes of 0.75 mm and 1.5 mm in diameter. These spot sizes were determined using formulae of geometric optics and verified with a series of index apertures.

For each power setting (5, 10, 20 Watts), lesioning energies of 5, 10, 20 and 40 Joules were achieved by varying the irradiation time, for a total of 12 operating points. Each of these operating points were repeated for the two specified spot sizes and the two wavelengths being studied. In order to establish experimental reliability, each of the 48 operating parameters were duplicated in different animals.

Forty-eight female, New Zealand white rabbits (weighing between 1.9 and 3.0 kg) were anesthetized and placed into a stereotaxic frame. Bilateral frontoparietal craniotomies were performed using a low-speed air drill. The dura mater was excised bilaterally. Brains exhibiting any surgical trauma were excluded. Each hemisphere was irradiated once in a relatively avascular region. These lesions were in different coronal planes.

Immediately following lesioning, 2% Evan's Blue (1cc/kg) was injected intravenously. This was done to indicate the extent of damage to the blood brain barrier.

Thirty minutes post-lesioning, the animals were sacrificed by intravenous sodium pentobarbital, the brains removed, photographed and fixed in buffered formalin.

Serial sections (100 μm intervals) in the coronal plane were made and stained using hematoxylin and eosin. Several sections adjacent to the center of each lesion were photographed and printed under constant magnification. Areas of histologically distinct zones were measured on the photographs using a Hewlett-Packard digitizer and mini-computer. In addition, the widths and depths of these zones were determined.

Results

In all cases of 1.44 μm irradiation, lesions were apparent prior to the injection of the Evan's Blue solution. However, with 1.06 μm radiation there was no visible indication of lesions at lower energies both before or after the Evan's Blue injection. For a given energy, the diameter of the blood brain barrier damage indicated by the staining was consistently larger for 1.44 μm radiation.

The lesions produced with 1.06 μm radiation (Fig. 3a) characterized by a conical area of coagulation necrosis which exhibited partial artifactual separation from a demarcating peripheral zone of rarefaction due to edema. Neurons within the central area of necrosis showed nuclear hyperchromatism and mild diminution of size. The cytoplasm was poorly defined. There was no evidence of linear distortion of nuclei. By contrast, neurons in the adjacent peripheral zone of edema exhibited marked increased staining affinities of both nuclei and cytoplasm. In addition, there was extensive pyknosis of cortical glia in this area. The lesions were further characterized by a narrow border of selective neuronal necrosis within the cortex adjacent to the edematous zone.

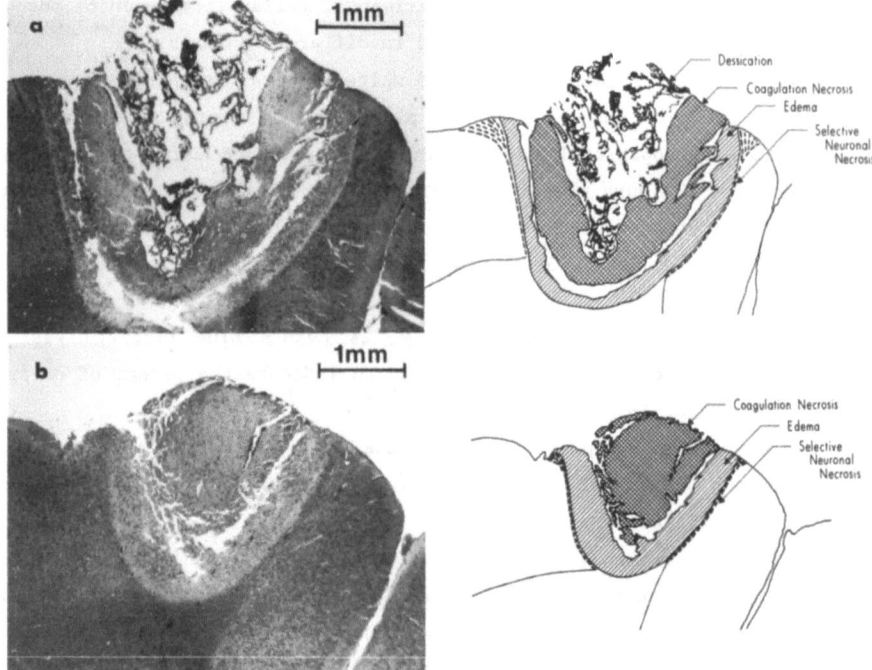

Fig. 3a 1.44 um @ 10 W, 4.0 sec., 0.75 mm dia. spot size (H+E X13)
 3b 1.06 um @ 10 W, 4.0 sec., 0.75 mm dia. spot size (H+E X13)

There was no evidence of inflammatory or histiocytic infiltration. No alterations were demonstrable in the subjacent white matter and no glial reactivity was present in the bordering cortex. By definition, the zone of coagulation necrosis in all lesions was measured to be inclusive of the zone of edema.

The alterations produced by 1.44 μm radiation (Fig. 3b) were dominated by a central zone of collapse of the conical area of coagulation necrosis. Apparent desiccation of this portion of the lesion resulted in reticular strands of partially conglutinated cortex in which occasional deeply staining neuronal perikarya could be identified. The cellular morphologic alterations were otherwise comparable to those of the lesions produced by 1.06 μm radiation in each of the defined zones of coagulation necrosis and edema. Comparable selective neuronal necrosis was present in a narrow margin of the cortex peripheral to the zone of edema.

For identical operating conditions, the lesions produced by 1.44 μm radiation were markedly different than those at 1.06 μm. For equivalent energies, the overall lesion area as indicated by the zone of edema was consistently larger at 1.44 μm. However at 1.06 μm, lesion areas were directly proportional to the applied power whereas, at 1.44 μm the areas were inversely proportional (spot size = 1.5 mm diameter)(Fig. 4). A larger component of conduction heating may contribute significantly to the inverse power relationship observed at 1.44 μm.

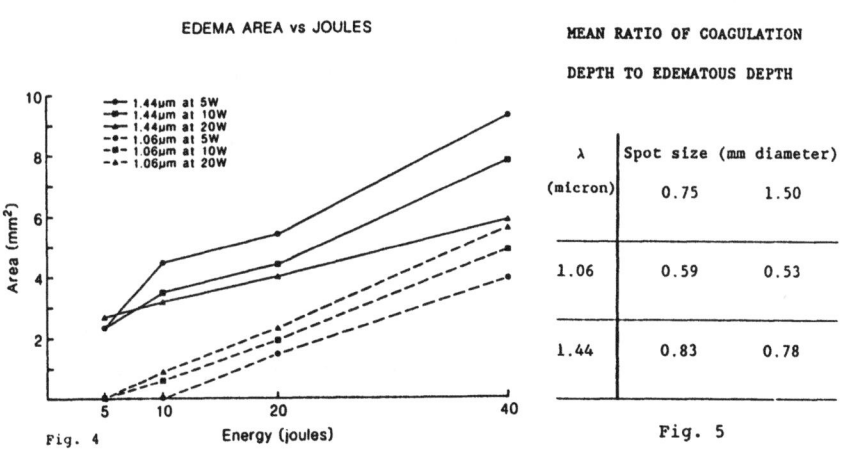

Fig. 4 — EDEMA AREA vs JOULES

Fig. 5 — MEAN RATIO OF COAGULATION DEPTH TO EDEMATOUS DEPTH

λ (micron)	Spot size (mm diameter)	
	0.75	1.50
1.06	0.59	0.53
1.44	0.83	0.78

A comparison of lesion width to depth ratios showed that all lesions, at both wavelengths, were greater in width than depth. In addition, these ratios were greater at 1.44 μm than at 1.06 μm. There was also a larger dependence of the ratio on spot size in the case of 1.44 μm irradiation. This can be attributed to the larger absorption coefficient of water at 1.44 μm, indicating that the radiation applied will be converted to thermal energy over a smaller distance than an equivalent power delivered at 1.06 μm.

The ratio of coagulated depth to edematous depth (Fig. 5) shows that coagulation extends to approximately 75% of the total lesion depth for 1.44 μm radiation while only 51% of the depth is coagulated at 1.06

µm. Similarly, the ratios of coagulation area to area of edema indicate that for 1.44 µm 66% of the lesion area is coagulated while at 1.06 µm only 37% is coagulated. Thus, for equal amounts of tissue coagulation the depth and area of peripheral edema is less at 1.44 µm than at 1.06 µm.

Conclusion

The lesions produced by 1.44 µm laser radiation in brain tissue differ from lesions produced by 1.06 µm radiation. These differences are summarized below:
1. For the same energy, the blood brain barrier damage (as indicated by Evan's Blue staining) is greater for 1.44 µm.
2. The cross sectional area of the lesions are larger for 1.44 µm under the same operating conditions.
3. The lesions made with 1.44 µm have shallower profiles.
4. For a given area of tissue coagulation, the depth and area of peripheral edema is less at 1.44 µm.
5. Evaporative tissue removal occurs with 1.44 µm radiation.

These demonstrable differences between the effects of 1.44 µm and 1.06 µm laser radiation can be explained by the greater absorption of the 1.44 µm radiation by the water in brain tissue.

Increased tissue effects at 1.44 µm mean that controlled photovaporization could be achieved with an Nd:YAG laser. The prototype laser has recently produced in excess of 50 Watts of 1.44 µm. This laser is also capable of producing radiation at 1.06 µm. As with this more conventional wavelength, the 1.44 µm radiation is transmissible via a standard optical fiber.

References

1. Zuev, V.E.: Propagation of Visible and Infrared Radiation in the Atmosphere, Appendix 2, pp 371-375, John Wiley & Sons, Ltd., Chichester, 1974.

2. Handbook of Marine Sciences, Vol. 1, F.G.W. Smith, ed. Table 3.2-5, Absorption of Radiation by Pure Liquid Water, CRC Press, Cleveland, Ohio, 1974.

Use of the Nd: YAG Laser in Microsurgery of Intracranial Tumors

H.R.Eggert, J.May

Neurochirurgische Universitätsklinik, D-7800 Freiburg,FRG

The Nd-YAG laser has been introduced to intracranial surgery by Beck in 1978 (1,2). But up to now, it has not been generally accepted as a microsurgical tool (3,5). In order to get an impression of its real value in intracranial microsurgery, records of operations were reevaluated with special regard to the type of tumors, surgical steps and irradiation parameters.

PATIENTS AND METHODS OF APPLICATION

From the beginning in 1983, each operation performed with the use of the Nd-YAG laser (4)(=1060 nm, medilas I, MBB-AT, München) was recorded in detail. The records included information on the surgical procedure done with the laser, irradiation parameters and the effects observed. In most cases, the laser was applied with a focussing handpiece (f=50 mm) or with a malleable applicator inside which the uncovered light guide is cooled by Ringer's solution. Since these applicators represent additional instruments on the instrument table, sometimes they are more troublesome than useful. The Nd-YAG laser could routinely be applied only when an adapter to the operation microscope became available. This adapter seems disadvantageous only in so far that it reduces the power of the pilot beam. Thus, the pilot beam may be visible only with difficulties when it is used in a defocussed mode in connection with halogen illumination of the microscope.

In most cases, the Nd-YAG laser was used in a continuous wave mode and the beam was moved over the area to be irradiated. Thus, the total energy released to a single spot was only small and could be changed as required according to the visible effect. From 1984 to 1986, 104 intracranial operations on brain tumors were performed with the help of the Nd-YAG laser (Tab. 1). This quantity corresponds only to 10 % of all operations on brain tumors performed within the same time period. This may give to understand that the Nd-YAG laser was introduced gradually with special regard to safety requirements.

Table 1. Laser assisted operations on brain tumors 1984 - 1986

MENINGIOMAS	N=55	CAVERNOMAS	N=4
GLIOMAS	N=17	PAPILLOMAS	N=2
NEURINOMAS	N= 9	HYPOPHYSEAL ADENOMA	N=1
ANGIOBLASTOMAS	N= 7	CHONDROSARCOMA	N=1
METASTATIC TUMORS	N= 7	AVM	N=1

RESULTS

In most cases, the Nd-YAG laser was applied in order to coagulate the surface of a tumor (Tab. 2).

Table 2. Frequency of Nd-YAG laser applications

	MENIN-GIOMAS	GLIOMAS	NEURI-NOMAS	ANGIO-BLASTOMAS	METASTATIC TUMORS	CAVER-NOMAS	PAPIL-LOMAS	N	%
COAGULATION OF TUMOR	40	6	6	7	4	4	2	69	66
HEMOSTASIS INSIDE TUMOR	27	8	3		5		1	44	42
COAGULATION OF INSERTION	23							23	22
DETACHMENT FROM INSERTION	14							14	14
DISSECTION OF ARACHNOID	14							14	14
(HEMOSTASIS AT THE BRAIN)	(8)	(8)		(2)	(2)			(20)	(19)
INCISION OF CRISTA GALLI	3							3	3

In extracerebral tumors like menigiomas, by this the volume of the irradiated part of the tumor was reduced and the tumor shrinked a little. Thus, dissection of the tumor from the surrounding brain was facilitated and, in some cases, the arachnoid together with small arteries and veins supplying normal brain tissue could be preserved which otherwise would not have been possible. However, due to the pale colour of some meningiomas, in 11 % of these cases this effect appeared insufficient. In gliomas as well as in metastatic tumors, coagulation of the surface of the tumor increased consistency and led to a better demarcation of the tumor from the surrounding edematous brain tissue. But this was observed in only few cases. In acoustic neurinomas, shrinking was insufficient in 22 % and coagulation of the surface of the tumor appeared to be not helpful. Coagulation of the surface of tumors was most satisfying in highly vascularized tumors like angioblastomas, cavernomas and papillomas. By shrinking of angioblastomas, small feeding arteries became visible and could be occluded selectively while the main arterial trunks supplying normal brain tissue could be spared. In these vascularized tumors rather low energy densities proved to be more useful than high output energies (Tab. 3). Irradiation of cavernomas led also to an excellent reduction in size with concomitant retraction of the tumors from the surrounding brain.

The other main application of the Nd-YAG laser was hemostasis during piecemeal resection of tumors. Usually, hemostasis could be achieved uncomplicated and faster than by bipolar coagulation. Only in feedeing arteries of more than 1 mm in diameter, bipolar coagulation was more effective and safer. Hemostasis within the normal brain tissue of the tumor layer was abandoned rather early. It appeared to be not economical and even hazardous in some cases.

Table 3. Irradiation parameters used for coagulation of brain tumors

MENINGIOMAS	30 - 50 W defocussed	METASTATIC TUMORS	30 - 40 W defocussed
GLIOMAS	30 - 50 W defocussed	CAVERNOMAS	20 W focussed
NEURINOMAS	30 - 40 W defocussed	PAPILLOMAS	20 W defocussed
ANGIOBLASTOMAS	10 - 20 W defocussed		

Other purposes of laser application were confined to intracranial meningiomas (Tab. 4). Tumors of the falx as well as of the skull base could be detached from their dural insertion by focussed Nd-YAG laser irradiation without hemorrhage. Thus, the main vascular supply of these tumors was interrupted. However, in most cases this aim could have been achieved by bipolar coagulation also. In 3 cases of olfactory groove meningiomas, the crista galli was transsected easily by focussed laser irradiation. Sometimes, this procedure may be troublesome due to severe hemorrhage if it is performed by other methods. In more than half of the meningioma cases, the site of dural attachment was coagulated after removal of the tumor if resection of the dura was not possible. The question if this measure will prevent from recurrences, can not yet be answered. Nevertheless, we observed in cases of parasagittal meningiomas that after irradiation of the sinus wall tumor tissue inside the sinus was completely denaturated.

Table 4. Laser application in microsurgery of intracranial meningiomas

SHRINKING OF THE TUMOR SURFACE	30 - 50 W defocussed
DETACHMENT FROM THE DURA	40 - 50(70) W focussed
TRANSSECTION OF CRISTA GALLI	50 W focussed
FINAL COAGULATION OF DURAL ATTACHMENT	20 W focussed - 40 W defocussed
HEMOSTASIS INSIDE THE TUMOR	30 - 50 W defocussed

In only one case, a complication (6) was observed which might have been due to the use of the Nd-YAG laser. The patient suffering from a unilateral falx meningioma developed a homolateral hemiparesis 24 hours after operation. Following removal of the tumor, the attachment of the tumor at the falx had been irradiated with an output power of 40 W and a slightly defocussed beam. In the postoperative CAT scan an area of low density within the opposite hemisphere adjacent to the irradiated falx was shown.

DISCUSSION

If microsurgical techniques and principles are applied to removal of intracranial tumors, the opinion of different surgeons about the usefulness of the Nd-YAG laser must be contradictory. Since the problems which can be solved by a laser have found other solutions before the introduction of the laser, the opinion of the surgeon will depend on his knowledge of microsurgical methods. The more a surgeon is experienced in applying microsurgical techniques the less he will realize the usefulness of a laser. Hence, we were not surprised that we did not find any tumor which could not have been removed with the same result without the Nd-YAG laser. On the other hand, we found a number of applications of the laser by which particular surgical steps became facilitated, safer and more comfortable. In general, these steps refer to the most important obstacles of microsurgery, impeded visibility due to hemorrhage and increased local pressure. Both of them may lead to inadvertant destruction of healthy brain tissue. The sensible use of the Nd-YAG laser may help even an experienced microsurgeon to overcome these obstacles. However, the basic requirements of safe application of a laser are a solid knowledge of optical properties of tissues the surgeon is dealing with and extensive training in a microsurgical laser laboratory.

REFERENCES

1. BECK OJ; Neurosurg Rev 3, 261-266,1980
2. BECK OJ; Neurosurg Rev 7, 151-158,1984
3. EDWARDS MSB, BOGGAN JE, FULLER TA; J Neurosurg 59,555-566,1983
4. FRANK F; Neurosurg Rev 7,145-150,1984
5. HANDA H, TAKEUCHI J, YAMAGAMI T; Neurosurg Rev 7,159-163,1984
6. JAIN KK; Neurosurgery 16,759-762,1985

Surgery and Plastic Surgery

The CO₂ Laser in Clinical Surgery: Past, Present and Future – State of the Art

I. Kaplan
Chilewich Chair of Plastic Surgery
Tel Aviv University
Ramat-Aviv, 69978 Tel Aviv, Israel

The CO_2 laser has a wavelength of 10.6 microns. This is the only laser beam which is entirely absorbed by water. Since the body tissue comprises between 75% to 90% water, it follows that if the CO_2 laser beam is focused on the body tissue it will cause a vaporisation of the tissue while at the same time, due to the release of thermal energy, the small blood vessels and lymphatics will be sealed. This results in a fine haemostatic incision leaving the residual tissue relatively undamaged so that one is not precluded from performing a primary repair of the residual wound, either by suturing or by skin grafting.

Using a defocused beam it is possible to perform accurate and controllable debulking of tissue by vaporisation thus providing a useful means of removing undesirable tissue from a distance. This can be achieved either by passing the beam through an endoscope or by operating under microscopic control.

It follows from the above that, theoretically at least, the CO_2 laser should have decided advantages over other known surgical "knives". Such advantages would include precise controllable haemostatic, non-touch atraumatic ablation, provided suitable instrumentation is available.

Early in 1972 we embarked on a two-fold project designed to investigate the application of the CO_2 laser in surgery as a whole, while at the same time attempting to develop an apparatus which would be human engineered and designed specifically for clinical surgery bearing in mind the physical conditions and requirements of the average operating room and the idiosyncrasies of the average surgeon, since what was available at that time was far from satisfactory for our purpose and required radical modifications in order to make it applicable to clinical surgery.

Accordingly, the prototype of what eventually became known as the "SHARPLAN" laser (Sharon + Kaplan) (Ref. 30) was produced. This laser, apart from enabling one to embark on clinical laser surgery of all kinds, eventually became the basis for the establishment of Laser Industries Ltd., one of Israel's best known science-based industries.

By the latter part of 1972, sufficient experience had been gained (1-4) to convince one that the hypothesis mentioned above was sufficiently well founded to justify embarking on a campaign of convincing others to adopt this modality.

Close cooperation between the surgeons and the industry gave rise to the introduction of various further modifications and the development of accessories designed to broaden the application of the Co_2 laser in order to encourage other surgical specialities to introduce this modality into their armamentatium. At the same time, publication of articles in professional journals, participation in congresses and symposia were all contributary to "spreading the gospel", (Ref. see bibliography) in spite of the natural scepticism of one's colleagues.

In 1975, the first international symposium on laser surgery was held in Tel Aviv (13) and this gave rise to the foundation of the International Society for Laser Surgery which has since held meetings every alternate year and whose membership has grown rapidly and steadily. This also inspired the formation of numerous regional and national societies throughout the world, with the result that many other lasers, each with its specific application, have been introduced into the medical field.

To date there are well over 1500 Sharplan CO_2 surgical lasers in routine use in 43 countries throughout the world in every field of surgery without ecxeption and it is estimated that approximately 8,000 surgeons are actively involved in laser surgery with this apparatus.

At the 4th Congress of the International Society for Laser Surgery, held in Tokyo in 1981, sixteen companies producing CO_2 lasers for surgery were represented. A sure indication one believes, that the CO_2 laser is an accepted modality in surgery.

Sufficient experience has been accumulated for one to determine where the CO_2 laser has a definite application in surgery and what advantages it has over other modalities.

This can best be classified under the following headings:

OPERATIONS WHERE THE ANTICIPATED BLOOD LOSS WOULD BE SIGNIFICANT

This could well encompass practically every surgical specialty, but is particularly well demonstrated by orthopedic and plastic surgery, where large excisions are involved. Mastectomies, mamaplasties, lipectomies, and other procedures of a similar nature have been performed by ourselves and other (20,49,55) whereas in hand surgery it is worthy of mention that not only is the saving of blood impressive in these cases, but the fact that the use of a tourniquet can be avoided reduces the postoperative morbidity and permits a more rapid return to function.

In neonatal and pediatric surgery the use of the CO_2 laser is, in the opinion of most of us, mandatory (52, 55) because of the vital importance of saving blood in these cases.

SURGERY PERFORMED IN HIGHLY VASCULAR AREAS OF THE BODY

Perhaps the best examples of this are tongue surgery and surgery of the scalp which are being performed routinely by ourselves and others by means of the CO_2 laser with impressive results (7, 14, 32, 55). The fact that the postoperative course in patients who have undergone partial or total glossectomies is almost entirely painless while postoperative oedema is negligible has in most cases made tracheostomies unnecessary and shortened the hospitalization considerably.

EXTIRPATION OF HIGHLY VASCULAR TUMORS

Many cases of cavernous hemangioma, Kaposi sarcoma, and hemangiosarcoma have been extirpated by us and others (15, 55). This enables us to avoid hypotensive anesthesia and ligation of feeding arteries.

SURGERY FOR MALIGNANT DISEASE

It is universally accepted by surgeons that the surgery of cancer should be performed with minimal opening of blood vessels and lymphatics and manipulation of tissue together with maximal visualization. Since the CO_2 laser seals the blood vessels and lymphatics during surgery, while at the same time permitting an almost nontouch extirpation to be performed, whereas the hemostatic effect enables the surgeon to distinguish accurately between pathologic and normal tissue, its application in cancer surgery is obvious. Those of us who have this modality at our disposal are using it routinely for the excision of accessible malignant disease in spite of the fact that our clinical follow-up is still too short to be able to reach definite conclusions regarding its applicability. Considerable experimental evidence exists, however (5, 16, 55), to indicate that the hypothesis upon which its introduction in cancer surgery is based is well founded. We have performed well over 200 wide excisions with primary skin grafting of malignant melanomata and have had no reason to regret having introduced this modality as a routine in our department.

OPERATIONS PERFORMED THROUGH HIGHLY INFECTED TISSUE

The excision of burns, synergistic gangrene, and decubitus ulcers are examples par excellence of the application of the CO_2 laser in this connection. The intraoperative sealing of blood vessels and lymphatics tends to eliminate the spreading of infection while at the same time the laser sterilizes the area of the debridement.

SURGERY PERFORMED ON PATIENTS SUFFERING FROM COAGULOPATHIES

The CO_2 laser has vitually revolutionised the surgical approach to these patients. In haemophiliacs, for example, it is possible to significantly reduce the amount of antihaemophilic factor administered pre intra and post operatively. This not only reduces the post-operative morbidity but makes the use of the laser very cost-effective.

CAVITATIONAL SURGERY

With the introduction of various laser endoscopes the CO_2 laser has become the modality of choice in many cavitational procedures, notably intra-abdominal, intra-thoracic, intra-articular and rectal.

MICROSURGERY

The addition of a micromanipulator has enabled the laser to be applied to various microscopic procedures, notably, in gynecology, otorynolaryngology, neurosurgery and

THE AMPULATORY TREATMENT OF CUTANEOUS LESIONS

In dermatologic surgery, the laser beam is used for the excision or vaporization of lesions. The procedure, which is generally conducted in an outpatient clinic, is rapid and uncomplicated, bloodless, sterile, almost painless, and well tolerated by children and the elderly. Postoperatively, there is no discomfort for the patient and no dressings are required; postoperative pain and infective complications do no occur. The treated areas heal rapidly because the skin appendages escape permanent damage. The cosmetic results of the treated areas are superior to those obtained by other methods and there is only minimal scarring.

COMPUTERIZED LASER DERMABRASION

It has long been felt that the treatment of extensive superficial lesions could be enhanced by the application of a CO_2 laser scanner. Accordingly, a computerized laser scanner was developed for this purpose and is used in our department for the dermabrasive treatment of large superficial lesions, such as port-wine stains and other extensive hemangiomas requiring vaporization, xeroderma pigmentosum, farmer's skin, Bowen's disease, post acne and burn scars, extensive pigmentation (giant nevi) Becker's nevi, nevus unius lateries, and decorative tattoos), large seborrheic keratosis, leukoplakia, pruritus vulvae and ani, crural and decubitus ulcers, and burn eschars. The system consists of a microprocessor control unit and an electric motor-driven scanner.

Method of Treatment

The surgeon can demarcate the area to be treated using the He-Ne laser guide light controlled by a joystick. The shape of the area to undergo dermabrasion is then stored in the memory. The laser is then set to work within the required limits and only the depth of the lesion requires further control. By depressing the laser "on" footswitch, the CO_2 laser beam is activated automatically, within the predefined boundaries in two directions, with preselected power level, speed, spot size, and line density. The debris is then wiped away with a wet pad and the depth of abrasion estimated. This can be repeated until the required depth is reached.

This procedure enables us to perform dermabrasion, with an accurate control of depth and extent, without bleeding, and without the scattering of debris and blood, more precisely and evenly than the conventional methods. The healing process is rapid with minimal pain and good cosmetic results.

MICRO-ANASTOMOSIS AND TISSUE WELDING

Since the CO_2 laser has been shown to seal blood vessels, lymphatics, bile cannaliculi, renal tubules, alveoli, etc. (this being a welding process and not coagulation) it is logical to assume that, provided the correct output and technique are adopted, one should be able to employ it for the purpose of welding tissue.

Micro-vascular anastomosis, as well as that of vasa deferentia, fallopian atubes, ureters, bowel and even welding of skin have been shown to be practical. This, therefore, has opened a new and exciting field of application of this versatile modality.

REFERENCES

1. Kaplan, I., Ger R. (1973) The carbon dioxide laser in clinical surgery - a preliminary report. Isr. J. Med. Sci. 9:1:79-83.
2. Kaplan, I., Ger R. (1973) Partial mastectomy and mammaplasty performed with CO_2 surgical laser - a comparative report. Br. J. Plast. Surg. 26:189-190.
3. Kaplan, I., Goldman, J., Ger R. (1973) Treatment of erosion of the uterine cervix by means of the CO_2 laser. Obstet. Gynecol. 41:795.
4. Kaplan, I., Ger R., Sharoñ, V. (1973) The CO_2 laser in plastic surgery. Br. J. Plast. Surg. 26:359-362.
5. Frishman, A., Gassner, S., Kaplan, I., Ger R. (1974) Excision of subcutaneous fibrosarcoma in mice - a comparative experimental sutdy of various methods. Isr. J. Med. Sci. 10:67:637-641.
6. Kaplan, I., Pariente, R., Baiani, G., Pochini, M., Tantillo, B., Toso, M., (1974) La resezion atipica sperimental di fegato mediante Laser al Biossido di Carbonio a flusso continuo. IL Policlinico - Sez Chirurgica 81:5.
7. Kaplan, I., Gassner, S., Schindel, Y. (1974) carbon dioxide laser in head and neck surgery. Am. J. Surg. 128:543-544.
8. Ben-Bassat, M., Gassner, S., Kott, I., Lavi, E., Kaplan, I. (1975) A comparison between the scalpel and the CO_2 laser beam in the healing of intestinal anastomosis. Proceedings of the 1st International Symposium on Laser Surgery, Dec. 1975. Jerusalem Academic Press, Jerusalem.
9. Kaplan, I., (1975) CO_2 laser surgery. Harefuah 89:6:243-4.
10. Kaplan, I., Peled, I. (1975) The CO_2 laser in the treatment of superficial telangiectases. Br. J. last. Surg. 28:214-215.
11. Kaplan, I., Peled, I. (1975) The carbon dioxide laser in plastic surgery. Rev. Iberoam. Cir. Plas. 1:4:35-45.
12. Peled, I., Kaplan, I., Mattos, S. (1974) Surgical uses of the carbon dioxide laser. Folia Med. 70:5.
13. Kaplan, I., (ed) (1976) Laser Surgery I. Jerusalem Academic Press, Jerusalem.
14. Ben-Bassat, M., Kaplan, I., Schindel, Y, Edlan, A. (1976) The CO_2 laser in surgery of the tongue. Laser Surg. 1:73-79.

15. Labandter, H., Kaplan, I., (1976) The treatment of haemangiomata using the CO_2 laser. Laser Surg. 1:109-111.
16. Peled, I., Shohat, B., Gassner, S., Kaplan, I. (1976) Excision of subcutaneous Lewis lung carcinoma in mice - a comparative experiment. Laser Surg. 1:66-69.
17. Morein, G., Kaplan, I., Gassner, S. (1976) Laser-induced epiphysiodesis. Laser Surg. 1:145-148.
18. Ben-Bassat, M., Ben-Bassat, M., Kaplan, I. (1976) Electron microscopic studies of soft tissue incision by means of CO_2 laser. Laser Surg. 1:95-100.
19. Ben-Bassat, M., Gassner, S., Kaplan, I., Kott, I (1976) The healing process in experimental bowel surgery. Laser Surg. 1:84-86.
20. Kott, I., Gassner, S., Ben-Bassat, M., Kaplan, I. (1976) The surgical knife and the CO_2 laser beam. Am. J. Proctol. Gastroenterol. Colon Rectal Surg. 27:2:31.
21. Labandter, H., Kaplan, I. (1976) Onychogryphoses treated with the CO_2 surgical laser. Br. J. Plast. Surg. 29:102-1-3.
22. Kaplan, I., Sharon, U. (1976) Current laser surgery. Ann N.Y. Acad. sci. 267:247-253.
23. Peled, I., Shohat, B., Gassner, S., Kaplan, I. (1976) Excision of epithelial tumors. CO_2 laser vs. conventional methods. Cancer Lett. 2:41-46.
24. Ben-Bassat, M., Ben-Bassat, M., Kaplan, I (1976) A study of the ultrastructural features of the cut margin of skin and mucous membrane specimens excised by carbon dioxide laser. J. Surg. Res. 21:77-84.
25. Taube, E., Glass, I., Motovitz, A., Kaplan, I., (1977) The CO_2 laser in veterinary surgery. Isr. Vet. Med. Assoc. 34:1:35.
26. Meiraz, D., Peled, I., Gassner, S., Ben-Bassat, M., Kaplan, I. (1977) The use of the CO_2 laser for partial nephrectomy. Invest. Urol. 15:3:252-264.
27. Kaplan, I. (1977) The Sharplan 791 CO_2 surgical laser in clinical surgery. In: Waidelich W. (ed) Laser 77 Opto-Electronics, IPC Science and Technology Press.
28. Labandter, H., Kaplan, I. (1977) Experience with continuous laser in the treatment of suitable cutaneous conditions. J. Dermatol. Surg. Oncol. 3:527-530.
29. Ben-Bassat, M., Levy, R., Kaplan, I. (1978) CO_2 laser in the treatment of Osler's disease. Br. J. Plast. surg. 31:157-158.
30. Kaplan, I. (1978) The Sharplan 791 Carbon dioxide surgical laser. Br. J. Clin. Equip. 227:229.
31. Ben-Bassat, M., Kaplan, I., Levy, R. (1978) Treatment of hereditary haemorrhagic telangiectasia of the nasal mucosa with the carbon dioxide laser. Br. J. Plast. Surg. 31:157-158.
32. Ben-Bassat, M, Kaplan, I., Schindel, J., Edlan, A. (1978) The CO_2 laser in surgery of the tongue. Br. J. Plast. Surg. 31 155-156.
33. Morein, G., Gassner, S., Kaplan, I. (1978) Bone growth alterations due to application of CO_2 laser beam to the epiphyseal growth plates - an experimental study of rabbits. Acta Orthop. Scand. 47:244-248.
34. Kaplan, I., (ed) (1978) Laser Surgery II. Jerusalem Academic Press, Jerusalem.
35. Kaplan, I., Ascher, P.W. (eds) (1980) Laser Surgery III. Jerusalem Academic Press, Jerusalem.
36. Kaplan, I., (1980) The Sharplan CO_2 surgical laser in clinical surgery. Laser Surg. 3:97.
37. Taube, E., Kaplan, I., Glass, I., Engelberg, M. (1980) Veterinary surgery by means of Sharplan CO_2 surgical laser. Laser Surg. 3:98-99.
38. Giler, S., Ben-Bassat, M., Kaplan, I. (1980) The use of the Sharplan CO_2 laser for lymph node dissection in cases of malignant melanoma. Laser Surg. 3:100-106.
39. Kaplan, I. (1980) The Sharplan CO_2 surgical laser in neonatal surgery. Laser Surg. 3:197-200.

40. Giler, S., Ben-Bassat, M., Taube, E., Kaplan, I., (1980) The surgery of pilonidal sinus with the CO_2 laser. Laser Surg. 3:201-203.
41. Giler, S., Gassner, S., Ben-Uri, R., Kaplan, I., (1980) The CO_2 laser in surgery of the pancreas - an experimental study. Laser Surg. 3:211-216.
42. Giler, S., Ben-Bassat, M., Gassner, S., Kaplan, I., (1980) The CO_2 laser in surgery of the spleen - an experimental study. Laser Surg. 3:217-233.
43. Giler, S., Kaplan, I. (1981) The use of the CO_2 laser for the treatment of cutaneous lesions in an outpatient clinic. Proceedings of 4th Congress of the International Society for Laser Surgery 1:1-4.
44. Giler, S., Kaplan, I., (1981) Multiple seborrheic keratoses treated with the CO_2 laser. Proceedings of 4th Congress of the International Society for Laser Surgery 1:5-8.
45. Segal, T., Nordenberg, D., Giler, S., Serebro, I., Kaplan, I. (1981) The effect of the Sharplan CO_2 laser beam on dental structure. Proceedings of 4th Congress of the International Society for Laser Surgery, 12:25-28.
46. Nordenberg, D., Segal, T., Giler, S., Serebro, I., Kaplan, I., (1981) The effect of the Sharplan CO_2 laser beam on dental caries: Sterilization a new approach. Proceedings of 4th Congress of the International Society for Laser Surgery 12:33-35.
47. Giler, S., Ben-Bassat, M., Taube, E., Kaplan, I. (1981) The use of the CO_2 laser in palliative surgery for cancer. Proceedings of 4th Congress of the International Society for Laser Surgery 23:12-15.
48. Giler, S., Kott, I., Ben-Bassat, M., Kaplan, I. (1981) The use of the CO_2 laser in anorectal surgery. Proceedings of 4th Congress of the International Society for Laser Surgery 23:36-38.
49. Kott, I., Reiss, R., Giler, S., Kaplan, I. (1981) The CO_2 laser in mastectomy: A comparative study. Proceedings of 4th Congress of the International Society for Laser Surgery 24:1-2.
50. Tadir, Y., Ovadia, J., Zuckerman, Z., Kaplan, I., (1981) Laparoscopic application of CO_2 laser. Proceedings of 4th Congress of the International Society for Laser Surgery 13:25.
51. Kaplan, I., (1982) Current CO_2 laser surgery. Optics Laser Technol. 41-42.
52. Kaplan, I., (1982) The Sharplan CO_2 surgical laser in neonatal surgery. Ann. Plast. Surg. 8:5:426-428.
53. Kaplan, I., (1982) Current CO_2 laser surgery. Plast. Reconstr. Surg. 69:3.
54. Kaplan, I., Sarig, A., Ben-Bassat, M. (1982) Le laser à CO_2 en chirurgie pediatrique. L'Information Dentaire 3/6/82 - No. 22 Special Laser 2141-2143.
55. Kaplan, I. Giler S. (1984) CO_2 Laser surgery. Springer Verlag.

Operative Treatment of Hemorrhoids with CO_2 Laser and Nd: YAG Laser Respektively

Ch. ARMBRUSTER, K. DINSTL, H. GREINER, A. TUCHMANN
1st Department of Surgery and Ludwig-Boltzmann-
Institut for Laser Surgery, KA Rudolfstiftung
Juchgasse 25, A-1030 Vienna

Introduction

Diseased hemorrhoids are usualy regarded as a simple disease and their surgical treatment as minor surgery. This is not true from the patients point of view. For the patient hemorrhoids are inconvenient, often painful, the postoperative course is marked by defecation problems and impaired healing.
Using a standardised surgical procedure, our intention was to shorten postoperative convalescence. Absence of pain and undisturbed healing after surgery are mandatory to achieve this goal.

Method

Since 1982 we employ laser in the surgery of hemorrhoids, Milligan-Morgans procedure is used generally. From 1982 to 1986 189 patients were operated on; 35 times using electrosurgical knife, 138 times carbon dioxide laser and 16 times Nd-YAG-laser (Tab. 1).
In a first series (1) 35 patients operated by electrosurgical knife were compared to 40 patients operated by CO_2-laser: in both groups a typical Milligan-Morgan procedure was performed. Operation was indicated in grade III and IV nodules, seldom in grade II cases. Laser operation was performed with a CO_2-Sharplan-laser using 20-30 watt.

Results

We summarize our results as follows (Tab. 2). The carbon-dioxide laser provides good peroperative control of bleeding, little postoperative pain was observed and no impaired or delayed wound healing occured. Late results as sphincterfunction, lack of symptoms and recurrence rate were comparable in both groups (2).
In consequence the next 98 operations were performed by CO_2-laser exclusively. We achieved the same favourable results, especially a reduced need for analgetics was evident.
Due to reports in literatur (3) about the use of Nd-YAG-laser in the treatment of hemorrhoids even in out-patients we performed 16 operations (Milligan-Morgan) with the Medilas 2 Nd-YAG-coagulation laser. The average output used was 20 Watt.

Whereas the peroperative control of bleeding was excellent, due to the high coagulation capacity, we had to observe less favourable results in the postoperative course.

In comparison to the above mentioned method (CO_2-laser) a markedly increased need for analgetics was evident. Whereas only 39% of the patients operated on by CO_2-laser and 65% of the patients operated on by electro surgical knife needed analgetic drugs, 100% in the group operated with Nd-YAG-laser required analgetic drugs.   Often pain occured only after discharge from hospital - averaging the 4th postoperative day. On postop. controls we regularely observed wound-necrosis which led to delayed healing.

Conclusion

Due to these results we left this method and returned to carbon dioxid laser for routine hemorrhoidectomy. In our experience this procedure satisfies the demands for patient security and minimal postoperative inconvenience for the patient.

Summary

189 cases of diseased hemorrhoids are reported. Carbon dioxid laser (138), Nd-YAG-laser (15) and electrosurgical knife (3) were employed to perform Milligan-Morgans procedure. Best results wer obtained by using the CO_2-laser (good control of bleeding, little postoperative pain and good healing tendency), whereas the use of Nd-YAG-laser resulted in woundnecrosis and increased postoperative pain. Therefore the use of CO_2-laser is recommended in Milligan-Morgan operation for diseased hemorrhoids.

Tab. 1.

Operationes for hemorrhoids 1/1982 - 12/1986	n	%
CO_2-Sharplan-laser	138	73
Medilas Nd-YAG-laser	16	8
Electrosurgical knife	35	19
	189	100

Tab. 2.

Advantage of CO_2-laser
1) excellent peroperative control of bleeding
2) little postoperative pain
3) good wound healing

References

1) Bastian L., Günter H., Härb H.J., Platthy G.: Die Operation nach Milligan-Morgan mit dem CO_2-Laser. Vortrag Laserkongress 1983 (München).

2) Greiner H., Günter H., Platthy G., Bastian L.: Spätergebnisse der Noduliope-ration nach Milligan-Morgan mit und ohne CO_2-Laser. Verhandlungsbericht der Deutschen Gesellschaft für Lasermedizin e.V. 1984; P. 30 - 33.

3) Eddy H.J., Yu J.C., Eddy E.C.: Total Hemorrhoidectomy with the Neodymium: YAG Laser - 300 Cases. Laser 1985 Opto-Electronics in Medicine, 1985; p. 348 - 350.

Endobronchial Laser Therapy in Pneumological Emergency

H.D.Becker
Thoraxklinik der LVA Baden
Amalienstraße 5, D- 6900 Heidelberg

The most frequent emergency situation in which the Neodym-YAG-Laser can be applied is the obstruction of central airways. Not only malignancies but also benign lesions - mostly membranes or granulomata after sugery or long-time intubation - may lead to dyspnea that is further aggravated by bleeding or retention of secretions.

As symptoms of imminent airway occlusion may run unnoticed for a long time, patients rather often are referred to our clinic in a state of acute decompensation with severe dyspnea and hypoxemia. Clinical sings frequently do not show the cause and extent of the stenosis and the critical state does not allow further investigation by non-invasive methods as hilar tomography for example.

Thus immediate endoscopy with the rigid bronchoscope under general anaesthesia has to yield exact information on the cause, location, and extent of airway obstruction.

The aim of treatment therafter is swift, extensive and stable desobliteration possibly leaving every option of definitive therapy.

The main problem in this procedure is sufficient ventilation which is further impaired by instrumentation and suction for removal of blood, secretions, and smoke.

In this situation to our opinion jet ventilation is essential for primary oxygenation. Moreover, frequently oxygen has to be added to the breathing air in high concentrations. Occasionally, in high-grade stenoses or difficulties in rigid intubation we apply a heat resistent jet ventilation tube that we developed recently. Laser resection can be performed fairly safely in the surrounding. During the procedure smoke is removed by continous suction. Thus burning of smoke and gases is prevented as well as toxic inhalation lung injury.

In addition, by low energy application of 30 to 40 Watts and short impulses of 1 to 2 seconds combustion is safely avoided even in resection close to plastic endoprothesis materials. Besides there is only a low risk of bleeding due to lesions of larger blood vessels or perforation of the tracheal or bronchial wall, however extensive the resection may be.

By this technique we were able to remove extensive stenoses in reasonable time of about 15 to 30 minutes sufficiently and mostly during the first session.

If relapse of symptoms occure due to retention of secretions or necrotic tissue after incomplete resection laser intervention can be repeated immediately for complete resection, without danger of perforation as necrosis does not penetrate deeply into the bronchial wall.

Now, is it worth while taking all the risks of this procedure, especially since most of the patients are of older age and suffer from fairly advanced malignancies?

TECHNIQUE OF EMERGENCY LASERBRONCHOSCOPY

RIGID BRONCHOSCOPE

GENERAL ANAESTHESIA

JET VENTILATION

HIGH OXYGEN CONC.

REMOVAL OF SMOKE/GASES

LOW ENERGY 30 - 40 W

SHORT IMPULSES 1 - 2 SEC.

Despite of the relatively high mortality in the short cause after laser resection - that is caused by complications of tumor or severe general impairment mainly - mean survival time is half a year, and not a few patients are living much longer under the ensuing definitive therapy.

In conclusion, endobronchial laser therapy in an emergency situation poses challenges to the skills of the endoscopist as well as the anaesthesiologist. In order to avoid risks in achievement of quick and sufficient palliation, to our opinion rigid bronchoscopy under general anaesthesia and jet ventilation are essential. As in many cases additionally high oxygen concentrations have to be added, we propose removal of smoke by continous suction and application of short laser impulses with low energies. By these proceedings not only burning but also severe bleeding and perforation are prevented.

Furthermore, every means of alternative emergency intervention as stenting of stenoses, blockage of bleeding or double lumen intubation, for example, should be familiar of cause.

Surgery of Breast Cancer with the CO_2 Laser – Report on 449 Operations

K. DINSTL, St. KRIWANEK, G. PLATTHY, A. TUCHMANN

1st Department of Surgery and Ludwig-Boltzmann Institut
for Laser Surgery, KA Rudolfstiftung, Juchgasse 25
A-1030 Vienna

Since 1975 1600 operations with the CO_2-laser (Sharplan 791) have been performed at the first surgical department KA Rudolfstiftung, Vienna. Most operations were done for diseases of the breast.

The use of CO_2-laser in breast surgery is based on the following characteristics (1):

1. reduced bleeding
2. reduced postoperative pain
3. reduced postoperative woundinfections
4. possibly reduced local recurrence

Reports on the results of laser surgery in cancer patients have been controversial. Therefore the following main points have been investigated (2):

1. Experimental investigations of the use of CO_2-laser versus scalpel or electric knife
2. Conduction of a prospective, controlled study on treatment of breast cancer in selected patients
3. Studies on CO_2-laser surgery treatment of breast cancer in all patients
4. Value of using CO_2-laser in patients with extensive tumors of the breast

Results

1. In an experimental study on CO_2-laser surgery in mice with Lewis-Lung carcinoma, there was no significant difference of survival time in animals operated on with laser or knife, but the incidence of local recurrence (independent of tumorsize) was significantly lower, the time between operation and recurrence was significantly longer.
The incidence of tumorgrowth was much lower in mice, when wounds had been exposed to CO_2-laser before swabbing tumorcells into them (2).

2. A prospective, controlled trial was started in 1981. The selection criteria were in 135 patients:

1. age less than 70 years
2. clinical tumor stage 1 or 2
3. pre or post menopausal state

Randomization was done by computer, a radical mastectomy was performed in all patients. Postoperative therapy was standardized according to hormon receptor state (either tamoxifen or chemotherapy). Until now we have not been able to find definitive results because the period of investigation has been too short (Tab. 1).

3. The follow up of 449 patients operated on because of breast cancer from 1975 to 1985 showed a reduced incidence of recurrence only when a radical mastectomy had been done (Tab. 2):

The incidence of recurrence tumor depended on kind of procedure used, but it seems that the use of CO_2-laser in breast cancer surgery gives an advantage against conventional methods relating to local recurrence (Tab. 3). The standardized axillary lymphnode dissection could not be done by laser because a dissection with laser would endanger axillary vessels or nerves.

Tab. 1.

	Follow up (6 years - 6 month)	
	Meta	+
L (n = 67)	3 (4%)	9 (14%)
ø (n = 68)	5 (8%)	8 (13%)

Tab. 2.

	Postoperative local recurrence after	
	n	Rec.
Lumpectomy	18	6 (33%)
Mod. Rad. Op.	15	6 (40%)
Rad. Op.	416	20 (4,8%)
	449	32 (7,1%)

Tab. 3.

	Radical Mastectomy (M_0)		
	T_1N_{0-1}	T_2N_{0-2}	$T_{3-5}N_{0-3}$
local rec.	3	10	7
ø	156	183	57
	159 (2%)	193 (5,2%)	64 (11%)

4. The advantages of CO_2-laser in the excision of extensive tumors of the breast are unquestionable.
Our experiences with 39 patients showed the following advantages of laser surgery compared to conventional procedures:

1. less bleeding
2. possibility of reducing the excision of skin to a minimum
3. significant reduction of local recurrence
4. less postoperative pain
5. possibility of primary skin grafting in exulcerated or infected tumors

A definitive statement according to survival time can not be made. Recently such cases of extensive breast cancer have been treated preoperatively by chemotherapy in our department. We found a significant reduction of tumors in patients responding to preoperative chemotherapy after 3 cycles.
We hope to prolong the survival of those patients by the additional use of CO_2-laser for the subsequent radical operations.
Nevertheless this procedure has yet to be proved for its value within the next years.

References

1. K. DINSTL u. P.L. FISCHER:
   "Der Laser"
   Springer-Verlag, Berlin Heidelber New York 1981

2. A. TUCHMANN, P. BAUER, H. PLENK,Jr, O. BRAUN, K. DINSTL
   Comperative Study of Conventional Scalpel and CO_2-Laser in Experimental Tumor Surgery
   Res Exp Med (1986): 375-386

The Combined 1.06 μm and 1.32 μm Nd: YAG Laser in Surgery

Horak, L.*, Fanta, J.*, Kabat J.*, Marek J.+

*IIl.rd Surgical Clinic of Charles University, Prague, Czechoslovakia
+Faculty of Nuclear Science and Physical Engineering, Technical University, Prague, Czechoslovakia

At present our surgical team of the IIIrd Surgical Clinic of Charles University Prague, tests the usage of Nd:YAG laser of Czechoslovak construction. Laser system was developed at the Faculty of Nuclear Science and Physical Engineering of Technical University of Prague.

This laser works at the classical wavelenght 1.06 micrometres at the output of 80 W and moreover at the wavelenght 1.32 um at the output of 40 W.

The technical setting of the appliance is able to change wavelenght 1.32 um any time during one single operation (1).

Before the actual using in clinical practice this laser appliance was tested on experimental animals, their liver, spleen, lungs, stomach, intestines, besides a wide scope of endoscopic performances. We presume its usage in clinical surgery in the domain of palliative operations of metastases into lungs and similary metastases into liver and palliative treatment of carcinoma of lower rectum.

We consider this usage of the laser to fully supplement the classical surgical supraselective proximal vagotomy from laparatomy.

We use both non-contact handpieces and contact saphire tips of our own Czechoslovak construction.

Both these wavelenghts have different absorption coefficient in water and different effect on tissue and organs (2).

The Nd:YAG laser with wavelength 1.32 um is suitable for vapourization of tissue. Both system with the CM and the NCM require only one-half of the energy needed for vapourization as compared with the 1.06 um Nd:YAG laser with the identical vapourization effect, the coagulation zone with the wavelenght 1.32 um is considerably wider than wavelenght 1.06 um. Therefore the 1.32 um laser appears more suitable for tumor treatment than for the coagulation of bleeding in the GI tract.

In intraluminal using the probability of damaging of intestinal walls, oesophagus or stomach is lower with 1.06 um wavelenght.

When we used wavelenght 1.32 um and power from 10-15 W on seroza of stomach or intestine we got coagulation zone only in seroza and muscle, not in submucosa and mucosa tissues. We need power output 50 W for the same effect with wavelenght 1.06 um then the risk of damaging of intestinal walls is higher.

There is no advantage in coagulation of liver and spleen between using wavelenght 1.32 um and power 40 W or wavelenght 1.06 um and power from 80 to 100 W.

We would like to demonstrate the advantage of using both wavelenghts in supraselective vagotomy.

In experiments with of laser on animals we have reached the same effect in supressing gastric secretion as in classical vagotomy. In comparison with classical vagotomy the time of operation with laser has been reduced by more than a half.

The usage of the wavelenght 1.32 um and low power from 10-15 W leads to denervation in a sufficient range and the procedure is safer when cutting on wavelenght 1.32 um than on wavelenght 1.06 um where we need higher power - 40W. In case of bleeding is better to change over from wavelenght 1.32 um to 1.06 um and to coagulate this bleeding vessels by this wavelenght.

References

1) K. Hamal, J. Marek, J. Kvapil, V. Skoda, :Combined 1.06/1.32um Nd:YAG Laser for Medicine, CLEO, Baltimore, USA, 27.4.-1.5.1987.
2) F. Frank, O.J. Beck, K. Haussinger, E. Keiditsch: Comparative Investigation of Tissue Reaction with 1.06um and 1.32 um Nd:YAG Laser Radiation, 2 nd International Nd:YAG Laser Conference, Munich, 1985.

Clinical Experiences in Laser Resection of Liver, Spleen and Kidney in Children – Indications and Morphological Results

H. Meier, K.H. Dietl, J. Morcate, E. Unsöld,
G.H. Willital
Kinderchirurgische Uni.-Klinik, Münster

Laser has found its application for research fields of medicine during the past years. In case of special indications laser application has already been accepted. Our study does not only reveal indications for laser therapy, and differentiates them from euphorc innovational indications, but shows when laser application is superior to conventional technique.

The newborn and the infant differ from an adult in terms of morphology and physiology. Therefore laser technique may be applied to the newborn and infant.

Here are the special morphologic and physiologic conditions:

1. Small organs.
2. Small diameter of blood vessels.
3. Less blood volume, e.g. a blood loss of 50 ml may lead to hemorrhagic shock.
4. Less tolerance in case of organ failure.
5. Malformation in the newborn require special therapy.

Special attributes of laser light

All types of laser have one principal of laser light development in commen:

There is a sumulant transmission of coherent monochromatic light. Multiple types of laser have been developed. They produce light on different wave lenghts. This development took place because of the availability of different laser media e.g. laser cristals, gas and liquid laser as well as the different types of energy delivery, the pumping, caused by light and gas, that is to say in an electric and thermodynamic way.

Following special attributes of laser light are important:
Minimal divergence, monochromasie and coherence lead to contactles transmission of energy to coagulate the tissue of parenchymal organs.

Coagulation of the tissue is due to the absorbed nonreflected laser light under low intensity. An area of carbonization remains under high intensity. A great distance from the site of absorbtion gives way to an hyperemic or edematous area which cells regenarate after the temporary destruction.

Experimental studies

In our experimental studies we perform subtotal resections of parenchymal organs like liver and spleen. The resulting areas necrosis were examined histologically and histochemically.

Temperature determinations were done in the neighbouring tissue. The various transmission systems and intensivities were compared. Determination of temperature in the neighbouring tissue were a hint for expected temperatures in each organ. This temperature was dependent on the distance between site of laser light application and the site of temperature determination. Critical increase in temperature was not observed with an intensity of 90 - 100 joules and a distance up to 7 mms.

The effect of laser was documented by histologic and histochemical staining. The first area is the area of carbonization or area of vaporization. In this area the tissue is heated up, vaporized and a tissue destruction remains.

The second area, the area of primary necrosis are coagulation, is described as the area where in the cells are heated up, coagulation takes place but vaporization is missing.

The third area, the area of secondary necrosis is characterized by an irreversible destruction of cells. Coagulation does not take place. This area should be small because it is not made use of in case of hemorrhage. Furthermore it enlarges the edge of necrosis.

The fourth area, the area of edema is characterized by a reversible destruction of cells; that is to say: a temporary edema is observed which results in an unaffected tissue after a couple of days.

Permanent occlusion of the blood vessels of the parenchymal organs at the site of resection was documented by rasterelectron microscopy. Right after organ resection by laser as well some weeks later we filled the blood vessels with Technovit ^{R} which became firm immediately then led to tissue maceration and resulted in an filling sample. Hence we were able to demonstrate the circulatory stop at the site of resection.

Considering the mentioned size of the organ permanent occlusion of the resection site was achieved without an additional ligature. The relative deep of the coagulation area caused by Neodym-Yag-Laser resection guaranties a permanent occlusion of the blood vessels.

On the other hand the body must restore this area of necrosis.

Hemisplenectomy – Hemithepatectomy

In 15 rabbits we do a hemihepatectomy and a hemisplenectomy. In non of the cases there was a bleeding postoperatively. None of the cases demonstrates a fistula of the biliary tree or an abscess. The histological examinations shows, that in 14 - 17

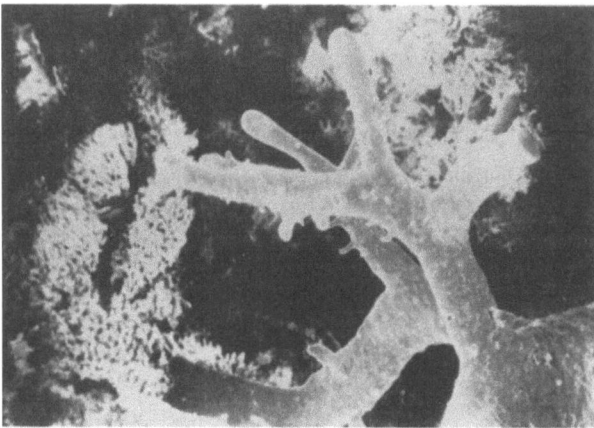

Fig.. Electro-microscopic investigations of the blood vessels of the liver. Complete closure of the vessels after laser resection is demonstrated

days fibroblasts have moved away from the periportal region and a neocapsular has been formed. 15 months later we were still able to demonstrate 1/10 of all necrotic cells.

Follow- up of the histologic section after 1 and 3 weeks as well as 3 months show a decrease in the amount of necrotic tissue and de-capsulation by the neo-capsula. In our experimental study we did not encounter postoperative hemorrhage, biliary tree fistulas nor and abscess. We found similar results after hemisplenectomy.

Clinical indications for laser resection of the spleen and liver are blunt abdominal injuries with splenic rupture, when an emergency splenectomy has to be executed and an irreversible hemorrhagic shock has to be avoided.

In case of superficial splenic capsular rupture alternative techniques like the infrared coagulation and fibrin glue are satisfying. However, in case of deep splenic rupture with arterial hemorrhage the above-mentioned alternative procedures fail.

There is a great danger of postoperative bleeding. Then partial splenic resection with Neodym-Yag-Laser is indicated. The large area of coagulation guarantees permanent occlusion of the vessels and the remaining splenic tissue is preserved. This is of great importance in the newborn and infant where the remaining splenic tissue has an immunologic function. Most of these cases do not have to undergo an autologicsplenic transplantation.

Partial liver resection and hemihepatectomy in children is necessary in accidents with hepatic rupture or tumor or undergoing diagnostic partial liver resection.

Laser-technique - it is a very bloodness procedure. We did not see any biliary fistulas, abscessformations or postoperative hemorrhage in any of the hemi-hepatectomies in animals.

In the last time we did partial liver resection in 4 children and hemisplenectomy in 1 children.

In 2 children a heminephrectomy was performed in cases of double pelvic system and double ureters and with permanent infections of the urinary tract.

Specific pediatric surgical problems such as the treatment of partial resection of the spleen, hemithepatecomy and heminephrectomy in newborns and infants represent new application possibilities for the laser. We have provided the basic for clinical use by means of extensive histological, electron-microscopical and histochemical studies and we have good results in clinical experiences with laser technique.

Postoperative Analgesia and Nd: YAG Laser Surgery

K.C. Moore, A. Steger, N. Hira
Oldham General Hospital,
OLDHAM, England, U.K.

Reports of reduced postoperative pain following Nd:YAG laser surgery have, to date, been mostly anecdotal. Following review of some 200 laser cases we have confirmed these reports and established the need for comparative clinical trials involving the use of low power contact Nd:YAG Laser and conventional operative techniques in body surface surgery, intermediate surgery (involving but not transecting muscle layers) and body cavity surgery.

Clinical Experience

Of the cases reviewed some 50% have involved operations on the body surface mostly for malignant pathology of the cutaneous and subcutaneous tissues. The most common operative sites have included tongue and oral cavity, breast, chest and abdominal wall, groin, perineum and vulva.
40% of cases involved the wide excision of primary tumour pathology (breast, tongue, finger, calf) or discrete metastatic tumour deposits (breast, chest, abdominal wall). The remaining 60% of cases required excision, cleansing and toiletry of sometimes extensive and frequently ulcerating and offensive secondary tumour deposits (breast, chest wall, lip, groin, perineum, vulva). This latter group of cases had failed to respond to conventional methods of treatment such as irradiation, chemotherapy and conventional surgical excision.
In spite of the frequently extensive nature of surgery, only 25% of all cases required any morphine derivative or its equivalent in the postoperative period.
 Analgesic needs for 50% of patients were satisfied by simple analgesics such as paracetamol, and the remaining 25% required no postoperative analgesia whatsoever.

Clinical Trials

To investigate and quantify the need for postoperative analgesia we have carried out three comparative trials involving the use of low power contact Nd:YAG Laser and conventional operative techniques in breast surgery, cholecystectomy and inguinal hernia repair. The operative protocol has previously been described in detail (1). Postoperative recordings included details of analgesic requirements, number of days to reach a zero pain score, time to mobilisation and duration of hospital stay.

The breast surgery trial involved either simple mastectomy or wide excision of primary breast malignancy. The results show a significant reduction in the need for postoperative analgesia in the laser group, only 20% requiring morphine related analgesics as opposed to 60% of the conventional surgery group. Perhaps as a consequence of this there was earlier mobilisation of the laser patients, 80% mobilised in under 24 hours as opposed to 50%, and the duration of hospital stay was some 36% shorter. Full details of this trial have already been presented (2). The inguinal herniorrhaphy trial showed a similar trend in reduced postoperative analgesia requirements, earlier mobilisation and reduced hospital stay for those patients undergoing laser surgery but not to such a significant degree as that of the body surface trial. The laser group reached a zero pain score (measured on a visual analogue scale) some 1.5 days (30%) earlier than the non-laser group, and there was improved mobilisation and a 15% reduction in hospital stay. The cholecystectomy trial showed very little difference between the two groups for analgesic requirements, time to zero pain score, mobilisation and hospitalisation.

Conclusion

The mechanism of pain suppression following the use of Nd:YAG laser energy is not clear. The precise nature of the contact low power method of application certainly reduces the trauma to adjacent tissues and is associated with less tissue oedema and tension in superficial structures. However, when musculo-fibrous tissue is transected, such as in body cavity surgery, the resultant postoperative pain shows no significant difference whichever surgical technique is used.

The only clear conclusion is that the use of the low power contact Nd:YAG Laser for superficial surgery is associated with a significantly reduced level of postoperative pain when compared with conventional surgical techniques.

References

1. Moore K.C., Steger A, Hira N: The operative care of patients for Nd:YAG contact laser surgery. In: Oguro Y, Atsumi K, Joffe S N (Eds): Nd:YAG laser in medicine and surgery. Fundamental and clinical aspects. PPS. Tokyo 1986 pp 124-127.

2. Moore K C: General anaesthesia for Nd:YAG laser surgery. In: Joffe S N (Ed). Advances in Nd:YAG laser surgery. Springer-Verlag, New York 1987. 38 : 634-645.

Application of the Laser Speckle Method for the Blood Flow Determination at Patients with Arterial Occlusive Disease

B. Ruth, D. Abendroth[*], L. Sunder-Plassmann[*], W. Waidelich

Gesellschaft für Strahlen- und Umweltforschung mbH München, Institut für Angewandte Optik, Ingolstädter Landstr. 1, 8042 Neuherberg, F.R.G.

[*]Chirurgische Klinik und Poliklinik, Klinikum Großhadern, 8000 München, F.R.G.

The blood flow in capillaries is essential for the nutrition of the tissue and the transport of the waste products. It is very useful to distinguish between micro- and macro-circulation, and therefore it is necessary to measure the microcirculation directly at the site of interest.

The skin of patients suffering on arterial occlusive disease is very sensitive and can easily be hurt. Therefore it is of great advantage to measure the blood flow realy without any contact.

The blood flow measurement with light is based on the penetration of the light into the skin with a mean penetration depth of 0.5 mm /1/. Most of the light is scattered and absorbed by the tissue. Only a portion of about 30% can reach the depth of the capillaries and may be scattered by the blood. At its way back to the surface the intensity of the scattered light is also reduced by the absorption. In this way only a portion of about 10% of the scattered light comes from the depth of the capillaries.
Light scattered by the arteriols in the deeper region of the skin cannot reach the skin surface again due to its high absorption on its long way back to the surface. Therefore, most of the light, scattered by the blood, originates from the capillaries.

The measuring principle can be explained in terms of the dynamic laser speckle effect. When laser light is scattered by an object surface it forms a granular structure, the speckles.
The only condition is that the surface is rough compared to the laser light wavelength and this condition is clearly valid for the scattering at the skin.

The speckles can be detected by an aperture in a certain distance to the laser spot with a diameter matched to the mean speckle width. A photodetector behind the aperture generates the signal I. When laser and object do not move, the speckles are stationary and the signal I is constant /2/.

With a moving object the speckles become time-dependent and the photodetector signal I reveals frequencies unequal to zero. It can be shown that the mean frequency is a measure of the blood velocity. The blood volume within the range of the laser light is represented by the mean intensity $\bar{I}$.

The measuring head used for the non-contact measurement of the blood flow is shown in fig. 1.

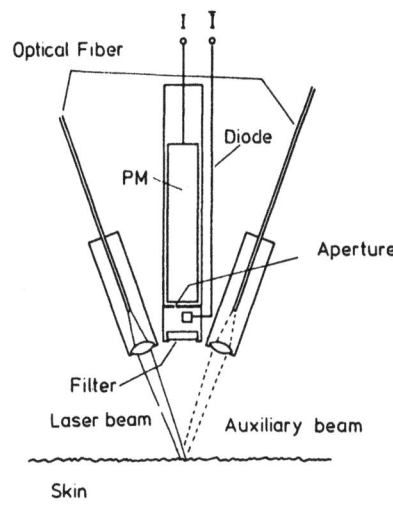

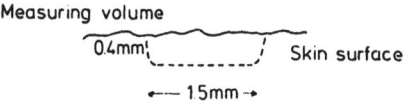

Fig. 1. Measuring head for the non-contact determination of the skin blood flow

The laser light diverges when it leaves the fiber and is focussed again by the lens and forms a spot at the skin with 1.5 mm in diameter. This diameter and the mean penetration depth of 0.4 mm define the measuring volume. The distance between skin and measuring head is about 6 cm. The light is detected by the aperture and the photomultiplier (PM) generates the signal I. The diode measures the mean speckle intensity $\bar{I}$.
The auxiliary light beam facilitates the adjustment of the measuring head at the correct distance.

The signals I from the photomultiplier and $\bar{I}$ from the diode are processed by an electronic circuit which is shown in fig. 2.

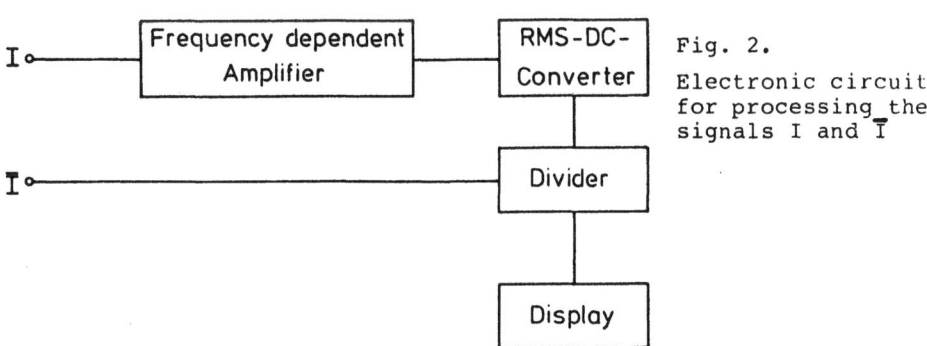

Fig. 2. Electronic circuit for processing the signals I and $\bar{I}$

The frequency dependent amplifier and the RMS-DC-Converter generate a signal which is a measure of the product of blood velocity and blood volume. That means, the output measures the blood flow /3/. The divider compensates the influence of the mean speckle intensity which can be varied by a change of the reflection conditions or the laser intensity. The measuring value, which is displayed, is called "blood flow parameter" (BFP).

In fig. 3 one example of a measurement at a patient (66 years) with arterial occlusive disease at the left side is shown.

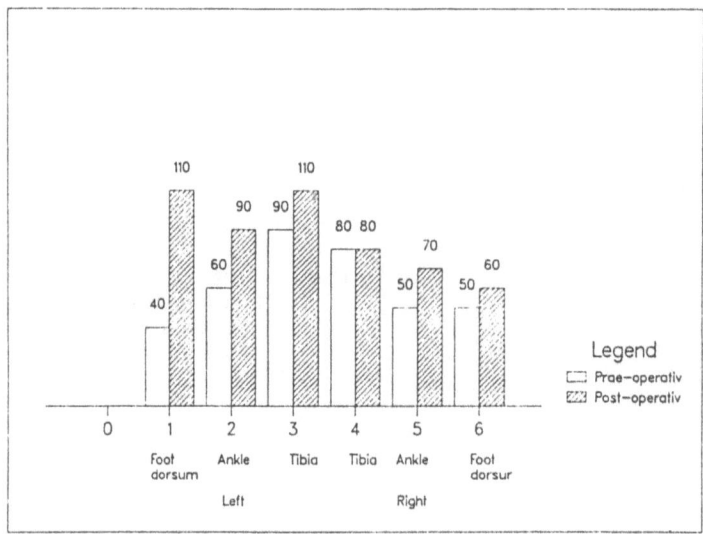

Fig. 3. Blood flow parameter (in relative units) of a patient with arterial occlusive disease before and after surgery

The measurements are taken from the foot dorsum, the ankle, and the tibia at both legs.
The blood flow parameter taken one day before surgery are indicated by the open columns and demonstrate that the BFP decline, when going from the tibia to the foot dorsum. Several days after surgery (by-pass) the BFP are given by the hatched columns and reveal a clear increase compared to the initial values. The relative decline between the measuring values at the tibia and the dorsum is obviously reduced. This accords well with the improvement of the blood flow in the left leg.

In fig. 4 a comparison is given between the laser speckle method, the skin temperature obtained by a recording of a thermo camera and the transcutaneous oxygen pressure.
All measurements are taken from nearly the same site at the foot dorsum. Again the measuring values before surgery are given by the open columns and the values after surgery are indicated by the hatched columns. All three methods reveal an increase of the measuring values.

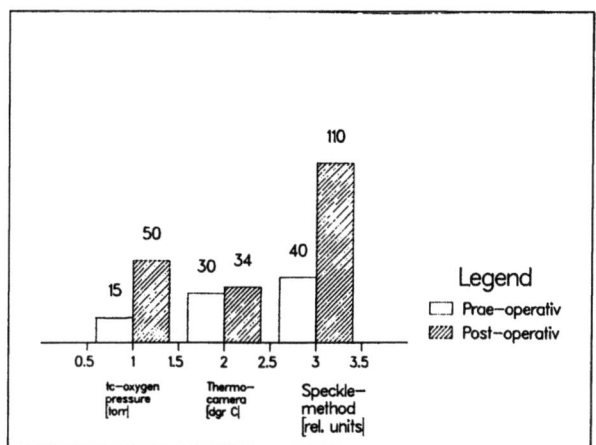

Fig. 4. Comparison of transcutaneous oxygen pressure, skin temperature and laser speckle method

In about 85 % of the cases an increase of the BFP and in 15% no change or a small decrease was obvious. The decrease may be due to the fact that the measurements are taken only a few days after surgery and therefore the improvement of the microcirculation cannot be seen at this time. Furthermore the measurements have shown that there are not only sites at the leg with a pronounced improvement but also other sites which show no change or a small decrease.

In conclusion, the laser speckle method has shown to be capable of measuring the skin blood flow of patients suffering on arterial occlusive disease. The main advantage is given by the non-contact procedure.

References

/1/ R.R. Anderson, J.A. Parrish: J. Invest. Dermatol. 77 (1981) 13.

/2/ J.C. Dainty: Laser Speckle and Related Phenomena, Springer Verlag, Berlin-Heidelberg-New York, 1975.

/3/ B. Ruth: J. Mod. Optics 34 (1987) 257.

Two Step Emergency Treatment of Malignant Tracheal Stenoses

H. Seibold, O. Sigg, D. Bunjes
Department of Internal Medicine and Otolaryngology, University of Ulm, FRG

Introduction
Neodym Yag laser treatment is widely used in urology, neurology, gastroenterology and pulmonology. In Pulmonology, laser therapy is usually limited to endobronchial processes when the perfusion of the afflicted lung is preserved, but there are essentially no restrictions to its use in cases of endotracheal obstructions not amenable to surgery or radiotherapy (1). Since these patients are frequently in a life threatening state with poor lung function and severe hypoxia the safe performance of the procedure usually requires general anesthesia with jet ventilation and the use of a rigid bronchoscope (2). In very rare cases the functional reserves of the patients are limited to such an extent that general anesthesia may be impossible. We would like to report the case histories of two patients whose treatment was particularly difficult due to severe restrictions of lung function testing.

Case reports
1. This 70 year old markedly overweight and multimorbid woman had had stroke 3 years ago. In addition to a chronic cough and stress induced angina pectoris and arterial hypertension grade 2-3, this woman developed increasing dyspnoea accompanied by stridor. 3 weeks before admission she had been intubated and mechanically ventilated in another hospital due to severe respiratory insufficiancy following a purulent bronchitis. She was tranferred to our hospital, because the stridor persisted after extubation.

Physical examination and status at admission
The patient was in respiratory distress with inspiratory and expiratory stridor, the lung sounds were low, the trachea was in the midline. The thyreoid was not enlarged. There were pretibial oedema and distended jugular veins. The lung function testing showed a severe obstructive pattern with a FEV1 of 750 ml in absolute terms. The flow-volume courve demonstrated a fixed stenosis particularly during expiration. The tomogram (fig 1) revealed a severe narrowing of the lumen of the proximal and middle part of the trachea.

Course in the hospital
After diuretics and prednisolone and theophylline the heart failure was compensated. Nevertheless the anesthesiologist felt that because of the poor condition of the patient a general anesthesia was not possible. Therefore rigid bronchoscopy was performed under topic anesthesia with 1% buprocain. We found a tumor on the left lateral

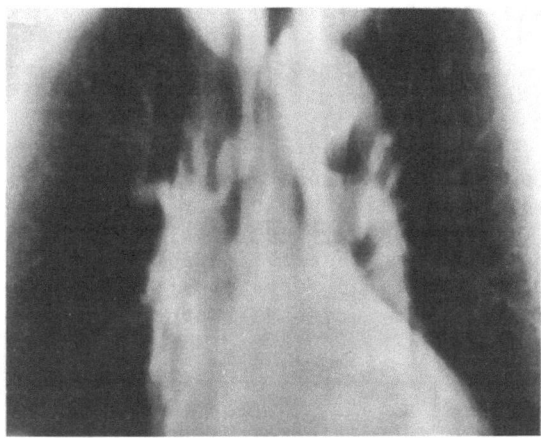

Fig. 1. Severe narrowing of the tracheal lumen by a tumor (length of the stenosis 3 cm)

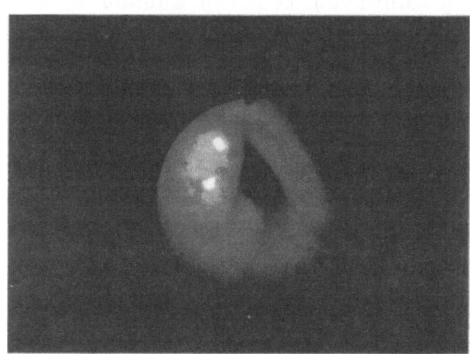

Fig. 2. Proximal view of the tumor (adenoid cystic carcinoma)

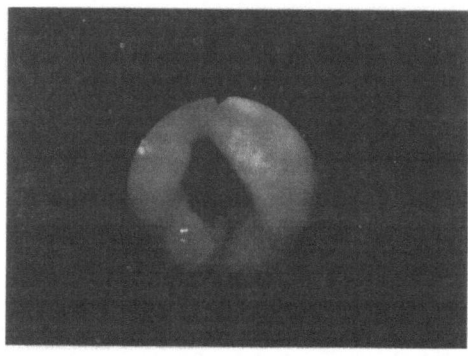

Fig. 3. Proximal view after laser evaporation

wall 3 cm distal of the plica vocalis. The tumor was pale with a
smooth surface and obstructed the lumen of the distal part more than
the proximal part Figure (2). Histologically the tumor was classified
as an adenoid-cystic carcinoma. An only 2o% reduction of the distal
stenosis could be attained by laser evaporation using 2o-5o watt
laser energy. As a result the FEV1 was 1200 ml. In a second step 70%
of the endotracheal tumor could be evaporated under general anesthesia and normofrequent jet ventilation with an inspiratory oxygen
concentration of 7o%. Following this procedure lung function was
perfectly normal. Figure 3 shows the endotracheal aspect of the tumor
after laser treatment. The procedure had to be repeated after 9 months
because of the tumor regrowth. It was also successful and the patient
is free of respiratory symptoms at present.

Case 2
This 60 year old woman suffered from a well diferentiated thyreoid
carcinoma which was treated by surgery and radiotherapy 8 years ago.
Diffuse nodular metastases of the lung were noticed 3 years ago which
were nearly constant in terms of size and number. Because of increasing stridor the patient was tranferred to our hospital for bronchoscopy and eventual laser treatment. Lung function testing showed a
combined restrictive-obstructive pattern with a vital capacity of only
50% of the predicted value and an airways resistance of 300% of the
predicted value. The paO2 was only 48 mmHg, the paCO2 was 34 mmHg.
A tomogram showed a 75% stenosis of the proximal trachea due to a
tumor originating in the left posterior dorsal trachea only 3 cm
below the vocal cords (Figure 4). The highly hyperemic tumor could be
partly resected under local anesthesia using a rigid bronchoscope. In
a second session under general anesthesia 2 days later profuse
bleeding occurred during coagulation with 20 watts. Because the lumen
was wider after laser treatment a 7 mm tube could be passed and ventilation was maintained without difficulty. It was then possible to
perform an upper tracheotomy. The tumor could then be removed by
surgery. Figure 5 shows the computer tomograms of the patient with
the peritracheal tumor masses and plastic tracheal cannula in situ.
There was no endotracheal tumor. The patient lived for 10 months after
the operation and died after thromboembolic episodes.

Discussion and conclusions
It seems clear that in both cases neither an operation nor radiotherapy were possible and that therefore laser evaporation was the
procedure of choice. Because of the localisation of the tumors in the
proximal trachea only a rigid bronchoscope could be used. The question as to whether a general anesthesia would have been possible as a
first step cannot be answered with certainty. A FEV1 of about 700 ml
is possibly borderline for Jet ventilation in cases of proximal to
mid tracheal stenosis. No value of FEV1 beyond which emergency
treatment is absolutely contraindicated has been defined to date,
but we believe that local anaesthesia plus sedation was safer in these
two patients than general anaesthesia could have been. On the other
hand we were surprised that during the second laser therapy in gene-

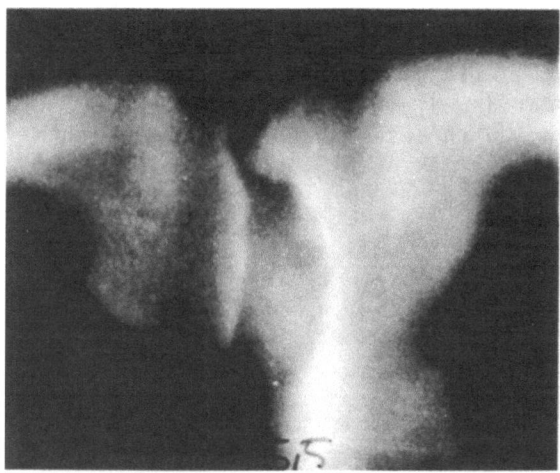

Fig. 4. Sagittal tomogram of the proximal trachea with a tumor obstructing the dorsal part of the trachea

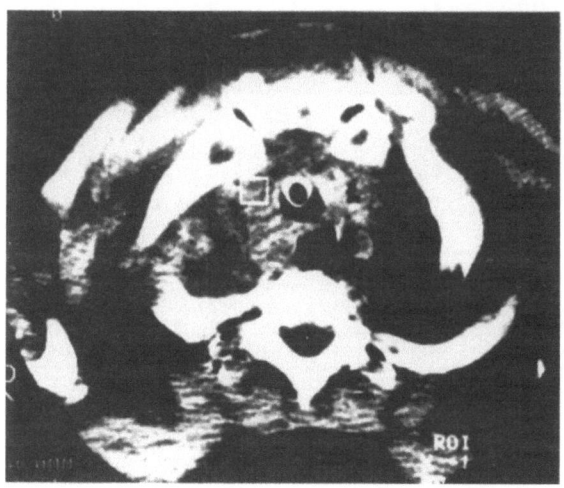

Fig. 5. CT scan of the tumor after tracheotomy and surgical resection with the plastic cannula in situ. Large tumor masses surrounding the trachea in the 2. ICR

ral anaesthesia jet ventilation was safe although the distance between the distal end of the bronchoscope and the main carina was 10 cm. Moreover, the oxygen saturation increased from 85% to 96% during laser evaporation in the patient with the adenoidcystic carcinoma reflecting an immediate effect on gas exchange. As to the second patient laser evaporation enabled us to intubate the patient and perform a cervical tracheotomy in a situation where a lower tracheotomy with sternotomy would have been impossible due to extensive peritracheal infiltration.

References
1. Dierkesmann, R., Huzly A.: Technik der endobronchialen Laser Behandlung. Prax. Klin. Pneumol 37 (1983) 211-215
2. Emslander HP., Prauer HD., Munteanu J. et al. Palliative endobronchiale Tumorverkleinerung durch Laserbehandlung. Behandlungsmodus-Sofortergebnisse-Langzeitergebnisse. Laser 1 (1985) 28-34

Morphological Peculiarities in Laser Wound Healing

V.I.Yeliseenko, V.E.Normansky

National Institute for Laser Surgery, Moscow, USSR

Biopsies of various organs of 2 000 patients were studied morphologically following operations with the aid of CO_2-, Nd-YAG and argon lasers in abdominal, purulent, plastic, hepatic and pancreatic surgery as well as endoscopic laser photocoagulation of acute gastric bleedings. The optimal power density of CO_2 laser irradiation for the resection of hollow organs in gastointestinal tract and liver, spleen and pancreas is about 3.10^3 Wt/mm^2. In the area of CO_2 laser incision of different tissues the coagulative necrosis about 60mcm takes place. The general width of thermal damages in biological tissues was about $132,7 \pm 18,3$ mcm. The peculiarities in laser wounds healind lies in the absence of leucocytic infiltration or edema of tissues ajaicent to the area of thermal necrosis. The application of CO_2 laser for surgical treatment of purulent wounds on soft tissues and in abdominal surgery gives a possibility to get the sterility and absolute hemostasis that results in healing these wounds in a type of an aseptic productive inlammation. This aseptic productive inflammation in healing process of the laser wounds leads to the shortening of treatment, and purulent wounds heal as clean surgical wounds. The macrophagal cells play an important role in the formation and progress of reparative processes. Their proliferation by the first day after operation was marked. The granulative tissue was formed by the 3rd day after laser incisions or endoscopic laser photocoagulation in acute gastric hemorrages. The whole regeneration of the mucous membranes of gastointestinal tract organs or epidermis was completed 30-45 days after exposure to laser and limited from the degree of the differentiation of the granulative tissue into the fibrous one.

Comparative Assessment of Conventional and Laser Treatment for Suppurative Wounds

O.K.Skobelkin, P.I.Tolstykh, V.I.Ryabov, V.A.Derbenev

National Institute for Laser Surgery, Moscow, USSR

Modern principles in the treatment of suppurative wounds are the following:(1)incision of devitalized tissues;(2) the primary or postponded suture;(3) utilization of a pulsed jet and a system of active aspiration. These methods are efficient in 85-90%. It satisfies the majority of surgeons. But thre are two things worth attention. First, the described scheme cannot be used in case of extensive flegmons, marked inflammatory changes around the purulent focus and when it has deep location near large vessels and nerves; when there is an extensive tissue necrosis and anaerobic flora. Secondly, the period of invalidity -with traditional methods being used - is unjustified in many cases. More effective therapy in extensive suppurative processes could be possibly reached with better management of a purulent focus and with the ameliorated influence on purufication and regeneration. For the latter one many surgeons are using enzymatic necrolysis. But natural proteinases turned to be not effective enough because of their rapid inactivation and withdrawing from the wound. Last years for treating purulent diseases we have been widely using three equally important modifications: laser treatment of a purulent focus, application of dressings with immobilized proteolitic enzymes and the stimulation of regeneration with helium-neon laser. The primary or postponded wound suturing is chosen depending on the location, the stage or extension of the process (Table 1).

Previously we used separate points of this programm as independent methods of treatment. Their combined effect has been studied lately on 300 patients. We cosider it necessary to perform the radical incision of devitalized tissues, to cut suppurative pouches with modulating a common wound cavity and to achieve good hemostasis. The excision is performed with a laser beam or with a steel scalpel. Then the wound is treated with a defocused CO_2 laser beam after modulating a common cavity. In case of a perifocal inflammatory process, and when it is impossible to put the primary suture or when

Table 1. The principal scheme for treating purulent wounds

operation	primary suture	postponded suture
Incision of purulent focus with laser	+	-
Laser debriment	+	+
Defocused irradiation	-	+
Irradiation with helium-neon laser	-	+
Dressing material with immobilized proteinaze	-	+
Suture material with immobilized proteinaze or antiseptic	+	+
Running lavage of the wound	+	+

Table 2. Comparative results of treating purulent wounds with different methods

Treatment with laser	Patients n	Supurrations %	Invalidity days
Primary suture	105	8,6	16,6
Postponded suture	99	4,1	20,8
"Open" wound	100	-	33,2
"Open" wound /no laser/	100	-	41,0

anaerobic infection is suspected, the wound is covered with dressing materials modified with proteinazes or antiseptics. In other cases the wound is closed with threads modified with immobilized antiseptics or enzymes. On the first or second postoperative day the wound is irradiated with a helium-neon laser with power density 20-40mW/cm^2 and exposure time 10 min. The secondary suturing is made after the inflammatory changes are irradicated on the second-fourth day, and after the repeated treatment with CO_2 defocused beam has been performed. Running lavage is used almost in all cases with a closed wound.

Thus, the period of purulent wounds' treatment can be considerably reduced when one combines CO_2 and helium-neon lasers with modified immobilized proteinazes. As we could conclude from our data the benefits of laser application are both in more perfect wound treatment and in stimulation of healing process. For example, studies of oxygen saturation in tissues at differet distances from the wound edges have shown that the healing process is more active when laser irradiation is applied.

12-Year Experience of CO_2 Laser Application in Surgeries on Hollow Organs of Gastro-Intestinal Tract

O.K.Skobelkin, E.I.Brekhov, G.D.Litvin, M.V.Smoljaninov, V.I. Ryabov

National Institute for Laser Surgery, Moscow, USSR

The laser as the surgical instrument has found an especially wide application in surgery on parenchymatous organs, in endoscopy, in pus surgery. The application of the laser scalpel on hollow organs is limited by the coplexity of laser beam manipulation in the depth of the wound, by the danger of damaging adiacent tissues and organs and by the overheating of tissues in the area of the incision. The tissue overheating takes place because the energy of the laser beam is absorbed by the blood flowing into the wound. Boiling blood leads to thermal damage of the surrounding tissue with the formation of large area of coagulation necrosis and with the inhibited regeneration processes. To avoid this we have developed a new and original technique of laser dissection of hollow organ's wall to which the blood supply is temporaly stopped with the help of special instruments. These latter have two jaws. Lower jaw serves as a screen and the upper onehas a through lengthwise slot for laser beam. The instrument permits an accurate gradual transmission of the light beam and allows to perform quick and bloodless tissue cutting. It causes minimal thermal tissue damage, asepticity and the so-called "the effect of biological tissue welding". The latter means tissue coagulation along the incision and layers' adhesion. The thin coagulation film on the wound surface prevents spreading of the infection and everting of the mucosa. It also gives better hemostasis. The laser surgical instruments protect simultaneously adjacent tissues and organs from laser irradiation. Nowadays we have developed sets of laser surgical instruments and suture devices for any surgery on lungs, esophagus, stomach and intestine. Contrary to usual devices the wall of the hollow organ sewed with the laser suture device is sterile, mechanically and biologically hermetical, blood is not oozing. This coagulation necrosis film prevents spreading of the infection in the depth especially along astaple. Starting from 1974 we have carried out experimental research work where we compared the healing process in laser wounds and anastomosis and in those performed with the traditional instruments. The specific feature of laser wound healing is rapid proliferative phase in inflammation and weak exudative process. It takes place because of an atraumatical incision, good hemostasis, absence of microbial invasion, coagulation nature of necrosis, short-term reaction of microvessels. Less number of postoperative complications is determined with the aseptical and productive nature of the inflammatory process. Up to now we performed 455 stomach resections with the laser instruments in patients with cancer and ulcer complications, 76 total gastrectomies, 116 resections of colon intestine. In the table there are the results of operations performed with Soviet laser instruments (CO_2-laser, laser surgical instruments and suture devices) and with the traditional instruments.

Table 1. Comparative Evaluation of Complications and Mortality in Laser and Traditional Surgeries

Operation		Number of patients	Complications %	Mortality %	Anastomosis insufficiency %
Total gastrectomy					
	with laser	76	25.0	6.7	3.9
	w/o laser	34	38.2	14.7	5.9
Stomach resection for cancer					
	with laser	252	11.9	2.4	0.8
	w/o laser	94	27.6	6.3	3.2
Stomach resection for ulcer					
	with laser	203	12.8	1.0	-
	w/o laser	71	21.3	2.8	-
Resection of colon intestine					
	with laser	116	17.2	4.3	1.7
	w/o laser	60	23.5	8.3	6.7
TOTAL	with laser	647	14.6	2.8	1.1
	w/o laser	259	26.2	6.9	3.4

As one can observe from the Table the surgical laser methods developed by us reduce the number of complications abd consequently, the number of deaths in 2-3 times.

Conclusions: 1. Laser scalpel in surgery of gastro-intestinal tract allows to simplify the process of the operation itself and to improve its quality. 2. Positive results and benifits from laser scalpel in gastro-intestinal surgery can be achieved only when it is used with special laser surgical instruments and suture devices. 3. Laser beam is reasonable to use only at key moments during the surgery, such as organ resection or anastomosis formation.

Morphologic Aspects of Nd:YAG Laser Application on Lung Tissue

Rolle A., E.Unsöld*, L.Ruprecht*, W.Permanetter**, F.Frank***
Chirurgische Klinik Innenstadt und Chirurgische Poliklinik der
Ludwig-Maximilians-Universität München, Pettenkoferstr. 8a und
Nußbaumstraße 20, 8000 München 2, und
Thoraxchirurgie Zentralkrankenhaus Gauting, Unterbrunner Str.85,
8035 Gauting (Direktor: Prof.Dr.med.L.Schweiberer)

Introduction

For nearly 10 years the Nd:YAG laser is used by several medical disciplines such as gastroenterology, urology, neurosurgery and pulmonology (2,8). The normally used wavelength of 1064 nm shows a good coagulation effect due to little absorption and high scattering in tissue. By resonance modification, a second wavelength of 1318 nm, at which water in particular, and highly vascularized tissue as well, demonstrate an absorption rate 10 times higher than that at 1064 nm, can be produced (fig.1,2; 1,3,4,9). Theoretically at this wavelength, one can expect a marked difference in the behaviour of parenchymal tissue, advantageous to clinical application, i.e. more precise tissue ablation and a superior degree of coagulation. Results of initial experimental studies examining use and effects of a Nd:YAG laser on leaver and splenic tissue can be found in the current literature (5,6,8). For the lung however such studies have not been performed, so that informations to application parameters as well as basic characteristics of the two wavelengths are not available. We therefore performed animal experiments evaluating the clinical application of the Nd:YAG laser in lung surgery.

Methods

The following questions were evaluated using anaesthesized beagles following a lateral, right thoracotomy, which in the dog, gives good access to all four lobes on the right lung:

1. The morphologic and histomorphologic effects produced in parenchymal lung tissue of the Nd:YAG laser as a function of wavelength, charge and energy density.

---

*GSF - Zentrales Laserlaboratorium Neuherberg b. München
**Pathologisches Institut der Universität München
***MBB Medizin-Technik Ottobrunn b. München

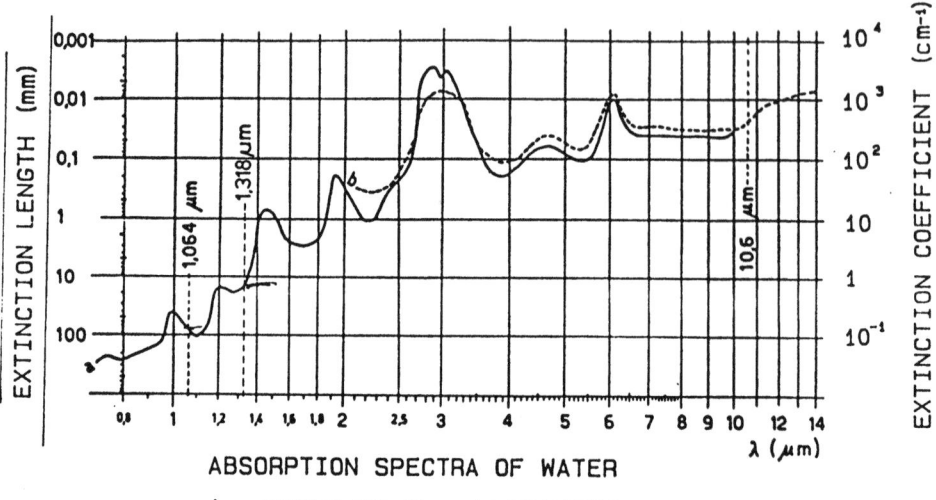

Figure 1. Absorption spectra of water (no additional text)

	ABSORPTION of 0.7% SALINE SOLUTION	EXTINCTION of HUMAN BLOOD
1.06 μm	0.07 cm⁻¹	34 ± 4 cm⁻¹
1.32 μm	0.73 cm⁻¹	12 ± 3 cm⁻¹

ABSORPTION OF SALINE SOLUTION AND
EXTINCTION OF BLOOD FOR 1.06 μm
AND 1.32 μm
(STOKES ET AL.)

Figure 2. Absorption of saline solution and extinction of
blood for 1,06 μm and 1,32 μm (no additional text)

2. The coagulation and cutting ability at both wavelengths (1064 nm, 1318 nm).

3. Whether adequate sealing of parenchymal lesions and fistulas can be achieved.

4. The practicability of the Nd:YAG laser as a thoracic surgical instrument in the spatial limitations of the thorax.

For our experiments the Nd:YAG laser in which both wavelengths could be applied via a light conductor was used. For other, later cutting and coagulation experiments, a defocussed beam was also used. As dogs do not have a mediastinum and do not tolerate thorax drains, maximal postoperative parenchymal sealing had to be achieved. Histological specimens were examined immediately after surgery and at the 6. postoperative day.

Results

Dotted rows of laser lesions, as well as cutting and coagulation experiments indicated that the 1318 nm wavelength caused steeper increases in necrosis width and depth. Therefore tissue effects identically to those observed upon laser application at 1064 nm could be produced at half the energy using the 1318 nm wavelength. The greater absorption rate, which is 10 times higher at 1318 nm creates a three-zone necrosis layer within lung tissue (fig.3). The central vaporisation crater is surrounded by an extended white zone of thermic denaturation with marked coagulation and hemostasis. The previous is inturn circumscribed by a hyperemic region. The 1064 nm wavelength, on the other hand, produces a two-zone necrosis. The previously described white zone surrounding the central necrosis crater which guarantees excellent hemostasis and sealing is absent. Instead, due

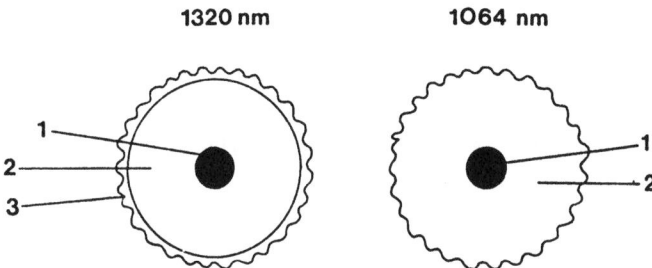

Figure 3. Zone structure of the Nd:YAG wavelengths 1318 nm and 1064 nm in lung tissue

    left: 1 = central vaporisation crater
           2 = wide "white" coagulation zone
           3 = hyperemic region

    right: 1 = central vaporisation crater
             2 = scatter zone with diffuse small hemorrhages

to high scattering, a white zone of diffuse small hemorrhages is present. These differences can be seen allready macroscopically. Although good cutting is possible at both wavelengths, the increased absorption at 1318 nm is responsible for the overall superior performance of this wavelength. The coagulation and sealing ability is markedly better. Attainance of a blood-free and air-tight incision is only possible when using the 1318 nm wavelength of the Nd:YAG laser. Lastly, the flexible laser scalpell proved very efficient, even if the lung was inflated. Using the Nd:YAG laser scalpell, a wedge shaped excision of the dog lung was possible without accessory instruments. At this wavelength as well, such excisions could be extended to an atypical segmental resection deep into the respective lobe. The segment bronchus supplying the region, however was closed with sutures. On the basis of these experiments, the 1318 nm wavelength must be considered most suitable for clinical applications in lung surgery, which had been started now.

References

1. Bayly IG, VB Karth, W.H.Stevence: The absorption spectra of liquid phase H_2O, HDO and D_2O from 0,7 µm to 10 µm. Infrared Physics 3: 211-233, (1980)

2. Beck O.J., F.Frank, E.Keiditsch, F.Wondrazek: Klinische und experimentelle Untersuchungen zur Erweiterung der Nd:YAG Laseranwendung in der Neurochirurgie. Laser Med u Chir 1: 13-18 (1985)

3. Bromson M.: Infrared Radiation. A Handbook for Applikation. New York: Plenum Press (1968)

4. Dinstl K., Fischer PL: Der Laser. Grundlagen und klinische Anwendung. Springer, Berlin - Heidelberg - New York (1961)

5. Frank F., O.J.Beck, S.Hessel, E.Keiditsch: Comparative investigations of the effects of the Nd:YAG laser at 1,06 microns and 1,32 microns on tissue. Laser in Surg Med 6: 546-551 (1987)

6. Godlewski G., P.Ginoves, J.M.Chincholles, E.Viel, J.P.Bureau, S.Rouv, H.Mion, A.Dubois, J.Fesquet: Hepatic resection with an Nd:YAG laser in pig. Laser in Surg Med 3:217-224 (1983)

7. Häußinger K., E.Held, R.Huber:
   Endobronchial laser therapy, differential therapeutic use and clinical value.
   Klin Wochenschr 62: 74-80 (1984)

8. Snider W.R., S.Li:
   Partial splenectomy with CO_2 laser. An experimental study.
   Laser Surg and Med 1: 357-360 (1981)

9. Stokes LF., DC Auth, D.Tanaka, JL Gray, C.Gulaesik:
   Biomedical utility of 1,32 µm Nd:YAG laser radiation.
   IEEE Trans Biomed Eng BME 28: 297-299 (1981)

Indication and Technique of Laserapplication in Pancreas-Resection in Children – First Results

G.H.Willital, H.Meier, M.Maragakis, G.Stöhr
University Clinic and Polyclinic for Pediatric Surgery Münster,
West-Germany

Surgical diseases of the pancreas in children

The most frequent pediatric surgical diseases of the pancreas (8,9) are: nontraumatic connatal and genetic determined diseases of the pancreas (6%), i.e. cystic alterations and stenosis of the branches of the pancreatic ducts (11,12); blunt abdominal trauma with damage to the pancreas tissue (19%); rupture of the pancreas (42%)(23); pancreas pseudocysts (18%); annular pancreas (8%) (14); alterations of the choledochal duct (4%) (15,22) and insulinomas (3%).

Indications for laserapplication in children

1. liver resections for liver tumors, echinococcus-cysts, rupture of the liver and diagnostic wedge resections
2. pancreas resections (fig.1) for pancreas tumors, ruptures and congenital alterations of the pancreatic duct (7,13,16,17,18)
3. spleen resections for a rupture and partial resection (trauma, Morbus Hodgkin)
4. kidney resections for a rupture or congenital anomalies which have to be corrected surgical
5. pilonidal-fistulae excisions creating absolute sterile conditions
6. hudge hydroceles in which laser surgery has the advantage that no alterations of the thin ductus and the vessels occur caused by the diathermy.

Indications for the use of laser must be restricted to those operative procedures, in which the laser really is a significant progress and has advantages compared to the standard operative procedures. We would not recommend and apply the laser as just an alternative surgical technique.

Indications for a pancreas resection (fig.2)

A survey of the frequency for pancreas resection in children out of our series from the last 16 years demonstrates that the frequency of insulinomas was about 6% (fig.3). The most frequent indication for a pancreas resection (3,4,5,6,19,20, 24,25) was the pancreas trauma with 82% and congenital alterations of the pancreatic duct in 12% (1,2,21). A survey of the different kinds of traumatic lesions of the pancreas is shown in fig. 4. For type 3 and 4 a pancreasresection or a Roux-Y-anastomosis is indicated. The Roux-Y-anastomosis is an organ preserving operation (pancreatico-jejunostomy) for a total rupture of the pancreas and an otherwise intact pancreas-

tissue (27,29). The guidelines to make a partial resection of the pancreas are
more   or less determined by the structure of the vessels (fig.5). Most important
for this is the arterial blood supply (1o,26).
The tissue in children differs very much from the tissue in adults:
the intracellular content of water in children is much more higher as in adults;
the collagen fibres are much more thinner, the quantity of these fibres is much
more less compared to adults; the vessels and the ductuli are much more smaller
as well as the thickness of the wall. A comparison of different resection techniques (fig.6) for the pancreas using the CO_2-laser, the neodym-YAG-laser, the
ultrasound method and the diathermy demonstrate that using the neodym-YAG-laser
respectively the ultrasound method a most sufficient occlusion of blood and lymph
vessels could be achieved (28).
An occlusion of the tissue itself was most save using the neodym-YAG-laser technique or the ultrasound technique whereas in cases of a CO_2-laser resection technique or using the diathermy more frequent fistulae of the pancreas occured.
The pancreatic duct itself could always be closed using a ligature. The thickness
of the tissue necrosis at the resectionline using the lowest intensity to cut the
organ is extremely small using the CO_2-laser, for the neodym-YAG-laser and the
ultrasound technique these tissue alterations were 2-3 mm and using the diathermy
usually a tissue damage over 3 mm is present.
Experimental studies have shown that the intraoperative use of an ultrasound probe
gives you the most informative pictures of the structure of the organ itself: the
borderlines of the tumor, the structure of the vessels, the borderlines of a cyst
and the topographic anatomical situation. This intraoperative analysis of a tissue
structure enables to perform a much more safer laser resection technique and enables furthermore to perform an organ preserving resection. Intraoperative ultrasound examination is a guide-line for the laser resection: laser-resection guided
by ultrasound: LU technique. Further clinical investigations are not available
at this point and one has to evaluate which advantage this technique will have
in the future.
The advantage of the application of the laser to resect parts of the parenchymatous
organs are:
1. Organpreserving resection technique with a reduction of postoperative bleeding
   and reduction of postoperative secretion from the tissue itself.
2. Being with the laser technique familiar a reduction of the operation time can
   be achieved (15-2o%). This is important in small babies and newborns.
3. Because a bleeding can nearly be completely avoided blood transfusion with all
   the disadvantage and dangers might be completely superfluous.

For literature 1 - 29 , please contact the authors.

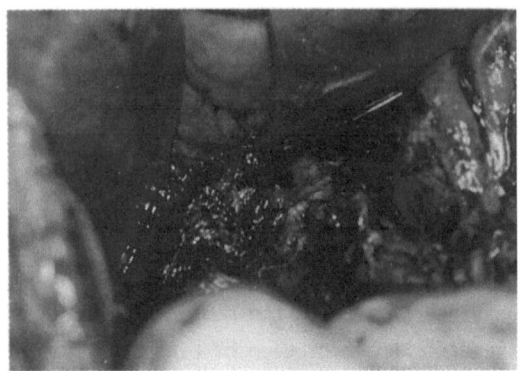

Fig. 1. Pancreasresection, following a pancreatic rupture with a complete damage of the pancreas tail and the corpus, leaving the processus uncinatus in place

Indikation zur Pankreasresektion im Kindesalter

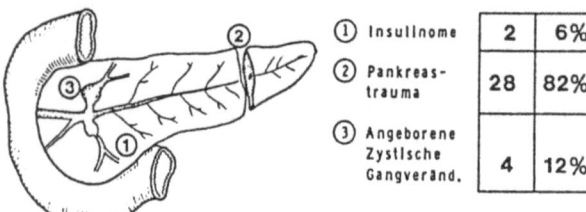

Fig. 2. Indication for pancreasresection in children

Überblick über die Lokalisation von Insulinomen bei Kindern

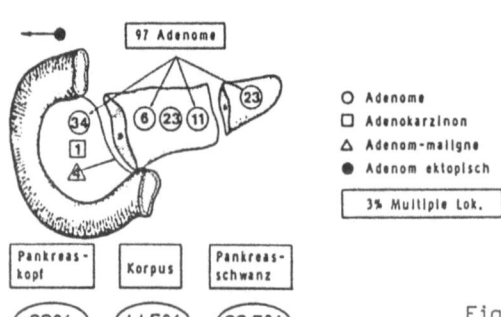

Fig. 3. Survey of the localization of insulinomas in children

INDIKATION ZUR ROUX'SCHEN-Y-ANASTOMOSE BEI
PANKREASRUPTUREN

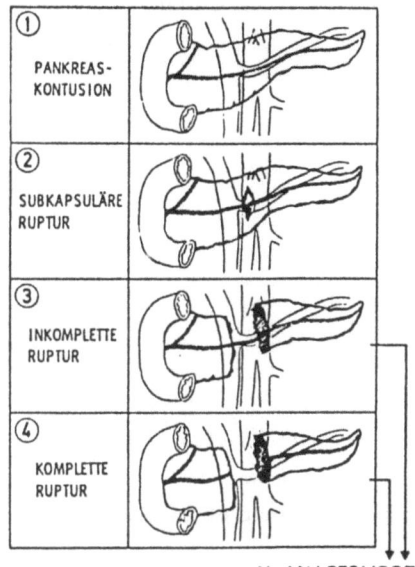

① PANKREAS-KONTUSION
② SUBKAPSULÄRE RUPTUR
③ INKOMPLETTE RUPTUR
④ KOMPLETTE RUPTUR

Y-ANASTOMOSE

Fig. 4. Indication for conservative and surgical treatment in cases of pancreastrauma in children and indication for a Roux-Y-anastomosis

Pankreassegmentresektionen entsprechend anatomischer Gegebenheiten

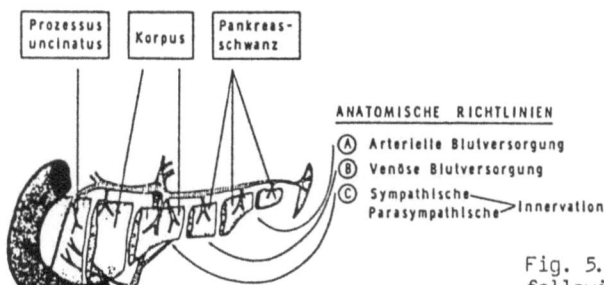

ANATOMISCHE RICHTLINIEN
Ⓐ Arterielle Blutversorgung
Ⓑ Venöse Blutversorgung
Ⓒ Sympathische / Parasympathische Innervation

Fig. 5. Pancreas-segmental resection following the anatomical-topographical arterial blood supply structures

Beurteilung unterschiedlicher Resektionstechniken beim Pankreas

	Blutstillung	Parenchymverschluß	Pankreasgang verschl.	Nekrosesaum	Bei Kindern besonders zu beachten
CO$_2$-Laser	−	+	−	<1 mm	① Höherer Wassergehalt des Gewebes
Neodym-Yag Laser	++	++	+	2-3 mm	② Weniger Bindegewebe
Ultraschall-messer	++	++	−	2-3 mm	③ Dünnwandigere und dünnkalibrigere Strukturen
Diathermie	+	+	−	<3 mm	

(soll chirurgisch erfolgen)

Fig. 6. Significance and evaluation of different resection techniques of the pancreas

Ultrasonographic Guided Lasertherapy for Liver Cancers – Experimental Temperature Measurements and Clinical Application

Daijo Hashimoto, Kiyotoshi Yabe, Yushio Uedera,
Shyunichi Yumoto, Yasuo Idezuki

2nd Department of Surgery, Faculty of Medicine

Tokyo University, 7-3-1 Hongo Bunkyo-ku, Tokyo, Japan

Introduction

Nd:YAG laser has been used for the treatment of tumors on the hollow organ through endoscopy, whereas, due to its property of recti-linear propagation, it has not been thought suitable for the treatment of tumors in parenchymatous organ.
Based on the supposition if spherically dispersed laser beam could make tumors in the parenchymatus organ be round coagulated tissues, we developed new laser therapy, in-depth radiation method for liver cancers.

Shape of the fiber tip

In order to obtain the optimum fiber tip for spherically dispersed radiation, computer simulation ray trace was exercised.
Optical ray trace by computer simulation was performed on each 20,000 rays with varying the conical angle.
Simulation data showed lateral radiation hardly could be expected with a single conical tip.
Computer simulation was exercised on double conical shape of tip. However at this time new parameters of theta 1, theta 2, radius of tip (R) were introduced, analyses of computer simulation results lead to the comparatively well balanced output radiation.
Based on the simulation result, probes with theta 1=70°, theta 2=30°, and R=0.3mm were manufactured.
Judging from the actual radiation pattern of this probe, computer simulation seemed to be satisfactory.

Optimal conditions for radiation

With the investigations of various shapes of coagulated tissues got by
animal experimentations, there were found out very interesting phenomena
in the relationship between laser energy power and coagulated shape.
As the laser power becomes higher the shape of tissue coagulated becomes
more spherical, whereas, as the laser power becomes lower the one
coagulated becomes more round.
From many experimentations, some 5 W continuous radiation energy was
proved to be optimum.
Applying 5 W continuous laser radiation, 500 Joule/cm proved to be enough
to get a round tissue coagulated in case of canine liver resected. As for
living canine liver, 1000 Joule/cm was necessary for the same size of
round tissue coagulated.
These different laser energy necessary for getting the coagulated tissues
seemed due to cooling effect of blood flow.

Gas evacuation device

During in-depth radiation, around the tip of the fiber probe temperature
beomes 200° - 300°C and mixed gases consist of CO , $H O$, melcapthane,
methylamine and aldehyde etc. were generated. As the temperature and
pressure of the gas was rather high, gas embolism in intra-hepatic vessels
or heat burn of intra-hepatic bile ducts might be caused.
By applying 15 cm $H O$ negative pressure, gas generated around the fiber
tip was completely removed.
This gas evacuatin device was made of a T shape tube. The T tube was
connected to a pump to apply negative pressure.

In-depth temperature measurement

We have developed a temperature measuring device to analyze in-depth
thermal distribution of irradiated tissues. This device consists of 37
thermocouples whose tips were placed in the shape of a regular triangle
with a side length of 7mm.
The informations of temperature measured by these thermo-couples were
processed by a computer through a data-logger interface and displayed on
a TV monitor.

In case of 5 W continuous radiation, expansion of iso-thermal contour map was observed as high echoic area got enlarged.
According to the in-depth measured data, the temperature of probe tip was some 240°C - 360°C that of white tissue coagulated was approximately 50°C - 60°C and that of layers carbonized was in the range of 100°C - 160°C.

Ultrasonographic observation

Proceeding with laser radiation, the enlargement of high echoic area of spheric coagulation was observed.
Owing to the histological examination, the size of the high echoic area was a slightly bigger than the utmost outer boundary which was visually white by some 2 mm.
Among the high echoic area, semi-spheric low echoic area existed and beneath it acoustic shadow was abserved.
The width of the acoustic shadow corresponded to the diameter of central vaporized zone. In case of no application of gas suction, scattering of tiny gas babbles could be observed, but with the application of gas suction no gas babbles were observed.

Clinical applications

A male patient of 54 years old who was suffered from hepato-cellular carcinoma, bone metastases to TH 12 and liver cirrhosis was admitted. In the upper posterior region of right liver, 2.7 cm diameter cancer was detected.
AFP value was 16250 ng/ml.
Hepatic malfuction of this patient was Child B grade.
In May 1984, in-depth radiation therapy was operated by applying 7638 Joule under laporatomy.
Resection of bone metastases were performed as well subsequently.
During and after in-depth radiation, neither bleeding nor bile leakage was observed.
As to after operation complications, slightly feverish symptom and hepatic coemzyme elevation were observed for the period of several days. AFP drastically dorpped into 77 ng/ml in two months.
The patient could return to work.
However he had gone seven months later due to rupture of esophageal varices. The AFP value just before his death was 150 ng/ml.

6 cases of hepato-cellular carcinoma with liver cirrhosis and 10 cases of meta-static liver cancers were treated successfully.

Discussion

Though with the recent progress in improvement of operation technique and in post-operation care, resections for hepatocellular carcinoma have been prevailed in CHILD A or B grade hepatic malfunction. In late stage hepatic malfunction such as the case of CHILD C grade or multiple liver cancers, TAE (Transcatheter Arterial Embolization) instead of resection has become available in recent years.
However, TAE should absolutely be avoided to apply on the case of main portal tumor thrombi because massive hepatic necrosis surrounding cancers are unavoidable.
Our new in-depth laser therapy is a kind of high local curable treatment for cancers, with minimum damage on surrounding normal tissues.
No bleeding and bile leakage during and post operation have been observed. This was supposed to be caused by surrounding thick coagulated zone made after vaporization of cancer. This supposition was proved to correct by observing microscopically that almost all the tiny vessels and bile canal in the coagulated zone were obliterated.
Aside from hepatic resection and TAE such local therapies as Cryosurgery, pure alchool injection therapy and microwave therapy have been tried so far.
Any one of these therapies has not been reported to get satisfactory treatment results. In general, laser therapy under laporatomy is most desirable from the stand point of radiation accuracy, in the risky cases, percutaneous transhepatic approach may be available.
Accordingly, our new therapy will become one of a hopefull and effective treatment method for liver cancers.

References

1. Hashimoto, D., Takami, M., and Idezuki, Y. ;
   In-depth radiation therapy by YAG laser for malignant tumors in the liver under ultrasonic imaging.
   Proceeding of the 4th meeting of the World Federation for Ultra-sound in Medicine and Biology. P. 78 1985

Application of the CO_2 Laser in Thoracic Surgery

H.R. Herrera, J.R. Hinshaw, R.J. Lanzafame
Department of Surgery and Division of Plastic
Surgery at Rochester General Hospital and the
University of Rochester School of Medicine
and Dentistry, Rochester, N.Y.

Advances in the management of median sternotomy infections over the past two decades have significantly reduced the morbidity and mortality of this major complication. The technique of open debridement introduced by Spencer[1] in 1961 and closed mediastinal irrigation with antimicrobial agents described by Shumacker and Mendelbaum[2] in 1963 made salvage of these patients possible. Recently, the use of muscle flaps, omentum, and CO_2 laser debridement for the reclosure of infected sternal wounds has improved the clinical outcome.[3-6]

We have now treated 10 patients with major sternal wound complications and some patients with empyema. Deepithelialized pectoralis major myocutaneous flaps and, when necessary, omental transposition have proved highly successful.

PATIENTS

Ten patients with major sternal wound infections were treated. All had purulent drainage from the sternal incision. Staphylococcus epidermidis, Klebsiella, Serratis, Proteus mirabilis, Escherichia coli, and Staphylococcus aureus were isolated in cultures. Following debridement, the wound was left open and packed with Betadine-soaked gauze until ready for final closure.

The total length of hospitalization ranged from 27 to 63 days, the average being 42 days. The length of stay from time of reclosure ranged from 7 to 27 days, averaging 15 days.

TECHNIQUE OF CO_2 LASER DEBRIDEMENT

The wound is debrided using the CO_2 laser with the 125mm lens at 30 to 40 Watts in a continuous mode until a satisfactory viable tissue is obtained.

TECHNIQUE FOR OMENTAL TRANSPOSITION

The technique of intrathoracic omental transposition has been well described.[4,6-10] The omentum is brought up through a small opening in the diaphragm just posterior to the sternum. Care must be taken not to rotate the omentum or cause traction on the stomach. Additional length, if needed, may be gained by dividing the left or right omental artery and unraveling the omentum based on its vascular arcade. Rarely, it may be necessary to dissect the omentum off the colon and stomach, dividing the left or right gastroepiploic artery.[11]

TECHNIQUE FOR ADVANCEMENT OF PECTORALIS MAJOR MYOCUTANEOUS FLAPS

We base our pectoralis major myocutaneous flaps on their thoracoacromial blood supply. H-incisions are made at both ends of the median sternotomy. The pectoralis major is dissected off the chest wall from medial to lateral. Counterincisions are made over the humeral attachments to the muscle, and the muscle is divided at its insertion. The flap is then deepithelialized medially for approximately 2 to 4 cm.

Several options are now available for closure of median sternotomy wounds. If the sternum has been closed, a single myocutaneous flap may be advanced across the midline to provide coverage of the sternotomy. If partial or total sternotomy has been performed, or if the sternum has been left open, the pectoralis major muscle flaps may be deepithelialized and turned into the wound. Drains are placed beneath the flap, and the skin and subcutaneous tissue are closed in layers.

DISCUSSION

Median sternotomy, because it provides safe, easy access to the heart and great vessels, has become the most commonly used incision in cardiac surgery. The reported incidence of major infections of this incision ranges from 0.5 to 5.0 percent.[1,12-15] It is, however, a very serious complication. The patients risk sepsis, graft thrombosis, disruption of the cardiac suture lines, and dessication of the mediastinal tissues.

Factors associated with an increased risk of sternal-wound infection include (1) a prolonged operative and perfusion time, (2) postoperative bleeding, (3) re-exploration, (4) external cardiac massage, and (5) low postoperative cardiac output.[1,12,16,17] In addition, Culliford et al,[16] have found an 8.5 percent increase in infection rate when bilateral internal mammary artery implants are used.

Experience has shown that early recognition and prompt initiation of therapy is crucial. Delay results in extensive soft-tissue and bony involvement, making eradication of infection more difficult. Purulent drainage is an obvious indication of a sternal-wound infection. More common but less specific signs include fever, leukocytosis, chest pain, and sternal instability.

Superficial infections may be treated with incision, drainage, and local wound care. Deep infections require exploration and thorough debridement.

Our management of deep sternal-wound infections now consists of open exploration, debridement of all infected soft tissue and bone, and removal of all foreign material. The wound is left open and packed. Dressings are changed frequently. Routine tissue cultures are performed, and appropriate systemic antibiotics are administered. When the wound appears clean and tissue cultures are negative, reclosure is attempted.

An earlier stratagem consisted of debridement and closed mediastinal irrigation with antimicrobial agents. However, the morbidity and mortality remained quite high, with one-third to one-half of patients not responding to this treatment. Recently, the use of muscle flaps and omentum in sternal reclosure has been advocated. Jurkiewicz,[3] reporting his experience with the pectoralis major muscle flap for those patients failing to respond to debridement and mediastinal irrigation, had success with this approach in 9 of 12 patients. We now use CO_2 laser debridement, muscle flaps and omentum in the initial reclosure of all major sternal-wound infections. Mortality with this approach has been nil, and morbidity and hospital stay have been reduced.

Several techniques for the rotation of the pectoralis major muscle have been described.[3,5,18] Jurkiewicz initially suggested basing it on its thoracoacromial blood supply and completely freeing it up to rotate it into the wound. More recently he has recommended basing it on its internal mammary vascular pedicle, dividing it laterally and folding it into the sternal defect. Both techniques require extensive dissection. The latter technique also requires an intact internal mammary artery, not always possible after coronary artery surgery.

We prefer to advance a myocutaneous flap and to deepithelialize the medial border. The flap is based on its thoracoacromial and lateral thoracic arterial blood supply, demonstrated by the anatomic studies of J.L. Freeman et al,[19] and is dissected free from the chest wall. Less dissection is needed, operative time is reduced, and adequate tissue is made available to fill the sternal defect.

The choice of closure depends on the sternal defect. If minimum debridement with the CO_2 laser has been performed and the sternum has been wired closed, a single pectoralis major myocutaneous flap may be advanced across the midline to provide additional covering for the sternotomy. If extensive sternal debridement has been performed and the sternum has been wired together, bilateral pectoralis muscle flaps are advanced to fill any defects and to provide stability to the chest wall. When partial or total sternotomy has been performed or the sternum cannot be wired together, omentum is placed over the sternal-xiphoid and heart, and bilateral pectoralis major flaps are advanced and turned into the sternal defect. This results in a stable chest wall with adequate tissue coverage for the mediastinum.

Our patients have no significant functional limitations. The appearance following these reconstructions is entirely acceptable. With the same principles, empyema cavities have been closed. The CO_2 debridement has provided precise excision, and reduction of bacteria in the contaminated field, and a good base for the reconstruction procedures.

SUMMARY

Closure of median sternotomy defects and empyema with CO_2 laser debridement, myocutaneous pectoralis flaps and omental transfer is presented. We think this technique provides adequate tissue, less dissection, and shorter operative time.

1. Engelman, R.M., Williams, C.D., Gouge, T.H., et al. Mediastinitis following open-heart surgery. Arch. Surg. 107:772, 1973.
2. Shumacker, H.B., and Mendelbaum, I. Continuous antibiotic irrigation in the treatment of infection. Arch. Surg. 86:384, 1963.
3. Jurkiewicz, M.J., Bostwick, J., Hester, T.R., et al. Infected median sternotomy wound: Successful treatment by -uscle flaps. Ann. Surg. 191:738, 1980.
4. Lee, A.B., Schimert, G., and Shatkin, S. Total excision of the sternum and thoracic pedicle transposition of the greater omentum: Useful strategems in managing severe mediastinal infection following open heart surgery. Surgery 80:433, 1976.
5. Arnold, P.G., and Pairolero, P.C. Use of pectoralis major muscle flaps to repair defects of anterior chest wall. Plast. Reconstr. Surg. 63:205, 1979.
6. Jurkiewicz, M.J., and Arnold, P.G. The omentum: An account of its use in the reconstruction of the chest wall. Ann. Surg. 185:548, 1977.
7. Samson, R., and Pasternak, B.M. Current status of surgery of the omentum. Surg. Gynecol. Obstet. 149:437, 1979.
8. Thompson, S.A., and Pollock, B. The use of free omental grafts in the thorax: An experimental study. Am. J. Surg. 70:227, 1945.
9. Goldsmith, H.S., Kiely, A.A., and Randall, H.T. Protection of intrathoracic esophageal anastomoses by omentum. Surgery 63:464, 1968.
10. Virkkula, L., and Eorola, S. Use of omental pedicle for treatment of bronchial fistula after lower lobectomy: Report of two cases. Scand. J. Thorac. Cardiovasc. Surg. 9:287, 1973.
11. Alday, E.S., and Goldsmith, H.S. Surgical technique for omental lengthening based on arterial anatomy. Surg. Gynecol. Obstet. 135:103, 1972.
12. Brown, A.H., Braimbridge, M.V., Panagopoulos, P., and Sabar, E.F. The complications of median sternotomy. J. Thorac. Cardiovasc. Surg. 58:189, 1969.
13. Jimenez-Martinez, M., Arguero-Sanchez, R., Perez-Alvarez, J.J., and Mina-Castaneda, P. Anterior mediastinitis as a complication of median sternotomy incisions: Diagnostic and surgical considerations. Surgery 67:929, 1970.
14. Thurer, R.J., Bognolo, D., Vargas, A., et al. The management of mediastinal infection following cardiac surgery. J. Thorac. Cardiovasc. Surg. 68:962, 1974.
15. Crmoljez, P.F., Barner, H.H., Willman, V.L., and Kaiser, G.C. Major complications of median sternotomy. Am. J. Surg.]30:679, 1975.
16. Culliford, A.T., Cunningham, J.N., Zeff, R.H., et al. Sternal and costochondral infections following open-heart surgery: A review of 2,594 cases. J. Thorac. Cardiovasc. Surg. 72:714, 1976.
17. Ochsner, J.L., Mills, N.L., and Woolverton, W.C. Disruption and infection of the median sternotomy incision. J. Cardiovasc. Surg (Torino) 13:394, 1972.
18. Brown, R.G., Fleming, W.H., and Jurkiewicz, M.J. An island flap of the pectoralis major muscle. Br. J. Plast. Surg. 30:161, 1977.
19. Freeman, J.L., Walker, E.P., Wilson, J.S.P., and Shaw, H.J. The vascular anatomy of the pectoralis major myocutaneous flap. Br. J. Plast. Surg. 34:3, 1981.

Use of Carbon Dioxide Laser in Genital System Corrective or Reconstructive Surgery

R. Pariente
University "La Sapienza"
Via Bruno Bruni 120, Rome, Italy

The reconstructive and corrective treatment of some congenital or acquired lesions in male and female genital apparatus, derives remarcable advantages from the use of Carbon Dioxide Laser.
This instrument, in fact, put us in a position to usefully effect surgery thanks to its characterictics, among which, preminently, that of sealing blood and lymphatic vessels while cutting them: and that of reducing tissue reactivity thus limiting oedema and consequently pain.
In particular, in breast reconstructive surgery, performed using a myocutaneous flap formed by the latissimus dorsi muscle, and in which it is necessary to make big subcutaneous underminings, extended to the whole interested hemithorax, Laser facilitates the processes and prevents minor bleeding which might originate lymphoematic scattering that would be very deprimental to the result of the Surgery. Laser affords analogous advantages in breast corrective surgery, both reductive and augmentative. In the reconstruction of the penis Laser is usefully employed in the remaking of both the missing urethra and in the reconstruction of the penile cylinder, as in preparing fitting material, by the use of a finrodermo-fat graft or a muscular flap from the rectus abdominis.
Also in the operations for hypospadias the above-mentioned properties of the Laser demonstrates their high usefulness.

To conclude, in the construction of the aplasic vagina, made following the Kirschner Wagner technique, which consists in forming a neovaginal cavity between the urethra and the bladder on one side, and rectum on the other one, and deepening to the Douglas, the Laser prevents the risk of the formation of lympho-hematic gatherings which would compromise the take of the skin graft applied on the neo-built cavity.

Laser Scalpel in Pancreatic Surgery

E.I. Brechov, G.D. Litvin, A.G. Kirpitchov,
V.V. Kalinnikov, A.N. Severtsev
Surgical Department, Hospital N 51
Alabjeva str., 7/33, Moscow, U.S.S.R.

At present operative treatment of pancreas gives the the great postoperative mortality rate and postoperative complications. This is due to the operative trauma of pancreatic tissue which gives rise to the acute postoperative pancreatitis and pancreonecrosis with further complications and to the development of specific postoperative purulent complications in the stump margin.

At present there are quite a number of papers both in the USSR [1,2] and in the West [3] showing the beneficial resuts of pancreatic transection using CO2 "laser-scalpel" both in case of its primary lesion and in case of the secondary lesion due to the stomach and colon cancer.

We report here our experiences in the management of patients who underwent CO2 laser resection for primary and secondary malignant lesions.

During 1980-87 we performed 35 pancreatic resection for malignant lesions of pancreas using CO2 "laser-scalpel" and special laser clamps. Of these, 5 underwent pancreatoduodenectomy, 28 underwent distal pancreatectomy (of these, 12 underwent sub-total pancreatic resection: body and tail of the gland, and 2 required a 95% pancreatectomy), and 2 patients had local excision (local resection) of the tumour of the ampulla of Vater using CO2 laser (of these, 1 patient had the special triangular laser cholecystojejunostomy: a bypass procedure).

35 patients in our group comprised 20 men and 15 women with the mean age of 52 1/2 years (ranging from 22 to 72 years).

We performed pancreatic resection in 25 patients with gastric cancer with direct overgrowth into the pancreas; in 5 patients with carcinoma of the ampulla of Vater; in 3 patients with pancreatic cancer, and 2 patients with colon cancer.

All surgical specimens were subjected to routine histologic study. Histological proof of the presense of carcinoma was available in all cases.

The postoperative mortality, defined as deaths within 30 days of surgery, was 20%. 7 of our 35 patients died. Of these, 2 had gastric cancer, 3 had pancreatic cancer, and 2 had colon cancer. The 7 deaths through surgery were due to cardiac and respiratory problems (3), peritonitis and septicaemia (2), pancreonecrosis and multi-system failure (1), and pancreonecrosis and a massive retroperitoneal haemorrhage (1).

All the anastomoses proved to be quite reliable in all 35 cases.

Clinically the acute postoperative pancreatitis was diagnosed in 13 cases. Of these, 5 patients were seriously ill (they had 3 or more positive prognostic signs as described by Ranson J.H.C. et al. [4]).

Laser transection time of pancreas ranged from 10 to 30 sec. in all cases. The mean operative time was 3 hours.

Specific postoperative complications of pancreas were noted in 11 cases (33,3%) /in 4 cases for combined operations/, in connection with this we noted: pseudocysts in 6 cases, pancreatic abscesses in 6 cases, pancreatic phlegmons in 2 cases, and pancreatic fistulas in 5 cases. Practically all these complications were corrected by the medical management. Only 3 cases were reoperated in order to correct these complications; external drainage having been used.

Main pancreatic duct was ligated in 5 cases (for 2 cases for gastric cancer). Other patients did not need this procedure since this duct was completely welded after using laser.

Conclusions

1. Laser resection of pancreas in case of its malignant lesions gives 20% decrease of postoperative mortality rate (about 14,3% for combined operations in advanced cancer of adjacent organs) due to the complete welding of its surface. This procedure excludes additional haemostatic measures and stops the leakage of pancreatic juice.

2. Specific postoperative complications of the pancreas happen in 33,3% (about 14,5% for combined operations in advanced cancer of adjacent organs); this is due to the fact that laser resection of pancreas makes operative treatment less traumatic.

3. This procedure helps save operative time during the stage of pancreatic resection.

References

1. Khromov B.M., Krylov K.I., Korotkevich N.S.: Comparative characteristics of operations performed using a laser beam, scalpel and electric knife. Vopr.Oncol. 20:106-107, 1974.
2. Korotkevich N.S., Mel'nikova A.P., Serebryakov V.A.: Effect of laser radiation on the pancreas: the use of optical quantum generators in modern sciene and technology. Leningdadski Dom Nauchno Tekhnychescoi

Propagande, 1973, p.90.
3.Orda, R., Barak, J., Orda, S., Wiznitzer, T.: Partial distal pancreatectomy with a hand-held CO_2 laser. Arch.Surg. 115:869-873,1980.
4.Ranson, J.H.C., Pasternack, B.S.: Statistical methods for quantifying the severity of clinical acute pancreatitis. J.Surg.Res. 22: 79-91, 1977.

Experience with the Use of CO_2 Laser and Infra Red Low Energy Laser in Aesthetic Plastic Surgery of the Face

R. E. AMAR (Marseille, France)

In our experience two Lasers were used since 1982 for many lesions, but the improvement of the technic and the quality of the healing process allowed a more specific utilisation in aesthetic plastic surgery where they became two outstanding tools for better results.
Since 1983, this presentation has been done in many scientific meetings to introduce them to the plastic surgeons in Europe, and also in Japan and in Brazil.

MATERIAL AND METHOD

The Lasers Apparatus used for this study are :
First : A Coherent CO2 Laser with a continuous power of 25 Watts. The Power setting range from 5 to 20 watts of continuous power according to the lesion.
The spot size was 1 mm for cutting effect, and a spot focus of 1 cm for tissue vaporization.
Second : a low energy laser was introduced to this study one year after to be tested.
A Gallium-Aluminium-Arsenid diodic Laser is acting with an impulse power of 15 milliwatts per square cm and is emitting within the Infra-red spectrum at 904 nanometers.
The Power supply is switching off automatically by the timer.

Since this infra-red light is invisible, an helium-neon red light helps define therapeutic areas as shown in a low motion picture.

PATIENTS

The CO2 Laser has helped to treat more than 300 patients for minor or major lesions as out patients in office surgery .
Here are some examples located in the face and neck .
1. numerous seborrheic keratosis were vaporized without local anesthetics. Only some light spots remain few months later.

2. Same result in a case of xanthelasmas

these two affections illustrate the necessity to clean the skin before face lifting or blepharoplasty.

3. an excellent result after treatment of naevus of the nasal groove and of the upper lip. The arrow point out the unconspicuous scars.
4. A naevus papillomatosus of the ciliary margin was vaporised. Care was taken to preserve the eye-ball by anesthesia of the conjonctive and protective spoon.
The same lesion in the nasal tip.

5. for some capillary hemangiomas the CO2 Laser can be used successfully . A test-patch on the margin must be done .
But the Argon Laser still remain the best for this kind of lesion.
The experience with the use of infra-red-diodic-laser in plastic and aesthetic surgery of the face is more recent.

A preliminary report was published in the french journal : les Annales de Chirurgie plastique in 1984.
Here is a representative case which is a good illustration of the low energy Laser biologic action.
1. a 53 years old patient presented a skin necrosis occuring immediately after a face lift. It was caused by a highly exeptionnal allergic reaction to a mercury containing pre operative antiseptic.
Three forty five minute laser sessions were needed to close in weeks the defect without any suture or skin graft.
Here is a closer view of the left side where the defect occured it looks as good as the other side.

Immediately after a face-lifting the low energy laser light help to relieve post-operative subjective syndrome, mostly after mobilisation of the SMAS : superficial musculo-aponeurotic system of the face.
* The first laser session is performed 4 days after intervention. One can observe less neck striction, less swelling and an improvement of the capillary vascularisation with reduction of ecchymosis on cheecks and neck.
* the best indications are patients older than 70 years because the subjective syndrome is maximum at that age .

DISCUSSION

It's more easy to explain the mechanism of action for the CO2 laser than for the low energy laser.
The process of vaporisation leave adnexal epithelium
within the dermis to re-epithelialize the surface. This controlled dermabrasion by a defocused CO2 laser is termed " LASERBRASION ".
Here is one case of rhinophyma where laserbrasion was used successfully. On these pictures you can notice the test patch on the root of the nose with perfect healing and on the next one the nose just after performing laser reduction.
15 days later one can notice the quality of the epidermisation.

This slide shows a case of acne scars after 2 chemical peelings and one dermabrasion. The laserbrasion performed under local anesthesia as outpatient in office surgery gave satisfaction to the patient. here are the result 15 days later and one month later.

The biological effect of the low energy laser is more controversial, but in our study one can unmistakably conclude that the infra-red diodic Laser light is a new therapeutic adjuvant in aesthetic plastic surgery with no side effect, no heat, no photoallergy and no phototoxicity.

IN CONCLUSION

These two kind of Lasers might be considered as new indispensable tools in the armamentorium of the aesthetic Plastic surgeon.

Hemorrhoidectomy and Fistulectomy with Nd:YAG Laser

S. Zhao*, Y. Chen**
*Beijing Heart, Lung & Blood Vessel Medical Center
**North China Research Institute of Electro-Optics
P.O. Box 8511, Beijing, PRC.

Hemorrhoids and anal fistulas have been the most common diseases among the Chinese. Since October 1985 724 of the number of the patients had received laser hemorrhoidectomy or fistulectomy, 314 had follow-up period of over 6 months: internal hemorrhoids 238, external 24, anal fistulas 52. Treatment parameters: laser working distance 5 mm, spot size $\emptyset$= 1 mm, power density 1910-3185 W/cm^2, M/F: 207/107, age ranged 9-82. 9 patients had been refused to give a routine surgical operation elsewhere because of being in the serious local infection stage, 12 because of accompanying hypertension, thyroidism, etc. Results: in most patients, 218 (92 %) for internal hemorrhoids, 24 (100 %) for external hemorrhoids, 52 (100 %) for anal fistulas both preoperative symptoms and physical signs disappeared; the symptoms of 20 (8 %) of internal hemorrhoids were improved because of various reasons. Complications: rebleeding 6 /1.9 %), severe pain 7 (2.2 %), dysuria 12 (4.1 %), anal sphincter spasm and skin bridge 5 (1.6 %), fissure inanal 5 (1.6 %). The advantages of laser operation, safer: bloodless or less bleeding during and after procedures, simple: out-patient treatment, no enema, antibiotics no formal dressing to be necessary, normal diet, bowels no limited, reduction days of work, 85 (27 %) patients didn't take rest post-operatively, less scar tissue formation, no infenction and less pain after operation, low cost.

The Effects of Laser Smoke on the Lungs of Rats

M.S. Baggish, M. Elbakry
Crouse Irving Memorial Hospital, Dept. of Obstetrics & Gynecology
736 Irving Avenue, Suite 308 W. Tower, Syracuse, New York 13210

Although laser surgery has gained increasing interest in gynecology during the past 10 years and a substantial volume of literature has been published in peer review journals regarding this modality of treatment, little data exists about the effects of the plume (vapor) by-products resulting from this surgery. The purpose of this study was to determine whether harmful effects might result if the vapor products of laser surgery were chronically inhaled.

The sequelae of the chronic inhalation of carbon dioxide laser smoke of ten white rats was studied in a three phase experiment. The fine particulate matter resulting from tissue vaporization was deposited in the animals alveoli producing a congestive interstitial pneumonia, bronchiolitis, and emphysema. During the smoke inhalation phase all rats exhibited similar behavior. At approximately 1 1/2 minutes, the animals became sluggish and stopped active movements. Activity resumed during the initial 2 minute rest period but stopped completely with subsequent smoke exposures. The pathology induced by laser plume are not dissimilar to those resulting from the chronic inspiration of other types of particulate matter. Utilization of an efficient smoke evacuator should offer substantial protection against these abnormal effects. To test the latter hypothesis five additional white rats were exposed to laser smoke but were protected by the interposition of an evacuation filter.

Orthopaedy

CO_2 Laser in Orthopaedic Surgery

P. Balasubramaniam
Professor of Orthopaedic Surgery
National University Hospital, Singapore

Though lasers have been in clinical use for the last twenty five years they have not moved into orthopaedic surgery. There was only one scientific paper in the uses of laser in orthopaedic surgery though a total of 319 scientific papers were presented at the 6th Congress of the International Society for Laser Surgery and Medicine in 1985. Does laser not offer any distinct advantage in orthopaedic surgery for it to have taken so long to get into orthopaedic practice? This paper describes our preliminary experience with CO2 laser in orthopaedic surgery. CO2 laser surgery was started at the National University Hospital, Singapore on 18 December 1985 and Professor Kaplan from Israel stayed with us for one week to start the programme.

Materials and methods

A Sharplan 60 watt CO2 laser machine was used for open laser surgery and a total of 56 cases were done during this period of one and a half years. Table 1 shows the types of orthopaedic procedures that were done with the CO2 laser.

Table 1. Orthopaedic Procedures Done with CO2 Laser

Procedure	Count
Squestrectomy and joint clearance	6
Open reduction and bone grafting femur	2
Arthrodesis of hip	1
Excision of tumours	20
Excision of bed sores and rotation flaps	6
Removal of bone cement from femur	2
Minor surgical procedures of the foot	17
Thoracotomy	2
TOTAL	56

CO2 laser was used in five groups of patients. They were for musculoskeletal sepsis, tumours of the limb, minor surgical procedures of the foot, thoracotomy and removal of bone cement from femur. Table 2 gives a list of procedures done with CO2 laser for musculoskeletal sepsis.

Table 2. CO2 Laser for Bone and Joint Infections

Chronic osteomyelitis and septic arthritis	6
Tuberculosis of the hip - arthrodesis	1
Carbuncle of the back	1
Rotation flaps for bed sores in paraplegics	5
Removal of bone cement from femur	2
TOTAL	15

CO2 laser was used for surgery of chronic osteomyelitis of femur. It was used from skin right down to the bone. Tensing the skin and muscles helps to cut and dissect them with the laser beam. The infected bed of bone and soft tissue was vapourised with CO2 laser (Fig 1) after saucerisation of the cavity in the bone with a gouge and curette.

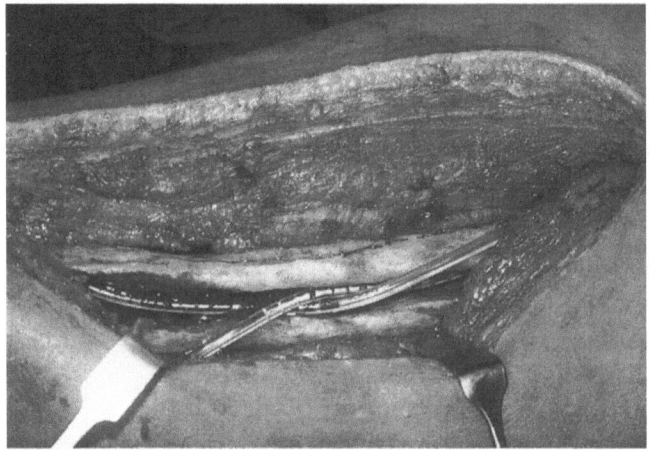

Fig 1 shows femur after saucerisation. The cut in the skin, fascia lata and muscle by the CO2 laser beam are sharp and clean.

CO2 laser was also used for excision of twenty benign and malignant tumours of the limb. One of them was a recurrent fibrosarcoma of the upper third of the thigh and a disarticulation of the hip was done with CO2 laser without any blood transfusion. There were three patients with extensive haemangioma of the lower limb and they had the tumour excised by CO2 laser under torniquet. CO2 laser does not coagulate blood vessels more than 0.5mm in diameter. An Esmarch bandage and a torniquet were therefore used to collapse the walls of the haemangioma. The collapsed walls of the haemangioma were then cut and coagulated with the CO2 laser beam. At the end of the surgery the tourniquet was released to check whether the blood vessels remain sealed.

Table 3 gives a list of the tumours that were excised with CO2 laser.

Table 3. Tumours excised with CO2 Laser

Fibrosarcoma of thigh	1
Extensive haemangiomas of the limb	3
Benign tumours of the limb	16
TOTAL	20

Minor surgery of the foot with CO2 laser was done in 20 patients and Table 4 give an account of the procedures that were done.

Table 4. Minor Surgery of the foot with CO2 Laser

Vapourisation of warts and ingrowing toenail	10
Desloughing for diabetic gangrene	4
Amputation of toes	3
TOTAL	17

A record of the amount of blood loss, blood transfusions and accidents with CO2 laser was kept for all the patients in this series. None of the patients in this series needed blood transfusion.

Discussion

The use of CO2 laser in orthopaedic surgery is relatively new and the present series is too small to make any analysis. A few facts seem to emerge from the experience.

In surgery of chronic musculoskeletal sepsis the problems are major blood loss and persistence of sepsis. The blood vessels in these chronic inflammatory conditions are surrounded by thick fibrous tissue and do not contract and they therefore keep on oozing blood. CO2 laser is effective in sealing these small blood vessels and helps to cut down the blood loss. The fifteen patients with chronic musculoskeletal sepsis who had CO2 laser surgery did not require any blood transfusion. The maximum amount of blood loss was 200ml.

Eradicating the sepsis is the other problem. The CO2 laser in the defocussed mode can be used to vaporise the infected bed in the bone and soft tissue. Removal of bone cement from femur was tried in two patients with CO2 laser. Special gouges were first used to break down the cement and the CO2 laser was then used to varporise the remnant cement. This method cuts down the operating time for vapourising the cement is a slow process.

Surgery of haemangiomas, especially the extensive ones is difficult. CO2 laser can only coagulate vessels up to 0.5mm in diameter. Therefore a new method was tried. The blood vessels were first emptied and their walls collapsed with an Esmarch bandage and a torniquet. When the walls of the haemangioma are collapsed their lumen becomes narrowed or obliterated and they can then be cut or sealed by the CO2 laser effectively. When the torniquet is released at the end of the procedure the blood vessels remain sealed.

The effectiveness of this method was well demonstrated in a patient who had extensive haemangiomatosis of his entire lower limb extending into the trunk and perineum. The patient also had a fibrous ankylosis of the knee and a deformed foot. A palliative supracondylar amputation through the haemangiomatous tissue was therefore done to fit him with a prosthesis. No blood transfusion was necessary for the patient.

Thoracotomy with CO2 laser without using any blood transfusion has been a valuable experience. Resection of the lobe of the lung was also done with CO2 laser and the lung tissue was effectively sealed by CO2 laser at 8 - 10 watts.

One accident with the use of CO2 laser has to be mentioned though it took place place during haemorrhoidectomy. It is customary for us to use diathermy to coagulate large vessels during CO2 laser surgery. The patient in this instance had paper towels beneath the surgical drapes. The laser machine was on when the surgeon was coagulating and he accidentally pressed the laser foot pedal though a finger-tip operated diathermy was used. The paper drapes caught fire and the patient had a burn. Laser safety and vigilance about fire hazard are important. To avoid this type of accident the laser machine must be on stand-by when the laser beam is not used.

Conclusions

1. CO2 laser can avoid or minimise the need for blood transfusions in orthopaedic surgery.

2. CO2 laser surgery may be useful in the treatment of chronic osteomyelitis and other bone and joint infections.

3. Extensive haemangiomas of a limb can be removed and coagulated by CO2 laser by collapsing the vessel walls first with an Esmarch bandage and a torniquet.

4. CO2 laser surgery is useful in thoracotomy for anterior spinal surgery.

Laser as an Operative Tool in Endoscopic Operations in Orthopaedic Surgery

Siebert W.E., D. Kohn, Breitner, S., H.J. Refior
Ludwig-Maximilians-Universität München, Orthopädische Klinik u. Poliklinik
Marchioninistraße 15, 8000 München 70

Introduction

Operations by means of endoscopy are nowadays being widely used as they have advantages, not least the minimal trauma they exert. The use of laser-surgery in urological, gynaecological and bronchial procedures has already become a routine procedure. In orthopaedic operations, such as for example meniscectomy or synovectomy, arthroscopic techniques have found an ever increasing use. Also in a spinal surgery, as well as in the operative treatment of a disc prolapse, microsurgical techniques as well as chemonucleolyses are progressively used. The aim of aur experimental investigations was to determine the effect of laser-operations on joints and intervertebral discs. This was done on tissue of corpses by means of exact infra-red thermographic measurements and histological examination of the tissues treated. Initially we investigated the possible means of employment as well as the suitybility of a CO_2-laser and a Neodym-Yag-laser (wavelength 1064 nm) for the treatment of disc-tissue, menisci, and synovial tissue. Following this we developed the application techniques and suitable instruments for the planned operations. Special attention was paid to temperature changes that occured. These were varied and optimized with regard to distance as well as timing, depending on the parameters of the instruments used. In our study we focused on the endoscopic treatment of meniscal and synovial tissue of the knee joint, as well as the so-called "nucleus pulposus vaporization". For the latter procedure we employed a technique similar to the well-known technique used for chemonucleolysis. We introduced a needle (1mm diameter) into the nucleus pulposus. By using an image intensifier, a 0,4mm thick light conductor was placed, through the needle, inside the nucleus pulposus. If one then adheres to the correct prerequisites, as they were developed by us, the nucleus pulposus can be vaporized effectively controlled, and without danger.

Results

Only the most significant results of our work will be mentioned here. At this given time and point of development, the CO_2-laser appears to be unsuitable for arthroscopic operations in the knee joint. It is dependent on a gaseous surrounding. Although it yields a good and rapid cutting-effect, bleeding and excessive smoke are troublesome. Problems result if suction is applied, especially as far as the maintenance of a constant gaseous pressure is concerned, which is needed for the arthroscopic procedure. In addition to the high expenditure, which indeed we did employ experimentally, the disadvantages of increased risk, poor sight, and missing suction remain. Therefore, we have now decided to use the technique by which the Neodym-Yag-laser is introduced into the knee joint by means of special instruments. Rapid resection of tissue is possible with the "pure" fibre even in water. Especiallsy degenerative threading of the meniscus can be melted away, leaving a resolving rim which is capable of bearing weight. In arthroscopic synovectomy the Neodym-Yag-laser acts complementary in controlling bleeding-points. More research is required into the effect which the Neodym-Yag-laser has on the rheumatoid synovial membrane, the histological changes that occur and whether the therapeutic effect is sufficient for the treatment of recurrent effusions. Fig. 1 shows the animal experiment in which we tested the arthroscopic procedures.

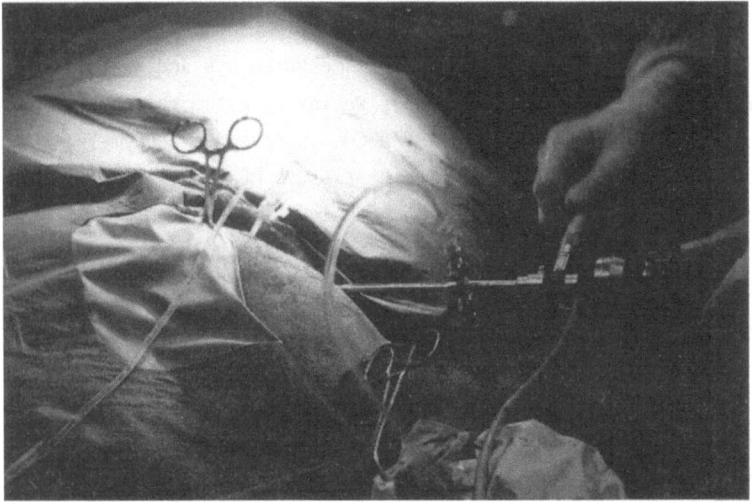

Fig. 1. Animal experiment with laser-arthroscopy (sheep)

Possibly this exemplifies an enrichment for the various arthroscopic procedures. Because of the aforementioned reasons, we do not regard the methods described by other authors as useful. (Whipple, Philandrianos).

The second focus of our study was directed towards the so-called "nucleus pulposus vaporization".

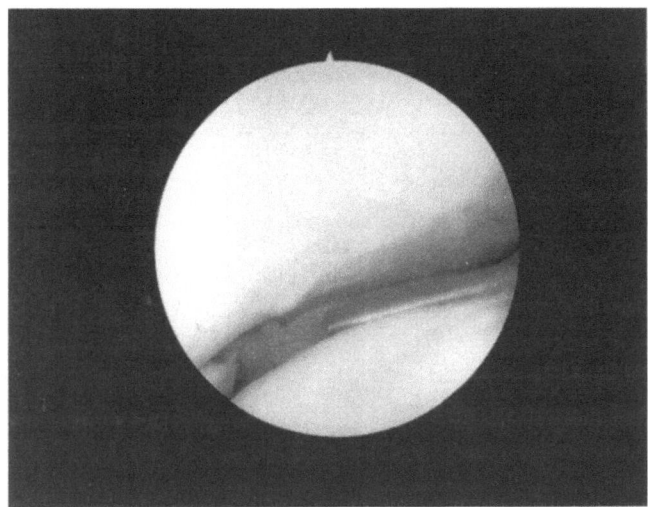

Fib. 2. Specific laser instruments which have been introduced into human knee joint during an operation on a meniscus

As mentioned above, we first develped suitable equipment for introducing the operating instruments. This was done by means of a technique related to that employed in chemonucleolysis, in which the instrument could be introduced into the disc without danger and with the use of the image intensifier. The use of thermography made it possible for us, employing various parameters, to exactly study the distribution of the temperature, the absolute height, as well as the changes in terms of time. As such as were able to develop safe and exactly reproducable prerequisites. For this purpose thermographic and histological examinations were performed on 160 dics from cattle. If one adheres to the prerequisites we worked out, the effect shown in Fig. 3 an Fig. 4 can be regularly obtained.

Discussion

The use of the laser in orthopaedic surgery will find wider employment not only in endocopic procedures. Through new techniques, such as the Erbium laser, and by using more specialized methods which do not only utilize the effect of heat (Ell, Wolleneck, Verhandlungsbericht), as well as through new and different instruments, the treatment of bone cement and certainly also of bony and cartilaginous tissue may become possible. In any event, there are definite advantages, in as far as nucleus pulposus vaporization and arthroscopic resecting-

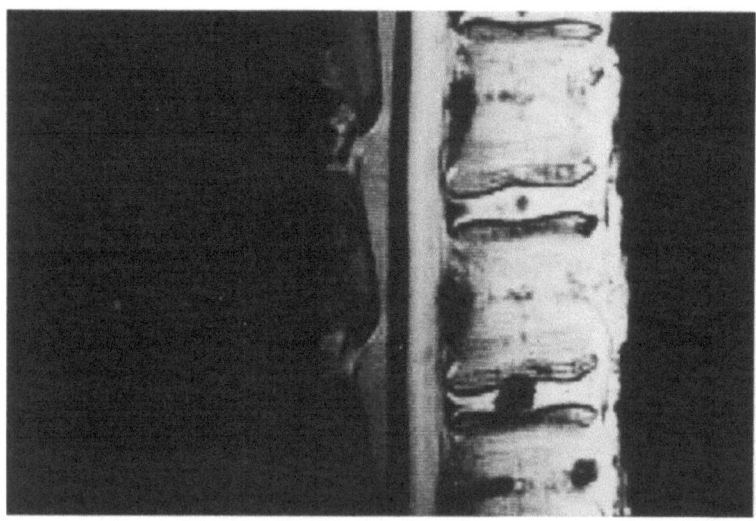

Fig. 3. MRI picture of a nucleus pulposus vaporization and a chemonucleolysis of an intervertebral disc from caudal to cranial. Effect of laser below, chemonucleolysis above

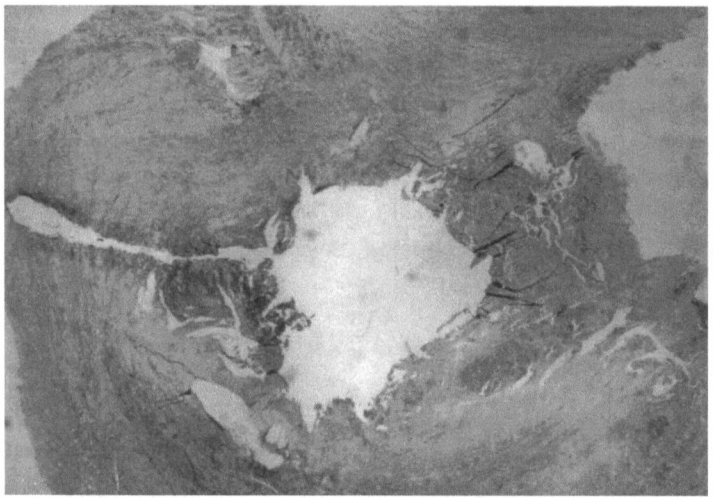

Fig. 4. Histological picture following a nucleus pulposus vaporization. Note: Minimal damage of the peripheral zone and the annulus fibrosus

techniques are concerned, which justify the clinical use of the laser. Especially in arthroscopic procedures, the effect of tissue welding might be used for the refixation of a torn meniscus or even the reconstruction of capsular and ligamentous structures. The disadvantages of chemonucleulysis, such as the danger of an anaphylactic reaction, the sometimes long interval before it becomes effective, and the resulting problems when a discectomy becomes necessary at a later stage, certainly make the nucleus pulposus vaporization a more favourable procedure. Work is still needed into whether there are advantages with the use of different wavelengths or different lasers, and also into the rate of reoccurance of symptoms. In the long run the orthopaedic use of the laser will also include the treatment of infections, as well as bony and soft tissue tumours, combined with the use of derivatives of haematoporphirin and other optically active substances.

Literature

1. Baumgartner, F.; Feyh, J.; Götz, A.; Jocham, D.; Schneeberger, H.; Stepp, M.; Unsöld, E.:
   Experimental Study on Laser-induced Fluorescence of Hematoporphyrin Derivate (HpD) in Tumor Cells and Animal Tissue.
   Laser 2: 4-9 (1986).

2. Bellina, M.D.; Joseph, H.; et al.:
   Analysis of electronically pulsed versus quasi-continous wave carbon dioxide laser in an animal model.
   American Journal of obstetrics and gynecology, St. Louis, 1984.

3. Choy, D.S.J.; Case, R.B.; Ascher, P.:
   Percutaneous Laser Ablation of Lumbar Discs. A Preliminary Report Of In Vitro And In Vivo Experience In Animal And Four Human Patients.
   33rd Annual Meeting, Orthopaedic Research Society, January 19-22, 1987, San Francisco, California.

4 .Ell Ch Wondrazek, L.; Frank, F.; Hochberger, J.; Lux, G.; Demling, L.:
   Laser-induced Chockwave Lithrotripsy of Gallstones.
   Endoscopy 18 (1986) 95-96.
   Thieme Suttgart-New York.

5. Frank, O.J.; Häussinger, K.; Keiditsch, E.; Landthaler, M.; Mexer, H.J.; Unsöld, E.; Wondrazek, F.:
Untersuchungen zur Wirkung der 1,32 ym Nd:YAG-Laserstrahlung auf Gewebe. s. Verhandlungsbericht der Deutschen Gesellschaft für Laser Medizin 1986.

6. Gamel, A.; Farine, J.; Horoszowski, H.:
Bone cement melting by a laser beam, gas analysis.
Laser and Electrooptic, 1, 12-13 (1981).

7. Müller, G.; Bader, H.; Greve, P.:
9,6 ym-CO_2-Laser für medizinische Anwendungen.
Laser 1 (1985) Nr. 2 - ORIGINALIA.

8. Philandrianos, G.:
Le laser à gaz carbonique en chirurgie arthroscopique du genou.
La Presse Mèdical, 30 novembre 1985, 14, n° 41.

9. Verhandlungsbericht der Deutschen Gesellschaft für Laser-Medizin e. V.1986 EBM GmbH,München;MZV AG,Zürich:1987

10. Whipple T.L.; Caspari, R.B.; Mayers, J.F.:
Arthroscopic Laser Meniscectomiy. In a Gas Medium.
Ther Journal of Arthroscopic and related Surgery. 1 (1) 2-7 (1985).

11. Whipple T.L.,Caspari R.B.,Meyers J.F.,
Synovial response to laser induced carbon ash residue
Laser Surg.Med.1984;3:291-5.

12. Wollenek, G.; Laufer, G.; Stangl, G.; Buchelt, M.; Wolner, E.;
Thermische Effekte der UV-excimer Laserstrahlung im biologischen Gewebe.
Chirurgische Universitätsklinik und Technische Universität Wien. s. Verhandlungsbericht der Deutschen Gesellschaft für Laser Medizin 1986.

Gastroenterology

Endoscopic Laser Treatment in the Gastrointestinal Tract – State of the Art

P. Kiefhaber, K. Kiefhaber, G. Nath
Stadtkrankenhaus Traunstein - Akademisches Lehrkrankenhaus der Ludwig-Maximilians Universität München -, D-8220 Traunstein, W-Germany

The most suitable laser wavelength for endoscopic use in the GI tract is a Neodymium-YAG laser with the wavelength of 1.06 μm and a power output of 100 W. The other wavelengths of 1.32 μm up to 3.4 μm are still experimental as well as eximer lasers and dye lasers used in tumours dotted with HPD. Pulsed Nd:YAG lasers and pulsed dye lasers have been tried endoscopically for destruction of biliary stones.

Feasibility of different laser transmission systems for different wavelengths delivered pulsed or continous are essential for efficiency of endoscopic laser treatment. Adaption of the laser transmission systems onto the endoscopes are further not totally solved problems.

Clinical indications for endoscopic laser treatment as accepted in many laser centers of the world are at present:

1. Acute gastrointestinal haemorrhage.
   Including all possible bleeding sources of the GI tract as varices, Mallory-Weiss tears, ulcers, carcinomas and erosions Nd:YAG laser coagulation showed a success rate of 94% in primary haemostasis. Compared to surgical results also mortality rate has been reduced markedly in patients suffering in acute haemorrhage. This has been proved in clinical studies of unselected patients and in controlled studies of selected, randomized patients.
2. Sealing of potential bleeding lesions as Osler haemangiomas and angiodysplasias resulting in a decreased necessity of blood transfusions.
3. Recanalization of obstructed tumours of the upper and lower GI tract as a palliative or preoperative measure. Obstructions causing dysphagia or aphagia can be recanalized to improve nutrition and quality of live. In combination with endoscopic Iridium afterloading treatment the medium survival time with carcinoma in the upper GI tract was 7.5 months (Dr. Bader, Munich).
4. Recanalization of peptic or scar stenosis.
5. Curative treatment of sessil, neoplastic but benign polyps in the upper and lower GI tract.

Endoscopic laser treatment needs in all fields a precise clinical indication and a clinical decision in each case where surgeons should be included in order to have the optimum of the possible treatment.

Endoscopic Nd:YAG Laserthermia: Experimental Study on Carcinoma-Bearing BDF₁ Mice

N. Kanemaki[1], H. Tsunekawa[2], C. Brünger[1], M. Nishida[1], H. Nishikawa[1], H. Kato[1], K. Hattori[1], N. Daikuzono[3]

1) Dept. of Internal Medicine, 2nd Hospital, Fujita-Gakuen Health University, Nagoya
2) Department of Gastroenterology, Meitetsu Hospital, Nagoya
3) SLT-Japan Co., Tokyo

Summary

Clinically laserthermia has proved to be safer and more reliable than conventional contact-laser irradiation in eradicating tumour tissue. Since the differences in the mechanism of tumour destruction are still not fully understood, we compared these methods in an experimental study using BDF1 mice and obtained the following results:

1) There are differences in the process of carcinoma cell destruction between laserthermia (low power, long time) and contact irradiation (high power, short time).
2) Laser-light itself has the ability to cause carcinoma cell destruction.
3) Changes due to laserthermia become detectable histologically 3 h after irradiation.

Introduction

In recent years, laser endoscopy has progressed rapidly, and especially contact laser irradiation with artificial sapphire probes has produced excellent results except in depressed early gastric carcinoma. Consequently, we have developed laserthermia as a safe and reliable method in which prolonged low power laser energy is applied through an interstitial probe for local hyperthermia. Several experimental studies using BDF1 mice inoculated with Lewis's lung carcinoma showed that a laser power of 2.0 W at the fibre tip produced the most desirable temperature curve, i.e. about 43-60°C at the irradiation site. Since the mechanism of tumour destruction by laserthermia is still not fully understood, we here report on further investigations.

Materials and Methods

We used the Nd:YAG laser model CL-50 with an attenuator and a computer control system (SLT-Japan) to obtain stable low laser power density. Thirty 3 week-old male BDF1 mice were subcutaneously inoculated with Lewis's lung carcinoma (1×10^6 cells/mm³), and divided into 3 groups (contact irradiation (A), laserthermia at 43-44°C (B), and at 39-40°C (C). After about two weeks, when the tumour had grown to a diameter of c. 1.2 cm, we performed either contact irradiation or laserthermia on the tumour. The tip of the quartz fibre was equipped with a conic probe (interstitial probe) made of artifical sapphire with a roughened surface, which was inserted into the centre of the tumour. The thermosensor for controlling the temperature was inserted 6 mm away from the laser probe (Fig. 1). Interstitial laser irradiation was carried out at 43-44 °C for 10 min with a laser output of 2.0 W. To further elucidate the mechanism of laserthermia, we performed ultrasonography before and after laserthermia (0 h, 3 h, 24 h, 1 wk, and controls without treatment). With a view to later clinical application we used endoscopic ultrasonography (EUS) with a 10 MHz head, which has the advantage of a very high resolution (Olympus-Aloka EU-M2). After EUS examination two mice from each group (A,B,C) were killed to obtain histo-pathological sections.

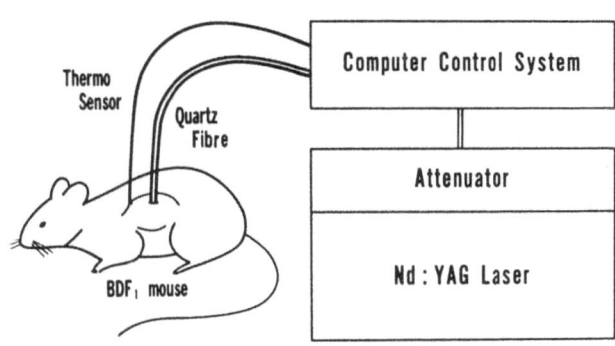

Fig. 1. Computer-controlled laserthermia system

We compared these ultrasonic and pathological findings with those obtained after contact irradiation with the tip type probe (30 W, 3.0 sec). Also, to clarify the effect of laser light alone, we examined histo-pathologically after laserthermia at 39-40°C for 10 min.

Results

1) Ultrasonographic findings

a) The course of laserthermia

The sonographic tumour image before irradiation showed a homogenous echogenic pattern without high or low echo spots (Fig. 2). Immediately and 3 h after irradiation, the ultrasonic image showed no change. But after 24 h, we observed irregular high echoic spots in the centre of the tumour, and after one week, the image changed to a mixed pattern with a predominantly hyperechoic structure and only a few slightly hypoechoic areas.

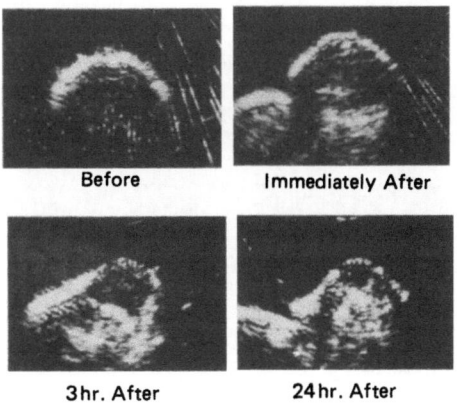

Fig. 2. Ultrasonic course of laserthermia

b) Comparison of laserthermia with contact irradiation

There were distinct differences immediately after irradiation (Fig. 3). Whereas the EUS image after laserthermia did not show any distinct changes compared to the pre-irradiation image, contact irradiation produced a uniformly high echo even at this early stage. One week after irradiation, laserthermia produced an evenly high echoic image with some low echoic spots, but contact irradiation showed a mottled pattern with high and low echoic spots. After two weeks, both images showed a similar mixed pattern due to renewed peripheral tumour growth.

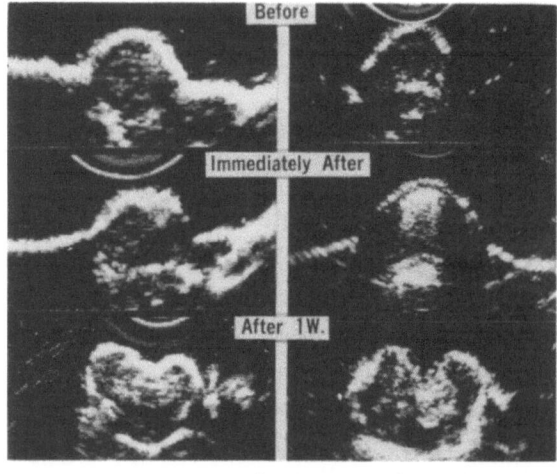

Fig. 3. Ultrasonic comparison of laserthermia (left) and contact irradiation (right)

2) Pathological findings
a) Laserthermia at 43-44°C

The tumour was characterized by a mass of dividing undifferentiated cells and scanty stroma (Fig. 4). Cell boundaries were relatively distinct and there was a high nucleus/cytoplasma ratio. Immediately after laserthermia there was marked dilatation and congestion of the blood vessels and a few areas of haemorrhage. Only minor degeneration of the tumour cells was apparent at this stage. After 3h, there were massive areas of marked haemorrhage and ruptured blood vessels. Tumour cells were undergoing degeneration, pyknosis and karyorrhexis. After 24 h, marked haemorrhagic necrosis that involved most of the central area of the tumour mass was visible. Most cells had been destroyed and cell boundaries become indistinct. Finally, after one week the irradiated area presented as a lake of necrotic debris.

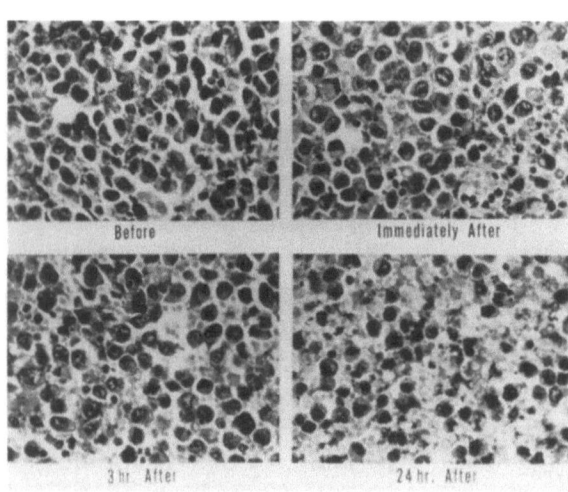

Fig. 4. Histo-pathological course of laserthermia at 43-44°C

b) Laserthermia at 39-40°C

   The process of pathological changes was approximately the same as after laserthermia at 43-44°C.

c) Contact-laser irradiation

   The irradiated areas immediately revealed distinct coagulation and degeneration, and after one week showed marked necrosis.

Discussion

Laserthermia is a new method of laser irradiation developed for indirect destruction of tumour tissue by applying local hyperthermia (43-44 °C) through low power laser irradiation. In our present experimental study, we observed the process of tumour destruction by laserthermia, and the differences between this and contact irradiation. Immediately after irradiation laserthermia produced only moderate congestion and minor degeneration without change in the EUS image. After 3 h, tumour cells were undergoing degeneration, pyknosis and karyorrhexis in spite of an unchanged EUS image. After 24 h, the EUS image changed with irregular high echoic spots, and pathological findings revealed marked congestion, degeneration and haemorrhagic necrosis. Seven days later, the pathological changes of necrosis and degeneration were correlated with a mottled pattern in the ultrasonic image. On the other hand, immediately after contact irradiation the tumour revealed a sonographically uniform high echo and marked degeneration and coagulation. After seven days, sonographic and histo-pathological findings showed a similar pattern to that of laserthermia. Significantly also, the pathological appearance of the tumour after laserthermia at 39-40°C was remarkably similar to that at 43-44°C.

These results suggest that marked histological changes due to laserthermia occur 3 h after irradiation, despite an unchanged EUS image, and that there is a difference between laserthermia (low power, long time) and contact irradiation (high power, short time) in the process of carcinoma cell destruction. Secondly, our results show a laserthermia effect even at 39-40°C, suggesting that laser light itself has the ability to cause carcinoma cell destruction. Consequently we propose that laserthermia is the synergistic effect of laser light and hyperthermia. We intend to continue our present investigations into the mechanism of tumour destruction by laserthermia.

References

1) Daikuzono N, Joffe S: Medical Instrumentation, 1985; vol.19/4, pp 173-178.
2) Tsunekawa H et al.: Laser Optoelektronik in der Medizin, Springer-Verlag, Berlin, 1985, pp 360-366.
3) Tsunekawa H et al.: Nd:YAG Laser in Medicine and Surgery, PPS, Tokyo, 1986, pp 105-109.
4) Kanemaki N et al.: Journal of the Japanese Society for Laser Medicine, vol.7/4, 1987, pp 47-48 (in Japanese).

Endoscopic Nd:YAG Laserthermia in Depressed Early Gastric Carcinoma

C.Brünger[1], H.Tsunekawa[2], N.Kanemaki[1], M.Nishida[2], H.Nishikawa[1], H.Kato[1], K.Hattori[1]
N. Daikuzono[3]

1) Dept. of Internal Medicine, 2nd Hospital, Fujita-Gakuen Health University, Nagoya
2) ·Dept. of Gastroenterology, Meitetsu Hospital, Nagoya
3) SLT-Japan Co., Tokyo

Summary

Laserthermia is a new form of treatment developed for indirect destruction of tumour tissue by applying local hyperthermia (43-44°C) through prolonged low-power laser irradiation. Since 1984 we have investigated this method in experimental and clinical studies. Here we report our clinical experience with 20 cases of depressed early gastric carcinoma (15 pre-operative cases and 5 inoperable cases, where treatment aimed at local cure).

In 12 of the 15 pre-operative cases, the bottom of the laserthermia-induced ulcer showed no residual cancer, indicating the efficacy of this treatment. Histo-pathological examination revealed that although laserthermia-induced degeneration was detectable down to the proper muscle layer, surface changes were confined to shallow ulceration. Of the 5 "curative" cases, one patient died after 13 months' follow-up. Autopsy revealed local cure achieved by laserthermia.

We have recently employed endoscopic ultrasonography to evaluate the depth of cancer infiltration and video endoscopy, to determine the extent of the lesion before treatment and to detect any cancer residue during follow-up. We believe, the combination of these techniques makes laserthermia the safest and most effective form of treatment for depressed early gastric carcinoma in inoperable cases.

Introduction

Endoscopic contact-laser treatment has proved very successful in the management of gastric borderline lesions (100%), GI polyps (100%), tumour stenosis (92%), GI bleeding (87%), and also in elevated early gastric carcinoma (100%). Results were, however, less encouraging for depressed early carcinoma (67%), probably due to the low total laser energy applied in order to prevent perforation. We therefore developed laser hyperthermia (hereafter called laserthermia), a system for transmitting low power Nd:YAG laser energy (2.0 W) through an interstitial probe (at 43-44°C). Since 1984 we have investigated this method in experimental (see previous paper: Kanemaki et al.) and clinical studies. Here we report our clinical experience with 20 cases of depressed early gastric carcinoma.

Subjects and Methods

1. Patients

Twenty patients with depressed early gastric carcinoma were selected for this study; 15 received pre-operative pilot-treatment, i.e. patients underwent gastrectomy approximately one week after laserthermia treatment. The remaining 5 patients received 2-8 laserthermia sessions (1200 - 3200 J) aimed at local cure, because they were judged inoperable owing to aortic aneurysm, congestive heart failure, etc.(Table 1). In fact, one patient died before treatment could be completed and another after 13 months' follow-up. The latter case will be discussed below.

Case	Age	Sex	Type	Location	No. of sessions	Total time	Dose (J.)	Biopsy	Follow-up
1	86	♂	IIc (por)	Angulus ~Body	2	10 min.	1188	(+)	†
2	83	♀	IIc (por)	Angulus Body	5	20	2376	(−)	15 ms.
3	72	♂	IIa (tub₂)	Body	8	42	3184	(−)	10 ms.
4	84	♀	IIc (por)	Antrum	4	30	2672	(−)	13 ms.†
5	77	♂	IIa + IIc (tub₂)	Antrum	6	23	2790	(−)	17 ms.

Table 1. Laserthermia in early gastric carcinoma: inoperable cases

2. Laserthermia system

Our computer-controlled laserthermia system in its present form is composed of an Nd:YAG laser (model CL-50, SLT-Japan) with an inbuilt laser attenuator and an attached computer control unit, which guarantee stable low power laser output. Laser energy is transmitted via a flexible quartz fibre, which is inserted into one channel of a double channel endoscope (Olympus GIF-T2) and tipped with an interstitial probe. A thermosensor, introduced through the other channel, is placed into the gastric lesion 8 mm apart from the interstitial probe, which is made of artificial sapphire and has a conic shape to supply uniformely dispersed laser light at the irradiation site. The thermosensor is connected to the computer, which keeps the temperature between pre-set limits (43 - 44°C) during irradiation over 5-10 min.

Results

Having established in preliminary experiments that a laser output of 2.0 W at the fibre tip yields the most satisfying results without fear of perforation, we applied endoscopic laserthermia to 15 pre-operative cases in 1-2 sessions of 5-10 min each.

Histo-pathological investigation of the resected stomach showed complete eradication of the carcinoma in 2 cases, and in 10 of the remaining 13 cases cancer residues were found only at the margin, but not at the bottom of the laser ulcer (Fig. 1). Although the effect of laserthermia reached down to the proper muscle layer, necrosis was observed only in the mucosal and submucosal layers, producing but shallow ulceration (Ul I-II).

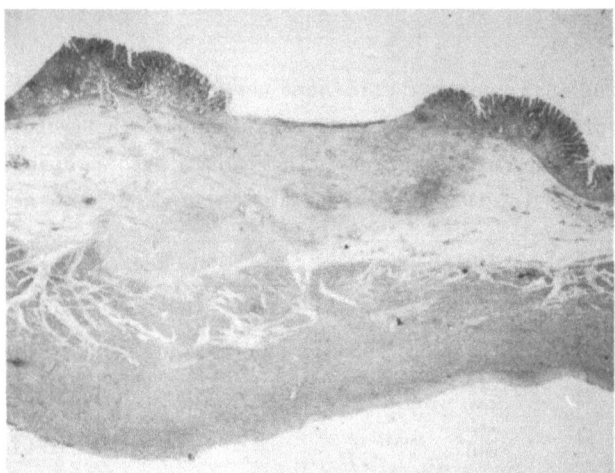

Fig. 1. Histo-pathology of pre-operative case: laserthermia effect down to the proper muscle layer, but only shallow ulceration

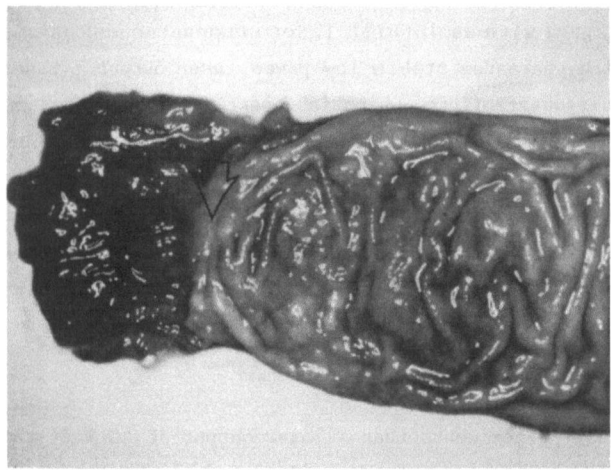

Fig. 2. Macroscopic aspect of laser ulcer scar (arrow) 13 months after cure by laserthermia

Of the five inoperable cases, one died due to a cerebral haemorrhage before his treatment could be completed and had at this point received only two treatments at 2.0 W for a total of 10 min. In the other four cases follow-up biopsies have been negative for 13-18 months. In case No.4 treatment was curative. A type IIc gastric carcinoma in the prepylorus disappeared completely after application of 2670 J in four sessions. We have previously reported the endoscopic course of this patient. She died of congestive heart failure due to combined valvular disease after a follow-up of 13 months. Autoptic examination demonstrated a complete cure both macro- and microscopically. Fig. 2 shows the gross specimen of the pyloric region, the antrum being to the right and the duodenum to the left. The arrow indicates the location of the laser ulcer scar. The histo-pathological section of the same area (Fig. 3) indicates only fibrosis under a normal regenerated mucosa (arrow). There is, however, no cancer residue. The proper muscle layer is notably unaffected.

Discussion

Surgical treatment of early gastric cancer has a success rate of almost 100%. As an alternative for inoperable cases contact-laser irradiation has been developed and is effective for elevated early carcinoma. Results with this form of therapy have, however, been less satisfactory in depressed types (IIc and III), probably due to the low laser power applied to prevent perforation.

To obviate these problems we have evolved the technique of laserthermia. It has to be said that the number of cases which we have treated is, as yet, rather small and the period of follow-up rather short. Nevertheless the results have been very encouraging. Namely, in the pre-operative cases laserthermia was effective down to the proper muscle layer, while confining necrosis to the mucosal and submucosal layers.

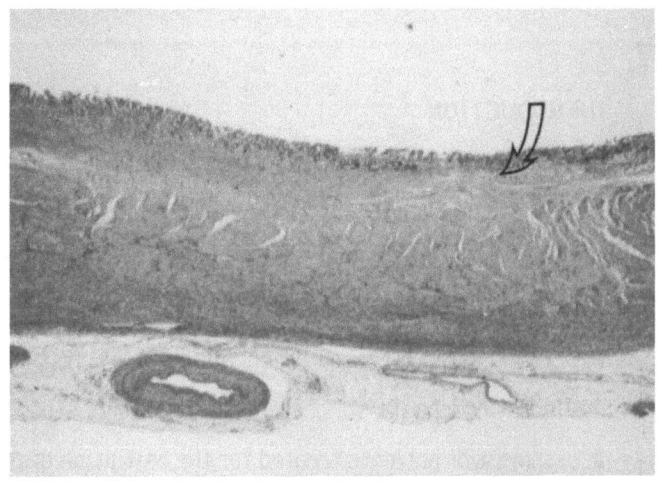

Fig. 3. Microscopic section of the laserthermia site shows fibrosis under normal mucosa, but no cancer

We have recently selected suitable cases for treatment using endoscopic ultrasonography to estimate the depth of cancer infiltration. We have used the same technique, along with endoscopy and biopsy, to detect any cancer residue during follow-up. To calculate the extent of the lesion we have utilized video-endoscopy. Computerized image-analysis of video films, and especially edge enhancement techniques, have enabled us to outline the lesion more clearly prior to irradiation. We hope to further employ and develop these methods for more accurate pre-irradiation assessment and for early detection of residual cancer tissue. We believe that the combination of these tools renders laserthermia both the safest and most effective method for treating depressed early gastric carcinoma in inoperable cases.

References
1) Tsunekawa H et al. in Waidelich and Kiefhaber (ed.): Optoelektronik in der Medizin, Berlin: Springer-Verlag; 1985, pp 360-366.
2) Tsunekawa H et al. in Oguro, Atsumi and Joffe (ed.): Nd:YAG Laser in Medicine and Surgery, Tokyo: PPS; 1986, pp 105-109.

Psychological and Quality of Life Analysis of the Palliative Treatment of Oesophageal Cancer

H. BARR AND N. KRASNER

Gastrointestinal unit, Walton Hospital, Rice Lane, Liverpool, England

INTRODUCTION

Palliative cancer treatment can not be assessed by using objective or 'hard' criteria such as mortality, recurrence of disease, or clinical data on the spread of disease. Emphasis has to be placed on 'softer' subjective data. There is little data of this nature on patients with oesophageal tumours treated by laser recannalisation or intubation for the relief of malignant dysphagia. We present a prospective study on the quality of life assessment of patients treated for the palliation of malignant dysphagia

PATIENTS AND METHODS

20 patients (7 women, 13 men) were assessed. They were either treated using the laser alone; that is initial laser therapy followed by laser endoscopy every 4 weeks until death to ensure no recurrence of dysphagia; or initial laser endoscopy followed by endoscopic intubation. There were 10 patients in each group. All had quality of life assessment by the QL index (1) and a Linear Analoque Self Assessment (LASA) (2). The QL index was designed for use by physicians and has been shown to have convergent discriminant and content validity among cancer patients (1). It is particularly useful in trials of the effectiveness of palliative care. It examines 5 variables : activity, daily living, health, support, and outlook on life. Each is scored 0,1,or 2, giving a possible maximum of 10.

The LASA consists of 25 Visual Analoque scales; 9 examined the effects of disease and treatment, 5 the psychological consequences of disease and treatment, 5 other physical indices, 5 personal relationships and 1 measured the patients self assessment of quality of life. The QL index was completed by the attending doctor and the LASA by the patient themselves on each visit to hospital (at least at every month).

Two doctors assessed the patients independently within 2 days to measure the interrater agreement of the QL scale. For 20 patients the interrater correlation coefficient was 0.77 ($p<0.001$, Spearman rank correlation). The Spearman correlation coefficient for LASA scores collected 24 hours apart was 0.865 ($p<0.001$).

RESULTS

The QL index before treatment was 4.9±1.86 for the laser only patients and 5.1±1.25 for those treated by intubation. The average post laser treatment QL index was 6.25±2.25 and the best achieved was 6.7±2.2. The average post intubation QL score was 5.9±1.3 and the best achieved was 6.6±1.4. The difference is not satistically significant although there may be a trend for the patients treated by the laser only to gain higher average post treatment score. The mean improvement following laser therapy alone was 1.35 and following intubation was 0.8. This trend is thought to reflect the difference in the number of patients developing recurrent dysphagia and complications following intubation and laser therapy. One patient developed perforation during laser therapy and 2 had episodes of recurrent dysphagia. However following intubation 2 patients had perforation and 4 had episodes of recurrent dysphagia. During these episodes the scores fell and this is reflected in the average QL score. The LASA scores reflected the same trend, the correlation coefficient of the QL to LASA was 0.84 ($p<0.001$).

DISCUSSION

The ideal method of treating inoperable malignant dysphagia has yet to be identified. Undoubtedly both intubation and laser therapy have a role.

However it is important to identify the best method of treating the majority of the patients referred. It is encouraging to note that the quality of life of these patients improved with improvement of the dysphagia. The trend identified showing the greater improvement in scores with laser therapy reflects the reduction in the score caused by more complications and recurrent dysphagia in the intubation group. We now are using laser therapy as first line treatment for malignant dysphagia and are present conducting a larger randomised clinical trial to see if the trend identified continues.

REFERENCES

1. W.O.Spitzer, A.J.Dobson, J.Hall, E.Chesterman, J.Levi, R.Shepard, R.N.Battista, B.R.Catchlove. (1981) Measuring the quality of life of cancer patients. A concise QL-Index for use by physicians. J. Chron. Dis., 34, 585-597.

2 T.J. Priestman, M.Baum (1976) Evaluation of qualty of life in patients receiving treatment for breast cancer. Lancet 899-900.

Nd: YAG Laser Treatment of Malignant Gastrointestinal Tumors

K. DITTRICH, Ch. ARMBRUSTER, K. DINSTL, H. GÜNTER
1st Department of Surgery and Ludwig-Boltzmann-
Institut for Laser Surgery, KA Rudolfstiftung
Juchgasse 25, A-1030 Vienna

Introduction

During the last years the treatment of malignant gastrointestinal tumors by Nd-YAG laser became of more importance (3,5). In the palliative treatment of tumors, the Nd-YAG laser has shown advantages that cannot be achieved with other forms of treatment (1,2,3,5). In particular cases according to a special indication and postoperative observation you can use the Nd-YAG laser in curative treatment (4).

Technique, patients and methods

General properties of our Nd-YAG laser: non contact Medilas 2 YAG, MBB-AT, Munich, W.Germany. Wave length: 1.064 nm, power 10-100 W, visible light: helium-neon laser 630 nm.

From 11.1985 until 5.1987 20 patients with malignant gastrointestinal tumors were treated with the non contact Nd-YAG-laser. Compared to all our patients (n=216) we used the Nd-YAG laser in 9,3%. 42 operations were performed, this means an average of 2,1 sessions per patient.

Most of the tumors were localised in the rectum (n=13) or in the anus (n=5) only 1 in the oesophagus and 1 in the stomach. All patients except 1 were of advanced age, the average age was 69,1 years (Table 1).

The palliative treatment (n=10) and the preparation for definitive surgery (n=3) were dominant, 7 times curative treatment could be performed (Table 2).

Above all the diagnosis was verified endoscopically and histologically in all cases preoperatively.

The following examples may show you indications and problems of the Nd-YAG laser application:

An 83 years old woman was treated with the Nd-YAG-laser to relieve the tumor obstruction of the oesophagus after the implantation of a tube had failed days before. 5 sessions were performed and now there is no sign of obstruction.

Because of significant cardiopulmonary disease and advanced age 4 patients with carcinoma of the rectum were unfit for surgery. The Nd-YAG laser offered the ability to vaporize these tumors and to restore patency of the lumen.

Since November 1985 an 86 years old man was treated 9 times because of rectal tumor obstruction, the last biopsy even did not show any evidence of tumor. 3 patients

Table 1.   Malignant gastrointestinal tumors
            Neodym-YAG laser treatment

Localisation	Number	Average age
Oesophagus	1	83
Stomach	1	61
Rectum	13	68
Anus	5	70,8
	20	69,1

Table 2.   Malignant gastrointestinal tumors
            Neodym-YAG laser treatment

	Number	Localisation
Curative surgery	7	4 Rectum 3 Anus
Palliative surgery	10	1 Oesophagus 1 Stomach 7 Rectum 1 Anus
Preparation for definitive surgery	3	2 Rectum 1 Anus

had recurrences at the suture line after anterior resection of the rectum combined with metastatic disease of the liver and the lung. The local situation could be controlled by vaporizing the tumor.

A female patient suffering from an anal carcinoma did not accept conventional radical surgery, therefore she underwent Nd-YAG laser surgery.

Preoperatively we recanalized an obstructive rectal carcinoma with the laser, an anterior resection with immediate anastomosis could be performed afterwards. 2 patients first did not accept radical surgery, the tumor ablation was done by Nd-YAG laser treatment. In one case three months later, in the second case five months later, both patients revised their decision and abdomino-perineal rectum-amputation could be performed. None did have metastatic disease and also the histological examination did not show any evidence of tumor.

Curative treatment was performed 7 times. 6 patients were not candidates for resection because of cardiopulmonary disease, a 22 years old woman suffered from rectal carcinoid with a tumor diameter of 1cm and could be treated with the Nd-YAG laser.

Results

No complication occured intra- and postoperatively.

During the follow-up period 3 patients died of their disease, local recurrence occured in 4 cases and up to now no evidence of tumor has been seen in 13 cases (Table 3).

On the other hand we do not want to make a final statement on the survival rates as the follow-up period is too short.

Table 3.   Malignant gastrointestinal tumors
                  Neodym-YAG laser treatment
          Follow-up: 1 - 18 months p.op. (∅ 8 months)

	Number	Localisation
No evidence of tumor:	13	8 Rectum
		5 Anus
Local recurrence (a.p.t.):	4	3 Rectum
		1 Oesophagus
Mortality (a.p.t.):	3	2 Rectum
		1 Stomach

Conclusion

The use of the Nd-YAG laser in gastrointestinal tract malignancies is limited. Curative treatment is reserved to special cases (4).

On the other hand palliative Nd-YAG laser treatment is of great importance (3). Patients with advanced disease or patients who are unfit for surgery because of significant coexistent medical disease or advanced age will have great benefit if Nd-YAG laser treatment is performed. The operation risk is low, the hospitalization is short and the quality of life compared to conventional surgical methods is better, especially if the consequences of colostomy can be avoided (1,3,5). Therefore we think being in line with other authors (2,3,5) that Nd-YAG laser treatment is a competitive alternative to palliative resection.

References

1) Bowers J: Laser therapy of colonic neoplasms, in Fleischer D., Jensen D, Bright-Asare P (eds): Therapeutic Laser Endoscopy in Gastrointestinal disease. Boston, Martinus Nijhoff, 1983, p. 139.

2) Fleischer D, Kessler F, Haye O: Endoscopic Nd-YAG laser therapy for carcinoma of the esophagus: A new palliative approach. Am J. Surg. 1982; 143:280-283.

3) Joffe S.N., Schröder T.: Lasers in General Surgery; in Mannick J.A. et all (ed): Advances in Surgery, Volume 20. Year Book Medical Publishers, Inc., Chicago-London, 1987; p. 125-154.

4) Oguro Y, Tajiri H: Present status of laser medicine and laser endoscopic treatment of GI-tract cancer in Japan, abstracted. Laser 85 Opto-Electronic, 1985, p 114.

5) Russin D.J. et al: Neodymium-YAG Laser: A new palliativ tool in the treatment of colorectal cancer. Arch. Surg. 1986; 121:1399-1403.

Clinic Experience in Endoscopic YAG Laser Therapy for Large Intestinal Polyps

(an analysis of 60 patients and 159 polyps)

Wang Rui-zhong, Wang Zhen-he, Wang Shu-shen
and Bai Yu-gang of the Shijiazhuang City
First Hospital
People's Republic of China

YAG laser is characterized by its strong perforative ability and the ability of cutting through human body tissues. Optical glass fiber led into human body by the endoscope can be used to resect the polyp in large intestine and treat them with gasification therapy. Since 1983, we have treated 60 patients suffering from large intestinal polyps with YAG laser made in China. 159 polyps were treated. 70 of them were cut and taken out intact. It was confirmed that the endoscopic laser is a reliable and effective therapy in treating large intestinal polyps.

1. CLINICAL DATA

So far, we have treated 60 patients suffering from large intestinal polyps. 159 polyps were resected. 44 of the patients were male, 16 were female. The oldest was 71 years old and the youngest was 4 years old. The largest polyp taken out was $1.5 \times 1.5 \times 2.5$cm. This paper is centered on talking about the practical techniques of how to cut the polyps.

2. THE THERAPY AND THE KEY TECHNIQUES

1) Case-selecting

All the cases of this group were diagnosed by colonofiberscope. Polyps with stems were to be cut and taken out. Polyps without stems but with bases were to be treated with gasification therapy.

2) Manipulation Techniques

As soon as the optical glass fiber got into the endoscope, helium-neom indicater should be lighted and aimed at the stem of a polyp in an angle of 70 - 80 degrees. It is the right time for the doctor to cut the polyp when the exportion end of the optical glass fiber is nearly to touch or touches it directly.

3) The Key Technique

The exportion end of the optical glass fiber can cut the tissues only when the power of the exportion end is above 40 watts.

While the cutting is going on, keep the exportion end directly touching or nearly touching the polyp stem. Either single or a return laser beam can be used.
The pedunculated polyps need to be cut at the juncture between the polyp and the stem. If the remaining stems are long, an additional gasification therapy is needed.
If the polyps are many, it is appropriate to have them cut in several times, once a month and 20 - 30 at one time.

3) THE RESULT OF THIS THERAPY

The deepest polyp in this group of the cases was located at ilium-caecum. Most of the polyps were 13 - 30cm. away from the anus.
58 of them were confirmed pathologically. 31 of them were adenomatous polyps, 18 were inflamatory polyps, 4 were juvenile polyps, 2 were hyperplasia polyps, and one was papillomtous polyp.

Besides, there were two adenomatous polyp cases. Both of the two were found malignant. They were transfered to the surgical department to be operated.

One of the 60 got a latent intestinal perforation 20 hours later after the polyps were cut. And after a surgical repair, the patient recovered and left the hospital. This perforation was caused by a too deep gasification on the base.

83 per cent of all this group of the cases were followed up in a period of six months by colonofiberscope after their therapy and were confirmed that there was no finding recurrance. And the polyp bases had already been re-covered by the normal mucous membrence.

4. DISCUSSION

It is recognized at present that large intestinal polyps are pathological changes before cancer. The data offered by Morson pointed out that half of the intestinal cancer patients originated from adenomatous polyps. And it is reported that 10 per cent of canceration is from the adenomatous polyps in 1 - 2cm. in diameter. The adenomatous polyps bigger than 2cm. in diameter have a 45 percent of canceration. So, the large intestinal polyps should be cut as soon as they are found. This should be considered as a rule.

Through the gasification treatment on the 89 intestinal polyps and through the 70 polyps cut and taken out, the evident effectness of the YAG laser therapy is positively confirmed. In comparison with the high frequency resection, it has its own original superiority. Occasionally a hemorrhage may happen when the blood vessels are damaged by high-frequency resection. Laser does not have electric currance to pass the tissue. So, we don't have to worry about the danger caused by the leakage of electricity. And it does not cause the patients to twitch. Laser can act on sealing the blood vessels and lymphoduct in the polyps.

Finally, I would like to remind you once again that YAG laser has a strong perforative ability. A slight inaccuracy and a slight over-gasification may lead to an intestinal perforation. Therefore, to operate the optical glass fiber through the endoscope demands a highly difficult technique. And to grasp a highly skilful technique on endoscopic examination and to operate it with a great care and patient are a vital important thing for the operator.

New Vascular Occulusion Method with Lateral Laser Aming Probe

Daijo Hashimoto, Hiroto Koyama, Kiyotoshi Yabe
Yushi Uedera, Shyunichi Yumoto, Yasuo Idezuki
2nd Department of Surgery, Faculty of Medicine,
Tokyo University, 7-3-1 Hongo Bunkyo-ku, Tokyo, Japan

Introduction

The primary disadvantage of the conventional forward aiming fiberprobe is the need to fire the laser parallel with, or close to the longitudinal axis of the gastrointestinal tract. Now, cancers and ulcers appearing on the wall of the gastrointestinal tract can be treated through laser radiation delivered by the lateral-aiming fiberprobe. After several years of study, we have succeeded in developing a lateral-aiming probe which incorporates a truncated quartz fiber tip protected by a micro-cap. Effective treatment of all lesions in hollow organs has become possible endoscopically with the ability to freely rotate the probe. We have successfully treated gastric cancers, bleeding duodenal ulcers and esopageal strictures which could not be effectively treated with conventional laser probes.
In this report we describe a new alternative to the treatment of vascular occulusion through the water balloon technique.

Method

Under laparotomy, laser radiation was delivered to canine mesentric vessels. Through a transparent ultra-thin latex balloon filled with water, mesentric vessels were radiated from approximately 1 cm separation by applying continuous 70 watts of laser energy through the lateral probe.

Results

70 watts laser energy of 5 second duration was delivered both directly and through a latex water balloon respectively. Vaporization, carbonization and vessel wall rupture leading to bleeding were observed with the direct technique. The balloon treatment produced good vessel wall coagulation

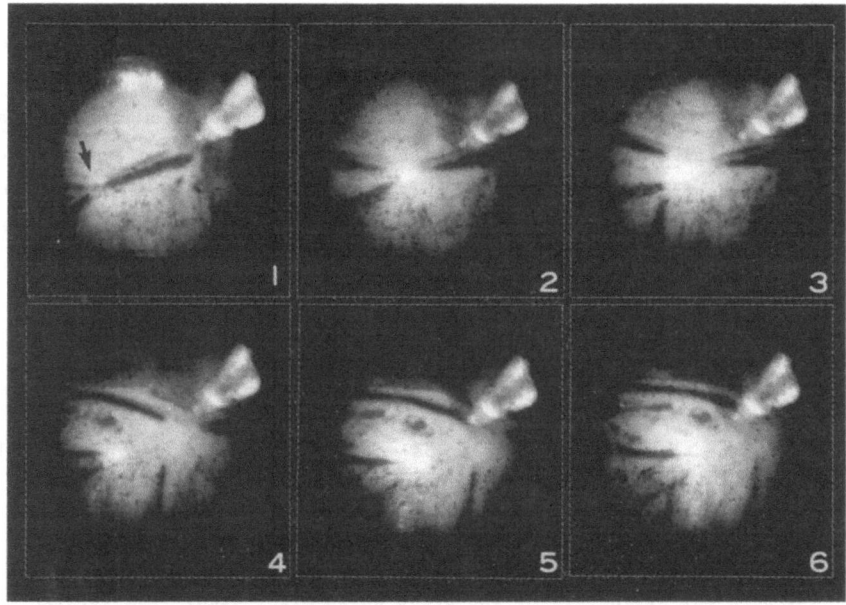

with slight carbonization. The same energy of 3 sec duration also led to damage of vascular wall and bleeding in the case of direct radiation. In the case of water-balloon radiation whitish vascular coagulation with neither vaporization nor carbonization was observed. On the basis of the histological observation, visually whitich coagulation was composed of the shrinkage of the vessels and intra-vascular coagulation. Based upon experimentation, 70 watts of continuous radiation at 3 second intervals was delivered to canine mesentric vessels through the lateral probe inserted into an endoscope of which the distal end was enclosed by a laxtex water balloon. Complete vascular occlusion approximately 4 cm in length was obtained by maneuvering the lateral probe to and fro coupled with the ability to freely rotate the beam along blood vessels.

Discussion

In recent years, sclero therapy for esophageal varicies has been effectivly applied on many cases, however, certain complications caused by sclerotic agents reported, such as drug induced esophageal ulcers which might bleed, lung embolism and lung abscess have been reported and in rare cases, paralysis of spinal axis has been described.

We have been developing a new fibrosing therapy for esophageal varices using the lateral fiber probe instead of injecting foreign matter such as schlerotic agents. As previously reported this new laser fibrosing therapy has excellent features that are free from lung complications and neulorogical damages. However, with even the lowest effective threshould of laser energy, thin wall varicous vein and/or vein rupture cases remain extremely difficult to treat. Based on Dr. Shimamura's treatment method of portal vein thrombus by using the water balloon and a forward-aiming fiber, we are investigating a new occlusion method of varicous vein in combination of the lateral probe and the water balloon. Several advantages of this new therapy could be considered as follows.

(1) As the target to be radiated is contacted with the thin latex filled with water, the temperature never rises higher than 100°C.
(2) By controlling the water temperature filled in the balloon, we could control the size of coagulation.
(3) Burn-out of the tip of the probe which might occur from foreign matter stuck on the protection cap easily can be avoided.

By using the balloon with thin transparent skin, we think ruptured varices will be able to be treated in the near future.

References
1. Hashimoto, D., Mihara, T., Yoshimura, K.
   A Lateral Radiation Probe in YAG Laser therapy.
   Gastro Intesinal Endoscopy vol. 32 (2) 124-125 1986

2. Hashimoto, D.
   Clinical Application of Lateral Radiation Probe in Laser Endoscopy.
   Lasers in Medical Science vol. 2:25 1987

3. Hashimoto, D.
   The Development of Lateral Laser radiation probes
   Gastrointestinal Endoscopy 33 (3) : 240-243, 1987

4. Terblanche, J., Northover, J.M.A., Bornman, P. etal.
   A Prospective evaluation of injection sclerotherapy
   in the treatment of acute bleeding from esophageal varices
   Surgery vol. 85 (3), 239-245, 1979

5. Colathur K.P., Abuabara S, Kraft A.R., and Jonasson O.
   Endoscopic Sclerotherapy in Acute Variceal Hemorrhage.
   The American Journal of Surgery 141:164-168, 1981

6. Seidman E., Weber A.M., Morin C.L., etal.
   Spinal Cord Paralysis Following Sclerotherapy for Esophageal Varices.
   Hepatology 4 (5) : 950-954, 1984

Nd: YAG Laser in the Management of Gastrointestinal Bleeding in Relation to Intensity

B.Jereb, R. Pulanić, V. Šalamon, M.Rosandić-Pilaš, B.Vucelić, N. Hadžić, S. Knežević, V. Borčić, F. Golem
Depts. of Medicine and Surgery, University Hospital Rebro, 41000 Zagreb, Yugoslavia

In 1984 we set up a new organizational programme for treatment of gastrointestinal bleeding at our Department of Internal Medicine, University Hospital Rebro, Zagreb, Yugoslavia. Namely, we opened a new Gastroenterology Interventional Unit. Immediately upon admission to our Unit, patients with upper GI bleeding are submitted to the urgent endoscopy followed by the appropriate endoscopic method, namely, photocoagulation utilized to stop the bleeding.
In some cases complications are encountered, the active bleeding cannot be stopped or rebleeding occurs. Such patients are then operated.
This new approach in the treatment of UGI hemorrhage claims a specific organization in the Interventional Unit. Therefore, an endoscopist is present in the Unit 24 hours a day. When a patient is admitted to our Hospital because of UGI bleeding, the endoscopic treatment is done immediately followed by the intensive medical management and continuos monitoring for eventual rebleeding which is immediately treated on the very onset. In the case of some of the patients, bleeding cannot be stopped and they are transferred to surgery for the operation. Such medical approach requires a team consisting of a gastroenterologist, surgeon, radiologist, anesthesiologist and transfusiologist available all the time.

Method

Photocoagulation is done by a neodim -YAG laser. We apply CO_2 insuflation only during the application of the laser beam and the application number of laser energy is 35-40 Joules. This enables us to apply a laser with a total energy above 1000 Joules per treatment with only a small amount of insuflated CO_2.
Between February 1984 and February 1987 laser photocoagulation in the treatment of the upper gastrointestinal bleeding was performed on 765 patients admitted to our Unit.
55,5% of the patients bled from the duodenal ulcer, 33,1% from the

gastric ulcer and the remaining 11,4% from the various other lesions.

87 patients or 11,37% had a severe underlying disease which was their primary problem, while upper GI bleeding was encountered as a complication. According to our own modification of Forrest's classification the bleeding lesions are divided into 4 groups according to their types: the arterial, venous and capillary (or the oozing from the ulcer rim) bleeding. At the same time, we subdivided the arterial and venous bleeding into three groups.

Type of bleeding		Operated from bleeding	Expired
1. Arterial bleeding	285	10	15
a) Active arterial bleeding	208	5	10
b) Coagulum on the artery	22	2	2
c) Visible artery	55	3	3
2. Venous bleeding	473	2	6
a) Active venous bleeding	206	1	3
b) Fresh coagulum on the vein	146	1	3
c) Visible vein	121		
3. Ulcer rim oozing	7		
4. Old coagulum in the ulcer base	∅		
N	765	12	21

Table 1. Type of bleeding

Statistical analysis of our results confirmed the value of this classification.

Results

The results obtained by the statistical analysis may be summarized as follows: the definite control of bleeding was achieved in 93,1% of the patients by photocoagulation only.

44 patients (5,6%) were operated. Surgery was indicated in 12 cases 1,4% because of unseccessful laser coagulation of bleeding lesions or because rebleeding was recorded more than twice within 48 hours after the initial treatment (10 of them from the arterial bleeding group and 2 from the venous bleeding group). The remaining 32 patients were operated after the successful laser coagulation due

to large and deeply penetrating lesions.
21 patients or 2,5% expired. 11 patients or 1,3% died after the surgical intervention and 9 patients or 1,2% died of the advanced age or associated severe chronic disease following the bleeding stopped.

Conclusion

We compared the patients treated for gastrointestinal bleeding in our Unit in the three year period and 1057 subjects who had an upper GI bleeding treated in our Hospital between 1979 and 1983.

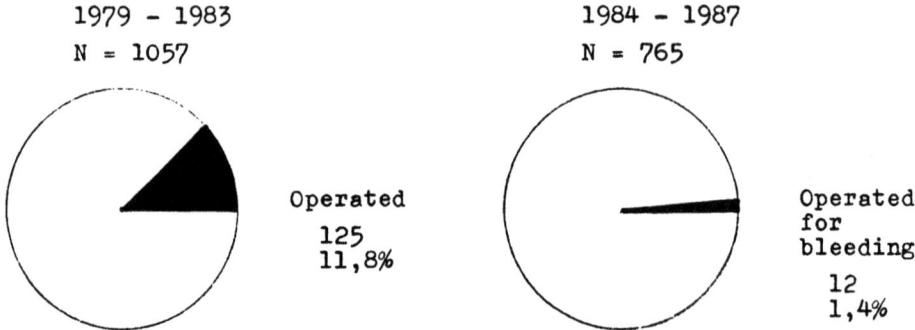

Table 2. GI bleeding in Departments of Medicine and Surgery

The use of photocoagulation reduced the frequency of surgery, so 11,8% of the patients were operated in the period prior to laser treatment, while only 5,6% were operated after the introduction of the laser technique, among this only 1,4% because of the bleeding.

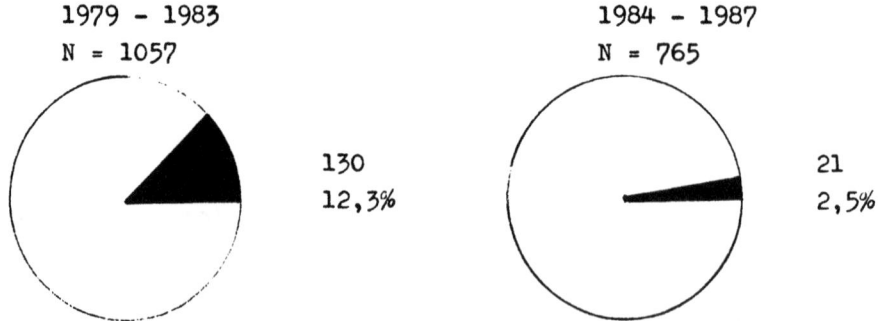

Table 3. GI bleeding in Departments of Medicine and Surgery

The decrease in the lethality rate from 12,3% to a 2,5% proves the value of the endoscopic photocoagulation in patients with the upper gastrointestinal bleeding.

Literature
1. Kiefhaber, P., K. Kiefhaber, F. Huber, G. Nath. Endoscopic Neodymium: YAG Laser Coagulation in Gastrointestinal Hemorrhage. Endoscopy 18 (1986) (Supplement 2), 46-51.
2. Salmon, P.R., C.P. Swain. Laser Photocoagulation - Results of a Randomised Controlled Clinical Trial. Endoscopy 18 (1986) (Supplement 2), 56-57.
3. Fleischer, D. Laser Photocoagulation for Upper Gastrointestinal Bleeding: The American Experience. Endoscopy 18 (1986) (Supplement 2), 52-55.
4. Auth, D.C. Animal Testing of Endoscopic Hemostasis with Lasers and other Devices. Endoscopy 18 (1986) (Supplement 2), 36-39.
5. Schönekäs, H. Wild, I. Trump, F. Bleeding Ulcers, Results with Nd-YAG Laser Coagulation. Proceeding of the 7th International Congress with 2nd International Nd:YAG Laser Conference 85. München. 317-322.

Lasers in Rectosigmoid Tumors

J.M. Brunetaud, V. Maunoury, J.P. Ancelin, D. Cochelard, A. Cortot, J.C. Paris, Multidiciplinary Laser Center, Hopital C. Huriez, and INSERM Unit 279, Lille, France

1 MATERIAL AND METHODS

1.1 Patients preparation
Patients were treated on an outpatient basis, without anesthesia or sedative medication. Patients were prepared with a small enema at the Laser Center and no special diet was required before the treatment. Patients were treated once or twice a week until functional improvement (advanced cancers) or until complete destruction of the tumor (1,2). Then they were followed up every two weeks until complete reepithelialization. Then patients with an advanced cancer were retreated every month, and the other patients were followed up and retreated if a recurrence or new lesions occurred.

1.2 Material for histology
The main disadvantage of laser photoablation is the lack of material available for a total histolgic study of the tumor. Before the treatment multiple biopsies have to be performed. For large tumors, a partial snare electroresection is perfomed when feasible. It has also the advantage of debulking the tumor and decreasing the laser treatment time. New biopsies are performed during and after the treatment.

1.3 Laser treatment modalities
Two types of laser are used for GI endoscopic treatment at Lille: the argon laser and the Nd:YAG laser. The argon laser is a 770 Lasersonics (Santa Clara, CALIFORNIA) with a 10 Watts maximum power output. The argon laser is used for vaporization of superficial tumor (until a flat surface was obtained as delayed necrosis is negligible) at a power of 8 Watts, a spot size of 1 mm (power density : 1,000 Watts/cm2) with a continuous beam. The Nd:YAG laser is the YM 101

CILAS (Marcoussis, FRANCE) with a 80 Watts maximum power output. The volume of delayed necrosis occurring after Nd:YAG vaporization can be difficult to predict from the macroscopic aspect of the tissue during the treatment (2). Therefore, the Nd:YAG laser is used at Lille only for coagulation (blanching) of the tumor and an interval of 2 to 3 days between two treatments allows the coagulated parts of the tumor to slough off. Reproducible effects without unexpected necrosis are obtained at 70 Watts, 2 mm spot size (2,000 Watts/cm2), and 0.7 s exposure time.

2. PATIENTS WITH A RECTOSIGMOID CANCER

Hundred and forty five patients with rectosigmoid cancer were treated from December 1979 to November 1986. All were non surgical. The average age of the patients was 79 (51-94). One hundred and twenty five patients were treated for an advanced tumor. The main symptom at the beginning of the treatment was abnormal rectal discharge in 108 patients and occlusion symptoms in 17. 20 patients had a small lesion. Small lesions were defined as a tumor less than 3 cm in length, with a circumferenrial extension of the base less than one third of the circumference, without sign of infiltration, and purely exophytic without ulceration.

Ninety percent of the patients with an advanced cancer were improved after an average duration of 18 days for the initial treatment (average treatments number 2.5). The treatment was ended in 72 and the average duration of improvement was 7.7 months (0.2-27.5). Life table analysis gives 39% of surviving patients at one year, 82% of them remaining improved. The improvement rate was higher in surviving patients with initial abnormal rectal discharges (95% at 6 months) than in those with obstructive symptoms (60%). An explanation of the failures was not found. The failure rate did not depend on the reasons for treatment, the localization, the circumferential extension, or the main symtom at the treatment beginning.

Negative biopsies were obtained in all the 20 patients with a small rectal cancer after an average treatment duration of 4.8 months. However one patient who had a metastases before the treatment died 8 months later. 2 patients deceased from another etiology and one was lost to follow up. The average follow up of the 16 patients who are still followed is 9.1 months (range 1-41).

Three complications occurred in the group of patients with an advanced rectosigmoid carcinoma (3% of these patients) : one perforation at the rectosigmoid junction (fatal), one perirectal abcess and one rectovaginal fistula.

3. LASERS IN RECTOSIGMOID VILLOUS ADENOMA

Two hundred and twenty three patients were treated at Lille from December 1979 to December 1986 for a rectosigmoid villous adenoma. The average age was 75 years (40-94). The indications for laser treatment were 1) non surgical patients (89 patients, 40 % of total), 2) small tumor which would require drastic surgery (67 patients, 30 % of total), 3) recurrent tumor after a previous non laser treatment (62 patients, 28 % of total) and 4) patient's refusal of surgery (5 patients, 2 % of total).

The treatment was not completed in 39 patients because 12 patients were lost to follow up, 14 died from another etiology during the treatment, and 13 are still under treatment. Results are available in the 184 remainig patients. Eleven patients (6%) had positive biopsies during the treatment. However, only 9 of this latter group of 11 patients had a true adenocarcinoma (4.9%). Two patients (1 %) could not be successfully treated : both had a circumferential lesion previously treated by a non laser procedure. The previous treatment was electrocoagulation in one which resulted in a very tight stenosis making any endoscopic treatment possible. Therefore only a diverting colostomy could be performed. The second patient had been treated by surgical transanal resection. He also developped a stenosis, but related to the laser treatment; the stenosis was not tight enough to require a colostomy, but made the endoscopic treatment impossible.

One hundred seventy one patients were successfully treated (93% of the patients with a completed treatment). Among them, 14 had a recurrence after an average period of 8.2 months. These were easily retreated. Eight developed a stenosis but only 2 stenosis were symptomatic and required endoscopic dilatations (1% of the patients with a villous adenoma). Among the 171 successfully treated patients, 41 are lost to follow up after an average follow up after laser treatment of 12.6 months (range 0.4-44.1), 3 died from another etiology after a follow up of 22.6 months (range 5.2-37.8) and 127 are still followed up since the end of the treatment for an average period of 20.3 months (range 0.9-69.2).

During treament with Nd:YAG some patients experienced warmth in the rectum when the tumor was close to the anus. For 2 or 3 days after a laser session, patients often had spotting with blood and evacuation of necrotic tissue. Two patients experienced fever to 38°C for 2 days unassociated with pain and this spontaneously abated. No perforations or massive hemorrhages were observed.

The circumferential extension was the main predictive factor which influenced the treatment duration until reepithelialization, the frequence of cancer, recurrences of lesion and stenosis development (table 1).

Table 1. Influence of circumferential extension of the tumor base on treatment duration, incidence of cancer, recurrence rate and stenosis development in patients with rectosigmoid villous adenomas. C1 indicates <1/3 circumference, C2 indicates between 1/3 and 2/3 circumference, C3 indicates ≥2/3 circumference.

EXTENSION	CANCER	Rx DURATION	STENOSIS	RECURRENCE
C1	2.2 %	2.9 mo	2.3 %	8.0 %
C2	4.2 %	4.7 mo	4.4 %	5.9 %
C3	17.4 %	9.5 mo	18.8 %	18.8 %
TOTAL	4.9 %	4.2 mo	4.8 %	8.2 %

REFERENCES

1. Brunetaud JM, Mosquet L, Houcke M, et al: Villous adenomas of the rectum: Results of endoscopic treatment with argon and Nd:Yag Lasers. Gastroenterology 1985;89:832-837.

2. Brunetaud JM, Maunoury V, Ducrote P, Cochelard D, Cortot A, Paris JC: Palliative treatment of rectosigmoid carcinoma by endoscopic laser photoablation. Gastroenterology 1987; 92:663-8

Endoscopic Electric Surgery and Nd: YAG Laser Therapy for Gastrointestinal Cancers

K.L. Wu, Tung-Chao Cheng
Tri-Service General Hospital, National Defence Medical Center
No. 622 Ding-Chow Road, Taipei, Taiwan, R. O. C.

Introduction

Surgery is the best available choice of treatment for the malignant gastrointestinal tumor. But in later stages of advanced obstructive cancer of the G-I tract most individuals are not good candidates for operation or irradiation. Implantation of endoprotheses for the stenotic G-I tumor has limiting factors that result in adverse conditions for some patients. Laser therapy is a palliative treatment in a lumen narrowing by G-T cancer by correcting obstruction and improving the patient's nutrition. Nd:YAG laser and electrocoagulation can both arrest G-I bleeding in the earlier years[1-5] In 1982, Fleischer first tried using the Nd:YAG laser to treat 5 patients with advanced obstructive esophageal cancer and their dysphagia was significantly improved.[6] A 63% effective palliative rate for the malignant tumor by Nd:YAG laser therapy was reported by Kobayashi in 1983[7]

The purpose of the present study is to evaluate the change in tumor size, and observe the clinical symptoms before and after therapy using electric surgery and irradiation with Nd:YAG laser.

Materials and Methods

A proven of 18 patients (14 males and 4 females) with gastrointestinal cancer were studied from Jan. 1985 to Dec. 1986. The average age was 53.2 years (40-75). The study of the G-I cancer patients included 5 with esophageal cancer, 9 with stomach cancer and 4 with rectal cancer. The involvement of cancer of the 5 cases of esophageal cancer, three had their tumors at the upper third of the esophagus. The other 2 had their tumors at the middle third and the lower third, respectively. The location of involvement in stomach cancer included 3 in the cardia, 2 in the body and 4 at the antrum. All 4 cases of rectal cancer were confined to the rectum. Dysphagia was characteristic of all 5 patients of esophageal cancer and 3 patients with cardia, stomach cancer. The remaining 6 patients of stomach cancer experienced abdominal distention and a poor appetite. The symptoms of those patients with rectal cancer were tenesmus and constipation.

An Olympus upper panendoscope GIF-Q or GIF-XQ10 or sigmoidfiberscope ITS (Japan) and a PSD-3 monopolar Olympus electrical surgical unit were used along with a Nd:YAG laser (Neodymium yttrium aluminium garnet laser) (West Germany). The patients were clearly informed of the operational procedure and prepared with topical anesthesia. An electrode or the laser catheter was inserted to approach the target by way of a biopsy channel with the endoscope. The electric surgery and laser therapy were carried out under direct vision.

The initial treatment by electric surgery was achieved by using an electrode directly appling 40-50 Watts to the stenotic area of the tumor. The treatment was continued until the narrowing lumen widened. The laser beam was circumferentially focused around the luminal opening and then continuously focused on the same side. Cavitation can form if the tip of the catheter was around 1 cm away from the tissue, and 60-80 Watts was applied. The destroyed tumor was removed by forceps, or aspiration. The treatment was successively applied to the next untreated tumor until the lumen was sufficiently opened to permit passage of the endoscope via the stenotic area of the tumor growth.

Whether it was necessary to perform the endoscopic therapy again, depended upon the repeated endoscopic observations 5-7 days after each treatment.

In our evaluation, the treatment was judged excellent if it resulted in the reduction of tumor size by 90% or better, and the patient was able to ingest solid food and showed easy passage of the stool. It was judged good if the reduction in tumor size was 50% to 90%, and the patient was able to eat semi-solid food. It was rated poor or judged as a failure if the symptoms were not relieved or the tumors remained.

Results

All 5 cases of esophageal cancer and 3 cases of cardia cancer of the stomach improved significantly after electric and laser therapy (Table 1) All the patients were relieved of dysphagia, and the endoscope was able to pass through the stenotic tumor very smoothly. The remaining 6 cases of stomach cancer had good results, with complete disappearance of abdominal distention (Table 1). The colonofiberscope could pass through the narrowing lumen easily in one case of rectal cancer after endoscopic therapy. All 4 cases of rectal cancer showed improvement in stool passage after therapy. One patient developed tumor bleeding after treatment. Thirteen patients died of causes other than those of electric surgery and laser therapy. Their average survival was 6.3 months.

Discussion

If there is any sign of obstruction in the late stage of advanced G-I cancer, neither surgical treatment nor irradiation therapy is useful. Thus, other methods of treatment must be employed. With electric surgery and laser therapy, the high energy can destroy the tumor to reopen the obstructive lumen and to improve the patient's nutrition. All 18 patients' symptoms improved, and the tumor size was reduced. Our results are similar to the 100% effectiveness reported by Flescher[6] and Buset[8] and the 90.9% effectiveness reported by Mellow and Pinkas[9], but better than that of Imaoka and Saniyo[10] Fleischer and Buset both recommended that laser irradiation be applied step-wise starting from the proximal margin towards the distal end.[6,8] The problem with this method is that the degree of stenosis and the natural course of the esophagus cannot be predicted precisely. Thus, the orientation of above method is more difficult. Ell et al suggested inserting the endoscope through the narrowing lumen and then directing the laser beam first to the distal margin of the tumor, then moving backwards to the proximal direction[11] The advantage of this method is that the risk of perforation can be reduced. However, the endoscope cannot pass through the stenotic area of tumor very easily. A third method was employed by Riemann, who recommended a combination of laser treatment with prior bougienage to dilate the narrowing lumen. He then passed the endoscope to the distal portion of the tumor, and applied laser irradiation backwards along the proximal portion[12] The disadvantage of this method is that more steps are necessary. In our work, we combined laser therapy with prior electric surgical treatment. Under endoscopic vision, the electrode was directly applied to the stenotic lumen as a guide probe to treat the growing tumor followed immediately by the laser beam at the proximal portion of the tumor until the narrowing lumen reopened.

Mellow and Pinkas[9] reported that a patient died of aspiration pneumonia secondary to esophagotracheal fistula, and another patient died suddenly 36 hours later after laser therapy. None of our patients developed fistula between the esophagus and trachea after treatment. The one case that developed tumor bleeding might have resulted from tumor necrosis and vessel disruption after laser therapy. Thirteen of our patients died, but the causes were not directly due to electric and laser therapy. The average survival time of 6.3 months was similiar to that which was reported by Mellow and Pinkas.

In conclusion, the combined electric surgery and Nd:YAG laser therapy can not be considered the best methods for treatment of advanced, obstructive G-I cancer, however, they can temporarily improve the nutrition and the quality of life for these patients.

Table 1. The results of electrocoagulation and Nd:YAG laser therapy for malignant Gastrointestinal tumor

G-I Cancer	Location	n	Therapeutic effect		
			Excellent	Good	Failure
Esophagus	U/3	3			
	M/3	1	5	0	0
	L/3	1			
Stomach	Cardia	3			
	Body	2	3	6	0
	Antrum	4			
Colorectal	Rectum	4	1	3	0
Total		18	9	9	0

References
1. Fruhmogen P, Bodem F, Reidenbach HD, et al. Endoscopic laser coagulation of bleeding gastrointestinal lesions with reports of the first therapeutic application in man. Gastrointest Endosc. 23(1976) 73-75.
2. Rutgeerts P, Vantrappen G, Broeckaert L, et al. Controlled trial of YAG laser treatment of upper digestive hemorrhage. Gastroenterology 83(1962)410-416.
3. Ohshita Y. Clinical effects of endoscopic laser hemostasis on upper gastrointestinal hemorrhage. Gastroenterol Endosc. (in Japanese) 25(1983)823-832.
4. Papp JP: Endoscopic electrocoagulation of upper gastrointestinal hemorrhage JAMA 236(1976)2076-2079.
5. Wu KL, Cheng TC: Endoscopic electrocoagulation for upper gastrointestinal hemorrhage J Formosan Med Assoc. 84(1985)113-116.
6. Fleischer D, Kessler F, Haye O. Endoscopic Nd-YAG laser therapy for carcinoma of the esophagus: A new palliative approach. Am J Surg 143(1982)280-283.
7. Kobayashi S. Laser treatment of gastrointestinal tumors. Gastrointest endosc. 29(1983)66-67.
8. Buset M, Dunham F, Baize M, et al. Nd-YAG laser, A new palliative alternative in the management of esophageal cancer. Endoscopy 15 (1983)353-356.
9. Mellow MH, Pinkas H. Endoscopic therapy for esophageal carcinoma with Nd-YAG laser: prospective evaluation of efficacy, complications, and survival. Gastrointest Endosc. 30(1984)334-339.
10. Imaoka W, Ida K. Application of YAG Laser irradiation toward digestive tract tumors. Gastroenterol Endosc (in Japanese) 24(1982) 1642-1644.
11. Ell CH, Riemam G, Lux G, Remling L. Palliative Laser treatment of malignant stenosis in the upper gastrointestinal tract. Endoscopy 18(1986)21-26.
12. Riemann JF, Ell CH, Lux G, Demling L,: combined therapy of malignant stenosis of the upper gastrointestinal tract by means of laser beam and bougienage. Endoscopy 17(1985)43-48.

Bleeding Ulcers Results with Nd: YAG Laser Coagulation

H. Schönekäs
Klinikum Nürnberg, Abtlg. f. Gastro-
enterologie
Flurstr. 17, 8500 Nürnberg, FRG

For a long time emergency endoscopy has proved to be of high diagnostic efficacy in bleeding of the upper digestive tract, concerning localisation, identification and activity of bleeding.

New methods of endoscopic hemostasis, developed in recent years, tried to transfer this high diagnostic efficiency into an effective treatment of patients suffering from gastrointestinal bleeding. They should all be judged by morbidity and mortality.

Conservativ techniques of fiberendoscopic hemostasis are based on application of medicaments, mechanical or thermic methods.

The eficacy of these techniques are to be measured by convenience in practice, effective hemostasis, safety of application and - last but not least - by the cost of staff and technical equipment.

While local application of medicaments and the use of hemoclips proved to be ineffective, good results have been reported from small groupes of patients treated by injection or sclerosing measures, bipolar electrocoagulation with or without a simultaneous jet and heater probes.

Contactless photocoagulation in bleeding of the upper digestive tract has been practiced since 1975 by the use of Argon- and Nd-Yag-laser.

The most important advantages of laser coagulation compared to conventional methods are the contactless application of energy, the exact direction of thermic reactions without losing control of the bleeding source and , above all, the effective hemostasis.

Encouraged by the results of KIEFHABER and his team we started in February 1978, to treat bleeding lesions in the upper digestive tract by Nd-Yag laser coagulation.

We use a Nd-Yag laser of 90 Watt output (Medilas, MBB, Munich), a laser endoscope in which a special triconis quartz fiber for transmission of laser radiation is installed (Nath, Munich), or a monoquartz fiber, developed by Frank a. Rother, which can be introduced into the biopsy channel of nearly all fiberoptic endoscopes.

In massive bleedings we prefer the transmission-system of Nath because of its better ability to suck off blood.

In our department we defined the following most important
preliminary conditions for an effective use of laser coagulation:

Necessities for laser coagulation of bleeding lesions in the
upper digestive tract.
- early emergency endoscopy
- early coagulation tests
- exact indications
- contraindications similar to emergency endoscopy
- skill and experience of the endoscopist
- avoidance of general anaesthesia
- avoidance of stomach lavage
- no limitation of coagulation time
- intensive care and medical therapy in an intensive care unit
  (proximity of the endoscopic department and intensive car unit)

In our hospital we are ready to carry out emergency endoscopy
24 hours a day. This makes it possible in our hospital for any
patient with upper G.I. bleeding to receive emergency endoscopy
within the first hour after initial shock control.

At the same time determination of clotting factors (platelets,
coagulation components etc.) is done - also for 24 hours a day -
and, if necessary, immediately substituted.

Indications for endoscopic blood staunching are active arterial
or venous-capillary bleeding and also visible or protuding
vessles - provided that not too big a layer of thrombotic material
covers the bleeding source.

Contraindications for laser coagulation exist - according to
our experience - only in those patients, who can not be examined
by emergency endoscopy.

Laser coagulation should bei limited to endoscopists with skill and
experience. They must have done at least a 1000 endoscopies and must
be able to identify and control bleeding within a short time.

To avoid aspiration, we use no pharyngeal anaesthesia, We also
regard general anaesthesia to be useless and even dangerous.
For premedication we use exclusively low doses of diazepam
(5 to 10 mg).

According to our experience Stomach lavage for identifying the
source of bleeding or carriing out coagulation is not necessary.

Continous coagulation by the laser is - also according to our
own experience - a better means of hemostasis than short single
impulses.

After treatment by laser coagulation patients need intensive care
and medical therapy in a gastroenterological intensive care unit
situated right next to the endoscopic department. The proximity of
the endoscopic department and intensive care unit enables us to repeat immediately a new laser coagulation if rebleeding should occur.

Under these conditions we carried out from February 1978 to December
1986 6.631 emeergency endoscopies for total number of 50.947 endoscopies.

In 1.221 patients we identified 1.456 active bleedings.

In 961 out of 1.456 patients the hemorrhage hat cost a loss of hemoglobin to at least 9 g%.

The most frequently identified sources of bleeding in the upper digestive tract were peptic ulcers, followed by bleedings from gastral or esophageal varices and Mallory-Weiss-tears.

From February 1978 to December 1986 we laser coagulated 320 patients with bleeding gastric-ulcers and 523 patients with duodenal ulcers.

92 % of active bleeding episodes in both groups were treated succesfully by Nd-Yag-laser. In lasering of peptic jejunal ulcers we had only one failure.

During an average of observation of 10 days rebleeding occured in 10 % of duodenal ulcers, in 14 % of gastric ulcers and in 10 % of peptic jejunal ulcers.

We saw rebleeding mainly in the first 48 hours after laser coagulation. In 77 patients the surgeons performed an elective operation.

From 1977 (before the introduction of laser coagulation) to 1985 the number of emergency operations in our hospital was reduced from 46 (8,5 %) in 1977 to 10 (1,0 %) in 1985.

The mortality rate of laser coagulated patients with bleeding peptic lesions (stage Forrest I a, I b and II) was 4,7 % in duodenal ulcers and 4,9 % in gastric ulcers in the years from 1981 to 1984. These 4,7 and 4,9 were exclusively old and primarily inoperable patients.

The average period of observation being 19 days.

The total lethality in duodenal ulcers, especially in gastric ulcers was essentially caused by high mortality of serious concomitant illnesses.

Mortality of laser-coagulated patients with bleeding ulcers
(1.1.1981 - 31.12.1985)

	Bleeding source (n)	Lethality (%)	Bleedings (%)	Concomitant illnesses (%)
Duodenal ulcer	252	9,8	4,7	5,1
Gastric ulcer	132	12,9	4,9	8,0

Zentrum für Innere Medizin, Klinikum Nürnberg
Abteilung Gastroenterologie

Complications in all our laser coagulations were rare, only three patients had to be operated because of perforation.

Based on our own experience and the results of random trials we think, that emergency endoscopy did not only prove high diagnostic efficacy but also succeeded beyond expectations in effective therapy of bleeding lesions in the upper digestive tract by means of laser coagulation with Nd-Yag-Laser.

In bleeding peptic ulcers (stage Forrest I a, I b and II) a laser coagulation by Nd-Yag-laser should be tried in every case.

In bleeding ulcers the rate of success with Nd-Yag-laser causing definitive hemostasis ist clearly better than all other methods.

The number of so-called "emergency operations", the number of rebleedings and the rate of lethality caused by severe bleeding of ulcers can be reduced decisivly.

Determination of clothing factors, intensive care and medical therapy, and close co-operation with the surgon will support a successfull laser therapy and help our patients.

Nd: YAG Laser Treatment in Early Gastric Cancer in our Institution

Hiroshi Fujimura, Ichiro Tanabe, Tatsuo Otani, Tsuyoshi Aibe, Takayoshi Noguchi, Yukinori Okazaki, Tadayoshi Takemoto*, Susumu Kawamura, Shigemi Ariyama, Tetsuro Sasayama, Mitsuhiko Tanabe and Hiroshi Kawano**

*The first Department of Internal Medicine, Yamaguchi university School of medicine, Ube, Japan, 755
**Department of Internal Medicine, Yamaguchi Rosai Hospital, Onoda, Japan, 756

Laser treatment cases of early gastric cancer

From December 1980 to June 1987, a total of 57 cases (63 lesions) of early gastric cancer were received laser treatment in our institution. Of them, 41 cases with 45 lesions were received follow-up examination for more than 3 months, 5 cases (5 lesions) were operated after laser irradiation, 7 cases (8 lesions) recieved follow-up less than 3 months which made impossible to evaluate therapeutic effect, and 4 cases (5 lesions) were drop-out (Table 1). The operated cases were shown in Table 2.

CASES OF LASER TREATMENT FOR EARLY GASTRIC CANCER

Less than 3 months follow-up terms	
alive	4 cases (4 lesions)
died of other disease	3 cases (4 lesions)
total	7 cases (8 lesions)
Over 3 months follow-up terms	
alive	25 cases (28 lesions)
died of other disease	16 cases (17 lesions)
total	41 cases (45 lesions)
Operation after laser treatment	5 cases (5 lesions)
drop-out	4 cases (5 lesions)
TOTAL	57 cases (63 lesions)

Table 1.

OPERATED AFTER LASER TREATMENT CASES OF EARLY GASTRIC CANCER

case	macroscopic type	depth	histological type	size	result
No. 1	IIa+IIc	sm	tub-2	15×15	cancer (−)
No. 2	I	m	tub-2	20×18	cancer (−)
No. 3	IIc+III	sm	sig	20×25	cancer (−)
No. 4	IIc	sm (pm)	tub-2	20×18	cancer (−)
No. 5	IIc	sm (pm)	sig	20×22	cancer (−)

( )= depth of laser effect judged by ultrasonic endoscopy
cancer (−)= no cancer cells are remained in the specimen

Table 2.

The results of follow-up group

The follow-up cases, endoscopy was undergone every 3 to 6 months. Recurrence of cancer was detected in 8 out of 45 lesions. As shown in Table 3, all the 8 recurrent lesions were detected during the first year. Beyond the first year, no recurrence to be found. Of the 8 recurrent lesions, 1 was operated, 3 were received other kinds of therapeutic endoscopy and 4 were re-irradiation. The incidence of recurrence was studied in terms of size, macroscopic type of early gastric cancer, histological type of cancer cell and depth of the cancer invasion.

Size of lesions and results of leser treatment

The recurrence was noticed in 2 out of 6 lesions which were over 20mm in diameter, and in 6 out of 39 lesions which were less than 20mm in diameter (Table 4). As a result, laser treatment was much effective in lesions less than 20mm in diameter.

FOLLOW UP TERMS AND RESULT IN THE CASES OF EARLY GASTRIC CANCER AFTER THE FIRST LASER IRRADIATION

follow up terms		cancer negative	cancer positive
5Y.~6Y.	1 cases (1 lesion)	1	
4Y.~5Y.	6 cases (7 lesions)	7	
3Y.~4Y.	5 cases (5 lesions)	5	
2Y.~3Y.	13 cases (14 lesions)	14	
1Y.~2Y.	4 cases (5 lesions)	5	
3M.~1Y.	12 cases (13 lesions)	5	8
TOTAL	41 cases (45 lesions)	37	8

Table 3.

RELATIONSHIP BETWEEN SIZE AND RESULT IN FOLLOWED UP CASES AFTER THE FIRST LASER IRRADIATION

size		cancer negative		cancer positive	
over	30mm (1 lesions)	1	4	0(0%)	2(33%)
	~30mm (5 lesions)	3		2(40%)	
	~20mm (31 lesions)	27	33	4(13%)	6(15%)
less than 10mm (8 lesions)		6		2(25%)	
TOTAL	(45 lesions)	37		8(18%)	

Table 4.

Macroscopic types and results of laser treatment

Early gastric cancer can be divided into 3 types, that is, elevated (I, IIa, IIa+IIc), flat (IIb) and depressed (IIc, IIc+III). In the elevated type, the recurrence was noticed in 1 out of 10 lesions only. While, in the depressed type, the recurrence was noticed in 7 out of 35 lesions. There have no flat type in the present series. The higher incidence of recurrence of the depressed type is probably due to difficult identification of the cancer invasion (Table 5).

Histological types and results of laser treatment

The recurrence was noticed in 12% of the well-differentiated type, 28% of the moderately-differentiated type and 40% of the poorly-differentiated type (Table 6). As a result, the therapeutic effect was related to the histological type, and laser treatment was much effective in well-differentiared or moderately-differentiated type.

RELATIONSHIP BETWEEN MACROSCOPIC TYPE AND RESULT IN FOLLOWED UP CASES AFTER FIRST LASER IRRADIATION

macroscopic type		cancer negative		cancer positive	
IIc	32	35 lesions	26	28 lesions	6(19%)	7 lesions (20%)
IIc+III	3		2		1(33%)	
I	1	10 lesions	1	9 lesions	0(0%)	1 lesions (10%)
IIa	7		6		1(14%)	
IIa+IIc	2		2		0(0%)	
TOTAL		45 lesions		37 lesions		8 lesions (18%)

Table 5.

RELATIONSHIP BETWEEN HISTOLOGICAL TYPE AND RESULT IN FOLLOWED UP CASES AFTER FIRST LASER IRRADIATION TO EARLY GASTRIC CANCER

histological type		cancer negative		cancer positive	
well dif. (33 lesions)		29	34	4(12%)	6(15%)
moderately dif. (7 lesions)		5		2(28%)	
poorly dif. (5 lesions)		3		2(40%)	
TOTAL	(45 lesions)	37		8(18%)	

Table 6.

Depth of invasion and result of leser treatment

With respect to the depth of invasion diagnosed endoscopically and radiologically, the recurrence was noticed in 3 out of 28 lesions in which cancer cells were located in the mucosal layer (type "m"). Of the 17 lesions which cancer cells seemed to invade to the submucosal layer (type "sm"). 5 recurrences were noticed (Table 7). The facts suggested that we needed more positive diagnostic tools for clarifing the depth of lesion and laser effect.

Evaluation of endoscopic ultrasonograpy (EUS)

Endoscopic ultrasonograpy (EUS) resolved this problems. When the cancer cells invaded the submucosal layer, disruption of the structure of normal layer is clearly visualized as a image by EUS. And the region of coagulared degeneration and necrosis after laser irradiation visualized as hyper-echoic on the image by EUS. Table 8 showed the list of cases examined by EUS and results of laser treatment. In conclusion, we considered that laser treatment of early gastric cancer should be evaluated particularly in inoperated cases. However, we needed more experience of laser treatment of early gastric cancer and diagnostic tool on metastasis to lymph node, if we intended to estimate laser treatment as the curative therapy to replace surgical method.

RELATIONSHIP BETWEEN DEPTH OF INVASION AND RESULT IN FOLLOWED UP CASES AFTER THE FIRST LASER IRRADIATION TO EARLY GASTRIC CANCER

depth of invasion		cancer negative	cancer positive
m	(28 lesions)	25	3 (11%)
sm	(17 lesions)	12	5 (29%)
TOTAL	(45 lesions)	37	8 (18%)

Table 7.

LASER TREATMENT CASES USING ULTRASONIC ENDOSCOPY TO JUDGE THE DEPTH OF LESION AND LASER EFFECT

Cases	depth of lesion and	depth of laser effect	macroscopic type and	histological type	size and result (cancer(−) or cancer(+), dead or alive)	
No. 1	sm	pm	IIc	group-4	10×12	3m.~1y. (−) dead
No. 2	sm	pm	IIc	sig	20×22	3m.~1y. (+) dead
No. 3	m	sm	IIc	group-4	8×9	4y. ~5y. (−) alive
No. 4	m	pm	IIc	tub-1	7×8	3y. ~4y. (−) alive
No. 5	m	sm	IIa	tub-1	8×9	2y. ~3y. (−) alive
No. 6	sm	pm	IIc+III	tub-1	20×25	3m.~1y. (+) alive
No. 7	sm	sm	IIc	tub-1	11×12	2y. ~3y. (−) alive
No. 8	m	sm	IIc	tub-1	12×15	2y. ~3y. (−) alive
No. 9	sm	pm	IIc	tub-1	20×22	2y. ~3y. (−) alive
No. 10	sm	pm	IIc	tub-1	20×21	2y. ~3y. (−) alive
No. 11	sm	pm	IIa+IIc	tub-1	12×15	2y. ~3y. (−) alive
No. 12	sm	pm	IIc+III	tub-1	12×14	2y. ~3y. (−) alive
No. 13	sm	pm	IIc III	sig	20×25	operation (−) alive
No. 14	sm	pm	IIc	tub-1	18×20	operation (−) alive
No. 15	m	pm	IIc	tub-1	12×15	3m.~1y. (+) alive
No. 16	sm	pm	IIc	sig	20×23	operation (−) alive
No. 17	sm	pm	IIc	tub-1	12×15	3m.~1y. (−) alive
No. 18	m	pm	IIa	tub-1	10×15	3m.~1y. (−) alive

Table 8.

A study on the metastasis to lymph node

We studied the metastasis of lymph nodes which surrounding the gastric wall with gastric cancer by EUS after oral administration of the emulsion. EUS was performed in 21 cases of gastric cancer after oral administation of 20% sesame o/w type emulsion (Table 9). Component of the emulsion was shown in Table 10. The ultrasonographic visualization rate of lymph nodes surrounding the gastric wall was 61% in the size of over 3mm in diameter and 79% in that of over 5mm in diameter (Table 11). The number of the lymph node shown in Table 11 means the localization of the lymph nodes surrounding the stomach based on the general rules for the gastric cancer study prescrived by Japanese research society for gastric cancer. Lymph nodes which had no metastasis histologically showed marginal and internal echo-enhancement after the administration of the emulsion. On the other hand, metastatic lymph nodes showed no enhancement inspite of administration. In the diagnosis of the metastatic lymph node by EUS using the emulsion, the sensitivity was 84%, and the specificity 91% in the lymph nodes of over 3mm in diameter. Moerover, the sensitivity was 90% and the specificity 91% in those of over 5mm in diameter (Table 12). EUS was thought to be very useful to diagnose the metastatic lymph node surrounding the gastric wall by using emulsion, despite some peoblems are still remained to be solved.

CASES OF GASTRIC CANCER IN WHICH EUS WAS PERFORMED AFTER THE ORAL ADMINISTRATION OF 20% SESAME O/W-TYPE EMULSION

early gastric cancer	m ;	5
	sm ;	5
advanced gastric cancer	pm ;	3
	ss ;	5
	s ;	3
TOTAL		21 cases

Table 9.

COMPONENTS OF 20% SESAME O/W-TYPE EMULSION

SESAME OIL	20.0 %
SURFACTANT	
HCO-60	2.4 %
MGS	1.6 %
SIMPLE SYRUP	15.2 %
PURIFIED WATER	60.8 %
TOTAL	100.0%

Table 10.

VISUALIZATION RATE OF THE LYMPH NODES SURROUNDING THE GASTRIC WALL BY EUS WITH 20% SESAME O/W-TYPE EMULSION

size / No.	3mm <	5mm <
No. 1	13/27 (48%)	9/12 (75%)
No. 2	2/10 (20%)	1/4 (25%)
No. 3	84/118 (71%)	55/61 (90%)
No. 4	56/85 (66%)	32/37 (86%)
No. 5	15/34 (28%)	11/19 (58%)
No. 6	28/53 (53%)	17/26 (65%)
TOTAL	198/327 (61%)	125/159 (79%)

Table 11.

ACCURACY RATE OF THE LYMPH NODE METASTASIS SURROUNDING THE GASTRIC WALL BY EUS WITH 20% SESAME O/W-TYPE EMULSION

	size of the lymph nodes	
	3mm <	5mm <
sensitivity	33/38 (84%)	28/31 (90%)
specificity	149/159 (94%)	86/94 (91%)
false negative	6/38 (16%)	3/31 (10%)
false positive	10/159 (6%)	8/94 (9%)

Table 12.

Nd:YAG Laser with Water Jet Stream – A New Transmission System with a Water-Guided Laser Beam

R. Sander, H. Poesl, F. Frank, P. Meister, M. Strobel, A. Spuhler, E. Unsoeld
I. Medizinische Abteilung, Städtisches Klinikum München Harlaching
Sanatoriumsplatz 2, 8000 München 90, FRG

Introduction

The transmission of laser light via flexible transmission systems is the prerequisite for the fiberendoscopic use of lasers in gastroenterology. Among the lasers that meet the necessary conditions, the Neodymium YAG laser has become widely accepted on account of its specific physical properties (1). Recently, changes in pulse quality, wavelength, and transmission system (2-6), have opened up the way to new forms of application. In the case of the Neodymium YAG laser, light is released either in the pulsed or continuous wave mode. For the pulsed laser, the wavelength 1.06 microns is always employed, while for the continuous wave laser (cw), two wavelengths are at present in use: 1.06 microns, and 1.32 microns. Light can be transmitted with or without contact with the tissue. The contact methods are differentiated in accordance with the material of the tip of the light guide. In the case of the non-contact procedures, a differentiation is made between fibers with coaxial CO_2 flow, and those with water flow.

Material and Method

We used a transmission system similar to the already known fiber system. It comprises a flexible, robust quartz glass monofiber with a teflon cover having a diameter of 600 μm. Light exits form the tip of the fiber at an angle of 10 degrees. Usually a coaxial flow of CO_2, contained by means of an outer teflon sheath, cools the apical metal jet which serves to keep free the exit portal of the laser light. The entire system has a diameter of 2.0 to 2.6 mm, and thus can be passed down the instrument channel of the commonly employed routine endoscopes. Here the coaxial gas flow is replaced by a water jet stream in conjunction with a pump (fig. 1).
At a throughput of about 50 cc/minute, the laser beam follows the water jet and is conducted via the latter, to the target tissue. The guidance of the laser beam through flexible fiber system is based on successive total internal reflexions of the light at the surface between 2 materials with different refractive indices. In the glass light guide the materials are quartz glass and teflon. Beyond the fiber tip the continuous water jet and air take over the role of quartz and teflon and direct the laser beam to the target tissue. Laser light of 1.32 μm basically is not well transmitted by the water jet system. This is due to the fact that its absorption in water is 10 times as high as with the 1.06 μm wavelength. We used the Nd YAG cw laser from MBB company, type MediLas 2, wavelength 1.06 μm. Transmitted maximum power 80 - 95 Watts.

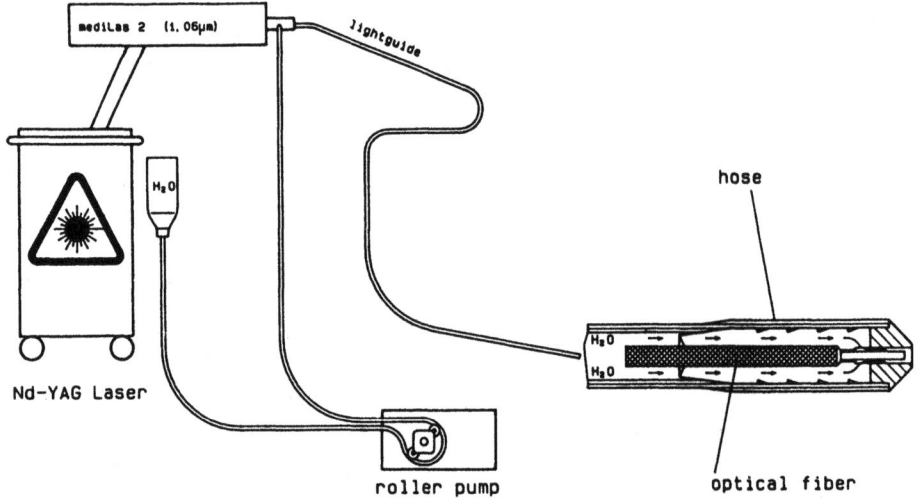
fig. 1. Water guided laser beam - principle of the system

Animal experiments were performed in 3 rabbits which were sacrificed whithin up to
1 hour after the laser irradiation of their stomach. Tissue coagulation was done
from different distances between fiber tip and target (1, 3, 5 cm) and with various
irradiation times (5, 10, 15 sec) while using a maximum power output of 90 Watts.
Owing the cooling of the irradiated area by water, the optical properties of the
surface of the tissue were not as much changed as with other application methods.
In our animal experiments we found after laser exposure of a rabbit stomach with
different amounts energy a slight whitening of a small area with a marginal haemorrhagic zone and a broad surrounding area of hyperemia alterations, which increased
in size proportionately to the distance and irradiation time. In the presence of
only slight backscatter of the light by blanching a deep volume absorption is
achieved. The histological changes are schematically shown in fig. 2.

Results

Between June 86 and January 87 we treated 8 patients, 5 female and 3 male, with 4
villous adenomas and 2 adenocarcinomas (T_1) in the colorectum and 2 adenomas in the
stomach, mean diameter 3 cm. The paint brush technique (laser treatment until a
slight whitening of the visible part of the tumor is achieved) similar to the gas
cooled non contact procedure was used. Maximum power output of 80-95 Watts was used.
The exposure time never exceeded 90 seconds/session, the duration of the single procedures of laser endoscopy was 5 to 15 minutes. No patient needed any special medications.
All tumors were completely eliminated after 1 to 2 sessions and energy of 3.000 -
5.000 Joule per patient and session. In the follow up period of 3 to 8 months (mean
5,8) there were no recurrences of the tumors or complications of the treatments.

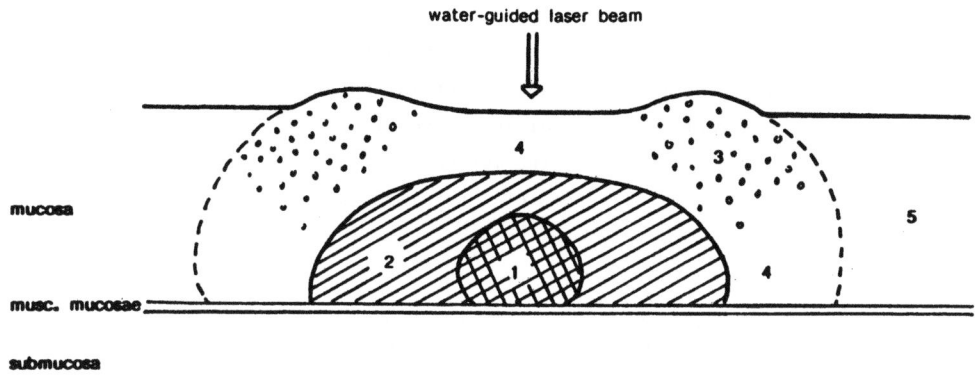

fig. 2. Histological alterations of the gastric wall of a rabbit after irradiation
with a water-guided laser beam.
Schematic cross view. 1 = complete necrosis
2 = partial necrosis
3 = hyperemia and hemorrhagic zone
4 = edema
5 = surrounding normal tissue

The scarring was only minimal, in most cases not visible.

Discussion

The new modus of laser application by using a water jet proved to be effictive in
destroying broad based adenomas. The treatment is painless as the organ is not
distended and no burning sensation is experienced in the rectum and esophagus unlike
the conventional systems, where most of the patients need sedative or analgetic medication, and it does not induce smoke. Both is advantageous to the patient and the
endoscopist. The average amounts of water inflow during the treatments are low,
approximately 250 cc per session. When longer procedures are required, intermittent
aspiration of water or continuous suction through a second channel keep the risk of
water intoxication or aspiration very low. If the water level raises, the target
can be kept in sight by suction and changing the position of the patient.

It opens new ways of deeper tissue effects which could be advantageous in the treatment of malignant tumors and (perhaps) hemorrhage. Especially adenocarcinomas with
deep invasion or tumors of the diffuse type can be treated in a more comprehensive
and therefore more efficient way. As the superficial layers of the irradiated tissue
are not as much destroyed as in the case of the usual application methods (7) better preconditions are given for a more natural reconstruction of the structure of
the organic wall by scar tissue when the treatment is finished. Although the damage
of the surface with this method is comparably low, a slight whithening of the irra-
dated area warns the endoscopist that for the moment enough energy has been applied
to that specific point of the tissue. Animal experiments and tumor treatments did

not indicate an increased risk of perforation. In hemostasis the slight damage of the lesion, i.e. a gastroduodenal ulcer, together with occlusion of blood vessels by edema and shrinkage of the tissue in the deeper layers of the wall, could improve both the hemostatic effect and the healing of the ulcer.

Further studies have to show whether the method is clinically more advantageous and efficient than the application systems of laser light which are already known.

References

1) P. Kiefhaber, G. Nath, K. Moritz, and A. Kreitmayr:
Der Einsatz des Neodym:YAG-Lasers bei der endoskopischen Blutstillung im Rahmen der Notfallendoskopie.
In Fortschritte der Gastroenterologischen Endoskopie (Hrsg. H. Lindner), Witzstrock Baden-Baden, Brüssel, 8 (1977) 226.

2) H. Hofstetter, F. Frank, E. Keiditsch, F. Wondrazek:
Intracorporale, laserinduzierte Stoßwellen-Lithotripsie (ILISL)
Laser 1 (1985) 155

3) F. Frank, D. Beck, S. Hessel, and E. Keiditsch:
Comparative Investigations of the Effects of the Neodymium:YAG Laser at 1.06 Microns and 1.32 Microns on Tissue
Laser in Surgery and Medicine 6 (1987) 546

4) R. Sander, H. Poesl, A. Spuhler, H. Hitzler:
Der Neodym-YAG-Laser: Ein effektives Instrument für die Stillung lebensbedrohlicher Gastrointestinalblutungen
Leber Magen Darm 11 (1981) 51

5) R. Sander, H. Poesl, A. Spuhler, F. Frank:
Neodym-YAG-Laser mit CO_2-jet-stream - Erfahrungsbericht
In Fortschritte der Gastroenterologischen Endoskopie (Hrsg. H. Henning), Witzstrock Baden-Baden, Köln, New York 11 (1980) 105

6) N. Daikuzono and S. Joffe:
Artificial Sapphire Probe for Contact Photocoagulation and Tissue Vaporization with the ND:YAG Laser
Medical Instrumentation 19 (1985) 173

7) M. Landthaler, R. Brunner, D. Haina, F. Frank, W. Waidelich, O. Braun-Falco:
The Neodymium-YAG Laser in Dermatology
Münchner Medizinische Wochenschrift 126 (1984) 1108

Laser Treatment of Colorectal Tumors – Initial Results of Clinical Studies with the Nd:YAG Laser, Wavelength 1318 NM

R. Sander, H. Poesl, A. Spuhler, M. Strobel, E. Unsoeld
I. Medizinische Abteilung Städtisches Klinikum München-Harlaching
Sanatoriumsplatz 2, 8000 München 90, FRG

Intruduction

The importance of the Nd YAG laser is expanding with its range of indications. New wavelengths have been developed with the goal of achieving more efficient laser treatments for localized tumors. After animal experiments in the rabbit stomach (1) a comparative, randomized and prospective study was initiated. This should help to clarify the effects of the 1.32 μm wavelength of the Nd YAG laser on colorectal tumors in clinical use - in comparison to the 1.06 μm wavelength which is commonly used.

Material and Method

Between January 1986 and March 1987 34 patients with colorectal tumors entered the study in 4 groups: Groups 1 and 2 contain 18 patients: with adenocarcinomas (10 pts) and adenomas (8 pts) treated with the 1.06 μm wavelength, groups 3 and 4 16 pts: with adenocarcinomas (8 pts) and adenomas (8 pts) treated with the 1.32 μm wavelength.

Indications for the treatment of malignant tumors were: The technical inoperability of the tumor, patients with serious underlying diseases and those who refused surgery, in a few cases patients in whom curative surgery was not possible. The therapeutic goals were: Achieving patency, reduction of the tumor mass with the possibility of a curative effect. In benign tumors we considered as an indication broad based villous adenomas which could only partially be removed by extensive polypectomy. Our goal was to destroy the rest of the tumor and to prevent recurrence. We used the Nd YAG laser MediLas 2 (MBB Ottobrunn, West Germany) with the two different wavelengths (1.06 μm, 1.32 μm: maximum power output at the tissue 95/35 Watts). The transmission system has a diameter of up to 2.6 mm and fits through the instrument channels of the commonly employed routine endoscopes. It is comprised of a flexible robust quartz glass monofibre having a diameter of 0.6 mm. A coaxial CO_2 gas flow cools the apical metal jet. Laser light application is effected, contact free, at a distance of up to 10 mm from the target tissue, with continuous, visually controlled exposure with no set time limit.

In case of malignant stenoses we use a circular vaporisation from the center to the margin and a step-by-step treatment of 2-3 cm recanalisation/session. In circumscribed tumors a paint brush technique of coagulation is used until a whitening of the tissue is achieved.

Results

The groupings basically were similar. The mean age of the 34 treated patients was 75.1 years, 14 of them were female, 20 male. The average follow up time was 6.8 months, the mean number of sessions per patient 5.4. The power setting for the treatment of adenocarcinomas was higher than for adenomas, also more medication was necessary when treating malignancies.

In general we found the following clinical differences between the two wavelengths: With the 1.32 /um wavelength we needed only 1/3 of the power setting, 50-60 % of the amount of energy per square cm tumor mass and only 2/3 of sedative or analgetic medication during the treatments, when compared with the 1.06 /um wavelength (fig. 1) In villous adenomas we finally achieved similar results using both wavelengths with a complete or nearly complete elimination of the tumor. In adenocarcinomas 3/8 patients were treated with the 1.32 /um laser which resulted in a local full or

	power (W)	energy (J) cm^2 tumor	medication % of treatment
adenocarcinomas			
I 1.06 /um (n=10)	80 - 95	635	98,5
III 1.32 /um (n= 8)	25 - 35	328	62,5
villous adenomas			
II 1.06 /um (n= 8)	30 - 70	748	46,7
IV 1.32 /um (n= 8)	15 - 25	421	34,4

Fig. 1. Laser therapy of colorectal tumors (- 3/87) results - success

	patients (n)	local success			
		complete	nearly complete	steady state	failure
adenocarcinomas					
I 1.06 /um	10	-	-	10	-
III 1.32 /um	8	2	1	3	2
villous adenomas					
II 1.06 /um	8	5	3	-	-
IV 1.32 /um	8	4	4	-	-

Fig. 2. Laser therapy of colorectal tumors (- 3/87) results - success

nearly full remission. None of the 10 patients with this type of tumor in the 1.06 µm group showed complete remission. On the other hand in 2 patients the wavelength 1.32 µm had to be changed because of a lack of efficacy in reopening the stenosis (fig. 2).

Discussion

The application of laser is based on the transformation of light energy into heat within the tissue. The extent and degree to which heat is generated is a function of the geometry of the beam and the energy of the radiated light, and also of the optical and thermal properties of the tissue.

The beam specific parameters are:
- spot diameter on the surface of the tissue
- beam power
- irradiation time

The thermal properties are:
- density
- specific heat
- thermal conductivity
- extent of blood circulation

The principal optical parameters are:
- absorption and
- light scattering

The absorption of the 1.32 µm wavelength in water is 10 times higher, in contrast blood has a 3 times lower extinction than in the case of the 1.06 µm wavelength (2). In connection with the fact that the transformation of laser light into heat takes place where it is absorbed we conclude that the efficacy of the 1.32 µm wavelength is higher in a tissue with a relatively high watercontent and that the presence of blood is not as significant as it is in the case of the 1.06 µm wavelength. This conclusion is supported by our animal experiments and clinical experience. Studies in layered tissue of the stomach of the rabbit revealed, that at identical radiation energies applied by the Nd YAG laser, the energy transmission was more efficient in the case of the 1.32 µm than in the case of 1.06 µm wavelength. We found a higher vaporisation (cutting) effect surrounded by broad zones of colaguation and edema. The zone of necrosis was smaller at equal parameters of energy, exposure time and shooting distance i.e. 2,5 mm in case of 20 W for 3 sec versus 4 mm when using the 1.06 µm wavelength. In respect to the 1.06 µm laser the coagulation zone was broadened and the small amount of ablated tissue was increased, when higher power or exposure times were used (1).

In clinical practice we found a better efficacy of the 1.32 μm wavelength in soft tissue of pink color. Problems arose in the treatment of indurated, far advanced carcinomas, tissues with low water and increased collagen fiber content, especially those with a white, grey or green colour of the surface. The latter fact gives a hint that the light backscatter plays another important role in the difference of the wavelengths. In order to treat this type of tumor with the 1.32 μm laser a higher output power would be required which from a technical standpoint is limited to 35 W. When treating colorectal tumors with 1.32 μm we required less power, less energy, and less medication for the same or in cases with soft tumors better effect in comparison to the 1.06 μm wavelength. Only when a clinical experience has been obtained, and further larger studies have been performed, a more accurate statement can be made as to possible improvements in the primary results through the use of the 1.32 μm laser in the treatment of colorectal tumors, and to further knowledge of physical and histological principles. Likewise, an assessment of the definitive results of treatment will be possible only on the basis of lengthy follow up periods. For a more effective use of the new wavelength an improvement in the laser power output is mandatory.

References

1) R. Sander, H. Poesl, M. Strobel, E. Unsoeld, F. Frank, A. Spuhler:
   Nd-YAG Laser in der Gastroenterologie - Erste Ergebnisse experimenteller und klinischer Studien mit der 1.32 μm Wellenlänge.
   Laser in Medicine und Surgery 2 (1986), 167

2) L. Stokes, D. Auth, D. Tanaka, J. Gray, C. Gulacsik:
   Biomedical utility of 1.32 μm Nd:YAG laser radiation
   IEEE Trans. Biomed. Eng. BME 28:297

Laser Treatment of a Stenosis After Continuity Resection of the Colon

T. Müller-Schwefe, P. Dreverhoff
Municipal Hospital Bielefeld-Mitte
Ölmühlenstr. 26, 4800 Bielefeld, Germany

The video clip of 12 minutes shows a case report of an 55 year old patient, who showed severe signs of illness in November 1983 and after he had been examined thoroughly was operated in an external hospital because of a tumor in the sigmoidal region, whose origin could not be cleared preoperatively.

The patient tells during an interview that he was told after the operation that an anus praeternaturalis had been applied because of a big inflammatory tumor, which already had involved the bladder and surrounding tissue, so it could not be removed during this operation. It was thought likely that the tumor was caused by a divertikutitis.

In January 1985 the patient was operated a second time and the now considerably smaller tumor was removed and the anus praeter sigmoidalis was closed and an anus praeter of the transversal colon applied instead.

A continuity resection of the involved sigmoidal segment was performed. The stapler suture of the anastomosis was insufficient and a stenosis resulted in this area after inflammation following insufficiency had disappeared.

The patient could eat everything after this second operation and took up normal work when wound healing was finished.

Because of the stenosis the stoma could not be closed as it was planned originally. Several controls of the stenotic zone with X-ray and endoscopic methods showed the constant stenosis. Pictures of the X-ray examinations are shown in the video.

In January the patient came to our hospital because he had heard that instead of a third operation to remove the stenosis we probably could help him by means of laser and set the condition to close the anus praeter.

X-ray contrast-examinations and endoscopy - both are shown in the video-show a stenosis of three to four millimeters in diameter in the

anastomosis area. A longer sequence shows the endoscopic procedure
in which we first used the neodym-YAG-laser, and then changed to the
papillotomy-equipment because very strong reflections of stapler
clamps from the stapler anastomosis seamed dangerous for the endoscope.
But the papillotomy probe could not be placed good enough in the
stenosis so we changed back to the laser and step by step cleared away
the stenosis. The passage of the endoscope through this area can be
followed in the video after the final laser shots are applied.
The X-ray control two days later showed a more than two centimeter
wide anastomosis.
Another two days later the anus praeter of the transversal colon could
be closed and the patient sent home after wound healing.
An endoscopic control of the treated area three months later is
demonstrated and shows no stenosis or inflammated districts, no signs
of the previous stenosis or of the laser treatment can be found.
The patient tells at the end that he now feels completely healthy,
has no complaints, no difficulties in digestion, no pain in defecation
and no flatulences and is satisfied with the result of the treatment
absolutely.

Gynecology

Laser Diagnostic Cylindrical Excision Versus Cold Knife Conization – A Clinical Experience of 60 Cases

Alex C. Wang, T.Z. Chang, Swei Hsueh[*], M.C. Kao[**]
Department of Obstetrics and Gynecology
Chang Gung Memorial Hospital
Taipei Taiwan, R.O.C.

[*] Department of Pathology
[**] Department of Surgery
  National Taiwan University Hospital
  Taipei Taiwan, R.O.C.

ABSTRACT

Laser conical excision of the uterine cervix is a much praised procedure in current gynecological practice. From March 1985 to February 1986, cylindrical excision of the uterine cervix by carbon dioxide laser was performed for 30 patients with abnormal papanicolau smears and colposcopic finding. During the same period another 30 patients with the same condition, underwent conventional cold knife conization, used as the control group. A comparison of the data of the clinical parameters between these two groups showed no significant difference. However, the comparison of the pathological parameters was as follows: specimen depth in laser cylindrical excisional specimen vs cold knife conical specimen was 6.43 mm $\pm$ 2.29 mm vs 4.68 mm $\pm$ 2.13 mm ($p < 0.001$), while the lesion distance in laser cylindrical excisional specimen vs cold knife conical specimen was 5.08 mm $\pm$ 2.65 mm vs 4.20 mm $\pm$ 1.67 mm $p < 0.01$. The aforementioned figures proved that the former procedure can remove a larger volume of tissue and include more definite extension of the lesion. The potential advantages of laser cylindrical excision in detecting a possible invasive lesion in the uterine cervix harboring CIN will be presented and discussed.

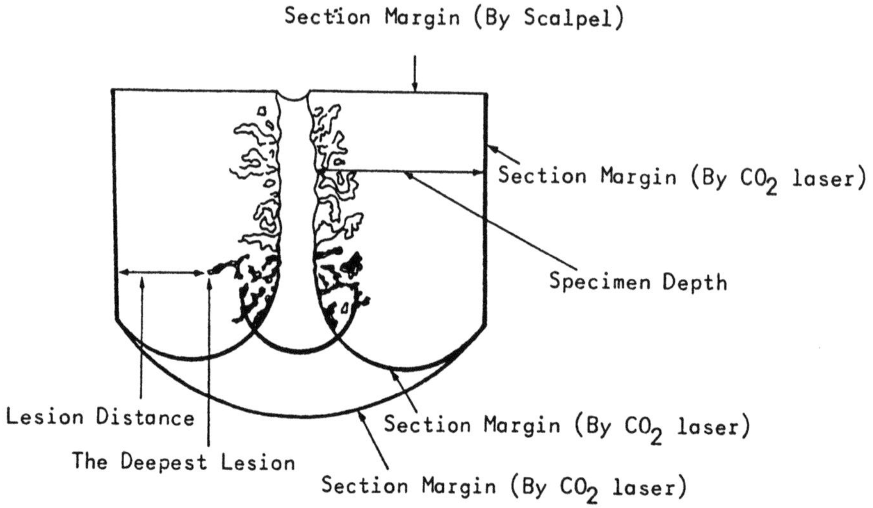

Section Margin (By Scalpel)

Section Margin (By CO_2 laser)

Specimen Depth

Lesion Distance

The Deepest Lesion

Section Margin (By CO_2 laser)

Section Margin (By CO_2 laser)

Fig. 1. Findings and 2 measurements of a section block

REFERENCES

1. Adelman H, Hajdu SI (1967): Role of conization in the treatment of cervical carcinoma in situ. Am J. Obstet Gynecol 98: 173.
2. Anderson MC, Hartley RB (1980): Cervical Crypt involvement by Intraepithelial Neoplasia. Obstet Gyneco 55 (5): 546-550.
3. Bellina JH (1978): Carbon dioxide microsurgery in gynecology. Int Adv Surg Oncol 1: 277.
4. Holdt DG, Allan AJ, Scott JC, Adam GM (1982): Diagnostic significance and sequelae of cone biopsy. Am J. Obstet Gynecol 143: 312.
5. Hsu CT (1986): Personal Communication.
6. Larsson G, Alm P, Grundsell H (1982): Laser conization versus cold knife conization. Surg Gynecol Obstet, 154: 59-61.
7. Marsden DE, Cavanagh D, Wishniewski BJ, Roberts WS, Lyman GH (1985): Factors affecting the incidence of infections morbidity after radical hysterectomy. Am J. Obstet Gynecol 152: 817-821.
8. Meandzija MP, Locher G, Jackson JD (1984): CO2 Laser conization versus conventional conization: A clinico-pathological appraisal. Lasers Surg Med 4: 139-144.
9. Prizybora LA, Plutowa A (1959): Histological Topography of carcinoma in situ of the cervix uteri. Cancer 12(2): 263-277.
10. Toaff R (1976): The carbon dioxide laser in gynecological surgery. In Kaplan I (ed): Laser surgery proc. of First Internat. symposium on Laser Surgery. Jerusalem: Jerusalem Academic Press, PP 129-132.
11. Wright VC, Davies E, Riopelle MA (1984): Laser cylindrical excision to replace conization. Am J. Obstet Gynecol 150: 704-709.

CO_2 Laser-Application in the Lower Female Genitaltract for Treatment of Cervical Intraepithelial Neoplasia, Bartholin Duct Cysts and Condylomata Acuminata

U.Heckmann . Dep.Gynecol.Obstet., Teaching Hospital University Muenster,Dortmund West Germany

The use of CO_2-laser can offer precision,bloodless field and accessibility to poorly visible areas.This report discribes the microsurgical techniques that can be performed by the CO2-laser in the lower femal genital tract.
New approaches in the treatment of cervical intraepithelial neoplasia (CIN) with the CO2-laser are intended to tailor the defect incorporating only the diseased tissue.Preserving normal tissue and maintaining an outer rim of the cervix,the regeneration will occur from all surfaces. In 145 cases CO2-laser treatments of cervical intraepithelial neoplasia were performed with a Coherent Model 450.
The technical data were as follows: a maximum power of 30 W, an objective focal length 30 mm, and an effective laser beam imprint of 1,5 mm (spot size).The power density was ranging from 400 - 600 W/cm^2 for the Vaporization and from 1,400 - 1,600 W/cm^2 for the excision of the tissue specimen.The laser was coupled to a Zeiss colposcope with a micromanipulator and a joystick used to direct the laser beam.
By instillation of methylenblue solution 1% into the cervical canal, the geometry of the cervical gland field,with involved crypts is under control of the colposcope.To ensure a bloodless operating field a vasoconstrictive solution (POR 8 Sandoz 10% in NaCl s.') a derivative of vasopressin, 1,5 cc was injected into each quadrant of the cervix.The peripheral extent of the cylinder is outlined by imprinting a series of circular spots on the portio.The initial cut is made into the cervix,usually with penetration to a depth of 5 - 8 mm. Then traction is placed on the cervical tissue by a laser hook. As the hook is moved around the periphery of the specimen,the laser beam simultaneouly freed up, usually to a height of 24 mm. The length of the cylinder is prepared in accordance with the cervical canal dimension measured prior to preparation.The apical pole of the cylinder is then cut at the endocervical margin with a sharp scalpel. The base of the cervical defect is treated by vaporization to a depth of 5 mm. The cylindrical specimen is removed to determine volume,diameter and length before it is send to the pathologist for further examination. This excisional procedure was performed with general anesthesia in a hospital.The patients were discharged after 2 to 5 days.
We chose the laser techniques based an lesion location,lesion size and need for a histological specimen.Cervical intraepithelial neoplasia grade I of ectocervical location was restricted to the vaporization procedure only, in 22 patients.
Regardless of disease severty, a laser cylindrical excision was performed in 123 patients.The mean age of the patients was 44,5 years varying from 18 to 77 years. The lesion location of CIN I was ectocervical overall in22.5%. For a disparty of smear,colposcopy and/or histology a cylindrical specimen of the endocervix was removed in 7.5%. The extent of the disease to the endocervix was 77.5% in total.Persistence of disease,that is disease present within the first 6 months of follow-up, was observed in 2/22 (9%) women with CIN I ectocervical after vaporization, and in 7/123 (5,6%)women with CIN II and III after cylinder dissection regardless of localisation of the disease.Recurrence of disease was seen in 2.4% of CIN grade II and III. In such cases,persistence was always present at the endocervical treatment margin.The percentage of patients with persistence of disease requiring hysterectomy was 7/123 (2.4%) with multifocal extent of the disease.In three patients hysterectomy was performed for other gynecological reasons

as Myoma and Descensus uteri.Recurrence of the disease after an interval of 8 to
15 Months had 3 patients (3/123=2.4%).This new disease was cured by laser retreatment.The laser cylinder dissection of the cervix required a mean time of 10 to 20
minutes depending on the mobility of the organ.The complication rate of the procedure is very low. 3 of 123 patients required the placement of a Sturmdorf suture
to control arterial bleeding.Six to twelth days after operation a vaginal gauze
pack was inserted in 4 of 123 patients to stop hemorrhage.

The volume of the biopsy specimen was determined in 40 patients.The average
excisional cylinder,measuring 16 mm in diamter and 24 mm in length, was of a mean
volume of 3.0 cc. A cylindrical specimen of the endocervix,not a cone shaped one,
will preserve more connective tissue and reduce the stroma defect.

The CO2-laser offers a rapid and effective method for the surgical management
of certain cyst structures in the lower reproductive tract.Bartholin duct cysts,
vaginal Mullerian cysts and sebaceous cysts of the vulva are successfully handled by simialar techniques.The anterior cystwall is incised using a spot size
of 1.5 mm and a power density of 1,000 W/cm^2. The incision should be long enough
to allow for complete drainage of cyst contents.A wet cotton tip applicator is
inserted into the cavity to elevate the anterior cyst wall. The vaporization of
the anterior cyst wall is performed over the wet cotton tip, using as a back
stop to protect the underlying tissue. A spot size of 1.5 mm is used with a power
density of 500 W/cm^2.The superficial wall of the cyst is not supplied with large
blood vessels and vaporization is bloodless.The posterior portion of the cyst
is exposed by two laser hooks.It contains the blood supply and, since only the
superficial lining is destroyed,large vessels are not surgically encountered.The
laser beam sterilizes the operating field.Thus ,the procedure is accomplished
either by primarily closing the wound or healing by granulation.The anatomy of
the vulva is restored after 10 - 14 days.The patients discomfort is minimized.
Thus the hospital stay is reduced to 4 - 6 days.In 15 cases of Bartholin duct
cysts and 5 patients of with sebaceous cysts of the vulva CO2-laser microsurgery
offered an advantage of the conventional techniques of excision.

The CO2-laser has contributed significantly to the treatment of the condylomata
acuminata and plana of the Vulva,Vagina and Cervix. In 65 patients the persistence
rate of the viral disease after the first laser treatment was approximately 30%.
Failures after the initial vaporization were treated by CO2 laser in combination
with the immunmodulator Inisoplex.Delimun: 6 tablets daily for 5 days repeated
3 times at intervals of one mounth .The first treatment was administered at the
time of the CO2 laser treatment.After a second theraypy in case of recurrence
were no failures seen.The combination of the local application of CO2 laser
and the systemic use of inosiplex is an effective form of treatment for the
recurrent condylomata acuminata.Simialar results are reported of b-Interferon
local injections into the lesion but more side effects are put into consideration.

New Methods in Treatment of the Portio Dysplasias by Carbon Dioxide Laser

L.Kovacs, A.Bartsch, P.Unk
Dept. of Gyn. and Ost. of Hungarian
People's Army
MN 1. Katonai Korhaz
H-1525 Budapest

On the basis several-year subject in connection with the gynaecoloqiccal control examinations and cancer screenings, according to epithelia lesions of different location and extension as well as seriousness, the authors suggest different laser surgical solutions taking the histological diagnosis of the lesion into consideration that is established from the result of the test-excision prior to the intervention in the cases where the screening examination proves an epithelia lesion going forward in the direction of malignancy.

On the vaginal portio of the uterus, on the surroundings of the external orifice of the uterus, there location of the transition between the cylindro-cellular cutis and the platecellular one viz. the transformation zona depends on the age and the hormonal staus of the woman as well as it depends on the change of the pH value due to an inflammatory process. The epithelia lesions recognized at the screening examinationscan set out from both the platecellular cutis and the cylindrocellular one, but most frequently from the transformation zonna. As regards their location processes setting out from the surface of the portio and processes setting out from the cervical channel are distinguished.

In the late decades frequency of the CIN increases according to the statistics. The incidence can be observed in younger and younger age. It is of the utmost importance that the treatment should not be more radical than it is necessary, but at the same time the treatment should remove surely the morbid tissue-portios.
In the cases when morbid epithelia was observed on the surface of the portio in the zona B we performed vaporization in connection with the control examination.

Principles of the laser vaporization
-The total lesion must be visible by means of a c lposcope.
-The total transitional zone must be viewed.
-The pointed biopsy taken from the lesion must prove that the lesion is not an invasive one.

— The CIN should not extended into the cervical channel.

Technique of the laser vaporization

- The total transformation zone including of course the morbid area too is drawn round.
- A power density of 750-1000 W/cm^2, a power of 20-25 W and a spot diameter of 2 mm are applied. The vaporization is performed up to a depth of 8-10 mm and in a width of 12 - 14 mm.
- In order to avoid closing of the path of the radius due to the blood or the tissue liquor flowing down the intervention starts from the direction of 6 o'clock.
- In order to avoid dangerous heat-effect the laser radius is driven quickly over the tissue to be removed in this way the wound-base remains suitable for histological examination.
- In order to avoid formation of wrinkle the radius should be driven in x, y and z directions.

The result will be a cathedral-shaped scar with straight edges, arched peak and a wound-base of smooth surface. The depth of the tissue destruction is of crucial importance too. Considering that injury of the cervical crypts in the dysplastic process can extend up to 6 mm distance from the surface /for non-invasive cases/, the vaporization should be performed at least up to this depth. The recidivation of CIN is in inverse ratio to the depth of the tissue destructions.

Depth of vaporization	CIN I recovery ratio	CIN II recovery ratio	CIN III recovery ratio
2 mm	50 %	14,3 %	9,8 %
5 mm	80 %	70 %	66 %
6-7 mm	100 %	91,7 %	88,5 %

The case is considered recidivation if after at least two negative colposcopic and cytologic diagnosis atypical cells are found after expiration of 12 months from the operation. The recidivation must be distinguished from remaining of tumor. In our examination we observed recidivation in 4-5 per cent of the cases. The literature reports the same ratio. The laser vaporization makes the ambulant treatment of the CIN possible. It is a rapid method, suitable for the patient and keeping conditions mentioned above it is a safe method. The early and the late complication is few.

In the cases when the lesion extends into the endocervical channel conization by CO_2 laser and cylindro excision respectively is performed.

The CO_2 laser conization is recommended in the following cases
- the colposcopic lesion extends into the endocervix but its upper edge is visible
- there are differences between the results of the cytology, the colposcopy and the biopsy
- sample to histological examination is needed.

Technique
- the demarcation line of the atypical epithelia is determined by Schiller's probe
- a ball catcher is placed transversally in the direction of 12 o'clock
- the stitches for arresting the bleeding are made in the direction of 3 - 9 o'clock
- infiltration by POR-8 solution
- in case of a laser held in hand a circular cut of 1 - 2 mm is made. The focal distance of the lenses are 50 - 125 mm, the spot diameter is 0,1 - 0,5 mm. The lateral distance should be at least 6 mm from the axis of the cervical channel.
- in case of a laser device built-in togethet with a colposcope the focal distance is 300 - 400 mm
- under use of smoke suction by power density of 1000 - 2500 W/cm^2 the morbid portio is cut conically
- a tissue section of 10 - 20 mm depth is removed, the axis of which passes in the middle of the cervix longitudinally.

The tissue section includes the external orifice of the cervix and a part of the endocervical channel in a length of 10 - 20 mm.

In the cases when the lesion extends to more deep, its upper edge is not visible or the histological results of the excision is more serious than the same for CIN I, so called cylindrical excision is performed by CO_2 laser instead of conization.

The volume of the cylinder is larger threefold than that of the cone. It is of very good efficiency in cure of all stages of the CIN.

The appropriate height of the cylinder is 18 - 20 mm from the external orifice of the uterus considering that generally the cervical intraepithelial lesions extend up to 10 mm depth into the cervical channel and only seldom extend to 20 mm.

Taking the aforesaid location of the CIN and its 5 - 6 mm lateral extension into account the significance of the cylindrical excision comparing to the conical one is understood. Namely at conization of lesion in such a height it can happen that cervical crypts containing morbid epithelia remain on the area of the peak of the excision.

Technique of the cylindrical excision
- the ectocervix is marked by a circle of 6 mm diameter
- pincers are placed at 6 and 12 o'clock, for larger areas to be excised at 3 and 9 o'clock
- pulling downwards the tissue section by means of the devices the surgeon drives the laser radius according to the mark
- after reaching the required 18-20 mm depth the tissue cylinder is removed at its upper pole by means of a scalpel
- the wound-base is vaporized.

Morbid tissue can remain only due to the following reason:
- the dept of the excision was not enough and morbid tissue remained in the channel
- the diameter of the marking circle was less than 6 mm and cervical crypts remained.

In our practice when cylinder excision is performed, in every case after removal of the cylindrical tissue section in a diameter of 6 - 8 mm and in a width appropriate to the ectocervical extension of the lesion respectively we vaporize in a depth of 6 mm. The cylinder shaped excision together with cathedral-shaped vaporization result a cowboy-hat form tissue-defect.

By this intervention besides keeping function of the organs close on a 100 per cent result can be achieved for CIN III too.

Recovery of the CO_2 laser conization and the cylinder excision respectively
- the 48th hour   erythema, rich flux, the necrose tissue is extruded
- the $48-96^{th}$ hour   coloured, purulent flux
- the $96-144^{th}$ hour   definite contout hollow covered with fibrin
- the $7-8^{th}$ day   the flux ceases
- the 10th day   intensive cuticularization can be seen
- the 14th day   the total surface is covered with a thin cuticule
- the 21st day   new platecellular cuticle can be observed
- the $28-35^{th}$ day   mature platecellular cuticle

Inthe cases when during period of 10-14th day the rate of cuticularization was not sufficient, in order promote recovery of the wound a biostimulation treatment was applied by means of a low-power He-Ne laser device according to the following description.

The extent of the operation performed by CO_2 laser determines the number of fields of the treatment. One treatment field was always 1 cm^2. The device was placed in such a distance from the patient that the the irradiation area according to the intended treatment field, taking the angular divergence of radius into account, was 1 cm^2. In our case the distance was 124 cm. The power density of the radiation got on every field was 1 J/cm^2. This power, taking the loss into consideration, was sent on an average during 3,5 minutes.

According to our experiences the low-power laser treatment speeded up effectively the recovery of wound. On the basis of earlier biochemical experiments performed by professor Kovacs in connection with He-Ne laser treatment of benignant epithelia lesions of the orifice of the uterus this kind of recovery process can be explained as follows.

The in vitro laser irradiation of the portio tissue segments got from a fresh operative preparation and followinng this determination of the protein biosythesis taking place in the tissues proved that the tissue segments covered with two kinds of epithelia /platecellular cutis or cylindro-cellular one/ rect to the irradiation in different way. The intracellular protein biosynthesis of the segments covered with platecellular cutis slightly increases while that of the segments covered with cylindrocellular cutis decreases by 50 per cent. Simultaneously the synthesis of proteins excreted from cylindrocells significantly decreases too. This reaction of the cylindrocells well explains shifting of pH of the vagina to acidic direction on effect of laser radiation as biosynthesis of cylindrocells of the ectopia decreases and the alcaline excretion will be less. The normalizing pH conditions stimulate further division of the plate epithelial cells.

In our opinion the results got from the above-mentioned biochemical experiments with increase of biosynthesis of the platecellular cutis well explain the favourable effect of biostimulation applied in the operational post-treatment.

Immediate, Short- and Long-Term Effects of CO_2 Laser Therapy on Cervical Epithelium

J.H. Faktor, E. Avram

Gynecological Cytology and Colposcopy Unit
Beilinson Medical Center, Petah Tiqva, Israel

In memory of the late Dr. A. Schachter

The management of benign and premalignant cervical lesions by CO_2 laser therapy has been widely discussed in the literature, but until now, few have described it in terms of cytological changes.

The present study was done with the purpose of following cellular modifications immediately after the application of the laser beam on a cervical lesion and during the healing process.

MATERIAL AND METHODS

From a consecutive series of 426 patients, cytologically, colposcopically and histologically investigated, 30 cases were selected for this study: 15 women with benign lesions (ectropions, vaginal discharges), and 15 with CIN 1 + 2 .

Cytological specimens under colposcopical control were obtained from 5 women before, immediately after, and 1, 2, 6, 12 and 24 hours after therapy. For all other cases cyto-colposcopical follow-up was scheduled at one week intervals for the first 3 months.

As short-term cellular changes, we considered those which characterized the smears during the first 4 weeks after treatment, and long-term cellular changes, as the entire healing process till the 12th week, the end of the study.

Any glandular tissue uncovered by mature squamous epithelium or CIN diagnosed by cytology, colposcopy or histology, more than three months after treatment was considered persistent disease or treatment failure.

RESULTS

In the 5 women in which smears were obtained during the 24 hours after treatment, certain criteria were used in order to assess the immediate cellular modifications. The target tissue is entirely destroyed and covered by carbon particles. Bizarre squamous and glandular cells were seen, even one day after treatment.

TABLE 1. **IMMEDIATE EFFECT OF LASER BEAM ON CERVICAL EPITHELIUM**
(0 - 24 hours)

CELLULAR FINDINGS	HOURS AFTER TREATMENT					
	IMMEDIATELY	1	2	6	12	24
CELLULAR DEBRIS	+++	+++	+++	+	+	-
CARBON PARTICLES	+++	+++	++	-	-	-
LEUKOCYTES	-	-	±	+++	+++	+++
ERYTHROCYTES	-	-	-	+++	+++	+
BIZARRE SQUAMOUS CELLS	-	-	±	+++	++	+
ELONGATED GLAND. CELLS	+	+	±	-	-	-
CYTOPLASMIC CHANGES	-	+	++	++	++	+++
NUCLEAR CHANGES	-	-	-	-	+	++

During the first 4 weeks after treatment, degenerative changes comprise: cytoplasmic vacuolization, bichromasia, large nuclei and cell distortion. Cellular reactions to the inflammatory process, such as perinuclear halo, binucleation and karyorrhexis, were present in 82% of the smears. Immature squamous metaplasia, as an initial healing process, was already found in 50% of the smears at the end of the second week post-treatment. Complete covering of the vaporized areas of the uterine cervix by mature squamous epithelium required 5 to 8 weeks in 95% of smears.

TABLE 2.
CELLULAR MANIFESTATION OF THE HEALING PROCESS AFTER CO_2 LASER THERAPY

CELLULAR FINDINGS	WEEKS AFTER TREATMENT							
	1 - 2		3 - 4		6 - 8		10 - 12	
	No.	%	No.	%	No.	%	No.	%
DEGENERATIVE	17	58	13	42	-		-	
INFLAMMATORY	16	52	9	30	4	13	2	5
IMMATURE SQ. MET.	15	50	14	45	2	5	-	
MATURE SQ. MET.	2	6	19	63	8	27	2	5
NORMAL EPITHELIUM	-		5	17	19	63	4	13
PERSISTENT DISEASE	-		-		-		2	7

As "persistent disease" we regard only the presence of immature metaplastic cells or columnar cells on the exocervical smear at the end of the follow-up.

DISCUSSION

The geometric configuration of the laser defect was described as a crater with Gaussian profile. The smears of the focal target tissue show, as expected, total necrosis. The distorted squamous cells and the elongated glandular cells, found even in the early smears, may represent the thermal effect of the laser beams on the surrounding tissue, as already suggested by Holmquist et al (1).

The short and long-term cytologic changes express the obvious response of cervical epithelium to the destructive action of heat, repairing and regenerative processes. The immature and mature squamous metaplastic cells were taken as parameters of the healing process. We saw initial healing one week after, and complete healing in 95% of cases in 5-8 weeks after laser therapy. This timing is consistent with other observations (1-4).

The cytologic follow-up during the first three months revealed a large spectrum of atypia, which was mainly related to benign regenerative processes. However, assessment of an underlying CIN process by cytology is unsatisfactory due to the mentioned atypia. Thus we adhere to Gondos and Ostergaard's opinion for cytological follow-up to commence at 3-6 months after treatment (5).

The healing process at the cellular level appears to be rapid and the damage to the adjacent tissue is minimal. There is general agreement as to the cytocolposcopical follow-up during the 2 years after treatment at three-month intervals, while the confirmation for a neoplastic process must be done cyto-colpo-histologically.

REFERENCES

1. Holmquist ND, Bellina JH, Danos ML (1976). Vaginal and cervical cytological changes following laser treatment. Acta Cytologica 14(7):386-9.

2. Bellina JH, Seto YY (1980). Pathological and physical investigations into CO_2 laser tissue with specific emphasis on cervical intraepithelial neoplasma. Lasers in Surgery & Medicine, 1:47-69.

3. Stafl A, Wilkinson EJ, Mattingly RF (1977). Laser treatment of cervical and vaginal neoplasia. Am J Ob Gyn 128:128-36.

4. Carter R, Krantz KE, Hara GS, Lin F, Masterton BJ, Smith SJ. Treatment of cervical intraepithelial neoplasma with the carbon dioxide laser beam (1978). Am J Ob Gyn 131:831-6.

5. Gondos B, Ostergaard DR (1973). Evaluation of cervical signs after cryosurgical treatment of CIN. J Reprod Med 11:68-73.

Treatment of Condylomata Acuminata by Means of CO_2 Laser

A.Bartsch, L.Kovacs
Dept. of Gyn. and Obst. of Hungarian
People's Army
MN 1. Katonai Korhaz
H-1525 Budapest

The condylomata acuminata is one of the most wide-spread sexual diseases. The pathogen is a DNA virus, the verruca vulgaris virus namely the human papilloma virus counted to the papova viruses (papilloma virus), that is known as the only member of papova viruses that is pathogic for human beings.

A certain inclination is required to coming into being of the infection caused by the human papilloma virus. Depending on the locatiotion of the sticking, the local circumstances (e.g. maceration by caused by hyperidrosis or fluor vaginalis) and the momentary immuno-status on different patients, sometimes on the same patient but on other skin area, the infection can produce different disease appearances those are called infectious epithelioma or acanthoma as well.

On the basis of the clinical appearance the following alternatives are distinguished: 1. verruca vulgaris, verruca plantaris, 2. verruca plana juvenilis, 3. condylomata acuminata.

Our lecture deals with the latter form occuring more and more frequently in the practice of women disease.

The papillomatosis caused by the human papilloma virus develops first of all in the epithelia soaked by the rich vaginal flux on the sexual organs and around the anus.

In 30-50 per cent of the cases a gonorrheal flux and in 50-70 per cent other origin one produces conditions of penetration of the virus. The gravidity as well as taking oral anticoncipients are predisposing factors.

In case of experimental inoculation the incubation period is approximately four months (1 - 20 months). The infection can be transmitted on the one hand in direct way (auto-inoculation and hetero-inoculation) and on the other hand in indirect way (collective bath and clothes, etc.) too. In our practice transmission of the infection most frequently occurs by sexual contacts.

In differential diagnostic aspect it should be distinguished from the condyloma latum (hypertrophized syphilisos papula) and the spinocellular carcinoma (this latter sits on a wide base, massive, occures at old people, quickly ulcerates).

Isolated, upwards widening, soft, reddish-brown tumors sitting generally on a thin, peduncle-like halve form. If the go dry their surface will be rough, massive and greish-white. Their size is variegated namely 0,15 mm to 100 mm. From time to time they unite into a cauliflower-like mass. On the surface of the large vegetations there necrosis easily develops and secondary bacteriologic superinfection can occur. Under the lobed and slashed surface bacteria will increase and smelly, purulent secretion will form. The numerous lesions taking place from time to time make the patient unsuited for the normal life-functions. Pruritus, bleeding, flaming feeling and pain will appear causing often urination and motion complaints. Schmauz,R.(6) reported that it was necessary hospitalize to empty the bowels only in narcosis. The urination complaints were solved by catheterization.

For years different agents have been tried for stopping the disease, e.g. Podophyllin of 20 per cent, trichloroacetic acid as well as freezing and electrocoagulation have been tried as well. These kinds of methods were painful and the recidivation was frquent. In addition to it on account of teratogenous effect of Podophyllin it was not permitted to administer in the first 12 weeks of the pregnancy. Considering localisation of the occurence the healing following the electrocoagulation and the cryotherapy caused serious problems; for women around the vaginal orifice, in the vagina, on the inner surface of the vaginal labium, on the perineum; for men on the inner lamella of the prepuce, in the sulcus coronarius.

Kovacs and Bartsch used a Hungarian surgical CO_2 laser device type TLS-60 for treatment of condylomal lesions. Their results came from treatments performed by vaporisation technique. 108 patients have been treated, all of the patients were woman. Of course prior to the first treatment for all patients careful examination of the vaginal secretion, if it was necessary bacteriological vegetation and according to it treatment of the vagina was performed.

After the first treatment sixty-three patients, 58 per cent of the cases, recovered. By three or more (maximum 5) treatments all the patients recovered. The patients were recalled after the lapse of 1, 2, 6, 12 and 18 months following the last treatment. Considering that from

time to time the incubation period of the virus is very long the
patients were regarded as recovered after 18-month symptomless.

The treatment was repeated altogether in 45 cases (42 per cent).
in 13 cases at two control examination following the first traetment
a further treatment was indicated because of local recidivation.
4 cases were recognized at the one month control and 9 cases at the
two-month one. Local recidivation was observed exclusively on the
perineum, around the vaginal orifice and after treatment of the lesion
located perianally.

In 32 cases because of a lesion macroscopically invisible at the
first treatment we repeated the laser treatment. These lesions were
recognized till the end of the third control examination namely till
the end of sixth month following the operation.

Thus in the cases when more than one treatment was applied, local
recidivation in 29 per cent of the cases and macroscopic lesion
previously invisible in 71 per cent of the cases necessitated the
repeated treatment.

At treatment of lesion of the **vulva** and perineum Procain was used as
anaesthetic. At treatment of complication-free lesions on the surface
of the portion anaesthesia was not needed.

In 35 cases condylomatic lesion was observed on the portion. Then
excision was performed prior to vaporization for histological examination. In three cases a lesion appropriate to CIN II. and in four cases
a lesion appropriate to CIN I. was in the histological finding.
Recently several researchers that there is a connection between the
HPV and the CIN, i.g. Baggish,M.(1),Colkins,J.W.(3),Reid,R.(5) and
Schmauz,R.(6).
Scott(7) treated 94 patients for condyloma. 83 per cent of the patients
were woman. 79 per cent of the patients suffered from chronic condyloma
with at leat a two-year anamnesis. For 37 patients excision was performed from lesion on the cervix. For 11 patients (11 per cent of the
cases) CIN II. was experienced.
In the material of Kovacs and Bartsch in 20 per cent of the condyloma
lesions observed on the cervix a histological lesion appropriate to
the CIN in the surroundings of the condyloma was experienced. In these
cases of course vaporization operational technique usual for epithelia
lesions of the portio was applied.

There were two pregnant women too among the patients got to treatment because of condylomatic lesion of the vagina. Later both pregnant women bore a child in vaginal way without complication.

Results

58 per cent of the patients recovered after the first traetment, but all patients recovered by three or more treatment. The patients were recalled for controll after 1, 2, 6, 12, and 18 months. The most frequent complication was the vaginal flux, in 18 per cent of the cases. Hospitalization and catheterization was not needed. It was not necessary to stop administration of anticoncipients. Of course of the partner should not be omitted as without this recovery will be hopeless.

Literature

1. Bagish,M.:CO_2 laser treatment for cond.acum. veneral infections. Obstet.Gynecol. 55/6 711-715., 1980.
2. Baggish,M.:Treating viral venereal infections with the CO_2 laser. J.Reprod.Med. 27/22. 737-742., 1982.
3. Colkins,J.W.:Management in cond.acum. with CO_2 laser. Obstet.Gynecol. 59/1. 105-108., 1982.
4. Hahn,G.A.:CO_2 laser surgery in treatment of condyloma. Obstet.Gynecol. 141/8. 1000-1008., 1981.
5. Reid,R.: Genital warts and cervical cancer. Evidence of an assotiation between subclinical papilloma virus infection and cervical malignancy. Cancer 50/2. 377-387., 1982.
6. Schmauz,R.:Condyloma acuminata and their possible relation to canceér of the uterine cervix. Case report and geographic observ. Acta Cytol. 27/5. 533-539., 1983.
7. Scott,R.S.-Castro,D.J.:Treatment of condyloma acuminata with CO_2 laser. A retrospective study. Lasers In Surgery And Medicine. Vol.4/2. 157-163., 1984.

The Use of Contact Laser Probe in Gynecological Endoscopy

J. Keckstein, A.S. Wolf, R. Steiner
Universitäts-Frauenklinik Ulm
Prittwitzstrasse 43, 7900 Ulm, FRG

Of the many lasers that have been used in surgical fields 4 have been introduced into gynecology: the CO_2, the argon, the Nd:YAG and the KTP-laser. Each of these lasers has a specific wavelength and thus different effects on the tissue.

In our hospital we started using the CO_2-laser in the beginning of 1986. Because of its specific properties we introduced also the contact Nd:YAG-laser.

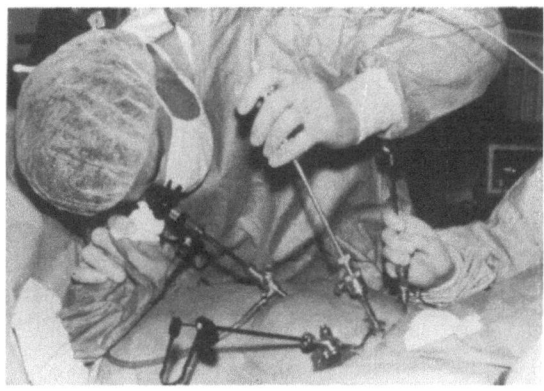

Fig. 1.

The operations are carried out with a Wolf laparoscope, a videa camera attached to.

Through the second, third and fourth puncture site we introduce the forceps, the scissors and the optical laser fiber. A special instrument with a movable tip improves the application of the laser by better guiding and manipulation of the optical fiber. The power density of the MBB-YAG laser ranges from 5 to 25 Watts. The SLT contact laser probes which are attached to the optical fiber by a connector are cooled with CO_2-gas or saline-solution.

Applications of Laser in Laparoscopy

UFK ULM

	CO_2	Contact	Nd:YAG
- Neosalpingostomy	X	(X)	(5)
- Salpingostomy	X	X	(15)
- Lysis of subovarian adhesions	X	X	(32)
- Vaporisation of myomas	X	X	(5)
- Abl. of lig. sacrouterinum	X	X	(5)
- Resection of lig. sacrouterinum	(X)	X	
- Resection of cysts and hydatids	X	X	(3)
- Treatment of polycystic ovarian syndrome	X	X	(3)
- Endometriosis			(7)
			75

Fig. 2.

X = operation possible with this laser

Until now we have used the ND:YAG contact laser in 75 patients. For different applications various shapes of the probes have been used: The conical, chisel, flat or rounded probe.

- 32 patients with postinflammatory <u>adhesions</u> underwent this contact laser laparoscopy. The adhesions were incised with low power density. The unwanted damage to healthy tissue was minimized. The precisely controlled focal point enables us to free the tube, the ovary or the bowel. Due to the flexibel fiber and the movable tip of the probe we get possibility of an operation technique like in microsurgery. Bleeding from bigger vessels can be stopped by coagulation with the rounded or chisel probe. Lysis of adhesions and coagulation of small vessels are done by the conical probe.

- <u>Distal tubal</u> occlusions could be opened in 5 cases. The "flowering" technique for the neosalpingostomy with the defocused CO_2-laser beam can also be done with the flat contact probe and low power density.

- 5 <u>uterine leiomyomas</u> were removed with the conical probe. Small fibromas were vaporised with the chisel probe. After removal of the leiomyomas hemostasis with the chisel or flat probe was achieved.

- <u>Ovarian cysts and hydatids</u> were treated in 3 patients.

- 7 cases of endometriosis could be treated. Especially very small implants can be vaporized or coagulated very precisely with the contact probe.

- The ablation or resection of the ligament sacrouterinum were done in 5 patients suffering from dysmenorrhea or unexplained chronic pelvic pain.

- The performance of ovarian wedge resection was the traditional treatment of polycystic ovarian syndrom, with the disadvantage of postoperative adhesions. Until now we have treated 3 patients endoscopically by opening the cysts and coagulation of the hormon producing cells with the contact probes. After this operation we achieved a decrease of the serum androgens and a higher ovulation rate.

- 15 tubal pregnancies could be operated with minimal tissue damage and preservation of the tube (figures below).

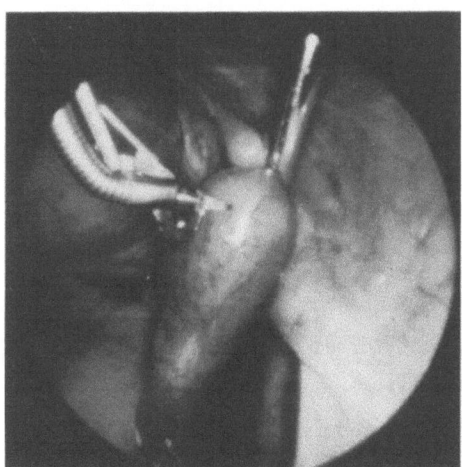 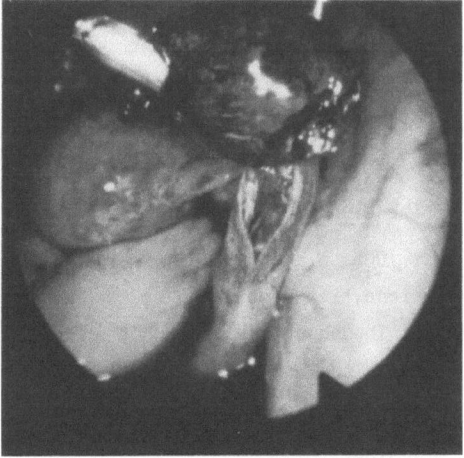

Fig. 3a. Salpingotomy with the laser contact probe in tubal pregnancy
Fig. 3b. Removing of the trophoblast

In summary

The advantages of this technique are:
1. The possibility of a more precise operation
2. Minimal tissue damage in comparison to the CO_2-laser
3. A very low complication rate

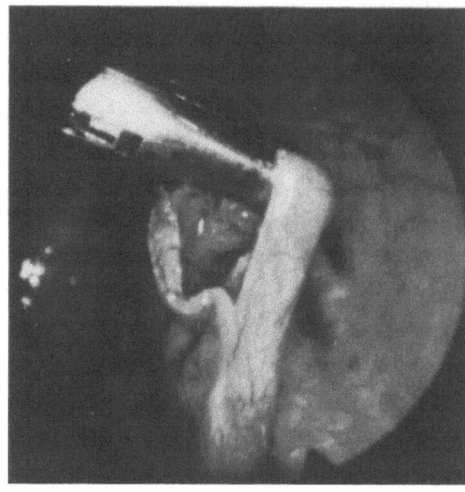

Fig.3c. Situs after operation: precise incision, no bleeding, complete conservation of the tube

4. No infection or postoperativ bleeding
5. Less smoke production
6. Less power requirement
7. Less backscattering
8. More mobility due to the flexible optical fiber
9. Less morbidity and faster recovery time

The disadvantages are:

1. Due to our limited experience and various technical problems we noticed tissue sticking to the probe.
2. Though the probe cannot break it may be deformed by power density being too high or by insufficient cooling system.
3. The changing of the probe during the operation is very time consuming.

Conclusions

We found that the contact Nd:YAG laser endoscopy has proved to be a safe and helpful procedure in gynecological surgery. To show the difference in outcome compared with other endoscopic procedures, a second-look laparoscopy should be performed. Literature by the author.

The Nd: YAG Laser Sapphire Tip in Reproductive Surgery, a Preliminary Report

D. Wallwiener, A. Morawski, D. Pollmann, G. Bastert/D

The CO_2 laser is used for several indications in operative laparoscopy. Many authors reported the advantages of CO_2 laser preparation. The open abdominal surgery with the use of laser is easy and relatively safe. The endoscopic operations-talking about the laser endoscopy we mean laser laparoscopy and laser hysteroskopy - in many cases are technically difficult, especially if rigid instruments are used. The main problem is the danger of damaging the neighbouring organs. It is also important to note the high costs of CO_2 laser equipment.

The recently developed "in-touch" technique of Nd: YAG-laser with sapphire contact probe allows using this laser system as a light scalpel.

Boodless cutting effect of the sapphire tip results from vaporisation and coagulation at the same time when using Nd YAG non-touch technique we can observe only esagulation.

We started with our research program wishing to find the answer to the question whether Nd - in - touch laparoscopy is the alternative method to CO_2 laser laparescopy. The main points of this study are the tissue effect by contact probe, the possibility of in-touch adhesiolysis and the laparoscopical application modes.

We are using Nd YAG laser - mediLas 40 N from MBB - which has integrated cooling system and is very stabile in low power range.

As we know, the power density results from relation between power output and spot size. In the case of contact tip technique the diameter of spot size is the same as the diameter of the tip of sapphire probe.

On the basis of our experiments performed on uterine horns of rats, we found the optimal cutting effect and the minimalized tissue damage in a power range of 15 watts per sec.
The cooling of the sapphire tips is possible by gas or liquid.
As the first, preclinica step for laparoscopical application of the sapphire tip we conducted several experiments on mini pig in order we find the optimal handling and optimal power range as well as to determine safety conditions.
In these experimets we applied a maximal energy on the sapphire tip without cooling and we have seen only overheating, but have never observed an explosion, or jump out of piece of sapphire tip.

For the laparoscopical clinical operations means of sapphire tip we have 3 various application modes.

1st: Single puncture laparoscope with a working chanel for the flexible light guide;
2nd: the rigid endoprobe for the second or third puncture for operations on organs relatively easy to reach;
3rd: we are studying actually the possibility of application of flexible instruments through second puncture. For this purpose we use the flexible Olympus hysteroscope with working chanel for the flexible fibre of Nd YAG laser.

The further experimets were conducted to find out whether the intraperitoneal adhesiolysis by means of contact technique gives comparable operarable operative results with those of CO_2 laser adhesiolysis. The laser adhesiolysis was performed on rats with artificially induced adhesions.

The ND YAG contact laser technique brought comparable results to CO_2 laser adhesiolysis.

As a result of experience gained in these procedures, 20 patients underwent operative laser laparoscopy by in-touch technique.

The following laparoscopical operations were performed: adhesiolysis, salpingo-oyariolysis, salpingostomy, salpingotomy (early tubal pregnancy).

In the cases of laparoscopic laser reproductive surgery no technical difficulty was noted and the procedure was bloodless by a sufficient coagulation effect.

The advantages of this method are: excellent handling by flexible fibres, precision of preparation and sufficient haemostasis, low risk of damaging other organs and comparable results to CO_2 laser adhesiolysis.

In spite of good operative results in the first second-look laparoscopies, the follow-up period of the cases is too short and the number of patients too low to enable us to reach any definite conclusions regarding the advisability of this technique, but we can affirm the procedure is relatively simple and safe and offers promise for the future.

Sapphire Tip in Treatment of Recurrence of Breast Cancer, of the Vulva and Tumor Reduction

A. Morawski, D. Wallwiener, G. Bastert/D

The CO_2 laser surgery in primary radical an palliative treatment of breast cancer and cancer of the vulva is recognized, since many years, as established method of treatment in several centres of the world. In the last two years, employing the new developed laser technique, we worked out in our research centre in the University of Saarland, further indications. We are using two surgical laser systems, CO_2 laser and Nd:YAG laser, for primary and secondary treatment of breast cancer and cancer of the vulva and, in the last period, for palliative surgery of recurrences of ovarian cancer. The comparison studies on mice (Lewis Loung carcinoma) are very well-known, and the results show indisputable superiority of CO_2 laser tumor excision over conventional cold knife surgery. In our own studies we compared additionally the results of CO_2 laser excision with the excision of the new developed Nd:YAG laser contact technique. We found out that the survival rate in both groups is similar. On the basis of our clinical studies we worked out following indications for the treatment of local recurrences of breast cancer:

By multiple, disseminated superficial metastases with a diameter of each less than 3 millimetres we are doing vaporisation by means of CO_2 laser with a power density of approximately 1500 watts/square centimetre.

In the next group, with subcutaneous mobile metastases we excise a tumor by means of CO_2 laser or Nd:YAG laser contact technique.

In the last group, with big immobile local recurrences, even in preirradiated area, we coagulated the tumor by means of Nd:YAG laser non-contact technique. The following pictures presenting examples of each situs.

The first one: disseminated skin metastases after CO_2 laser vaporisation, the second one: situs after Nd:YAG laser non-contact coagulation.

The next two pictures show, on the left side, excision by means of CO_2 laser and, on the right side, excision with sapphire tip.

On the basis of our clinical experience we found out that the Nd:YAG laser with both techniques (contact and non-contact) is more universal in secondary treatment of breast cancer, but for the primary treatment, the CO_2 laser still plays a very important role. In treatment of cancer of the vulva we are using the laser for radical vulvectomy, palliative vulvectomy, as well as for the treatment of local recurrences.

As a first example I would like to present a palliative vulvectomy in a 90 years old woman with a big exophytic cancer of the vulva. The operation, done by means of CO_2 laser was almost bloodless and we reached very rapid primary healing of the wound. Even in cases without primary closure of the wound, the secondary healing was very good.

As comparison of two laser systems in treatment of local recurrences of cancer of the vulva, I would like to present an example of a 79 years old woman. 10 years after primary vulvectomy with, let us say, "permanent local recurrences", a CO_2 laser vaporisation was done the first time. And we observed within a very short time a new recurrence. Second time, we used Nd YAG laser non-contact technique. A high power coagulation was successful as presented in the next picture.

In several cases we have done excisions of local recurrences by means of CO_2 laser or Nd:YAG laser contact-technique. Here we found a superiority of Nd:YAG laser contact-technique, especially in the cases, where tumor was unfortunately located very near to urethra or anus.

The new indication in the gynecological oncology which I would like to present, is a much promising application of sapphire tip for intra abdominal palliative reduction of the tumor mass, especially in recurrences of ovarian cancer.

Unfortunately, the follow-up period is too short for final evaluation of this new technique, but I believe that first clinical experiences authorize to note several advantages. They are: less traumatic procedure, oncological sterilisation of the wound bed, lower recurrence rate, minimal bleeding, high operative precision, possibilities of more aggressive intra abdominal surgery and good wound healing.

Nd: YAG Laser Sapphire Tip in Operative Hysteroscopy – A Preliminary Report

A. Morawski, D. Wallwiener, G. Bastert
Universitäts-Frauenklinik, D-6650 Homburg (Saar)

The subject of my report is contact laser technique in operative hysteroscopy. It is my opinion that this newly developed laser technique will play a very important role in future operative hysteroscopy. To make my point clear I would like at the beginning to recall the known indications for operative hysteroscopy. They are: septa, synechia, polyps, myopas and, as fifth indication, bleeding, in my opinion, impossible to treat by means of conventional methods. At present we have following methods for intrauterine surgery: for conventional methods we can use sharp cutting instruments often combined with electrocautery. The instruments are: known in urology resectoscopes and electrosurgical cutting loop. To exclude the danger of insufflation of CO_2 in blood vessels we have to use during operative hysteroscopy liquid distension medium, for example, Hyskon or 5% glucose with continuous or interrupted flow. All hysteroscopists know exactly how uncomfortable is this technique. Because of danger of bleeding the conventional operative hysteroscopy requires very often vasoconstrictors; for proper coagulation we need the electrosurgical unit with a power of 50 watts. A possibility of transcervical intrauterine operation eliminates in many cases the need for an extended abdominal operation.

The other advantage of operative hysteroscopy is the use simple and inexpensive instruments. Still, we can't forget several problems connected with the conventional operative hysteroscopy methods: first of all, danger of bleeding, then the great tissue damage by electrocautery, the uncomfortability because of fluid distension medium and the necessity of using the intrauterine balloon as precaution against intrauterine adhesions.

As mentioned above, the treatment of bleeding is impossible by means of conventional methods. It is, however, possible since 1980, since the time when Milton GOLDRATH performed his first Nd:YAG laser

vaporisation of endometrium by excessive bleeding. The number of
patients undergoing permanent marcumar therapy is steadily increasing.
In this group operative high risk cases, laser hysteroscopy is the
method to choose. In our clinic we are using a MediLas 2 Nd:YAG
laser with a maximum power of 110 watts. The Nd:YAG laser - vaporisation of endometrium is performed under following conditions: the
5% glucose plays a double role, first as distension medium and second
as a cooling system. The laser light guide has a diameter of 0.9 mm,
therefore, we need a flexible or rigid instrument with a working
channel of 1 mm.

Most of the operations were performed with the average power range
of 60 watts. It is a painfree procedure and because of that general
anaesthesia is not required. We noted the following advantages of
Nd:YAG laser: non-contact irradiation gives very deep and wide tissue
defect. That is the reason why in many cases we can observe something similar to ASHERMAN syndrom. On the one hand, in this way we
can successfully treat the uterine bleeding, on the other, very precise and accurate preoperative histological diagnosis must be reached
to exclude endometrium carcinoma and his further uncontrolled and
silent growth.

This excellent method of treatment of excessive bleeding is contraindicated in young women in reproductive age because of, as demonstrated, big tissue damage. The recently developed Nd:YAG contact
technique allowed to use this laser-system for the first time as a
light scalpel. The tissue damage was minimal. In our clinic we are
using the Nd-YAG laser with the sapphire tip for following indications:
intrauterine septum where the cutting is very precise and we should
also note the absence of bleeding; even very wide and long intrauterine septum can be removed in one session. The operation takes
very short time. It is also an excellent method for treatment of
intrauterine synechia. We observed also very good handling and good
results in cases of pendiculated myomas; the removal of submucous
myomas with a wide basis is questionable because of very big endometrium defect.

In these cases, precise coagulation of blood vessels is probably a
better method. The operation of endometrium polyps is very easy by
means of sapphire tip. The conditions of laser contact hysteroscopy:

the light guide has a diameter of 1.2 mm and, therefore, we can use
flexible or rigid instruments with a working channel of 1.3 mm. This
condition is fulfilled in, for example, Olympus flexible hysteroscope
with a diameter of 5 mm. With this laser technique we can use for
the first time the CO_2 as a distension medium; since the sapphire tip
at the same time cuts and closes the blood vessels, there is no danger
of insufflation unit. Only in this way it is possible to control properly the intrauterine pressure and the flow. All our operations we
reconducted with a normal flow of pressure. The CO_2 is insufflated
through the laser light guide and plays a double role: on the one
hand, as a distension medium, on the other, as cooling for the
sapphire tip. Because of normal gas flow we have to limit the applied
energy - the used energy was between 6 and 9 watts, which means we
were working in low power range. For this reason we selected the
newly developed MediLas 40 N which is very stable in this range.
Because of safety we performed the physical, chemical and toxycological analysis of the sapphire tip. The results authorize us to say
that safety conditions were fulfilled. Regarding our material:
We have done operations of septum with the sapphire tip in 4 cases,
in 2 cases operations of synechia, also 2 cases of myoma, and in one
case we performed an operation of endometrial polyps. For evaluation
of this method we performed control hysteroscopy in 6 cases and we
found normal uterine cavity in all of them. 2 of our patients are
pregnant and till now we have no complications. To sum up the advantages of the newly developed Nd-YAG laser hysteroscopy by means of
sapphire tip: we can use CO_2 as distension medium, the technique is
very precise and it is a bloodless procedure. We observed easy
handling because of the possibility to use flexible instruments. We
hope that it will be possible to employ this technique as outpatient
procedure.

Histological Differences in the Tissue Effect; As well as the Healing Process After the Uterotomy Performed on Rats with the Use of CO_2 Laser (Sharplan 1060) – Super-Pulsed Wave Versus Continuous Wave

D. Wallwiener, A. Morawski, R. Damböck, G. Bastert

The recently developed CO_2 laser technique, the electronically superpulsed CO_2 laser beam shows until now unknown abilities of tissue preparation. In this study, we would like to present our first results of experiments performed on rats comparing tissue defect, thermal injury of tissue and healing process after incision of uterine horn by superpulsed and continuous-mode. We used CO_2 laser Sharplan 1060.

This unit can operate in both CW and pulsed modes with rated peak power outputs ranging up to 500 W, maximum pulse repetition rates (PRR) up to 990 pps, and PW ranging from 0.1 to 0.9 ms. CW power outputs extend from a low to 1 W to a maximum of 60 W.

Laser surgery was carried out as follows

The uterine horns were exposed in the presented way. The uterotomy was performed by means of a laser microscanner, fixed on an operation microscope, for electronically drived laser beam, with a focal lens of 30 mm and a spotsize diameter of o.53 mm.

The velocity of motion of laser beam by microscanner was kept accurately constant.
3 variations of sp mode (2, 4,8 W/sec) were compared with the same number of cw settings.

Of the animals undergoing horn incision, ten were immediately sacrificed, ten lived for 2,5,7,14 and 21 days, then were sacrificed.

All study tissues were freshly removed after in-viva perfusion by BOUIN solution. After fixation tissue was blocked in Metacrylat and stained with RACHINOW-GIEMSA (WITTEKIND) solution.

Tissue defect and zones of injury were calculated with the use of double-headed light microscope coupled to Interactive Digital Analysis System (IDAS Kontron).

It is a versatile image analysis system that derives measurements and statistics from images traced on a digitizing tablet. When interfaced to a computer, this system allows for multiple parameters to be measured and accurately calculated electronically. A computer printout translates these measurements into quantified data. The wounds and the areas of necrosis were tabulated in square millimeters.

RESULTS

1. Tissue defect or wound

The typical "super-puls-wound" in lower power range is as presented with an indented cut edge and finger-shaped off-shoots from the zone of necrosis with the greatest indication of thermal damage at the wound base. The typical "super-pulse-defect" in higher power range is funnel-shaped. The "continuous-tissue-defect" is TUP-SHAPED.

2. Calculation of necrotic zone

The calculations of the areas of necrosis show average values with increasing of damage zone corresponding to power range for both settings (sp + cw). The calculated difference between square millimeters of damage between comparable average power settings is significant in the area of the wound base. A 3 time reduction in the area of thermal necrosis occured when sp was substituted for cw.

3. Healing

In relation to healing progresses, the early prolonged healing of "sp-wounds" is compensated by faster healing of " sp. wounds" later on.

DISCUSSION

The results of this study are comparable to results of other authors especially to the investigations of BAGGISH.

In relation to comparison of sp and cw mode of CO_2 laser, it was hypothesized that superpulsing would allow cooling of tissue between each pulse and diminish necrosis. They very high peak power attained would diminish laser time on tissue, thereby reducing peripheral heat damage.

But, interestingly, we can show that the geometric pattern of the wounds by means of sp-wave mode in several power ranges, lower power range on the one hand and higher power range on the other hand, are completely different.

CONCLUSION

In conclusion, we can say that sp-wave mode in significantly diminishing tissue defect and tissue injuring, but the most important fact is the correct choice of power range for this application mode of CO_2 laser.

In further studies we should like to present the completes results of super-pulsed CO_2 laser tissue effects.

Complementary Laser Application in Gynaecology

U. Herrmann
Charité-Frauenklinik, Laserabteilung
Schumannstr. 20/21, 1040 Berlin, GDR

Partially the application of CO_2 laser surgical method is of a complementary character, i.e., the application of CO_2 laser surgery forms an essential part of the operation process or the spectrum of surgical methods of the type of operation respectively. The reason for the essential nature has to be seen in the special effect of the CO_2 laser beam on certain tissue. The complementary character, however, consists in the limitation of the CO_2 laser surgical effect as far as the whole complex of methods used in a certain type of operation is concerned. The complementarity of the CO_2 laser surgical method consists in its alternating effect with the electro-micro-surgical, micro-surgical and macro-surgical method.

The tables show the following types of operation as far as the complementary application of CO_2 laser surgical method is concerned: ovariolysis, salpingolysis, adhesiolysis, salpingostomy, isthmo-isthmical tubal anastomosis, tubo-cornual anastomosis, utero-tubar implantation, ovarioplasty, uteroplasty, conservative intervention in case of ampullar pregnancy.

<u>Ovariolysis</u>

In carrying out the ovariolysis the CO_2 laser surgical operating step consists in eliminating massive and tightly sticking adhesions on the ovary surface by laser vaporization (fig. 1). The complementary scheme of methods consists in applying laser-micro-surgical, electro-micro-surgical resp. micro-surgical methods. On 35 patients both sides ovariolysis with complementary CO_2 laser surgical application were carried out. The rate of success of this procedure was found out 6 - 18 months post operationem by laparoscopy and was of 89 %.

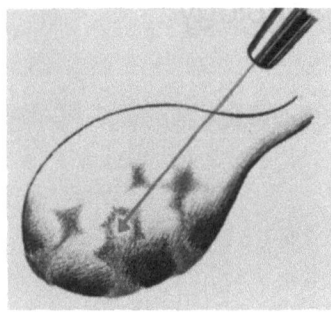 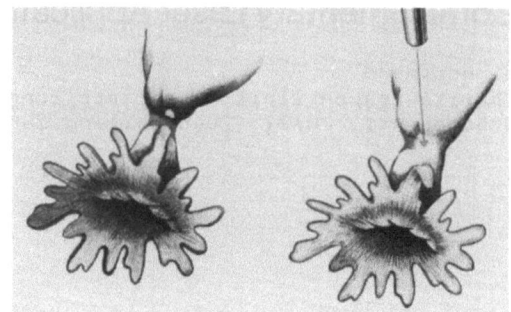

Fig. 1.   Fig. 2.

fig. 1. CO2 laser surgical operating step in cases of ovariolysis

fig. 2. CO2 laser surgical operating step in cases of salpingolysis

Salpingolysis

The complementary CO2 laser surgical operation step in the case of salpingolysis consists in eliminating strictured tightly sticking adhesions on the tubal surface (fig. 2). The complementary method scheme corresponds that of the ovariolysis. On a total of 22 patients salpingolyses of this type were carried out. The criterion of a successful intervention was to set tubes free, which was examined 6 - 18 months post operationem by laparoscopy. The rate of success was of 91 %.

Adhesiolysis

In the case of adhesiolysis the complementary CO2 laser surgical intervention consists in disconnecting vascularised adhesions. The whole complex of methods consists in utilizing laser-micro-surgical, electro-micro-surgical and micro-surgical methods respectively. On a total number of 41 patients adhesiolysis were carried out in this way. The proof of the rate of success was done indirectly by examining the colour of the liquid sucked of the drainage which was put on the intraperitoneal area intra operationem. The rate of success was 81 %.

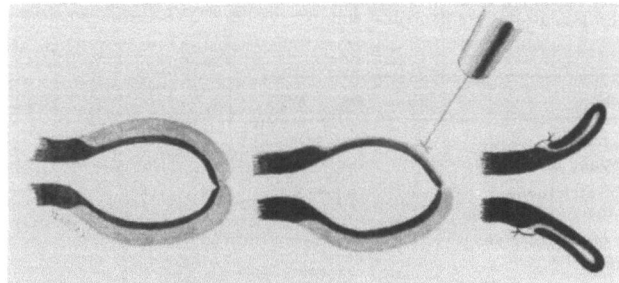

fig. 3. CO2 laser surgical operating step in cases of salpingostomy

Salpingostomy

In carrying out the salpingostomy the complementary CO2 laser surgical operation step consists in the massive ablation of the fibrotically modified tubal wall of the eventration area (fig. 3). The different types of methods comprise laser-micro-surgical, electro-micro-surgical or micro-surgical methods. The rate of success of the CO2 laser surgical application was found out by laparoscopy 6 - 8 months post operationem with 78 %. The criterion was a remaining eventration effect.

Isthmo-isthmic tubal anastomosis

The complementary CO2 laser surgical operation step in the case of isthmo-isthmic tubal anastomosis, consists in a partial radiar incision of the tubal wall in the framework of resectio tubae. The whole scheme of methods is based on laser-micro-surgical, electro-micro-surgical and micro-surgical method respectively. A total number of 45 patients underwent this operation. The success rate was found out by laparoscopy and salpingography 6 - 12 months post operationem. It was of 89 %.

Tubo-cornual anastomosis

The complementary CO2 laser surgical operation step in the case of tubo-cornual anastomosis consists in laying open the locked part of the intramural tubal area. The complex of methods is the same as in the case of the isthmo-isthmic

Tab. 1. Types of operation, laser surgical interventions, complementarity of laser (micro)surgical, electro (micro)surgical, microsurgical and macrosurgical methods

operation	ls intervention	ES	mS	MS
ovariolysis	vaporization of massive adhesions on the ovary surface	+	+	−
salpingolysis	vaporization of stricturing adhesions on the tubal surface	+	+	−
adhesiolysis	disconnection of vascularised adhesions (type B)	+	+	−
salpingostomy	ablation of fibrotically modified tubal wall of the eventration area	+	+	−
ithmo-isthmic tubal anastomosis	incision of the tubal wall (resection tubae)	+	+	−
tubo-cornual anastomosis	laying open the intra-mural tubal area	+	+	−
utero-tubal implantation	tunnelling of the uterus wall	+	+	+
ovarioplasty	vaporization of endometriose centres	+	+	−
uteroplasty	vaporization of myomas (diameter up to 5 mm)	+	−	+
conservative intervention in cases of tubal pregnancy	coagulation of the placenta placenta bottom	+	−	+

(ls - laser microsurgical, ES - electro microsurgery, mS - microsurgery, MS - macrosurgery)

tubal anastomosis. Tubo-cornual anastomoses of this kind were carried out on 18 patients. There was a success rate of 72 %, found out by salpingography 6 - 18 month post operationem, the tubes showing a normal passing through capacity.

Utero-tubal implantation

The complementary CO_2 laser surgical operation step in the case of utero-tubal implantation consists in the tunnelling of the uterus wall (fig. 4). The methods comprise laser-micro-surgical, electro-micro-surgical, micro-surgical and macro-surgical application. 8 patients underwent this operation. The control of the results was carried out by salpingography. In 86 % of the cases a free passing through of the tubes was achieved.

Ovarioplasty

As far as the ovarial endometriosis is concerned, the complementary CO_2 laser surgical operation step consists in eliminating the endometriosis implants

Tab. 2. Laser (micro)surgical interventions, the number of patients, methods to prove results, criteria and rate of success

Is intervention	number of patients	proof	success rate
vaporization of massive adhesions on tubal surface	35	laparoscopy	free ovary surface: 89% (30)
vaporization of stricturing adhesions on the tubal surface	22	laparoscopy	free tubal surface: 91% (20)
disconnecting of vascularized adhesions	41	redon drainage	light-coloured liquid of drainage 81% (35)
ablation of the fibrotically modified tubal wall of the eventration area	9	laparoscopy	constant eventration effect 78% (7)
incision of the tubal wall	45	laparoscopy salpingography	free tubal permeability 89% (40)
laying free of the intramural tubal area	18	salpingography	free tubal permeability 72% (14)
tunnelling of the uterus wall	8	salpingography	free tubal permeability 86% (7)
vaporization of endometriose centres in the ovary	7	laparoscopy	constant ovary dimension 100 % (7)
vaporization of myomas (diameter less than 5 mm) in the myometrium	9	laparoscopy hysterography	constant dimension of the uterus and cavum 78% (7)
coagulation of the placenta bottom in cases of ampullar pregnancy	8	salpingography	free permeability, free of residuous parts 100% (8)

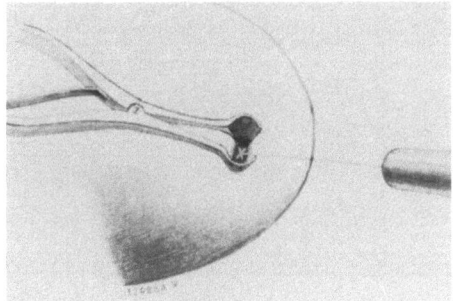

fig. 4. CO_2 laser surgical operating step in cases of utero-tubal implantation

within the ovarial tissue. Laser-micro-surgical, electro-micro-surgical and micro-surgical methods are applied. This operation was carried aut with 7 patients. The control of the results was made 12 months post operationem by laparoscopy. The criterion was the constant dimension of the ovary. There was a rate of success of 100 %.

Uteroplasty

The complementary CO2 laser operation application in the case of the uteroplasties with uterus myomatosus consists in eliminating myomas with a diameter up to 5 mm. The methods consist in laser-micro-surgical, electro-micro-surgical and macro-surgical application. The operation was made on 9 patients. The control of the results was carried out by means of laparoscopy and hysterography 9 - 12 months post operationem. The criterion was the constant dimension of the cavum and the corpus. The rate of success was 78 %.

Conservative intervention in cases of tubal pregnancy

The complementary CO2 laser surgical intervention with the conservative technique consists in the coagulation of the placenta bottom. Methods are the laser-micro-surgical, electro-micro-surgical and macro-surgical intervention. The operation was carried out on 8 patients. The control was made in the form of salpingography and ß-HCG-determination. There was a success rate of 100 %.

Clinical Experience of CO_2 Laser Treatment of Vaginal and Vulval Diseases

W. Albrich, A. Götz, H. Hepp, K. Richter, W. Waidelich
Department of Obstetrics and Gynecology,
Klinikum Großhadern, University of Munich,
Marchioninistr. 15, D 8000 München 70, FRG

Introduction

In recent years the laser has become a very useful tool for the treatment of different gynecological diseases.
In condylomata acuminata of the vulva, the vagina and the cervix CO2-laser radiation is the treatment of choice because of the low recurrence rate and the rapid and nearly scarless healing.

In the United States, the increasing incidence of HPV induced dysplasia of the vulva, vagina and cervix in young women first led to the search for conservative operating procedures.
Many authors experienced good results with the CO2-laser vaporisation of intra-epithelial neoplasias of the lower genital tract, whereas the intrauterine and intraperitoneal laser treatment is still in an experimental stage; as is hysteroscopic coagulation of the endometrium, laparoscopic vaporisation of peritoneal endometriotic implants or laser therapy of tubal sterility.

Patients and treatment

We have been using the CO2-Laser for the treatment of different diseases of the vulva and vagina since 1981 (Table 1). The incidence of condylomata acuminata and intra-epithelial neoplasia of the vulva in our department is low. Twenty-six patients had 27 procedures because of condylomata acuminata, 5 patients suffered from different benign diseases of the vulva such as fibroma, hemangioma etc. Six patients with carcinoma in situ of the vulva had 7 operations. Due to the diagnostic dilemma of laser vaporisation we have not yet treated cervical intra-epithelial neoplasia.

In contrast to the literature we have used the CO2-laser in treating invasive carcinoma of the vulva, as well as in selected cases of other malignant tumors e.g. melanoma or metastases of cervical and endometrial carcinomas.

Table 1.
Indications for CO2-laser treatment

Disease	N° of procedures	N° of patients
Condylomata acuminata	27	26
other benign diseases	5	5
Ca in situ vulvae	7	6
invasive carcinoma of the vulva	36	33
other malignant tumors of the vulva and vagina	9	9
	84	79

Table 2.
CO2-laser vulvectomy in patients with invasive carcinoma

	N° of patients	age range years	average age years
primary treatment	30	34 - 83	70.6
treatment of recurrences	6	43 - 82	65.0

From 1981 to 1985, 36 patients with invasive carcinoma of the vulva were treated by CO2-laser resection (Table 2). Thirty patients had primary therapy. Six procedures were performed for recurrences, 3 after different primary therapies in other clinics, 3 were failures after laser treatment in our department.

The youngest patient was 34 years, the oldest 83 years old. The average age in the group with primary therapy was 70.6, in the group with recurrences 65 years.
The age distribution demonstrates the well known fact that most patients present in the seventh and eight decade (Figure).

The staging was based on the histopathological examination (Table 3). Nine patients had tumors of under 2cm diameter, 16 had larger tumors.

Table 3.
Stage of disease of patients primarily treated
by CO2-laser vulvectomy for invasive carcinoma:

local tumor stage	N° of patients	Metastatic involvement of inguinal lymph nodes	N° of patients
T 1	9	N 0	19
T 2	16	N 1	2
T 3	5	N 2	6
		N x	3
	30		30

In 5 patients the tumor reached the urethra, vagina or the anus.
In 19 patients the regional lymph nodes were free of disease, 8 patients had uni- or bilateral groin metastases. In 3 patients the inguinal lymph nodes were not resected because of reduced general condition.

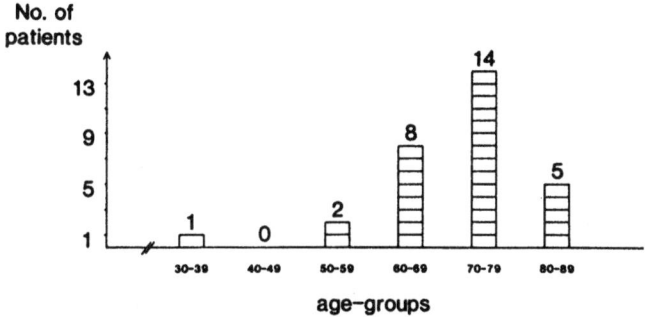

Figure. Age distribution of patients primarily treated by
CO2-laser vulvectomy for invasive carcinoma (n=30)

Procedure

Our procedure of laser vulvectomy is based on the electroresection method described by Berven and Weghaupt: Firstly the vulva is resected by the focused CO2-laser beam. That way, the specimen is available for histologic examination. After vulvectomy the wound is coagulated by the defocused laser beam.

The specific laser effect leads to a visible shrinkage of the wound reducing postoperative hemorrhage. Healing occurs by open granulation. The patient carries an indwelling urinary catheter for 10 to 14 days. After that time the patients can be discharged. Complete re-epithelisation usually takes about 6 weeks.

Results: (Table 4)
After a follow up of between 7 and 59 months, 17 patients remained free of local diseases. Four patients suffered from local recurrences. One patient died tumor related, 3 patients died of unknown cause and another 3 of different diseases. Three patients were lost to follow up.

Table 4.
Results of primary CO_2-laser therapy in patients with vulva neoplasia

Follow up	N° of patients	length of follow up mths	Median follow up mths
free of local disease	17	7 - 59	31
local recurrences	4	9 - 42	20
died of recurrence	1	23	--
died of unknown cause	3	1 - 42	14.5
died of other disease	3	5 - 27	18
lost to follow up	3	--	--

Discussion and conclusion
In our experience the CO_2-laser shows advantages and disadvantages in the treatment of invasive vulva neoplasia when compared with other surgical procedures:

The healing period is shorter than after electroresection of the vulva. The local tumor control is comparable with the latter method (KUCERA, 1980) or with radical vulvectomy (BARTHOLDSON et al., 1982; CALLIES et al., 1984) in our limited experience of only 30 cases. Disadvantageous are the extended operating time, and the high cost of the laser equipment.

The most important and disappointing complication was often a troublesome stenosis of the vaginal introitus. Possibly the coagulation of the vulva after resection causes this embarrassing outcome.

Summary

Report on 84 gynecological Co2-laser operations performed for condylomata acuminata (27), benign tumors of the vulva (5), preinvasive carcinoma of the vulva (7) and malignant tumors of the vulva and vagina (45).
Of 30 patients with invasive carcinoma of the vulva 17 were free of local disease, 4 suffered from local recurrences and one died tumor related. The CO2-laser vulvectomy needs an extended operating time compared with electroresection. A troublesome complication is the tendency to stenosis of the vaginal introitus. The healing period is shorter than after electroresection. The local tumor control is comparable to that after electroresection or radical vulvectomy.

References

Bartholdson, L, J. Eldh, E. Eriksson, L.-E. Peterson:
       Surgical Treatment of carcinoma of the vulva.
       Surg. Gynec. Obstet. 155 (1982) 655

Berven, E.: 117 Fälle mit primärem Vulvakarzinom
       Acta radiol. 22 (1944) 99

Callies, R., U. Kock , G.X. Zeller, U. Sickmann, U. Schulz,
H. Ludwig: Behandlungsergebnisse beim Malignom der Vulva,
       eine retrospektive Analyse an 119 Fällen.
       Zbl. Gynäkol. 106 (1984) 440

Kucera, H.: Die Behandlung des Vulvakarzinoms an der I. Universitäts-Frauenklinik Wien (386 Fälle)
       Strahlentherapie 156 (1980) 598

Weghaupt, K.: Elektroresektion und Elektrokoagulation als Therapie des Vulvakarzinoms.
       Fortschr. Med. 96 (1978) 1629

Laser Technique for Non-Surgical Female Sterilization and Reversal of Sterilization by Tissue Welding

E. Lachman, A. Shulman, C. Bahari, D. Aravot, S. Giler, I. Kaplan, D. Sagie, J. Kagan, Y. Kalisky

An attempt to develop a new, simple, safe and effective non-surgical method of sterilization and a possible way of reversing this procedure was made using the Holmium Laser technique.

The need for a non-surgical, safe method has come from couples who have completed their family circle in both the western societies and the third world communities. Hulka has estimated that 600,000 female sterilization procedures are performed annually in the United States alone. From this high figure it is estimated that 1-2% of these patients require reversability of their operation.

At the moment there are four main ways of performing sterilization:

a) Via the abdomen.
b) Via the laparoscope.
c) Via the vagina.
d) Via the hysteroscope.

The first three procedures require hospitalization, theater time, trained personnel and obviously are expensive and therefore limited.

The fourth type is tubal occlusion by chemicals like silicon, quinacrine hydrochloride or methyl cyanoacrylate, that are placed in the fallopian tube ostium, through the uterine cervix with the guidance of an hysteroscope, or an intra-uterine contraceptive device.

This last procedure is an office procedure and is done under paracervical block anesthesia. The main disadvantage of this technique today is the failure rate and the need of highly qualified personnel. In the case of an experienced hysteroscopist we can expect to succeed in placing bilateral effective plugs in 85% of patients (Houck and Cooper).

Here is our report on animal experiments using the Holmium Laser with a view to developing a new non-surgical method of tubal sterilization. The Holmium Laser emits a wavelength of 2.1 microns. This mid infrared beam falls between the neodymium: YAG (1.06 microns) and the CO_2 (10.6 microns; both of which are well established today as lasers with clinical applications. Based on measured data of light interaction with several organs through the relevant spectrum - the Holmium Laser has the advantages of both laser: cutting almost like a CO_2 laser and photocoagulating like the Neodymium:YAG laser. The other prominent advantage of the Holmium Laser is its ability to deliver this laser light through a standard commercial optical fiber.

In our experiments we took advantage of the wavelength and the fiber optic delivery potential. The experiments were run under two main subtitles. The first experiment was: Evaluation of the efficiency of tubes and cavities occlusion and blockage via the fiber optic laser energy transfer, examining also the flexibility of the fiber optic while progressing through the cavities with blind introduction. The second experiment was the evaluation of the efficiency of the tissue welding ability.

I) **Cavities and Tubes Occlusion Using the Penetration Ability**

These experiments were performed initially by a direct and open technique. We opened the research animal, identified the uterine horns, punctured them with a venflow and introduced the fiber via this route. At a later stage having gained experience with the fiber, we managed to introduce it "blindly" via a speculum through the bitch's vagina up to the uterine horn, (Fig. I) and perform the blockage at different sites (Fig. II). We have also used human uterii after removal due to benign conditions. The fiber was easily introduced through the human utero-tubal ostium to the tube in order to perform blockage at the mid-tube segment or the ostium. The first for possible future reversal of occlusion, the second for more permanent blockage, thus demonstrating the unique characteristics of this method of the Holmium Laser and showing its potential by operating with minimal invasion.

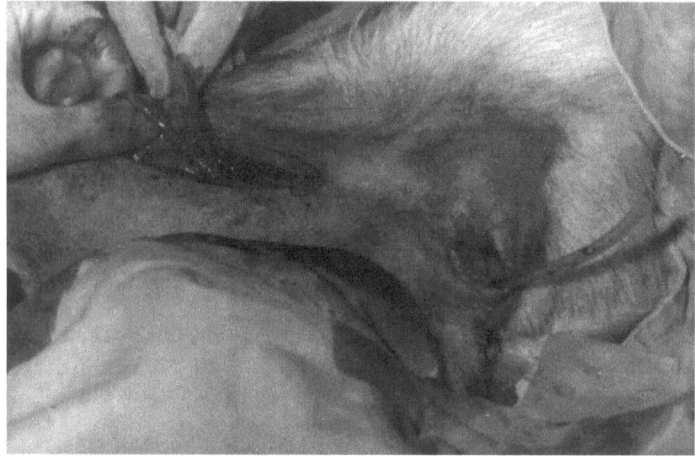

Fig. I. The fibre being introduced via the bitch vagina up to the uterine horn

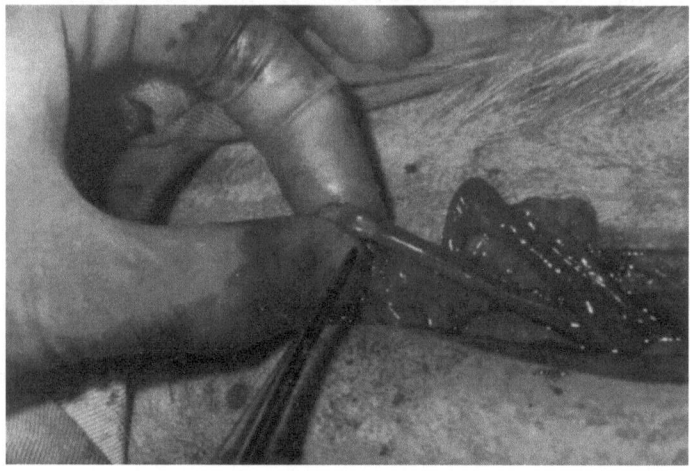

Fig. II. The uterine horn obstruction with the laser technique

II) **Tissue Welding Technique**

Experiments were performed mainly on the bitch's uterine horn as a model for the human tubes obstruction. The horns were cut with or without the removal of a short segment and then reanastomized. The first step was to introduce a fiber optic up to the discon-

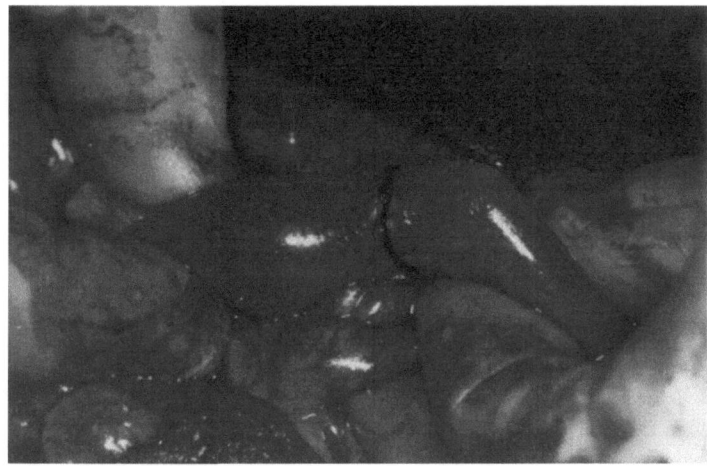

Fig. III. The uterine horn after the tissue welding

nected segment to act as a guide and to keep the cavity open, then two or three "holding stitches" were placed and the tissue welding technique commenced (Fig. III). All were rechecked up to 1 year by X-ray showing patency.

SUMMARY

In performing the above mentioned experiments we have managed to show three qualities of the Holmium Laser with the fiber:

I.   Flexibility and penetration.
II. Cavities obstructions.
III. Tissue welding.

In the fields of obstetrics and gynecology the message is clear. Tubal litigation is a highly effective contraception method, much in need in the western countries as well as in the third world population.

The reanastomosis technique in tubal reconstruction after sterilization can also take advantage of the Holmium Laser. Primarily the damage to the tube with laser use is very limited and that portion can be easily resected and the tube reanastomized. Obviously any other form of partially damaged tube can be removed and reanastomized by the tissue welding technique. Future considerations are unlimited including management of ectopic pregnancies, polycystic ovarian disease, etc.

Urology

Lasers in Urology – State of the Art

A. Hofstetter, Department of Urology, University of Lübeck,
Ratzeburger Allee 160, D-2400 Lübeck 1

15 years of experimental and clinical use of laser technology have the effect that lasers are not only known in urology but meanwhile firmly established in many sectors of this field (table 1). Moreover, there are new indications in diagnostics and therapy which have not yet exceeded the experimental state. (table 2/3).

Tumor destruction was worked out by our group experimentally from 1972 to 1976. Till today, we have treated more than 1500 patients with superficial and infiltrating bladder tumors by applying the Neodym-YAG laser. With this mode of treatment the local recurrence rate is remarkable low compared with the transurethral resection. This is presumably connected with the total, contact free destruction of the tumor-bearing vesical wall area by simultaneously sealing the blood and lymphatic-vessels (7,10). Apart from this, the excellent view during the endoscopic tumor coagulation should not be underestimated because there is no or only an unimportant bleeding.

Table 1. LASERS IN UROLOGY

Aim of treatment	Laser	Indication (sured)
a) Tumordestruction	Neodym-YAG	superficiale kidney- and Ureter-, Bladder-, Urethra-, Penile Cancer Tumors of the external genitalia
	Dye	superficiale Urinary Bladder Carcinoma
b) Lithotripsy	Neodym-YAG Dye	Ureter- and renal pelvical stones
c) Suppression of Inflammation	Neodym-YAG	Interstitial, radiogenic Cystitis

Prospective, controlled and randomized studies on bladder carcinoma also prove the superiority of the Nd:YAG laser over the transurethral resection (10). Here, it was clearly shown that the laser reduces the incidence of relapse rate and prolongs the recurrence-free intervals. The long term results of the so called "cystectomy cases" provide special proof of the efficiency of the Nd:YAG laser in the treatment of bladder carcinoma (Fig. 1).

Photodynamic therapy of superficial bladder carcinoma and carcinoma in situ is rich in promise according to the reports of BENSON, DOUGHERTY, JOCHAM and ROTHAUGE (1,4,12,15), included our own experience. In this context it should be emphasized that due to the photodynamic qualities of the laser there is a wide field of research for us in order to optimize the current procedures and to search for alternatives.

The application of the Nd:YAG laser in connection with prostatic cancer and superficial urothelial carcinomas of the upper urinary tract also showed amazing results as exemplified by BEISLAND (2) and our own experience.

Tumors of the exterior genitals - first of all condylomata acuminata and penis carcinoma - as well as tumors of the urethra also allow a satisfactory treatment with the Nd:YAG laser by saving the affected organs as far as possible (7,10,16).

Different groups in UK (WATSON), Austria (SCHMID-KLOIBER) and Germany (HOFMANN) are working in lithotripsy (6)

We have also been working on laser-induced shockwave lithotripsy LISL) since 1978. In the meantime we were able to develop two different methods - using the Q switched Nd:YAG laser and one employing a flashlamp pumped Dye laser (9,13). These methods constitute further steps forward not only in endoscopic urology but also in general endoscopy if one considers our results in stone destruction of bile- and pancreatic duct calculi.

The antiphlogistic and analgetic effect of the laser irradiation was demonstrated with patients having interstitial and radiogenic cystitis. These results were confirmed by SHANBERG and others (18).

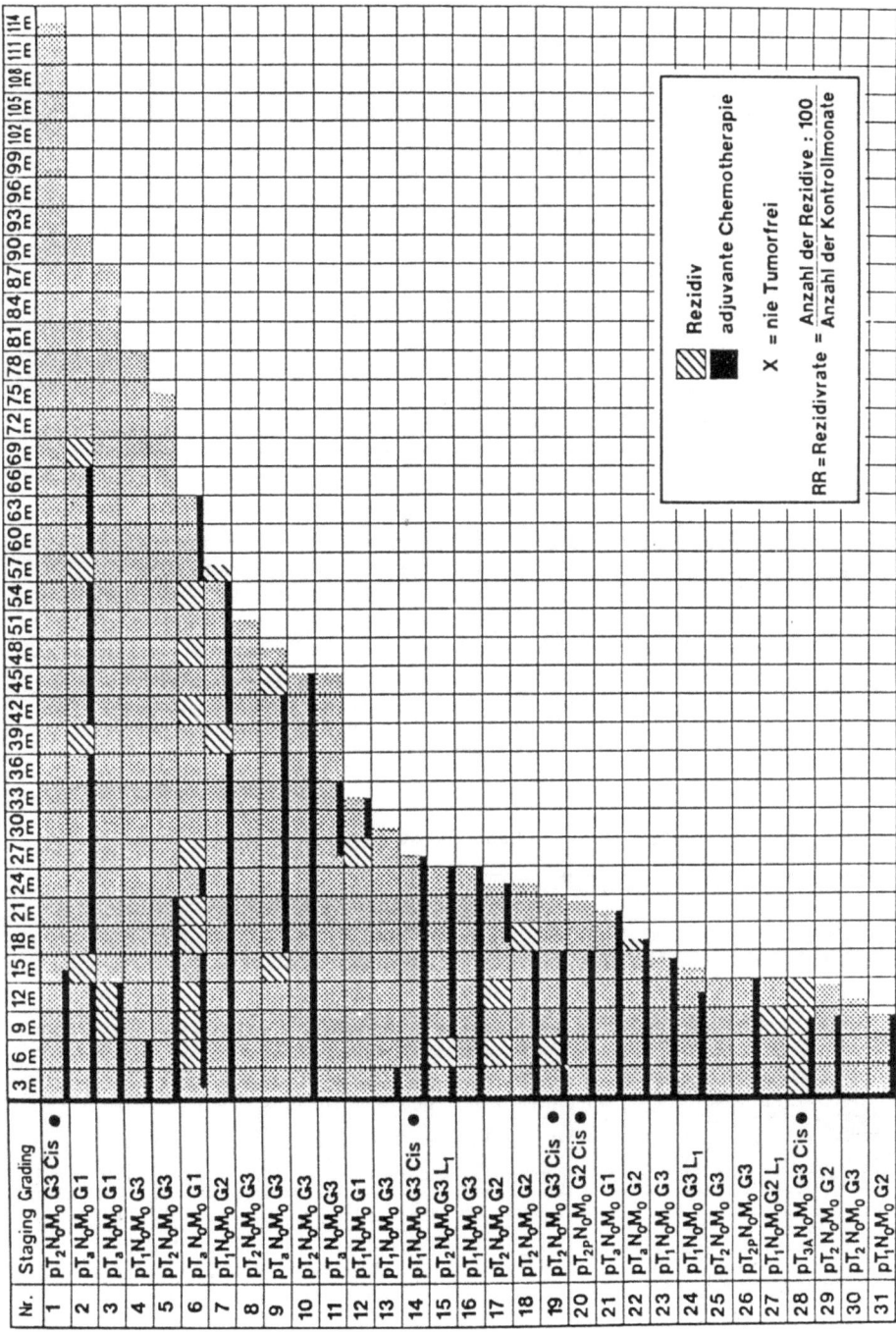

Fig. 1: Survival time after laser treatment of patients with bladder tumors, who refused cystectomy

These are in short the possibilities and results of laser application in urology, as it is considered and assured today.

Now we are testing (table 3) the significance of laser application in the recanalization of arteries, for instance renal and small pelvic arteries, with different thermal and non thermal methods.

Endoluminal ureteral occlusion combined with percutaneous urinary drainage is a possible palliativ treament for cloaca formation after pelvic tumor irradiation (14).

Table 3. LASERS IN UROLOGY

Aim of treatment	Laser	Indication (clinical trial)
a) Removal of Strictures	Neodym-YAG Argon CO_2	Urethra- and Ureter-strictures
b) Angioplasty	Neodym-YAG Dye Argon Eximer CO_2	Revascularisation (art. renalis, iliaca, obturatoria, penis)
c) Closing of Ureter	Neodym-YAG	Stopping Urine-Passage

ROTHAUGE (15) uses the Argon laser for the stricture removal. By virtue of its excellent cutting effect the CO_2 laser would preferably be qualified to split strictures. Flexible transmission systems for endoscopic application of this laser are in experimental use now. New solid state lasers with variable infra-red wavelenghts might combine advantages of both CO_2 and Nd:Yag lasers. The combination of the cold cut with the urethrotome and coagulation of the sectional edges with the Nd:YAG laser would also appear to be of value. The long lasting necrosis after Nd:YAG laser coagualtion could prevent the postoperative bouginages.

As far as diagnostical laser application is concerned we have up former experiments for the definition of tumor spreading in the bladder wall with the aid of interferometric holography (5) (table 2).

Table 2. LASERS IN UROLOGY

Diagnostic	Laser	Indication (Experiment Station)
a) Interferometric Holography	Rubin	Tumorinfiltration
b) Photochemical Processes	Dye	Cis-Recognation

Photodynamic proceedings cannot be used for the tumor destruction alone but also for identification of carcinomata in situ. These examinations, are of course still in the experimental phase; they are being reviewed and checked presently at the Medical Laser Center Lübeck.

I believe that this short summary of already established and possible future methods of using lasers in urology is interesting enough to find general attention and deserves to be carried on. Lasers are multi functional tools which in view of their physical characteristics are well qualified to open new ways in diagnostical and operative medicine.

In conclusion I should like to say that whatever may be technologically feasable at present and in the future we should nevertheless lose the sight for the relation between the makeable and the sensible.

Literaturverzeichnis

1.) Benson, R: Use of HpD in the Treatment of Neoplastic Diseases.
    Eur. Urol. 12: suppl. 1, (1986)

2.) Beisland, H., O., Sander, St.: Experience with treatment of localized prostatic carcinoma using the Nd:YAG laser.
    Eur. Urol. 12: suppl. 1, 37 (1986)

3.) Bőwering, R., Hofstetter, A., Keiditsch, E., Frank, F.:
    Irradiation of prostatic carcinoma by Nd:YAG laser.
    Optics Photonics appl. Med.: 211, 16 (1979).

4.) Dougherty, T., Gomer, C., Weishaupt, K.:
    Energetics and efficiency of photoinactivation of murine tumor cells containing hematoporphyrin.
    Cancer Res. 36, 2330 (1976).

5.) Grünwold, K., Vachutka, H., Hofstetter, A., Bőwering, R.:
    Interferometric investigations of the rabbit urinary bladder.
    In: Holography in Medicine and Biology,
    G.v. Bally, Optical Sciences, 18, Springer, Berlin, Heidelberg, New York (1979).

6.) Hofmann, R., Schütz, W.: Zerstörung von Harnsteinen durch Laserstrahlung
Urologe A, 23, 181 (1984)

7.) Hofstetter, A., Frank, F.: Der Nd:YAG Laser in der Urologie.
Editiones Roche, Basel (1979)

8.) Hofstetter, A., Böwering, R., Keiditsch, E. Frank, F.:
Zerstörung von Uretertumoren mit dem Nd:YAG Laser.
Fortschr. Med. 101, 625 (1983)

9.) Hofstetter, A., Frank, F., Keiditsch, E., Wondrazek, F.:
Intracorporale, laserinduzierte Stoßwellen Lithotripsie
Laser 1, 155 (1985)

10.) Hofstetter, A.: Treatment of Urological Tumours by Neodymium YAG Laser
Eur. Urol. 12: suppl. 1, 21 (1986)

11.) Hofstetter, A., Schmeller, N., Pensel, J., Arnholdt, A., Frank, F., Wondrazek, F.:
Harnstein Lithotripsie mit laserinduzierten Stoßwellen.
Fortschr. Med. 104, 654 (1986).

12.) Jocham, D., Schmiedt, E., Staehler, G.:
Laser photodynamic Therapy of Multifocal Bladder Carcinoma using Hematoporphyrine Derivative as a Tumour Photosensitizer.
XXth Congr. Soc. Urol., Vienna (1985)

13.) Pensel, J., Frank, F., Rothenberger, K.H., Hofstetter, A.:
Stone Destruction by Laser Application
Proc. 1th Congr. Intern. Soc. Laser Surg. and Med.
Tokio (1981)

14.) Pensel, J., Schmeller, N., Unsöld, T., Kriegmair, M., Hofstetter, A.:
Percutaneous Ureter Occlusion with Nd:YAG Laser
Laser 85 Opto Elektronik, München (1985).

15.) Rothauge, C.F., Röttger, P., Kraushaar, J., Nöske, H.D.:
Die Phototherapie des Blasenkarzinoms in Licht der Histologie.
Diagnostik, Intensivtherapie 8, 17 (1983).

16.) Rothenberger, K.H.:
Value of the Nd:YAG Laser in the Therapy of Penile Carcinoma.
Eur. Urol. 12, suppl. 1, 34 (1986).

17.) Schilling, A., Böwering, R., Keiditsch, E.:
Use of Nd:YAG Laser in the treatment of ureteral tumors and urethral condylomata acuminata.
Eur. Urol. 12, suppl. 1, 30 (1986),

18.) Shanberg, A.M., Baghdassarian, R., Tansey, L.A.:
Treatment of interstitial cystitis with the Nd:YAG laser
J. Urol. 134, 885 (1985).

Laser Assisted Urethrotomia Interna

A. Schilling, A. Friesen, R. Böwering
Abtlg. f. Urologie, Städt. Krankenhaus München-Bogenhausen
Englschalkinger Straße 77, 8ooo München 81, BRD

Unfortunately cold knife urethrotomy of urethral strictures has only a very limited succsess rate. Recurrences are seen in 5o to 7o % of the cases.
In order to improve our results we combined the cold knife incision with a debridement of the scar tissue by Nd. YAG laser coagulation.

Material an methods

Only male patients with 2 or more local recurrences of their urethral stricture during 12 month of observation after simple cold knife incision were admitted to this study (tab. 1). The strictures did not exceed more than 1 cm in length.
In 11 patients with an average age of 51,2 years (37 - 64 years) laser assisted cold knife incision of the urethral strictures was performed. The cold knife incision was done in a star- shaped manner. The sagittal Nd. YAG laser coagulation of the strictural scar tissue was done either before or after the cold knife incision using 4o Watts over a period of 2 - 4 seconds. A 24 F. silicone catheter was placed postoperatively for 24 hours.

Results

6 patients remained free of a recurrent stricture during the observation period (6 - 23 month; average 13,3 months).
Using the conventional treatment, 24 repeat surgical procedures were necessary in 132 patient- months. Using the combined treatment, only 6 repeat procedures were needed in 13o patient - months (tab. 1).

Table 1. pre- and post-op. recurrences as well as number of surgical procedures requised for stricture treatment

recurrencies during 12 mo.	total no. of preceding surg.proced.	observation after laser (month)	recurr. strict. after laser
2	3	6	∅
2	2	6	∅
2	2	8	∅
2	3	11	1 after 7 mo.
2	2	12	2 after 3 and 7 mo.
3	2	12	1 after 9 mo.
2	2	16	1 after 13 mo.
2	3	17	∅
2	2	18	∅
2	3	18	1 after 12 mo.
2	2	23	∅

Discussion

Treatment of urethral strictures using the CO_2 - laser was reported as well by ROTHAUGE (4) and BÜLOW et al (1) in 1979 as by CAMEY and LE DUC in 198o (2). However this method could not be established as an accepted treatment modality. Promising results using the Nd. YAG laser were reported by PEREZ- CASTRO and MARTINEZ - PINEIRO (3). Less enthusiastic experiences were mentioned later in 1984 by SMITH an DIXON (5). Since we believe that one of the reasons for stricture recurrence is the readhesion and closure of the excessive strictural scar tissue which was only opened by a linear cut, a debridement of this tissue combined with the urethrotomy should result in better results. From this point of view the use of a Nd. YAG laser should be superior to a CO_2 laser because of it's good tissue shrinking effect, whereas the CO_2 laser provides only a good cutting quality.

Moreover, Nd. YAG laser coagulation leaves the collagenions structures of the organ intact thus providing good conditions for the reepitheliasation (4).

Our preliminary results indicate the superiority of the combined treatment to the standard cold knife urethrotomy. Because of the promising results we feel the application of the laser assisted urethrotomy is justified in cases where more than one local stricture recurs in a short period of time. However the time of observation is too short to allow a final judgement of the value of this new treatment modality.

Summary

Cold knife urethrotomy was combined with laser coagulation of the strictural scar tissue. Because of its good tissue depletion effect the Nd. YAG laser was used instead of the CO_2 laser. In 11 cases with recurrent strictures 6 patients remained free of recurrencies during the follow-up period of 6 - 21 month. Before the combined treatment 24 surgical procedures had to be done in 132 patient-months, whereas with the combined treatment only 6 reinterventions were needed over a period of 13o patient- months. These preliminary results indicate a superiority of the laser assisted urethrotomy to the standard cold knife incision. However for a final judgement, more cases and a longer period of observation are necessary. We are convinced that, despite the improvements that this method may bring, urethral strictures will remain a major problem in urology.

Literature

1.) Bülow,H., U. Bülow, H.G.W. Fromüller: Transurethral laser urethrotomy in man: preliminary report; J. Urol Vol 121,3, 286- 287 (1979)

2.) Camey,M., A. Le Duc: Preliminary study of the action of the YAG laser on canine prostatic adenoma and experimental urethral stenosis; Eur Urol. 6, 175- 179 (198o)

3.) Pèrez- Castro,E., J.A. Martinez- Pineiro: El làser en urologia; Archivos Espanoles de urologia 6, 413- 422 Nov. u. Dez. (1981)

4.) Rothauge, C.F.: Possibilities of application of the laser in urology; in Laser Surgery III, proceedings of the 3 rd international congress for Laser surgery Graz 24-26, September 1979

5.) Smith, J.A., J.A. Dixon: Neodymium: YAG laser treatment of benign urethral strictures; J. Urol. Vol. 131,6, 1o8o-1o81 (1984).

6.) Stern,J.: J. Zimmermann, F.Frank, E. Keiditsch: Restitution der transmuralen Koagulationsnekrose nach Neodym YAG Laser-Bestrahlung, pp 129- 135, Zuckschwerdt, Munich 1983).

Contact Nd:YAG Laser Surgery in Urology

Eric J. Sacknoff, M.D., F.A.C.S.
Mount Auburn Hospital
300 Mt. Auburn Street, Cambridge, Massachusetts, U.S.A.

The Neodymium:YAG laser produces a 3-5 mm. depth of thermal damage in the bladder due to protein denaturation with preservation of mechanical stability of the bladder wall stroma.[1,2,3] Until recently the non-contact method of delivering laser light to the bladder, urethra and, on occasion, the upper urinary tract, has been the primary method of delivery. This non-contact technique may play a role in decreasing the rate of recurrence due to implantation.[4,5]

Contact laser probes have been made of a physiologically neutral, synthetic sapphire crystal which has mechanical strength, low thermal conductivity, and a high melting temperature at 2030-2050°C. These probes are used in direct contact with tissue allowing precise tissue manipulation with tactile feedback to the surgeon. The geometrical configuration of the probe determines whether primarily contact cutting or coagulation will occur. The contact probes deliver high power directly with reduced backscatter, allowing lower power of laser energy to be used. Whereas, non-contact urologic laser surgery equipment requires up to 50 watts of power to adequately coagulate, vaporize, and administer interstitial irradiation.

The aim of this equipment was to evaluate whether laser energy delivered via contact probes could produce an effect similar to non-contact laser energy on these tissues at lower power levels in the bladder and prostate of the dog. Light microscopy of the specimens was used to substantiate the penetration of laser energy in tissue at various dosimetry schedules.

MATERIALS AND METHODS

Cystoscopy under general anesthesia was performed on two male mongrel dogs weighing 55-65 lbs. Nd:YAG laser energy (Cooper LaserSonics, Model 8000, Santa Clara, CA) was delivered via a 0.6 mm. diameter quartz fiber through a 21 Fr. ACMI cystoscope sheath with an Albarron bridge to deflect the fiber light guide. A chisel-shaped contact laser tip (Surgical Laser Technologies, Malvern, PA) was connected to the standard optical quartz fiber using a universal metal connector.

An exploratory laparotomy was performed to expose the bladder, prostate and bulbous urethra. The urethra was surgically mobilized as far distally as possible to provide transurethral access with the cystoscope.

Areas of the dog bladder were randomly irradiated in vivo with 5, 10, 15, and 20 watts of Nd:YAG laser power at a 4-second pulse passed through the chisel probe in direct contact with the bladder mucosa. An irrigating solution at room temperature was used to maintain visual clarity and cool the interface between the quartz flow and the sapphire probe.

Nd:YAG laser energy was applied circumferentially to the right lateral lobe of the dog prostate with the chisel probe at 20 watts power in 5 second pulses to enlarge the prostatic urethral diameter. Well-defined areas of tissue destruction resulted as the tip of the probe was placed at precise points against the target tissue. No bleeding was encountered in either the bladder or prostate with the contact method. Immediately after laser photocoagulation, a cystoprostatectomy was performed. Dog bladder tissue samples at various power levels were placed in separate coded jars of 10% buffered formalin for histologic examination. Longitudinal and cross-sections of tissue were stained with hematoxylin and eosin and masson trichrome. The light microscopy was interpreted by an independent observer. Color photography was taken of all histologic specimens with a Leitz Laborlax 12 photomicrography system.

RESULTS

BLADDER: Microscopic examination of bladder irradiated specimens revealed increasing depth of penetration with increased power. The 4 second pulse duration was used one time only for each respective power level of Nd:YAG laser irradiation. Histologic section through the bladder revealed discrete areas of necrosis in the mucosa and lamina propria. In order to obtain necrosis in the muscularis layer, 20 watts power with a 4 second pulse was necessary. Coagulative necrosis was clearly present at all power levels with the greatest depth of damage being present at 20 watts power with a 4 second pulse. Only minimal thermal damage of the superficial bladder mucosa was found at 5 and 10 watts of Nd:YAG laser power. At all power levels, a well-defined homogeneous area of focal coagulation necrosis was seen at the site of contact between the probe and the adjacent tissue.

PROSTATE: The diameter of the prostatic urethra was slightly larger than the 21 Fr. cystoscope sheath, indicating an 8 mm. urethral diameter preoperatively. Resection of the right lobe of the dog's prostate was easily accomplished by making repetitive deep grooves in the tissue with the chisel probe. Enlargement of the diameter of the prostatic urethra was easily observed as the operation progressed on the right lobe. Blood loss could not be accurately measured but was minimal and, at no time, were any bleeding vessels encountered.

Following cystoprostatectomy, the transverse diameter of the prostatic urethra of each dog was measured from the mid portion of the intact left lobe to the opposite mid portion of the resected right lobe. After resection of the right lobe with the chisel probe, the postoperative urethral diameter increased from 8 mm. to 17 mm. and 18 mm. respectively

A 50% increase in the diameter of the prostatic urethral channel was obtained after resecting only one lobe. Histologic sections of the dog prostate demonstrated superficial coagulation necrosis of glandular tissue without deep areas of necrosis at 20 watts of Nd:YAG laser power at 5 second pulses.

DISCUSSION

The major use of the Nd:YAG laser is to treat small, superficial low-grade bladder tumors. The laser is also used palliatively in those patients with localized invasive bladder cancer unfit for radical cystectomy or external beam radiation therapy. Since 1976 the technique of endoscopic Nd:YAG laser surgery in the treatment of bladder tumors was non-contact. Dosimetry studies indicated that if the laser beam was moved slowly across the tumor at a power of 45 watts for 3 seconds, tumor coagulation was achieved to a depth of 3-5 mm. without perforation to the serosal surface. A characteristic blanching on the tumor surface indicated coagulative necrosis of the lesion. This non-contact method of tumor destruction is performed with the tip of the quartz fiber light guide approximately 3-5 mm. from the surface of the tumor. Whether non-contact techniques contribute to a decreased incidence of heterotopic recurrences remains to be proven.

The aim of this study was to examine the histologic effect of Nd:YAG laser energy on the dog bladder and prostatic tissue delivered through the contact sapphire probes. Light microscopic examination of the bladder showed a direct relationship between the depths of coagulation necrosis and power used. A well-defined, localized region of coagulation necrosis was achieved at the tip of the contact probe with only 20 watts power at 4 seconds' duration. This represents half of the conventional power of 40-45 watts used in non-contact laser bladder surgery. The precise placement of less laser energy at the target to achieve the same desired result produces less forward scatter and less chance of perforation or injury to the adjacent tissue.

The fact that contact laser surgery proceeded easily in a bloodless field made the use of the chisel probe in the prostate even more attractive. Histopathologic examination of the prostatic urethra showed a precise thermodestruction of the prostatic glandular tissue with excellent hemostasis at only 20 watts power with 5 second pulses. Resection and division of prostate tissue in a forward direction with the chisel probe of 1.8 mm. diameter was unusual for a resectionist accustomed to drawing an electrocautery loop from distal to proximal in a backward direction. Future changes in the geometrical designs of the contact probes into a scoop shape might thermocoagulate a larger volume of tissue in a shorter period of time.

SUMMARY

The sapphire contact laser probes provide the delivery of a high focus of laser energy within a target tissue at lower power levels. There was a relationship between depth of tissue damage and power levels in the bladder wall. The prostatic urethra was easily enlarged with the chisel-shaped probe (20 watts at 5 second pulses) without bleeding or deep necrosis of tissue. The prospect of transurethral laser resection of prostate tissue with complete hemostasis and shorter recovery time remains a distinct possibility.

1. Hofstetter, A., Frank F.: The Neodymium YAG Laser in Urology. Basel: Editiones Roche, F. Hoffman-LaRoche and Co., Ltd. pp. 24-30, 1980.
2. Staehler, G., Hallsdorsson, Th., Laugherhole, J., Bilgram, R.: Endoscopic Applications of Nd:YAG Laser in Urology: Theory, Results, Dosimetry. Urol. Res. 9:45-51, 1981
3. Stein, B.S.: Urologic Dosimetry Studies with the Nd:YAG and CO_2 Lasers: Bladder and Kidney. Lasers in Surgery and Medicine. 6: 353-363, 1986
4. Walzer, Y., Matheny, R. B., Blatnik, A.F., Soloway, M.S.: Urothelial Trauma-A Mechanism of Tumor Promotion? World J. Urol., 1: 100-102, 1983
5. Soloway, M., Masters, S.: Urothelial Susceptibility to Tumor Cell Implantation: Influence of Cauterization. Cancer, 46:1158, 1980
6. von Eschenbach, Andrew C.: The Neodymium-Yttrium Aluminum Garnet (Nd:YAG) Laser in Urology. The Urol. Clinics of No. America; 13:3, 381-391, August 1986
7. Sacknoff, Eric J. : Neodymium:YAG Laser in Urology. In Joffe, Muckerheide, and Goldman (eds.), New York: Elsevier Science Publishing Co., Inc. pp. 106-117, 1983
8. Smith, J. A., Middleton, R. G., Bladder Cancer. In Smith, J.A., Jr. (ed.) Lasers in Urologic Surgery; Chicago, Yearbook Medical Publishers, Inc. pp. 52-62, 1985
9. Pensel, J., Hofstetter, A., Frank, F. et al: Temporal and Spatial Temperature Profile of the Bladder Serosa in Intravesical Neodymium:YAG Laser Irradiation. Eur. Urol. 7: 298, 1981

Value of the Nd: YAG Laser in the Therapy of Penile Carcinoma

Rothenberger K.H.
Städt.Krankenhaus Landshut
Robert-Koch-Straße 1
8300 Landshut

Squamous cell carcinoma of the Penis accounts about 1 % of all malignancies in men in Europe in contrary to some countries in Africa where a rate of 10 % is found.

The high recurrance rate after conventional therapy (table 1) was reason for trying the Neodymium-YAG-laser in a man with metastatic disease by Hofstetter and Staehler 1976.

Carcinoma of the Penis therapy of Stage T_1 to T_2

Method	Rate of Relapses
local excision	40 % (Hanash 1970)
partial amputation (tumor-free margin of about 2 cm)	10 % (Gursel 1973)
irradiation therapy	15 % (Pointon 1975)
Bleomycin	50 % (Ichikawa 1977)
Iridium-192-Moulage	8 % (Salaverria 1979)
Neodymium-YAG-Laser	

Table 1.

The good local result encouraged for further laser treatments in local penile cancer in the stage T_1 to T_2.

Local tumor therapy

As a rule we use a tourniquet in the form of a small red rubber catheter around the base of the shaft. Under bloodless conditions the macroscopically visible carcinoma is removed with a scalpel. The tumors base and a margin of 0,5 cm is treated with the laser. In small superficial tumors we first use the laser and perform the excision of the coagulated tissue in a second step. We aim to achieve a reproducible, homogeneous end deep necrosis to ensure complete devitalization of any remaining tumor cells with the Neodymium-YAG-laser. In this indication the laser is used purely for coagulation and not for ablation or cutting. The laser light is transmitted through a flexible teflon-sheathed quartz-glass fiber light guide into a hand-held applicator with a focussing lens system. The latter permits the beam diameter to be changed, depending on the distance from the target. In order to achieve the maximum necrosis depth of 3 mm without water cooling, a power output of 45 W must be applied for approximately 3 s. The depth of necrosis achieved can then be easily estimated on the basis of the white discoloration of the tissue surface. There is a point beyond which it is no longer possible to shorten the exposure time by increasing the laser power owing to superficial tissue changes, e.g. desiccation and carbonization. Carbonization increases tissue energy absorption by a factor of about 40, resulting in massive overheating of the surface and vaporization of the tissue. Thus, the actual depth of penetration is not increased. If the tissue surface is covered with blood, a similar effect occurs, since the absorption of laser energy by blood is also about 40 times greater than that of normal tissue. In this case the depth of penetration is even reduced.

If the tissue surface is cooled with water, rapid superficial tissue change is delayed, so that the coagulation temperature can also be attained in deeper zones without tissue ablation. In this manner necrosis depths of 6 mm can be achieved.

Specimens of the tumors base and margin are removed with the biopsy forceps to determine the therapeutic success. After removing the tourniquet occasional isolated bleedings can be stopped by the focussed laser.

The healing phase usually lasts 6-8 weeks, daily penis baths for example with camomile are usefull.

In every case an exact tumor staging including lymphadenectomy is done.

Results

So far we have treated 14 patients in the stage T_1 and 8 patients in the stage T_2 without metastases. Another two patients with removable local inguinal positiv lymphnodes were treated in the same way. The patients were aged between 26 and 86 years. In two cases we found in the first year a carcinoma in situ. After a second laser therapy these patients remained tumor-free.

Neodymium-YAG-Laser Therapy
in Carcinoma of the Penis

$T_1 N_0 M_0$	n=14
$T_2 N_0 M_0$	n= 8
$T_1 N_1 M_0$	n= 1
$T_2 N_1 M_0$	n= 1

Follow up 7-89 months (∅ 4,5 years)
Mortality 4,2 % (n=1, 4,5 years
    after treatment, no local relapse)
Relapse rate 8,4 % (n=2, T_{IS} in
    the first year)

June 87 Rothenberger   Table 2.

One patient died (4,2 %) after 4,5 years on metastatic disease, there was no local tumor relapse found (table 2).

The mean observation period is 4,5 years, its range lasts from 4 months to 7,5 years.

In the diagram (table 3) the individual observation periods can be seen. Some patients were treated in the last months. We can see that the survival rate after 5 years is about 95 %. In the literature we find survival rates between 50 % an 77 %. In conclusion we can say today, that the combined laser treatment with the Neodymium-YAG-laser is the best treatment for local penile cancer.

Table 3. NEODYMIUM-YAG-LASER THERAPY IN PENILE CANCER

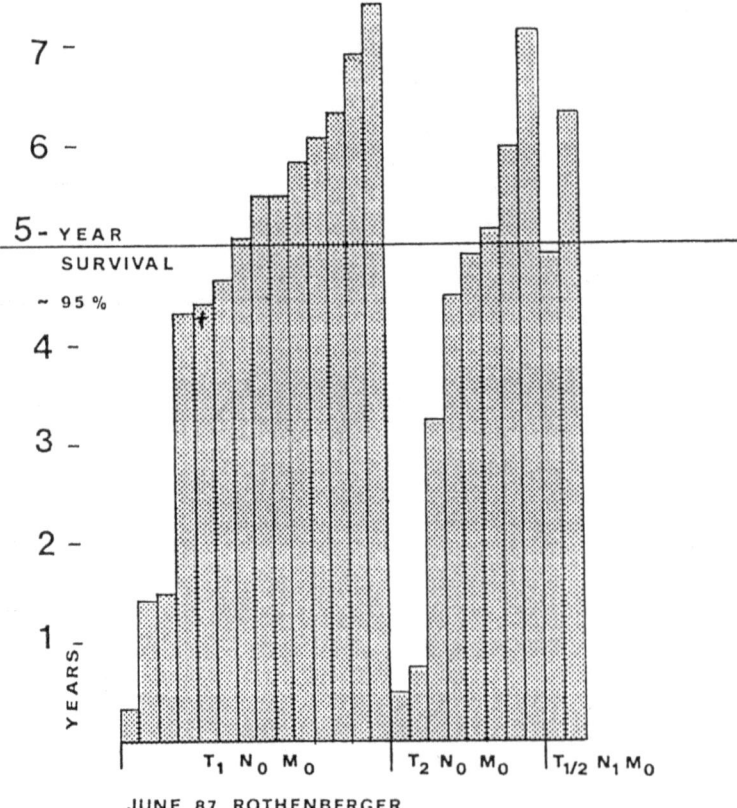

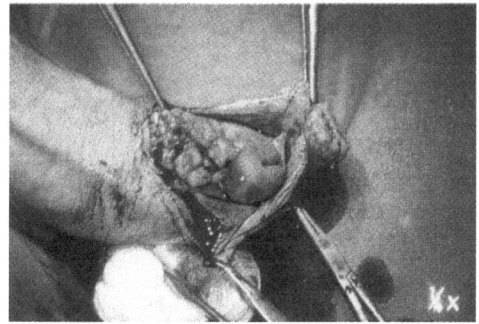 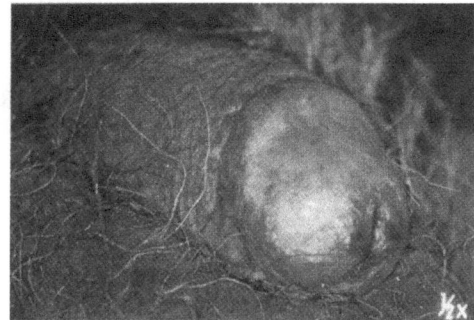

Fig. 1. A.S., 58 years old. Highly differentiated keratinizing squamous cell carcinoma.

Fig. 2. A.S., 58 years old. 3.5 years after laser therapy.

Induratio Penis Plastica: Laser-Chemo-Therapeutic Treatment

D'Ovidio M.; Leonelli G. -CENTRO TUMORI UNIVERSITA' DI ROMA

Many therapies have been tried for Induratio penis plastica but many of them have failed.

Local injection of drug antiflogystic provoque pain, risk of infections and possibility of haematomas.

The use of jonoforsis is preferable and more accetable by the patients. The contemporary application of the laser give better results but is neccessary select the indicated laser.

The analisis of the various type of laser suggest the IR diodic laser as the best.

Ninety patients have been treated with that metodique with good results.

Transurethral Laser Surgery for Bladder Tumor. With References to Tumor Recurrence

K. Okada, S. Kiyotaki, H. Asaoka, A. Nakano.
Department of Urology, Nihon University School of Medicine
30-1, Oyaguchi, Itabashi-ku, Tokyo, Japan.

I. Introduction

Nd:YAG laser surgery has a lot of advantage propagated as a non-contact destruction and complete necrotization of the tumor tissue[1]. Therefore, transurethral Nd:YAG laser surgery (abbreviated TULS) would be an ideal method for the treatment of bladder tumor in this point of view. However, the indication of TULS was limited to only a small tumor. The bulky tumor should be applied with standard TUR prior to TULS[2].

For the past seven years, over 200 patients with bladder tumor were treated with TULS. Though most of the papers in terms of laser surgery showed the minimal tumor recurrence[3], it is still controversial whether laser is able to prevent the tumor recurrence. The object of the present study is to demonstrate the technique of TULS performed in our department, to show the background factor of the patients undergone with each techniques, then to clarify the tumor recurrence of the present series and to estimate the efficacy of this modality.

II. Method

As a hard wear, MediLas YAG was used with 50w power output. Two kinds of delivery fiber were utilized depend upon the tumor shape and size. Straight type means standard quartz fiber with 5-degree angle of divergence. The other is dispersed type fiber. The tip of the quartz fiber is attached with sapphire, from which laser beam is dispersed to 120-degree angle. When the Helium-Neon beam is applied through the dispersed type fiber, the large spot of red light of Helium-Neon beam could be obtained. straight type fiber is able to project a spot size of 2mm at a distance of 1cm, while dispersed type fiber will get a spot size of 45mm at the same distance.

With regard to endoscope, rigid cystoscope has a disadvantage in terms of the angle in the bladder. To eliminate the disadvantage a flexible cystoscope is employed for the treatment of bladder tumor, especially those in the dome and anterior wall. The tip of the flexible endoscope is able to bend approximately to 120-degree during the insertion of the delivery fiber.

III. Irradiation techniques

Two kinds of techniques are advocated, non-contact and contact methods. Generally, tumor surface irradiation is started with non-contact method. After the eradication of the tumor, it is also irradiated with lower power of laser beam as non-contact method. On the other hand, if the tumor is middle sized or large, intra-tumoral irradiation is performed with contact method. Direct pedicle irradiation is carried out with contact method in cases of pedunculated tumor. 50w and 5sec. irradiation was used as one unit.

To avoid the complication during the irradiation of middle sized tumor, we have utilized ultrasonography with transabdominal sector scanning. After the application of the fiber, echogram reveals linear shadow of the delivery fiber. It is interesting to note that a mass of the bubble like a signal fire appeared during the intratumoral irradiation. Thus, TULS could be performed safely by virtue of the transabdominal sonography.

IV. Materials
The cases of this study were selected to evaluate the definite tumor recurrence and the efficacy of this modality. 117 cases with low stage and low grade tumor were chosen and the cases used transurethral electrocautery were excluded for the present investigation. They were consisted of 72 of primary cases and 45 of recurrenct cases with histories of the bladder tumor. They were also divided into 36 treated with non-contact and 31 with contact method (Fig. 1).

V. Result
The following analysis was shown according to the each treatment. As to the tumor shape, 34 of 96 pedunculated tumor were treated with non-contact and 62 with contact method. But 2 of 21 sessile tumor were treated with non-contact, 19 with contact method. Thus, sessile tumors were easily treated with contact method(Fig. 2).

With regard to the number of the tumor, there was no significant relationship between the number of the tumor and the treatment method. But in case with multiple tumor, contact method would be faster to finish the operation than non-contact method.

Clearly result could be obtained in terms of the tumor size. Of 36 treated with non-contact method, 31 belonged to small tumor less than 1cm in diameter. On the other hand, middle sized and large sized tumors were treated with contact method. That is, non-contact method was a tendency to be limited to small tumor group, while contact one expanded its indication to the middle and large tumors (Fig. 3).

As far as the tumor recurrence of the primary cases was concerned, one year non-recurrence rates of non-contact and contact methods were 71.4% and 75.5%, respectively. Therefore, tumor recurrences were not significant different between two groups, and 1 of 4 patients shows the tumor recurrence in one year even after laser surgery (Fig. 4).

The location of the recurrence and the recurrent rate of primary cases were shown herein. Orthotopic and heterotopic recurrences were found in cases of non-contact method, while heterotopic recurrences were significant in cases of contact method. But recurrence rates of both non-contact and contact methods were 1.74 and 1.84, respectively. Therefore, laser surgery could minimize the tumor recurrence in comparison with the data in other paper performed with transurethral electrocautery (Fig. 5).

In the recurrent cases with histories of bladder tumor, it seems to show high rate of tumor recurrence. Orthotopic and heterotopic recurrence occurred in both method, and recurrence rate of total cases showed 5.12. It would be quite difficult to prevent the tumor recurrence in the recurrent cases even with the use of laser surgery.

IV. Summary
From the present study we summarize the following comment. As to the indication of the treatment madality, small tumor could be treated with non-contact, while middle sized tumor is managed with contact method. In sofar as the location of the recurrence is

PATIENTS

1. Selected cases·········117
     Bladder tumor Ta Tl, G0-G2
     Laser only (not used electrocautery)

2. Background factor

	Non-contact	Contact	Total
Primary cases	22	50	72
Recurrent cases	14	31	45
Total	36	81	117

Fig. 1 . Patient selection

SHAPE OF THE TUMOR

	Non-contact	Contact	Total
Pedunculated	34	62	96
Sessile	2	19	21
Total	36	81	117

Fig. 2 . Shape of the tumor

SIZE OF THE TUMOR

	Non-contact	Contact	Total
Small	31	39	70
Middle	5	40	45
Large	0	2	2
Total	36	81	117

Fig. 3 . size of the tumor

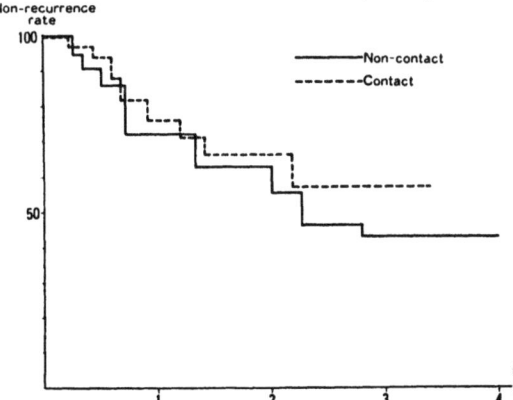

Fig. 4 . Non recurrence rate of primary case

RECURRENCE OF PRIMARY CASES

	Non-contact	Contact	Total
No.	22	50	72
Recurrence	11	14	25
orthotopic	4 (36%)	2 (14%)	6
heterotopic	5 (45%)	11 (79%)	16
mixed	2	1	3
Rec. rate	1.74	1.84	1.79

Fig. 5. Recurrence of primary cases

concerned, non-contact and contact method tended to occur orthotopic and heterotopic recurrence. However, from the results of low rate of tumor recurrence of primary cases, TULS could minimize the tumor recurrence, but could not prevent completely.

REFERENCES
1. Pensel, J., Hofstetter, A., Frank, F., Keiditisch, E. and Rothenberger, K. : Temporal and spatial temperature profile of the bladder serosa in intravesical neodymium-YAG laser irradiation. Eur. Urol., 7, 298-303, 1981.
2. Staehler, G. and Hofstetter, A. : Transurethral laser irradiation of urinary bladder tumors. Eur. Urol., 5, 64-69, 1979.
3. Staehler, G., Chaussy, C., Hocham, D. and Schmiedt, E. : The use of neodymium-YAG lasers in urology; indications, technique and critical assessment. J. Urol., 134, 1155-1160, 1985.

Argonlaser-Urethrotomy in Male: Results and Problems

Noeske,H.D.,Kraushaar,J.,M.Wolf and Rothauge,C.F.
Dep.Urology,Justus Liebig-University Giessen

The benign urethra stricture disease in male at all times presents a challenge to the surgeon thus justifying the development of ever new methods of operation.The problem involved is neatly summed up by HELMSTEIN in 1964: "Once a stricture,always a stricture! As early as 1880 the Viennese Leopold von DITTEL had thus characterized the difficulties of therapy:Neither incision nor dilation result in radical cure,whereas urethrotomy solves the problem more quickly and recidivation takes longer.
As today 80 % of all strictures are iatrogenic,i.e.the result of invasive urological techniques;stricture prophylaxis is more important than unsatisfactory therapy.
The generally practised internal urethrotomy (SACHSE) is undisputed a relatively safe procedure in the hand of the urologist. But the experience over 15 years has shown a high rate of recurrence.In our opinion clinical studies do not sufficiently take into consideration the different forms of strictures with regard to their etiology,localisation,degree of severity and foregoing treatment.The postoperative periods of observation are often too short.In this context we want to point out KONAKs statement,that a follow up on patients treated for strictures should last as long as they live and not just for several months.

Because of the limitations of conventional modalities new ways of therapy are opened up with different kinds of medical lasers since 1977.The effect of laser in strictured urethra rests on the removal of the stricture tissue by vaporisation and thermal coagulation of the fibrous area,destroying the whole stricture and not only incising it in one or several places.Theoretically a re-epithelialisation of the urethra takes place with more elastic properties and less fibrous contraction and scarring.

The neodymium-YAG laser was tried out by BÜLOW first on dogs later on humans.In 1984 SMITH and DIXON from Salt Lake City report poor results in 17 patients with foregoing conventional treatment.In 11 cases recurrent strictures developed during follow up of only six months after irradiation.For them the use of neodymium-YAG laser offers no benefit over conventional techniques.We believe, that the relatively deep penetration of this kind of laser can produce further periurethral fibrosis and recurrent stenosis.
Carbon dioxyde laser (CO_2) is potentially the most promising for urethrotomy.The physical principles of this laser enable it to a precise tissue removal by intense heating and vaporisation with minimal bleeding.The strong absorption of his energy by water

and the lack of transmission systems, however, forbid its endoscopic application in the lower urinary tract (urethra and bladder). The argonlaser has certain advantages over the neodymium-YAG laser because of a more immediate tissue vaporisation and

smooth recanalisation of the urethra.

Therefore, since 1978, we treat all urethral strictures with an

30 watts argonlaser from SPECTRA PHYSICS. The laser energy is delivered via a 600 μ fiber. The operation is performend under spinal anesthesia through a 21 F urethroscope. Either the light conductor finds the way through the stricture on its own or a

small ureter-catheter is inserted as guide through the stricture lumen into the bladder. After opening up the stricture the borders

must be smoothed and the so called "hanging formations" must be removed by careful irradiation. Postoperative 24 F silicone catheter-drainage is used for two days.

All the patients were able to void excellently immediately after this treatment. Nobody had any significant problems with bleeding.

We hoped, that a precise removal of the fibrous stricture tissue by argonlaser vaporisation would be much more effective than the simple incision achieved with conventional urethrotomes.
1983 we have demonstrated here 27, two years later 79 and now we

can report conclusions about 208 stricture-patients.
In cases of foregoing conventional treatment - most of them in other medical centers - our results are disappointing. The patients

had undergone multiple urethral dilations and internal urethrotomies. Because of advanced scarring in the strictured area the

incidence of recurrence is as high as before. The average follow up is 18 months; early recurrence in the time between 6 to 12 months is almost the rule. In spite of repeated laser operations

the recidivation don't took longer.
Untreated patients show better results because of early, superficial scarring in only a short distance. No difference in the

stricture localisation could be observed. Recidivation takes longer, the rate of recurrence is 30 %.

To sum up the results:
1. The argonlaser is suitable for urethrotomy. Because of its

unique physical properties and tissue effects this laser offers theoretically advantages.
2. The simple stricture - untreated before - has a relatively good chance of being removed finally.

3. The complicated advanced stricture with foregoing treatment can be removed even under adverse conditions but it shows a high

rate of recurrence.

Endoscopic YAG-Laser Therapy for Localised Carcinoma of the Prostate

T.A. McNicholas, C.Charig, S.StC.Carter, J.E.A. Wickham and E.P.N.O'Donoghue.
Institute of Urology, London WC2H 8JE, U.K.

We have further developed a method extending the role of endoscopic surgery in the treatment of early prostatic carcinoma. An "extended" transurethral resection of the prostate (TURP) under ultrasound (U/S) control reduces the prostatic tissue to a thin residual prostatic capsule suitable for subsequent coagulation by endoscopic YAG laser. 26 patients with apparently early disease were entered into the pilot study. Three were excluded after staging (2 ToA and one found to have involved lymph nodes on pelvioscopy - T2 N1 Mo). 17 have received a full course of treatment. Mean follow up so far is 6 months (1-14). Two early patients with excessive residual tissue had positive biopsies and underwent second treatments with subsequently negative biopsies. Two other patients have positive biopsies. No tumour has progressed. Complications have been minimal. One patient has reduced frequency of erections and one required bladder neck incision for symptomatic bladder neck stenosis. There were no other effects on potency or continence.

Carcinoma of the prostate is the commonest urological cancer and is the fifth commonest malignant tumour of males worldwide (Parkin et. al., 1984). In the United Kingdom it characteristically presents to urologists at a late stage with metastases. The natural history is such that once a patient presents with M1 disease his median life expectancy is approximately two years and this is unaffected by hormonal manipulation (Parker et. al. 1985). Despite the recent interest in new methods of hormonal therapy there is no evidence that they confer improved survival over orchidectomy and they should be regarded as palliative rather than curative. Therefore, if attempts are to be made to improve the outlook for this disease attention must be focused on early disease.

The range of treatments for early prostate cancer range from radical prostatectomy through radical radiotherapy and extend to radioactive seed implants. Survival rates for radical surgery and radical radiotherapy are similar at the 5 to 10 year level, but surgery seems to show an advantage at the 15 year level. Seed implantation is a relatively new technique and sufficiently long term follow up is not readily available, although at shorter follow up it seems to have disease free survival rates slightly below that of radiotherapy

However, both radical surgery and radical radiotherapy have significant complications and side effects. Radical surgery is frequently associated with impotence and incontinence although recent developments in methods of surgical removal of the gland, sparing the neurovascular bundles, have contributed to a reduction in the incidence of serious side effects (Walsh 1984). Radical radiotherapy commits the patient to a 6 - 8 week course of daily treatment, and even in the hands of the most experienced in this form of treatment a significant complication rate of 10 - 12% has been reported (Ray and Bagshaw 1975). In addition the patient feels generally unwell during the treatment period and for a period afterwards.

Therefore, there is room for an alternative method of treatment. Ideally, such treatment would be endoscopic rather than requiring major open surgery, able to deal with prostatic tumour within any part of the gland, would have an acceptable incidence of side effects, and have limited effects on potency or continence.

In the early 1980's a novel technique was reported (Sander and Biesland 1984). This combined a radical resection of the prostate to remove the bulk of tissue and "de-bulk" the tumour, followed by photocoagulation of the remaining prostatic capsule with the Neodymium-YAG laser in an attempt to sterilise any remaining cancer cells in the capsule. Their initial results were encouraging in terms of disease free survivals and there were no instances of impotence or incontinence(Biesland and Sander 1986).

We have utilised this technique and adapted it in the light of our own experience, particularly by incorporating new ultrasound techniques to define the extent of resection required, in an attempt to determine whether the boundaries of the endoscopic treatment of localised carcinoma of the prostate could be extended further.

Patients who appear to have disease localised to the prostate undergo a second look or "extended" TURP carefully done in planned and mapped segments. The purpose of this is firstly to debulk the prostate gland under ultrasound control aiming to leave a residual rim of prostatic capsule 6 mm or less in depth. Secondly, this procedure allows further staging pathologically. All chips are examined and results for the number of chips involved, the weight resected and the Gleason histological scoring both per segment and overall are then obtained.

Ten weeks following the "extended" TURP the patient undergoes laser coagulation of his prostatic capsule using the YAG laser. The energy is passed through a fine quartz glass fibre that is passed down the cystoscope or resectoscope and the whole of the capsular walls are irradiated using a power of 50W. slowly moving over the surface of the prostatic capsule in an attempt to evenly coagulate the whole area. The laser beam rests on any particular site for not more than 3 - 4 seconds at a time giving a depth of penetration of the laser energy of approximately 6 mm.(Pensel et. al. 1981). Rectal temperatures are monitored by means of a thermocouple held against the anterior wall of the rectum behind the prostate. Adequate access is possible to the posterior prostatic capsule, the anterior tissue and to the bladder neck. However, for good access to the apical regions a suprapubic approach is necessary. We have adapted the well-known techniques of percutaneous access to the kidney to allow the creation of a dilated track into the bladder followed by the passage of a specially designed access cannula through which a range of endoscopes can be passed into the bladder and into the resected prostatic cavity allowing excellent access to the apical regions of the prostate. The urethral catheter is removed after a minimum of 36 hours and the patient goes home usually on the fourth day.

Patients were assessed at one month to confirm that they were progressing satisfactorily and were admitted for a full assessment at 3/12, 6/12 and one year following treatment.. Potency was assessed and serological tests for SAP, PAS and alkaline phosphatase were performed. They underwent examination under anaesthetic and endoscopy to monitor the healing of the prostatic capsule, in particular the bladder neck. "Blind" transrectal Tru-cut prostatic biopsies of each lobewere taken as well as biopsies taken under ultrasound control. Subsequently they are seen in the prostate clinic with an annual bone scan.

Twenty-six patients have been enrolled in this pilot study. As a result of the staging procedures three have been excluded, one because of lymph node involvement found at pelviscopy, and two with T0a disease confirmed on second look TURP in relatively unfit men .17 men have undergone the treatment since April 1986. The average age of all patients was 63.5 ± 8.2 years, range 39 - 76 (n = 26) and of the laser patients 62.4 ± 7.6 years, range 39 - 75 (n = 17)

RESULTS Immediate post-TURP complications were minor. The average in-patient stay was four days. One patient was noted to have a degree of bladder neck obstruction.

After laser treatment several patients described perineal discomfort.. These patients had all received much higher energy doses than previously. Three patients had a large amount of slough in the prostatic cavity which was removed with the resectoscope loop. This tissue was avascular and did not bleed. Two patients were noted to have a mild bladder neck stenosis and two had a more marked bladder neck stenosis requiring bladder neck incision.

At the present state of follow up two patients have had positive biopsies. In both cases clinical, ultrasonic and endoscopic evidence suggested that an excess of tissue had been left. They have both undergone further debulking TURP and second laser treatments with negative biopsies subsequently. On ultrasound assessments we have found that the appearances can be very confusing as a result of the effects of often two TURPS and laser treatment with frequent hyperechoic regions particularly at the urethral surface. Again clinical examination is also difficult as a result of the procedures that have been performed. At present two patients have clinical and pathological evidence of remaining disease. However, in no case has disease apparently progressed.

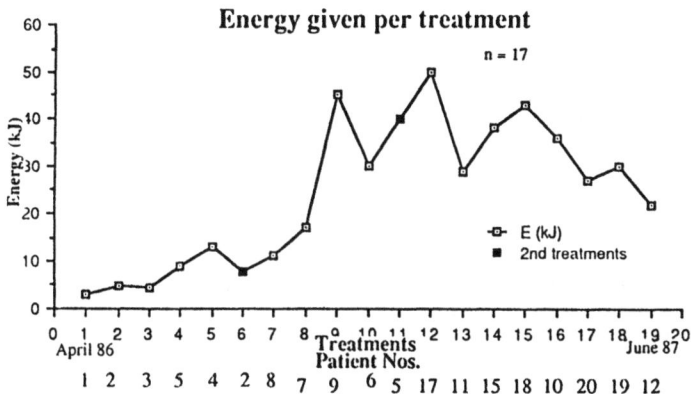

It can be quite clearly seen from the graph above that the technique is evolving with greater experience. In effect however this does mean that the early patients have been undertreated and any real effect from the treatment will only be possible in those treated later in the series. At present the technique holds promise as an alternative for those relatively young men with an apparently localised malignant prostate gland who can expect to be at relatively high risk of disease progression (Haapiainen 1986).

References
Beisland H.O. and Sander, S. (1986). First clinical experiences on neodymium-YAG laser irradiation of localised prostatic carcinoma. Scand.J.Urol.Nephrol. 20:113-117.
Haapiainen R., Rannikko S., Makinen J., Alfthan O. (1986). T0 carcinoma of the prostate: influence of tumour extent and histologic grade on prognosis of untreated patients.
Eur Urol. 12: 16-20
Hald T.and Rasmussen F.(1980). Extraperitoneal pelvioscopy: a new aid in staging of lower urinary tract tumours. A preliminary report. J Urol. 124: 245-248.
Lindholt J.and Hansen T.P.(1986) Prostatic carcinoma: complications of megavoltage radiation therapy. Br. J. Urol. 58: 52-54.
Parker M.C., Cook A., Riddle P.R., Fryatt I., O'Sullivan J.and Shearer R.J. (1885) Is delayed treatment justified in carcinoma of the prostate? Br. J. Urol. 57, 724-728.
Parkin, D. M., Stjernsward,J.and Muir C.S. (1984). Estimates of the worldwide frequency of twelve major cancers. Bull. W.H.O., 62, 163-182.
Pensel, J., Hofstetter A., Keiditsch E. and Rothenberger K. (1981). Temporal and spatial temperature profile of the bladder serosa in intravesical neodymium YAG laser irradiation. Eur.Urol.,7, 298 - 303.
Ray G.R.and Bagshaw M.A. (1975). The role of radiation therapy in the definitive treatment of adenocarcinoma of the prostate. Ann. Rev. Med. 26:567.
Ritchie A.W.S. et. al. (1985). Prediction of response to radiotherapy for localised prostatic cancer.
Br. J. Urol. 57: 729-732.
Sander S. and Beisland H. O.(1984).Laser in the treatment of localised prostatic carcinoma. J.Urol.132: 280-281.
Walsh, P. C.and Mostwin J.L. (1984) Radical prostatectomy and cystoprostatectomy with preservation of potency: Results using a new nerve sparing technique. Br. J. Urol. 56:694-697

Carcinoma of the Penis Treated with the Nd: YAG Laser

Terrence R. Malloy, M.D.
Alan J. Wein, M.D.
Victor L. Carpiniello, M.D.

ABSTRACT

Eighteen males with squamous cell carcinoma of the penis were treated primarily with the Neodymium YAG Laser. Six patients had TIS, 10 patients had T1 tumors, and 2 men had T2 carcinoma. All patients had refused traditional therapy of partial penectomy and received informed consent as to the investigational nature of the Neodymium YAG Laser photoradiation therapy.

Circumcisions and deep tissue biopsies were performed on all patients prior to tumorcidal Neodymium photoradiation treatment. The patients were followed from 12 to 36 months.

In followup, 6 patients with TIS had no evidence of recurrent cancer. Of the 10 males with T1 squamous cell carcinoma of the penis, 7 patients (70%) were tumor free at a mean followup of 28.6 months. The 2 men with T2 carcinoma of the penis had reduction of the tumor mass but were not cured.

The obvious advantage of the Neodymium YAG Laser in treating carcinoma of the penis is preservation of the penis eliminating disfiguring amputation and its psychogenic sequelae.

INTRODUCTION

The Neodymium YAG Laser has been effectively utilized in urologic surgery since Hofstetter's pioneering work in 1976.(1) Benign and malignant lesions of the external genitalia, urethra, bladder, ureter, renal pelvis and kidney have been successfully treated.(2)

Cutaneous lesions of the penis were ideally suited for laser therapy. Both the CO_2 and Neodymium YAG Laser were used in benign and malignant lesions of the penis.(3, 4) Hofstetter in 1980 reported on 3 patients treated with the Neodymium YAG Laser for carcinoma of the penis.(1) Rosemberg in 1986 reported on 4 patients with squamous cell carcinoma of the external genitalia treated with the CO_2 and Neodymium YAG Laser.(5) Hofstetter in 1986 reported on 17 patients with penile cancer treated with the Neodymium YAG Laser.(2)

Commencing in 1983, a study was undertaken at the University of Pennsylvania to treat squamous cell carcinoma of the penis with the Neodymium YAG Laser. Eighteen males were entered into an investigational protocol for diagnosis and treatment.

MATERIALS AND METHODS

From March, 1983 until September, 1986, 18 males with squamous cell carcinoma of the penis were treated primarily with the Neodymium YAG Laser. Six patients had TIS, 10 patients had T1 tumors and 2 men had T2 carcinoma. The TNM classification of penile carcinoma was used to stage the penis Table 1. (6) Diagnostic evaluation was accomplished following the criteria listed in Table 2.

Table 1. TNM Classification of Penile Carcinoma

T = Primary Tumor

TIS Preinvasive carcinoma (carcinoma in situ)

To No evidence of primary tumor

T1 Tumor 2 cm or less in its largest dimension. Strictly superficial or exophytic.

T2 Tumor larger than 2 cm but not more than 5 cm in its largest dimension with minimal infiltration.

T3 Tumor more than 5 cm in its largest dimension or tumor any size with deep infiltration including into the urethra.

T4 Tumor infiltrating neighboring structures

N = Regional lymph nodes

N-0 No palpable nodes

N-1 Moveable unilateral nodes
    N1a Nodes not considered to contain growth
    N1b Nodes considered to contain growth

N-2 Moveable bilateral nodes
    N2a Nodes not considered to contain growth
    N2b Nodes considered to contain growth

N-3 Fixed nodes

M = Distant Metastases

M-0 No evidence of distant metastases

M-1 Distant metastases present

Table 2. Minimal Diagnostic Criteria for Carcinoma of the Penis

T = Primary Tumor
    1. Clinical examination
    2. Incisional or excisional biopsy of lesion

N = Regional Lymph Nodes
    1. Clinical examination
    2. CAT Scan
    3. Superficial femoral node biopsy (Optional)
    4. Lymphangiography (optional)

M = Distant Metastases
    1. Clinical examination
    2. Chest x-ray
    3. Biochemical determination (Liver function studies, Calcium)
    4. CAT Scan, Bone Scan (optional)

All patients were given informed consent as to the investigational nature of the use of the Neodymium YAG Laser in cancer of the penis. Traditional therapy consisting of partial penectomy were offered to all patients. If Neodymium YAG Laser was unsuccessful, all patients were informed that conventional therapy should then be utilized.

All patients had received deep penile biopsies and circumcision prior to the utilization of the Neodymium YAG Laser photoradiation therapy. The YAG Laser photoradiation was applied with the focusing hand piece. Iced saline was applied to the lesion as laser therapy was delivered to provide surface cooling, prevent carbonization on the surface of the tumor, and promote deep penetration of the carcinoma with the Neodymium YAG Laser phototherapy. All patients were evaluated for possible metastatic foci with careful physical examination, CAT scans, and/or lymphangiography. Three of the patients received ilioinguinal lymphadenectomies.

RESULTS

Six patients with TIS had no evidence of recurrent cancer followed for an average of 28.6 months (Range 18-36 months). Of the 10 males with T1 squamous cell carcinoma of the penis, 7 patients (70%) were tumor free at a mean followup of 24 months (Range 15-37 months). One patient required 2 treatments. Three patients had ilioinguinal lymphadenectomy performed with 2 men showing no evidence of metastasis and 1 male showing 2 positive inguinal nodes but negative iliac nodes.

The 2 patients with T2 carcinoma of the penis had reduction of the tumor mass but were not cured. One patient developed a urethrocutaneous fistula in the area of the treatment. Otherwise there were no complications from laser therapy in this group of patients.

DISCUSSIONS

Thy physics of the Neodymium YAG Laser show that the effect of photoradiation in tissue produces maximum scattering of the energy within the tissue penetrating 4 to 6 mms. depending on the power utilized and time of application.(7, 8) Photoradiation energy delivered to carcinoma of the penis can be enhanced by the application of iced saline to the surface as the Neodymium YAG Laser is applied to the cancer. The iced saline cools the surface of the cancer, preventing carbonization on the surface and enhancing the depth of penetration of the laser beam.

The CO_2 laser is maximally absorbed at the surface, allowing it to be used for cutting or excising cancers. However, it will not obtain deep tissue penetration as is possible with the Neodymium YAG Laser. The optical scattering of the Neodymium YAG Laser permits deep thermal destruction of the carcinoma of the penis. The necrotic tissue produces slough in the post-operative period. This primary attribute of the laser allows the patient the retention of his glans and penis. The disabling sexual and psychological dysfunction associated with partial penectomy can be avoided.

The power and time application of the YAG Laser depends on the size and depth of the carcinoma. The surgeon must gain experience with tissue effects produced by the YAG Laser so that he can determine when the cancer has been adequately treated. In this series of patients power settings of 25 to 38 watts were utilized with the focusing hand piece. Total energy in joules delivered to the lesions is only a rough estimate of the tissue effect.

The success of the Neodymium YAG Laser in treating carcinoma of the penis was shown in Hofstetter's series of 17 patients (p T1-pT2, N-o, M-o) followed from 3 to 6 years. Only 1 patient died of metastatic disease.

In our present series of patients it is obvious that the Neodymium YAG Laser is extremely effective in patients with TIS (100% cure rate). In those men with T1 cancer of the penis, 70% of the patients were tumor free at an average of 24 months followup.

Obviously in the 2 patients with T2 cancer (2-5 cm. primary lesion) the results were not successful.

Further evaluation in multiple urologic centers is needed to evaluate the proper power, time and energy applications in utilizing the Neodymium YAG Laser in treating carcinoma of the penis.

REFERENCES

1. Hofstetter, A., Frank, F.: The Neodymium YAG Laser in Urology. Basle, Switzerland, Hoffman-LaRoche & Co. 1980.

2. Hofstetter, A.: Laser in Urology. Lasers in Surg & Med: 5:412, 1986.

3. Rosemberg, S.K., Jacobs,H.: Continuous-wave carbon dioxide treatment of balanitis xerotica obliterans. Urology 19:539, 1982.

4. Rosemberg, S.K., Fuller, T.A.: Carbondioxide rapid superpulsed laser treatment of erythroplasia of Queyrat. Urology 16:181, 1980.

5. Rosemberg, S.K.: Lasers and squamous cell carcinoma of external genitalia. Urology 27:430, 1986.

6. Schellhammer, P.F., Grabstald, H.: Tumors of the Penis. In: Campbell's Urology, Edited by Walsh, P.C. Gittes, R.F., Perlmutter, A.D., Stamey, T.A. Philadelphia, W.S. Saunders Co., Vol 2, Chapter 34 p. 1583-1606, 1986.

7. Fuller, T.A.: Laser Physics, In: Lasers in Urologic Surgery. Edited Smith, J.A. Chicago, Yearbook Medical Publishers. Chapter 1, p. 1-15, 1985.

8. Smith, J.A., Dixon, J.A.: Tissue Effects of lasers in the Genitourinary System. In: Lasers in Urologic Surgery. Edited by Smith, J.A. Chicago, Yearbook Medical Publisher, Chap. 2 p. 16-31, 1985.

Ultrasound Guided Lasertreatment of Urothelial Tumors

A. Baumüller, R. Vannahme
Dept. of Urology
Karolinenhospital Hüsten, 5760 Arnsberg 1, FRG

The use of the Neodym-Yag-Laser for the treatment of superficial urothelial tumors alone or in combination with other treatment modalities has proved its value during recent years.
Especially smaller tumors with little or no infiltration into the muscular wall can be treated with great success.
The advantages of this method are well known and need not be discussed again.
During the Lasertreatment of larger or deeper infiltrating tumors with stage T2 - T3 complications due to lacerations of adjacent organs outside the bladder were reported. The worst case was a lethal small bowl fistula originating from perforation of the Laser beam throu the bladder wall and the small bowl.
The non-touch-technique with the Laser led to the misjudgement of the depth of the infiltration with the Laser beam, which can only be estimated very roughly.

We herein report a simple and easy to perform method to help estimate the danger of destruction of perivesical organs by a too deeply infiltrating Laser beam.

Technique

For better estimation of the bladder configuration and the thickness of the bladder wall as well as tumor size and location we routinely perform suprapubic ultrasound with one of the common Realtime scanner.
Besides the aforementioned advantages we are also able to see if any part of the bowl ore other intraabdominal structures are in the direction of the Laser beam and thus jepardised.
In case the tumor area cannot be located directly with the ultrasound the area can be pointed out with the cystoscope and thus marked.
If the bladder wall is very strong (e.g. in case of intravesical obstruction due to BPH) it is sometimes better to fill the

bladder in order to extend the wall. We hereby also differenciate between regid and flexible parts of the bladder, giving some indication of possible tumor involvement.
In some cases the filling of the bladder pushes the intraperitoneal structures cranially allowing the complete destruction of tumors at the vesical fundus.
The suprapubic ultrasound makes it therefore possible to treat tumors at locations and in deeper layers of the bladder wall that otherwise cannot be reached be standard laser treatment.

Results

Since August '85 216 patients were treated by laser, 60 of them female, 156 male. Alltogether 352 procedures were done, 212 cases with laser only and 140 combined with TUR. The majority of cases was done in tumorstage pTis - pT2, but 2 cases belonged to stage pT4 and 3 to stage pT3. In these cases lasertreatment was only a palliative procedure.
In no case gastrointestinal irritations were seen nor did we notice any specific symptoms due to laser lesions to perivesical structures.

Discussion

With the routine suprapubic ultrasound during endoscopic lasertreatment of urothelial neoplasms an additional tool to improve intraoperative safety is given.
Lesions to other perivesical organs or structures (e.g. small bowl perforations etc.) could be avoided completely.
In addition to greater safety, larger tumor areas as well as deeper infiltrating neoplasms can be treated when the bladder wall is extended by greater filling volume. This streching can be controlled easily by suprapubic ultrasound and also an estimation of the thickness can be given, enabeling us to adjust the depth of infiltration of the laser beam.
Since normal ultrasound scanner are available even in small hospitals and suprapubic scanning of the bladder and prostate is done frequently for other reasons, our method - as presented here - means nothing but a consequente application of readily available hospital equipement.

Histopathological Findings of Biopsies Gained from Urothelial Tumors Following Laser Therapy

G.E.Schubert, A. Baumüller, R. Sonnenberg
Institute of Pathology, Municipal Hospital of Wuppertal and
University of Witten / Herdecke
Heusnerstraße 40, D 5600 Wuppertal 2 / FRG

The treatment of urothelial tumors with endoscopic application of the Nd: YAG-laser has gained increasing importance during recent years. After laser - radiation biopsies from tumors are altered and thus the question arose if such material is useful for determination of stage and grade in these particular cases. To evelute this problem, biopsies from 89 patients were investigated.

The treatment of the tumors was by endoscopic Nd: YAG - application and consecutive electroresection or cold knife biopsy. Our material consisted of 71 male (mean age 68.4 years) and 18 female (mean age 65.7 years) patients. The various tumor stages and grades are listed in table 1. 194 biopsies were evaluated. The material was fixed in 4 per cent formaldehyd embedded in paraffin sectioned in 6 µ slices and stained with hematoxylin and eosin. We determined tumor grade, depth of invasion and nine more histological parameters: Coagulation necrosis, nuclear pycnosis, dissociation of epithelial cells, detachment of non-invasive epithelial cells from the basement membrane, indistinct structures of the cytoplasm and / or nuclei, cytoplasmic vacuolisation of epithelial cells in particular above the basement membrane in normal epithelium an in non-invasive tumors (pTa and pTis), hydropic degeneration of the cytoplasm and nuclei, lack of epithelium with denuded basement membrane.

Typical coagulation necrosis as defined by classical standards was observed only in 17 biopsies from 14 patients (15.7 per cent of all patients) . These necroses were always focal. In all these specimen enough material without necrosis was available to allow exact grading and staging. In 64 biopsies (33.0 per cent of all biopsies) nuclear pycnosis was found.

Dissociation of intercellular connections were found in 101 (52.1 per cent) biopsies. Detachment of the normal epithelium

	G1	G2	G3
pTis	0	5	5
pTA	19	3	1
pT1	0	8	5
pT2	0	6	11
pT3	0	0	10
pT4	0	1	3
pT0	10		
pTX	2		

Table 1.

or the epithelium of non-invasive cancers from the basement membrane could be seen in 59 biopsies (30.0 per cent). Indistinct structures of the nuclei and the cytoplasm appeared in 181 probes (93.3 per cent). The extent of these "indistinct structures " varied considerably : In 13 biopsies more than 80 per cent; in 4 specimen 50 - 80 per cent ; in 10 biopsies 20 - 50 per cent; in 43 biopsies 5 - 20 per cent and in 108 specimen less than 5 per cent of the epithelium was involved. Vacuoles between the basal layer of the urothelium and intermediate cell layers or the basement membrane appeared in 25 biopsies. Hydropic degenerations of the cytoplasm showed up in 102 specimen (52.6 per cent).
These various lesions are obviously signs of thermic alterations of the cells by the laser beam.
In 30 patients (33.7 per cent of all patients) with 40 biopsies (20.6 per cent of all biopsies) the histological assessment was impaired. In 15 patients (16.9 per cent) a significant, in 9 (10.1 per cent) patients a mild and in 6 (6.7 per cent) a minimal impairment of the diagnosis was noted. In most cases a loss of the epithelium with denuded basement membrane was the reason for this.
In twelve cases due to this effect no tumor tissue was found, in 5 patients a flat carcinoma in situ was altered hereby. In spite of these lesions an invasive carcinoma could be excluded in those cases. The smaller the specimen, the more of it was altered. In spite of the various lesions mentioned above, a sufficient judgement in 86 patients was possible to aid in determining the further treatment.
Only in 3 patients no sufficient assessment was possible due to lack of enough biopsy material. Most difficulties origined from the detachment of the epithelium, especially in pTa - G_1 - G_2

and pTis tumors. PT_2 - G_2-G_3-tumors usually contained enough well preserved cells in the deeper layers to allow histopathological grading . These deeper cells apparently had not been destroyed by the laserbeam.

The staging of the tumors was not impaired, compared to "normal" transurethrally obtained material. Denaturation due to laser-application obviously causes devitalisation of the cells in most cases but does not result in a coagulation necrosis.

Although cold punch biopsies are better for exact grading and staging of tumors, specimen taken out transurethrally after laser application as described before are in most cases sufficient for histopathological work-up in order to help for further therapeutic steps, provided the pathologist is aware of the specific alterations and pitfalls due to laser-beam-denaturisation of urothelial tissue.

Frank, F. Beck, O.J., Hessel, S., Keiditsch, E.
Comparative Investigations of the Effects of the Neodymium:
YAG Laser at 1.06 Microns and 1.32 Microns on Tissue
Lasers in Surgery and Medicine 6 : 546 - 551 (1987)

Frank, F., Hofstetter, A. Böwering, R., Keiditsch, E.
Endoscopic Application of the Nd: YAG Laser in Urology, Biophysical Fundamentals and Instrumentation
Proceedings of the Society of Photooptical Instrumentation Engineers 211 : 9 (1979)

Keiditsch, F., Hofstetter, A., Zimmermann, I., Stern, J., Frank, F., Babaryka, I.
Histological Investigation to Substantiate the Therapy of Bladder Tumors with the Neodymium - YAG - Laser
Laser 1: 19 - 23 (1985)

Smith, J.A.
Lasers in Urologic Surgery
Year Book Medical Publishers, INC, Chicago pp 63 - 81 (1985)

Laser Application in Pediatric Urology

H.-P. Berlien, W. Biewald, J. Waldschmidt, G. Müller

Laser Medizin Zentrum Berlin and Pediatric Surg. Dep.
Klinikum Steglitz Freie Universität Berlin
Krahmerstr. 6-10, D-1000 Berlin 45

Diseases of the urologenital tract in childhood are very different from these of adults. At adults mostly we have tumors, at children there are in addition to that congenital malformations and also traumatic conditioned diesease. This wide spectrum of diseases in pediatric urology performs a manifold use of different laser systems, where especially the Nd:YAG laser became qualified because its radiation can be transmitted by fiber without any problem (Fig. 1).

Indications for laser in pediatric urogenitialtract	Ar^+	Ar^+-Dye	Nd:YAG	Nd:YAG non contact	CO_2 contact
intraabdominal fusion, ligaments					
congenital	+		(+)	++	
acquired	+		(+)	++	+
endometriosis	+		(+)	+	+
ovarian cysts	+			+	+
epithelial dysplasias					+
leucoplakia					++
M. Bowen				(+)	++
cervical dysplasia				(+)	++
carcinoma in situ		+			+
condylomata	+	+		(+)	+
verrucae	+	+		(+)	+
urethral-, uretric stenosis					
congenital	+		+	++	
acquired	+		+	++	
diverticulum				++	
tumors of the bladder			++		
resection of the kidney				++	

Fig. 1. Indications for laser therapy in the urogenital tract and the types of lasers which we prefer

The radiation of the Nd:YAG laser in the near infrared with 1.06 um has a high penetration depth into the tissue, mainly followed by a wide coagulation zone. This laser performs an ideal instrument for working bloodless and for the tumor destruction. For a fine, microsurgical working he was regarded as unsuitable. This was the domain of the CO_2 laser even the fact that it was impossible to couple the radiation into the fiber and a working with flushing system, as it is usual in urology, not possible. An essential advance was the development of the sapphire contact tips. Due to the high energy densities at the needle point and the special beam geometry a very exact working by formation of a small coagulation zone of just about 1,5 - 2 mm is possible (Fig. 1). This instrumentarium can always be used for surgery at outer genitals if an accurate laser application is needed. There are for example the recanalisation of the hymenal- and vaginalatresia as well as in surgery of chloacal malformations. Mainly at recidives of rectourethal or rectovestibulous fistulas another application of the sapphire contact tips has proved. Using the cylindric sapphire or the spheric sapphire the fistula mucosa can be denaturated by laser radiation with an output about 10 W in cw and slow pulling of the fiber through the fistula with following shrinking of the perifistular tissue. In this way risky recidive operations can be avoid (Fig. 2+3).

Nd:YAG cw   wavelength = 1.06 μm   P = < 100 W

quality	tissue interaction	effectivity coagulation	effectivity cutting	indications	accessories
volumeabsorption	coagulation	++	+	bleeding	fiber, handapplicator,
				tumorstenosis	touch probes
				resection of paren-	rigide endoscope
				chymatous organs	flexible endoscope
				congenital ligaments	operationmicroscope
				abscessmembranes	micromanipulator
				adhesiolysis	
				congenital stenosis	
				hemorrhoids	
				analektropium	
				hemangiomas	
				condylomatoma	
				portwine stains	
				(teleangiektasia)	
				(pigmental anomalies)	
				skintumor, verrucae	

Fig. 2. Quality and indications for the Nd:YAG laser

Fig. 3. Traditional the advantage of the CO2 laser is the exact cutting and of the Nd:YAG laser the homogeonous coagulation with haemostatic effect. Due to the progress in contact method specially using the sapphire tips it is also possible to make an exact cutting with small focal necrosis by the Nd:YAG laser in the contact method

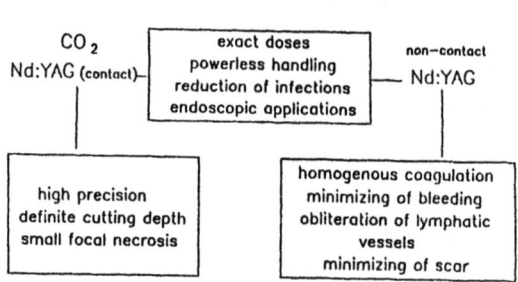

These sapphire tips cannot be used for cystocopy in childhood, because by coupling with the fiber a too large diameter of the system is the result which cannot be lead through the infant endoscope. But in using short exposition times of 0.2 - 0.5 s you can work with the bare fiber without destroying of the fiber. This is very helpful for the treatment of urethra diverticula with following shrinking of the diverticula, but also for the destruction of the urethral valves.

Fig. 4. In pediatric urology we cannot use the Sapphire touch probes. In these cases we use the bare fiber under saline solution for shrinking for fistula and diverticulum

Laserapplication, contact
Nd:YAG laser 1.06 μm
—bare fiber—, sapphire touch—probes

shrinking (fistula, diverticulum)
power   : 10 watts
pulse duration : 1 — 2 sec/area
speed   : 0.5 — 1 mm/sec

Remark: only retrograde procedure;
if necessary use fibringlue

At congenital or scary urethral stenoses an incision and recanalisation with even shorter exposition times of 0.1 - 0.2 s and an output of about 30 W in contact method with the bare fiber can be achieved without transmural necrosis of tissue and following destruction of the urethra wall. It appears that not always a complete removal of the tissue has to occur, but that by repulsion of the developing coagulation necrose finally a sufficient large lumen results (Fig. 5-7).

Laserapplication, contact
Nd:YAG laser 1.06 μm
—bare fiber—, sapphire touch—probes
(congenital, benign malformations)

    coagulation
    power   : 10 watts
    pulse duration : 0.2 – 0.5 sec
    incision
    power   : 15 – 35 watts
    pulse duration : 0.2 – 0.3 sec

Remark: take care of overheating
         and coagulation necrosis

Fig. 5. Also for coagulation and incision in the urethra we use the bare fiber during cystoscopy

Fig. 7. With higher power density and short pulses it is also in the non-contact method possible to make an incision with small focal necrosis

Laserapplication, non contact
Nd:YAG laser 1.06 μm
—bare fiber—
(congential, benign malformations)

    coagulation
    power   : 15 – 25 watts
    spot size   : 1.5 mm
    pulse duration : 0.2 – 0.5 sec

Remark: take care of overheating
         and coagulation necrosis

Fig. 6. For the treatment of intravesical and urethra structure it is also possible to use the non-contact method for coagulation. Sometimes it is not necessary to remove all tissue due to the spontaneous absorption of tissue

Laserapplication, non contact
Nd:YAG laser 1.06 μm
—bare fiber—
(congential, benign malformations)

    incision
    power   : 40 watts
    spot size   : 1.5 mm
    pulse duration : 0.1 sec

Remark: take care of overheating
         and coagulation necrosis

The good haemostatical and coagulation effect of the Nd:YAG laser can be utilize especially for kidney resections. By using high exposition times of more than 100 W and a focus handpiece a bloodless parenchyma resection can be made in order to achieve sufficient high power densities. To do so a clamping of the kidney vessels is not necessary. If necessary extravasating blood out of the resection surface will be intermittent rinsing and sucking by saline solution. This is important as in the haemoglobin the complete radiation will be absorbed and therefore a sufficient cutting effect doesn't result anymore. By slightly spreading apart of the resection surface a clean, precise cut can be achieved. Just larger vessels around the pyelon have to be ligated, mattress sutures are not necessary. They represent a additional risk by cutting into the parenchym. The pyelon takes special note. Larger dissections of the pyelon have to be closed either by a primarily suture or by omentum- or peritorium interposition. Surgery in the hilus area for example tumor enucleation or similar need attention that the renal pelvis doesn't get injured due to a coagulation necrosis. This can lead to a perforation under performing an urine phlegmone after several days of latence (Fig. 7).

The experiences we got from other fields of the pediatric surgery like for example the endoscopic surgery of the upper orotracheal and the oesaphogogastrointestinal tract, and the experiences of the laser surgery at angiomas, we could use with success in the pediatric urology (Fig. 9). It has shown that on one hand by minimizing the output energy and short expostion times uncontrolable disstructions of the surrounding tissue can be avoid, on the other hand that for a sufficient organ resection with the Nd:YAG laser a high output is necessary. Regarding some few manipulations this method proved to be a bloodless, organ protecting proceeding. This is of high importance for the surgery in childhood as blood loss of 50 ml or more can lead to a severe haemorrhagical shock at infants and children.

Resection
tumors, parenchymatous organs
Nd:YAG laser 1.06 µm

power	: 100−120 watts
spot size by focussing handpiece	: 0.5 mm
pulse duration	: cw
speed	: 1 mm/sec

Remark: continuously aspiration and intermittent rising with high−pressure saline solution during the resection

Fig. 8. Procedure of kidney resection with the Nd:YAG laser a high power density and a slow resection speed is necessary for a good result.

Resection of parenchymatous organs and tumors

− lung
− liver
− spleen
− pancreas
− kidney
− tumors esp.:
 soft tissue sarcomas
 neuroblastomas ⟨intrathoracal / intraperitoneal⟩
 teratomas
 invasive bone tumors
 vascular tumors

Fig. 9. The experience in the pediatric surgery with the whole endoscopic and open surgery in other organs are very helpful also in pediatric urology. These means especially the tumor surgery of large retroperitoneal tumors.

Comparative Study of Microvascular Anastomosis Using a CO$_2$ Laser, a Nd: YAG Laser and Conventional Suture Techniques

R.A. Bürger, C.-D. Gerharz, P. Küppers, U. Engelmann, R. Hohenfellner
Department of Urology and Institute of Pathology, Medical School Mainz
Langenbeckstrasse 1, 6500 Mainz, Federal Republic of Germany

Application of microsurgical laser techniques have been made in an attempt to minimize tissue trauma and to facilitate and speed up small vascular and vas anastomosis (1,2,4,6). In this study, we will compare laser-assisted microvascular anastomosis (LAMA) performed with a microsurgical CO$_2$-laser[1], with a 1.32μ Nd:YAG-laser[2], and also with conventional microvascular suture anastomosis (CMSA).

Material and Methods

End-to-end anastomosis of the femoral artery, using either CMSA or LAMA was performed on ninety-four male Sprague-Dawley rats weighing 300-350 g. The conventional sutured anastomoses were done with approximately 8-10 interrupted sutures, using 10/0 nylon.

In LAMA, three 10/0 interrupted nylon sutures were placed at 120° intervals using the triangulation technique (5). Everting sutures were used for Nd:YAG-LAMA. In CO$_2$-LAMA, short pulses (0.1 sec) of laser energy (300-380 mW) with a spot size of 0.5 mm were applied. The Nd:YAG-LAMA were welded, applying pulses of 0.1 sec duration, 0.2 mm spot size and 5.5-7 W. The completion of the anastomosis was accompanied by a light brown-yellow discoloration of the welded tissue.

----

[1] Sharplan 1060, Sharplan Lasers, Inc., Allendale, N.J., USA.

[2] MBB-Medizintechnik GmbH, München, FRG.

Postoperative investigations

The patency was assessed immediately postoperatively, 30' p.o. and at the time of necropsy, which was done at various time intervals (3 days, 2 weeks, 4 weeks, and 8 weeks p.o.). Gross observations were made with special notice of the formation of connective tissue around the anastomoses. Specimens for light microscopy were stained with H&E and van Gieson (Elastin), and tensile strength measurements of the anastomosed arteries were done on an Instron material tester (series 6000[3]) at 293° K with a test-speed of 20 mm/min. Statistics: Statistical differences between the 3 groups were assayed, utilizing analysis of variance (ANOVA) with two factors.

Results

The time needed for completion of the anastomosis in group 1 (CMSA) was 15-25 minutes, while in groups 2 (CO_2-LAMA) and 3 (Nd:YAG-LAMA), it was considerably less. Group 2 required 8-13 minutes and in group 3, 10-15 minutes were needed. When harvested, all anastomoses were patent. At all intervals, tensile strength was significantly higher for sutured anastomoses, while differences between the CO_2- and the Nd:YAG- laser groups were not statistically significant.

Histology: Day 3: In CMSA and LAMA, the intima was denuded of endothelium up to 2 mm proximal and distal to the anastomosis. Minute deposits of fibrin were occasionally seen adhering to the exposed lamina elastica interna; however, patency was not affected. In CMSA and LAMA, a complete necrosis of the media was observed, having an extension of up to 2 mm on both sides of the anastomosis. The structural integrity of the lamina elastica interna and externa was preserved, except at the site of sutures or vessel transsection. Nd:YAG-LAMA exhibited small gaps at the site of the anastomosis which were filled with fibrin plugs, which were not seen in CMSA and CO_2-LAMA. Coagulation necrosis of the adventitia was evident in LAMA. In CMSA and LAMA, sparse infiltration of polymorphonuclear and mononuclear cells was present in the adventitia adjacent to the anastomotic site.

Day 14: The endothelial lining on the intimal surface had been restored,

---

[3] Instron International Limited, Offenbach, FRG.

and a layer of endothelial cells also covered the anastomosis. The circumferential proliferation of intimal cells, resulting in thickening of the intima, only moderately decreased the size of the lumen. In Nd:YAG-LAMA, the small anastomotic gaps were now filled by proliferating intimal cells. In CMSA, the necrotic media had almost completely been reconstructed, whereas in LAMA, there were still remnants of media necrosis, evidenced by a deficit of nuclear staining. Coagulation necrosis of the adventitia was still present in Nd:YAG-LAMA, but not in CO_2-LAMA. Predominantly mononuclear cells and foreign body reaction were present around sutures in CMSA and LAMA.

Day 28: Wound healing had been completed. On the luminal side, the anastomosis was completely covered by a broad proliferation of intimal cells. In CMSA and LAMA, the site of the anastomosis could hardly be detected and was only marked by sutures or by the persistent discontinuity of the lamina elastica. The proliferation of the intima did not reduce the lumen significantly. Small aneurysms that could only be detected microscopically were seen in CMSA (1/4) and in LAMA (1/6). The nonabsorbable suture material in CMSA caused a foreign body reaction.

Day 56: In CMSA and LAMA, the thickening of the intima layer did not increase, but the atrophy of the media, already noted occasionally on day 28, was more marked, and was most intense in areas with broad intima proliferations. A persistant foreign body reaction with chronic inflammatory infiltrations adjacent to the suture material was seen in CMSA.

Discussion

The use of laser welding techniques for microvascular anastomosis can reduce clamp time significantly, and anastomoses can be completed much faster. Neblett, et al. reported a reduction in clamp time from 15-20' to 5-10' in rats, Jain from 15' to 5' also in rats and Frazier, et al. from 30' to 20' in miniature swine (2,3,5). Our own results confirm the data: 15-25' for CMSA and usually half the time for LAMA. LAMA is technically easy to perform. There are few reports on tensile or bursting strength measurements of LAMA: Neblett, et al. found tensile strength (t.s.) to be variable with t.s. of CMSA being slightly greater than t.s. of LAMA (5). Quigley, et al. studied bursting strength of femoral artery anastomoses in rats and found LAMA to burst at consistently lower pressures than CMSA with statistically significant differences on day 1, day 3, and 1 week p.o. (7). We found the tensile strength of CMSA to be consistently and significantly higher than t.s. of LAMA. However, at 4 weeks p.o., CMSA and CO_2-LAMA had nearly the same tensile strength. CO_2- and Nd:YAG-laser groups did not show any statistically significant differences in tensile strength measurements. Frazier could describe less fibrotic reactions around laser-anastomoses when compared to conventional anastomoses in minipigs, while others found no marked difference (2). Our results indicate that there are less external fibrotic reactions in LAMA, probably due to less foreign body material. Neither in gross observations nor histologically could we find any significant differences between CO_2- and Nd:YAG- laser groups.

In urology, the potential applications for microsurgical laser systems are numerous: microvascular anastomoses in the treatment of erectile dysfunction, in pediatric urology and for free bowel-, omentum- and composite grafts in reconstructive urology. Furthermore, we are currently investigating the use of laser systems for sutureless, watertight anastomosis of the pyelon, ureter and urethra with a potential application in pediatric reconstructive urology.

References

1. Engelmann U., Morris J., Gray K., Lynne C., Neblett C. (1985) Die Laser-unterstützte mikrochirurgische Vasovasostomie und Gefäßanastomose. Verhandl Dtsch Gesell Urol 37. Tagung (1985) p. 426-428 1986 Thieme Verlag Stuttgart New York.

2. Frazier O.H., Painvin G.A., Morris J.R., Thomsen S., Neblett C.R. (1985) Laser-assisted microvascular anastomoses: Angiographic and anatomopathologic studies on growing microvascular anastomoses: Preliminary report. Surgery 97: 585-590.

3. Jain K.K. (1980) Sutureless microvascular anastomosis using a neodymium- YAG laser. J Microsurg 1:436-439.

4. Lynne, C.M., Carter M., Morris J., Dew D., Thomsen S., Thomsen C. (1983) Laser-assisted vas anastomosis. Lasers Surg Med 3:261-263.

5. Neblett, C., Morris J.R., Thomsen S. (1986) Laser-assisted microsurgical anastomosis. Neurosurg. 19:914-934.

6. Rosemberg S.K., Elson., Nathan L.E. (1985) Carbon dioxide laser micro- surgical vasovasostomy. Urol 25:53-56.

7. Quigley M.R., Bailes J.E., Kwaan H.C., Cerullo L.C., Brown T., Fitzsimmons J. (1985) Comparison of bursting strength between suture- and laser- anastomosed vessels. Microsurg 6:357-365.

Laser Surgery of the Bladder Neck and Prostate

Roger S. Warner, M.D.   Marc S. Cohen, M.D.

New York, New York, U.S.A.

Sixty patients with proven urologic outlet obstruction were studied. Each patient had cystometric studies, cystoscopy and uroflometry. A total of forty-one males underwent photoirradiation of the bladder neck while 19 patients underwent treatment for prostatic adenoma; some in combination with bladder neck contractures. All patients were screened with transrectal ultrasonography of the prostate and were eliminated from the study with any suggestion of abnormality. Procedures were accomplished using a 100 watt Neodymium:YAG laser with type of delivery source varying from contact probes at low energy to bare fibre in direct contact at watts ranging from 60-80 watts. The procedure that seemed most effective was bare fibre, high energy contact therapy. Patients were followed up from 3-30 months and though early in the observation period, some conclusions appear clear from our results. Patients underwent all procedures under local anesthesia or intravenous sedation with Diazepam or occasional Demerol in the office setting as outpatients. Patient's ages ranged from 49-88 years. Results can be divided into two groups: laser therapy of the bladder neck for contracture and laser prostatotomy.

LASER THERAPY OF BLADDER NECK CONTRACTURE

NUMBER OF PATIENTS	41
TIME PERIOD (AVG. MONTHS)	3-30
JOULES DELIVERED	2-9,000
AVERAGE	4,200
S/P TURP	26
S/P OPEN PROCEDURE	15

Patients undergoing bladder neck therapy with Neodymium:YAG laser totaled 41 with an average observation period of 3-30 months. The number of Joules delivered varied from 2-9,000 with an average of 4,200. The etiology of the contractures was thought to be surgery in all cases. Twenty-six were status post transurethral resection and fifteen after suprapubic or retropubic prostatectomy.

RESULTS OF LASER TREATMENT FOR BLADDER NECK CONTRACTURE

NUMBER OF PATIENTS	41
IMPROVED SYMPTOMS	38
IMPROVED UROFLOW	39
RECURRENCE (AVG. 1½ YRS.)	3
FAILED TUR OR INCISION	10
COMPLICATIONS	6
EPIDIDYMITIS	1
BLEEDING	4
SEPSIS	1

Of 41 patients studied, 38 had improved symptoms and 39 had improved uroflow. The criteria for improvement in uroflow was at least a three-fold increase in the flow rate. There were three recurrences with an average of 1½ years post resection and of interest, were patients whose procedures utilized the lowest energy levels, averaging 2,600 Joules. Of forty-one patients studied, ten had failed a prior transurethral resection or incision of the bladder neck. Complications numbered six. Epididymitis was present in one patient who also developed sepsis and required hospital admission and intravenous antibiotics. Four patients developed postoperative bleeding; none required hospitalization and no patient was catheterized following his procedure.

RESULTS OF LASER PROSTATOTOMY

NUMBER OF PATIENTS	19
IMPROVED SYMPTOMS	16
IMPROVED UROFLOW	17
RECURRENCE (TURP	1
COMPLICATIONS	2
BLEEDING	1
REOPERATION	1

Laser prostatotomy was attempted in 19 patients and the vast majority of these were patients who had prior transurethral resection and residual tissue amounting to 10-15 grams. Improved symptoms were observed in 16 patients and improved uroflow in 17 patients. One patient had an approximately 40 gram prostate which we were unable to accomplish using current technology and who required admission to the hospital for transurethral resection of the prostate. Complications included bleeding in one patient and subsequent reoperation. All patients who underwent laser prostatotomy required the use of a #18 or #20 Fr, Foley catheter left in place overnight. Again, however, they were treated as outpatients and returned the following day for catheter removal. The period of observation of this group was 3-24 months and an average of 6 months. The number of Joules delivered was 4,000-19,000 and averaged 10,000 Joules.

LASER PROSTATOTOMY

NUMBER OF PATIENTS	41
TIME PERIOD (MONTHS)	3-24
AVERAGE	6 MONTHS
JOULES DELIVERED	4-19,000
AVERAGE	10,000
S/P TURP	9
S/P RADICAL PROSTATECTOMY	2

Nine of these patients had been status post transurethral resection of the prostate and two were status post radical prostatectomy with recurrent disease. Significant improvement in both symptoms and uroflowmetry was observed in 56 of the patients studied. Minimal complications were reported and only two patients to this point have required hospitalization and the procedure appears to be safe. It is too early, however to evaluate the long-term results of laser prostatotomy using present technology; further technological advances permitting use of laser therapy on larger prostates with advancements in delivery-system technology will be studied as they become available. We now feel the procedure of choice for bladder neck contracture is contact laser therapy.

BIBLIOGRAPHY

1. Shanberg, A.M., Chalfin, S.A., Tansey, L.A.: Neodymium:YAG laser: new treatment for urethral stricture disease. UROLOGY 24:15 (1984)
2. Staehler, G., Chaussey, C., Jocham, D., Schmiedt, E.: The use of Neodymium:YAG lasers in urology. Journal of Urology 134: 1155 (1985)
3. Smith, J.A. Jr. (Ed): Lasers in Urologic Surgery, Chicago, Yearbook Medical Publishers, 1985.
4. Smith, J.A. Jr.: Unpublished data, personal communication, 1985
5. Shanberg, A.M.: The use of the Neodymium:YAG laser in prostatotomy. AUA Presentation, 1985
6. Shanberg, A.M.: Personal Communications. 1985-1987.

BLADDER NECK CONTRACTURES

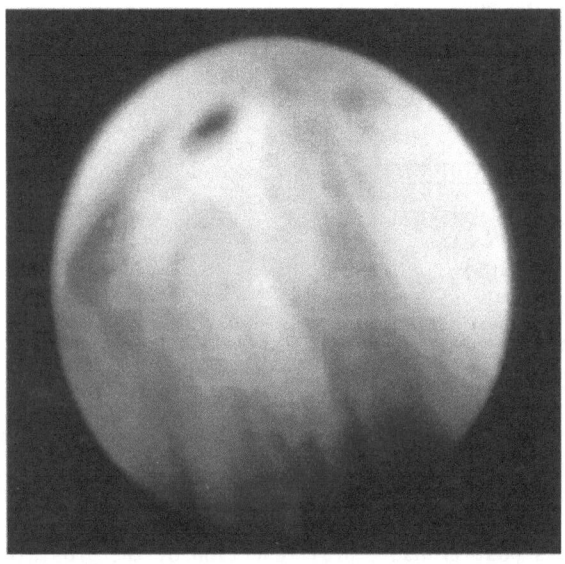

A TYPICAL BLADDER NECK CONTRACTURE AS VIEWED FROM THE PROSTATIC FOSSA PRIOR TO CONTACT PHOTOIRRADIATION.

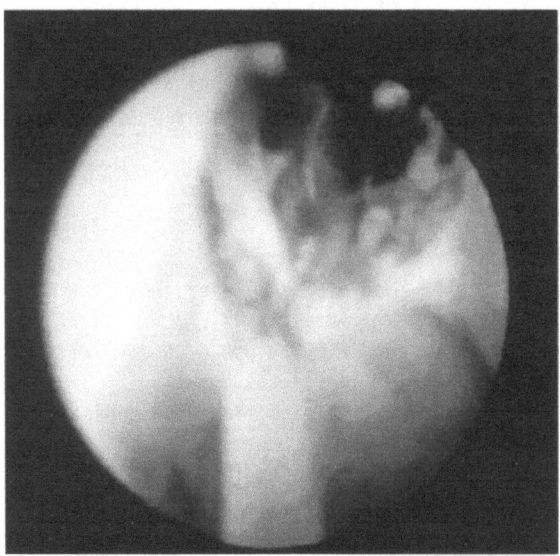

OBTAINED MIDWAY THROUGH THE 360° TREATMENT OF THE BLADDER NECK.

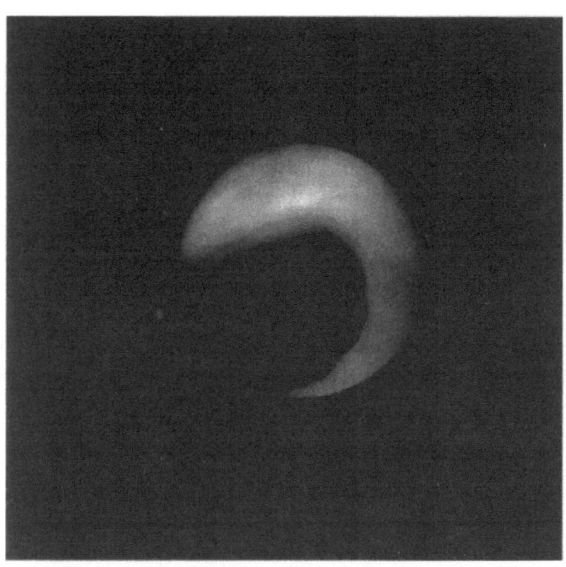

A THREE-MONTH FOLLOWUP AFTER THE
INITIAL PROCEDURE SHOWING A WIDE-OPEN
BLADDER NECK.

LASER PROSTATOTOMY

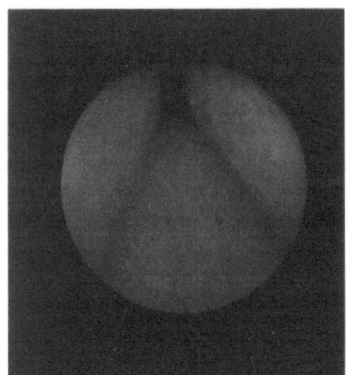

A TYPICAL BLADDER NECK OBSTRUCTION AND RESIDUAL
PROSTATE OF MEDIAN BAR VARIETY.

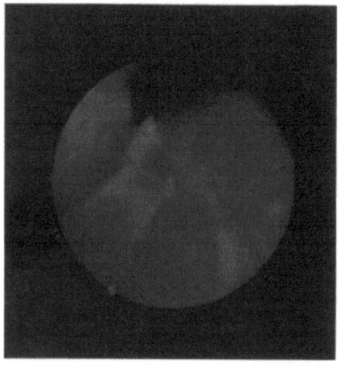

DEMONSTRATES VAPORIZATION OF THE OBSTRUCTING TISSUE BEGUN AT THE MIDLINE.

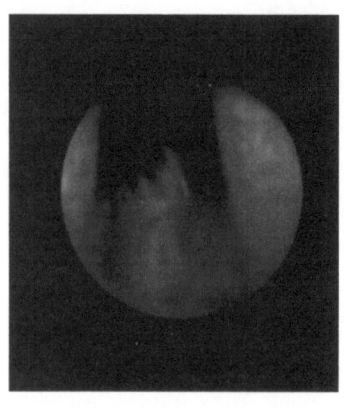

SAME AREA VIEWED MIDWAY THROUGH THE LASER VAPORIZATION PROCEDURE.

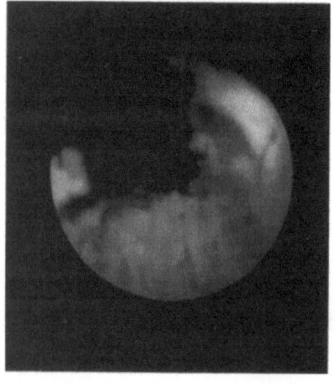

DEMONSTRATES THE OPEN PROSTATIC FOSSA OBTAINED AFTER COMPLETION OF THE MEDIAN LOBE LASER VAPORIZATION.

Laser Neodymium-YAG in Urology

Raul A. Olmedo, Pedro M. Minuzzi, Pedro G. Minuzzi,
Federico G. Minuzzi, Susana I. Minuzzi, Juan A. Saenz
Laser Center, Hospital Espanol of Cordoba, Argentina

From the opening of the LASER Center in the Hospital Espanol of Cordoba, I have made some treatments in several urological pathologies, following the protocols of the International Bibliography and in particular the experiences of Prof. A. Hofstetter.

Thanks to agreements signed between the German firms M.B.B., KARL STORZ and RICHARD WOLF, we have equipment of LASER Neodymium Yag and Endoscopics for urological applications.

I think it is necessary to repeat some basic concepts about the biological action of the different kinds of LASER which justify its use and the therapeutic advances that the photocoagulation with the LASER ND Yag have meant comparatively with the TUR of electric resection and coagulation.

The experimental studies and the clinical experiences which have been made in Cistectomy that previously went through photocoagulation with LASER or electrocoagulation, show a great difference in the histological aspect.

In cases where electrocoagulation was used, the final result is an irregular area of fibrosis without precise limitation; sanguinous and lynfatics vessels kept permeable. On the other hand, the photocoagulation with ND:YAG LASER produces a reaction that is characterized by an homogenic fibrosis of the whole vesical wall and what is more important, it produces a true scaling of the sanguinous and linfatic vessels as it is shown in the works of F. Keiditsch and collaborators. Our experience is shown in the next slide where there is a high percentage of applications in bladder tumors and there is a small number of applications in urethral stenosis.

LASER ND:YAG also is used in external applications in genital lesions as penis chondilome cavernous, anghiome of penis, and in open surgery of residivaded tumors of vesical origin with methastatis in surgery scar and deepening danger of the abdominal wall.

Recently we have begun to use the laser ND:YAG in stenosis of the urethral meatus and carrying out cunciform resection in the fibrosis area and reconstructing with the FLAP of the skin, with good transitory results.

In superficial bladder tumors, the immediate results are good although we cannotmake comparative studies because it has passed only a short period of time since then.

In infiltrated tumors (T2-B1-B2) if they are the only injuries, the results superpose to the ones we got with the TUR, until now after a year of experience.

In bladder infiltrated tumors (T3-T4-C-D) most patients have gone through the photocoagulation with palliative intentions because the tumoral stage did not allow to make a valid ancological therapy with surgery criteria. In these cases, the ND:YAG LASER alone or accompanied by the TUR of big tumors allow the patient to be comfort and avoids the saving cistectomy, dissapearing the hematuria. We have had the opportunity of putting a patient through resection and photocoagulation of an urethral tumor through Urethroscopy, getting good results, keeping the function and having the opportunity of making urological checking. In urethral stenosis, we associate the photocoagulation to the cold urethrotomy with sachse but reversing the order of applications of other authors (Martinez Pineiro). First we make the photocoagulation of the area which will be sectioned and in this way we avoid the formation of hematoma and inflammatory granuloma which is the reason of a great number of recidives.

If we think that this does not require the post surgery catheter, and in this way we get a rather good results, to which we will value adequately in time.
In external applications in genitalia injuries, our experience is limited only two cases of penial chondilome, a case of a boy with a cavernous angiome of GLANDE, and two cases of glande carcinoma and the last experiences of urethral meatus.

ND-YAG LASER

TREATMENTS

PATHOLOGY		APPLICATIONS
VESICAL TUMOR	46 patients	68
URETHRA STENOSIS	9 patients	11
URETER TUMOR	1 patient	1
ACUMINATE CHONDILOMA OF PENIS	3 patients	5
PENIS CANCER	2 patients	2
URETEROCELE	2 patients	2
STENOSIS OF URETHRAL MEATUS	3 patients	3
TOTAL	66 patients TOTAL	92 applications

BLADDER TUMORS
STAGE

T1-T2	12 patients
T2-B1-B2	11 patients
T3-T4	23 patients
TOTAL	46 patients

BLADDER TUMORS
BLADDER PLUS TUR

T1-A	16 applications
T2-B1-B2	11 applications
T3-C-D	26 applications
TOTAL	53 applications

LASER (MONOTHERAPY)

T1-A	15 applications
TOTAL OF APPLICATIONS	68 applications

URETHRA STENOSIS

TOTAL NUMBER OF PATIENTS	9	
No. OF APPLICATIONS	7 patients 1= 7	
	2 patients 2= 4	TOTAL 11 appl.
LASER PLUS SACHSE		
LASER (MONOTHERAPY)	1	

Lithotripsy

Laser-Induced Shock Wave Lithotripsy (LISL)-Biologic Effects and First Clinical Application

R.Hofmann, R.Hartung, H.Schmidt-Kloiber[*], E.Reichel[*]
Department of Urology, Technische Universität München, Klinikum re.d.Isar and*
Institut for Experimental Physics, Karl-Franzens-University, Graz, Austria

Continuous wave lasers induce thermic lesions in an irradiated tissue by transformation of the laser energy into heat. Laser energy from a pulsed Nd-YAG laser with a pulse duration in the nanosec. range is changed into mechanic energy as shockwaves by creation of a localized plasma. This procedure-laser induced breakdown-can be used for disintegration of concrements (e.g. urinary calculi)(1).

A prerequisite for uncomplicated application of laser energy in the urogenital tract is to evaluate the possible tissue damage by inadvertent irradiation of the urothelium.

Material and methods: laser light from a Nd-YAG laser(1064nm, 8nsec pulse duration) was irradiated either as a single pulse or a pulse series(20Hz). Single pulse energy ranged between 50-120mJ and was significantly higher than later used in patient treatment(35mJ).

Energy variation was performed with gray filters in the laser beam. The horizontal laser beam was reflected 90° down with a mirror and focussed directly on to the tissue surface with a small "focussing device". This sterilizable apparatus was built of a biconvex lens in a cylindrical tube and a fixed up "plexiglas-cone". The opening of the cone on the lower side was set upon the tissue and with the help of the red light of the Helium-Neon pilot laser, the laser beam focussed exactly on to the surface. The interior of the device could be filled with sterile solution (e.g. sodium chloride 0.9%). Additional experiments were accomplished with focussed irradiation of the urothelium directly out of the laser fibre. Laser induced breakdown was created with an energy of 30mJ at the fibre tip.

Biologic effects of laser irradiation were evaluated by irradiation of cell cultures, whole blood and urothelium of bladder, ureter and kidney parenchyma in pigs.

1. Irradiation of various tissue cultures was performed(fibroblasts-short time cultures of allogeneic renal cancer cells-xenogeneic kidney tumor cells). Pulse energy varied from 50-84mJ with up to 600 pulses. The cell culture monolayers were stained with Methylene blue for vital cells.

2. Irradiation of whole blood was performed by focussing the laser beam into a flask, filled with 20ml blood.

3. Kidney, ureter and urinary bladder in pigs were exposed transperitoneally. The ureter and the bladder were opened, the lumen held open with threads and the urothelium exposed to radiation.

**Experimental setting for energy variation and focussed irradiation
with Nd-YAG laser pulses on the tissue surface**

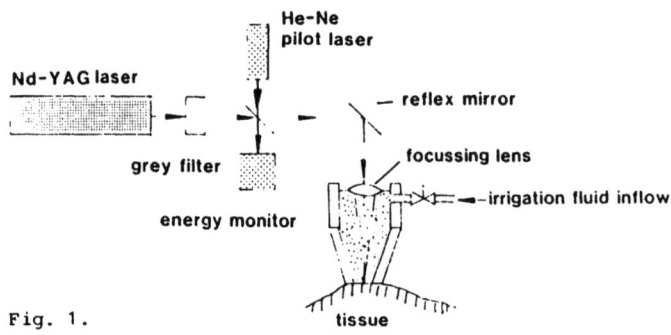

Fig. 1.

a. Urothelium was irradiated in 3 pigs to study the immediate effects of radiation. Laser energy varied from 50-84mJ with 20 pulses and in a second series 75mJ with 1,10,20 and 60 pulses for evaluation of the depth of the lesion. These animals were put to sleep immediately following irradiation. The exposed areas were enclosed by non-resorbable threads for easier histologic identification of the lesion.

b. Late effects were studied in another 4 pigs with laser irradiation of 60 resp 80mJ single pulse energy for 10 and 30 seconds and 30mJ for 10 and 30 seconds out of the laser fibre. The exposed tissue was examined 2,4,8 and 12 days thereafter. Electron-microscopic and histologic evaluation was performed using Elastica-van Gieson and Elastica-Ladewig staining.

Results:1. Tissue culture irradiation: only directly hit cells in the focus were destroyed and flushed away, while all cells surrounding the focus were vital and growing further in the culture.

2. Irradiation of whole blood showed no significant hemolysis after laser exposure for up to 15 minutes.

3. immediate effects of nanosec laser pulses: macroscopically the area of irradiation could be found sometimes as a tiny point in the urothelium. 4 of 18 tissue sections showed a small rupture cone with a maximum depth of 40μm. The electron microscope revealed a cone-like defect of about 40-50μm depth and 100μm width(fig 2 and 3)
Late effects of nanosec laser pulses: No macroscopic change could be seen on the pig urothelium 2,4,8 and 12 days after laser irradiation. Serial cuts of 5μm in the exposed area showed no histologic change, especially no thermic damage, necrosis or hemorrhage. Electron microscopy also did not reveal any tissue alteration.

Clinical results: At first stone disintegration was simulated in a mock system of an irrigation bag simulating the ureter. A urinary calculaus was impacted in the outflow of the bag and laser stone disintegration performed.

Starting patient treatment just recently in June 1987, 5 patients with ureter and kidney

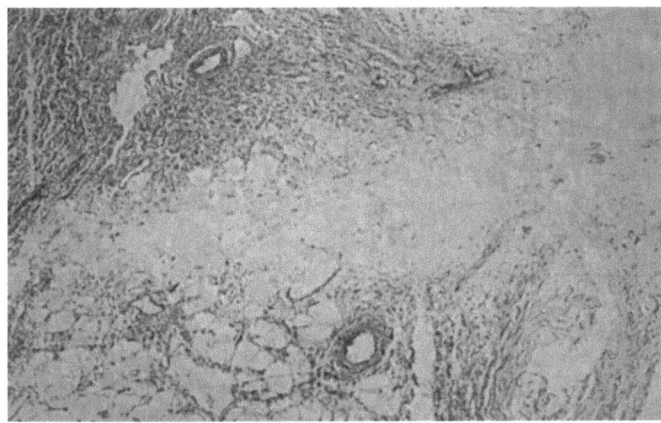

Fig 2. histologic section of rupture cone following irradiation with 8nsec, 84mJ and 20 pulses. The depth of the rupture cone is 40µm.

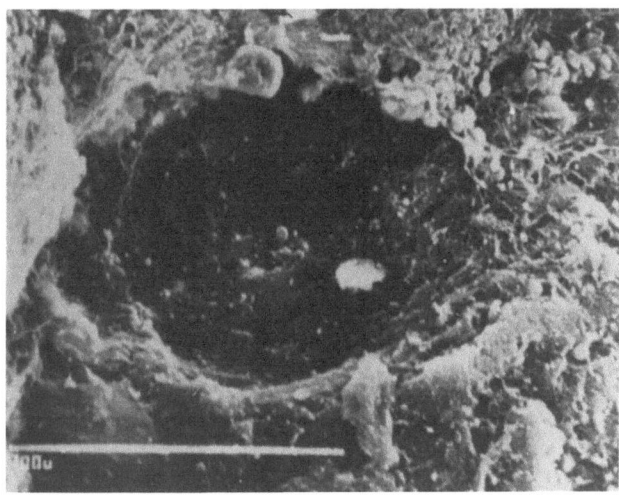

Fig 3. electron-microscopy of the lesion (see fig 2). The depth of the lesion is 40µm and 100 µm width. No necrosis or thermic effects are found

stones were treated. Only stones which did not pass spontaneously out of the ureter and kidney stones not suitable for ESWL treatment were exposed to laser irradiation. The laser beam of the Nd-YAG laser with 8 nsec pulse duration, 20 Hz repetition rate and 35mJ energy at the tip was coupled to a highly flexible 600µm quartz fibre by means of a specially designed tube. The fibre is either passed through the rigid ureteroscope(11.6 F) or nephroscope, using the percutaneous approach. The laser fibre is advanced close to the stone, so that the focussed laser light could disintegrate the stone from the surface. The procedure is done under constant vision, using an irrigant solution. The tiny stone fragments are sucked off close to the fibre tip through a 500µm channel. 3 obstructing ureteral stones and 1 kidney stone were completely fragmented and washed out within 2-5 minutes laser irradiation time. One kidney stone could only be disintegrated partly; the residual stone was removed by forceps. Stone analysis revealed calcium oxalate monohydrate and -dihydrate composition of the stones. So far clinical results are very prominsing, laser stone disintegration being a fast, effective and secure procedure, creating tiny stone fragments or even "stone powder". No additional measures to remove stone parts (e.g. forceps, ultrasound probe...) from the kidney or ureter are necessary. With small flexible probes for ureterorenoscopy, the advantage of a highly flexible and thin (600 or 400 µm) laser fibre can be ideally combined. No thermic side effects or damage of the tissue can be found with laser energy from a Nd-YAG laser with nanosecond pulses (2)

Literature

1. R. Hofmann, R. Hartung, K. Geißdörfer, R. Ascherl, W. Erhardt, H. Schmidt-Kloiber, E. Reichel, H. Schöffmann
   Morphologische Untersuchungen des Urothels nach Einwirkung intensiver Nanosekunden-Laserpulse- Urologia internationalis in press

2. H. Schmidt-Kloiber, E. Reichel, H. Schöffmann
   Laser-induced shock wave lithotripsy (LISL) - Biomed. Technik 30, 173 (1985)

Laser Lithotripsy: Measurement of Pressure and Shockwaves in Stones

Th. Meier, E. Keckeis, R. Steiner

Institut für Lasertechnologien, Universität Ulm

Postfach 40 66, D-7900 Ulm/Donau, F.R.G.

Introduction

Opto-mechanical effects induced by short pulsed lasers are widely used for disruption or disaggregation of biological structures like e.g. kidney stones and gall stones.

The destruction process is due to the shockwaves resulting from a laser induced micro-explosion. This may be an optical breakdown in pure liquids or a plasma generation similar to that in the ablation process on the surface of solids.

In order to get a better understanding of the generation of shockwaves and their propagation in stones we measured pressure waves in water and inside the stones. This can help to find the best laser parameters for the destruction of stones (laser lithotripsy).

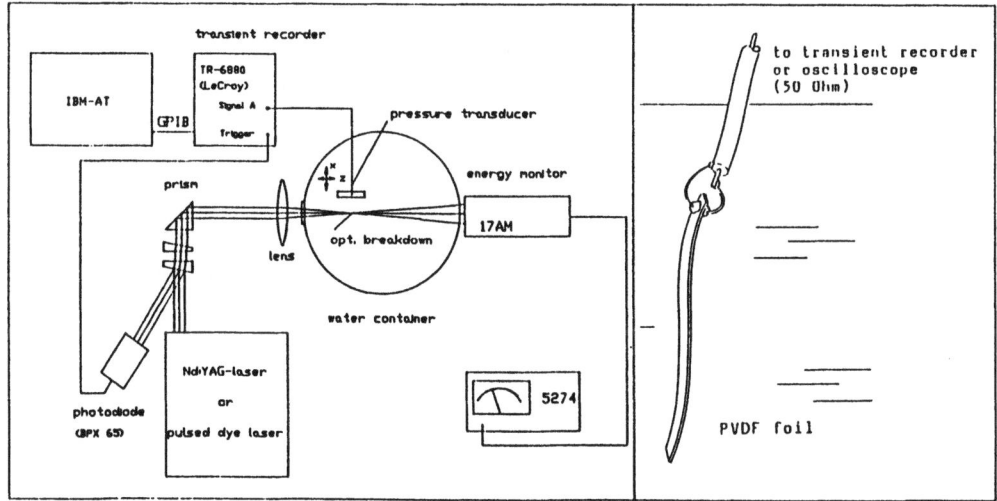

Fig. 1. Experimental set-up. The pulsed laser was focused either in water or on a stone with embedded pressure transducer

Fig. 2. PDVF pressure transducer in 'strip geometry'

Experiments

The experimental set-up is shown in Fig. 1. The laser beam was focused either in destilled water while the pressure transducer was placed in the vicinity of the optical breakdown or on the surface of the stone when the transducer was embedded in the stone. Two lasers were used: a Nd:YAG laser (JK lasers, Q-switched) and a flashlamp pumped dye laser (Candela SSL 500, T (pulse) = 500 ns, λ = 590 nm).

The pressure transducer consisted simply in a piece of piezo electric foil (PVDF). This material is widely used for measuring shockwaves. Normally, the sensitive area is kept very small (appr. 1mm^2 or less) to get a high spatial and temporal resolution. In contrast, we used a rather extended geometry ('strip geometry'), which is easy to handle and well suited for being embedded in stones. It follows from simple geometrical considerations that a plane PVDF-foil and a sharp spherical shockwave results in a signal not very different from those obtained with more sophisticated arrangements.

For the measurements inside the stones, the stones were cut into two parts and then glued together with the PVDF-foil in between. First experiments with biological concrements (kidney stones) resulted in signals which where hard to interpret, without the typical shockwave formation and not reproducible. We decided therefore first to perform some measurements on a more homogeneous material as e.g. limestone.

The electrical signal was fed into a transient recorder with a risetime less than 1.5 ns (Le Croy, Mod. 6886).

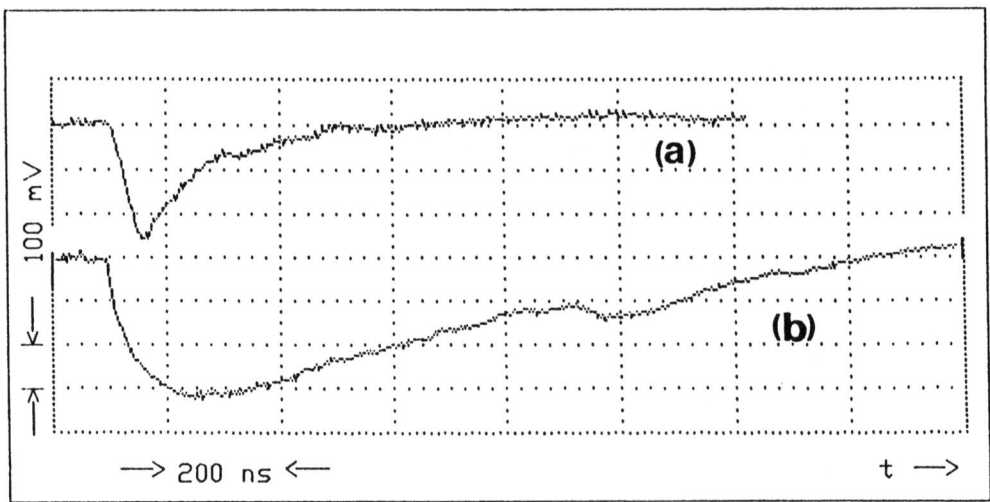

Fig. 3. Pressure transducer signal, in Volts, from a shockwave in water after optical breakdown induced by the Nd:YAG laser (a) and by the pulsed dye laser (b). The polarity depends on the accidental connection to the cable

Results

As a first check we recorded the pressure wave after an optical breakdown induced by the 10 ns Nd:YAG laser pulse (Fig. 3 a). Risetime and pulse duration clearly indicate the existence of a shockwave. Fig. 3 b shows the corresponding signal from a 500 ns dye laser pulse. While the risetime is still short the rest of the pulse is a reproduction of the laserpulse. When we focused the Nd:YAG laser on the surface of the stone we could still

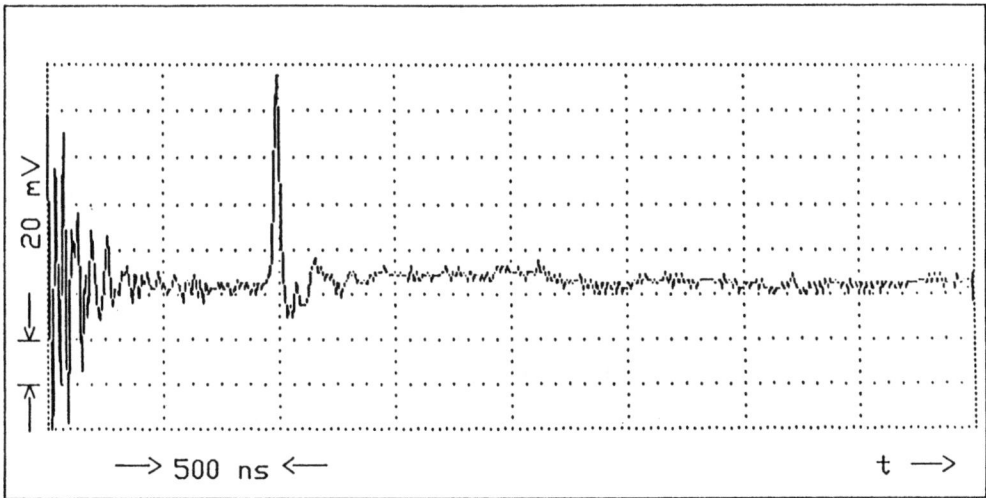

Fig. 4. Shockwave signal induced with the Nd:YAG laser and measured with a transducer inside the stone. The strongly fluctuating signal in the first time division is electrical noise from the laser ignition. The distance d (stone surface-PVDF-foil) was 6 mm

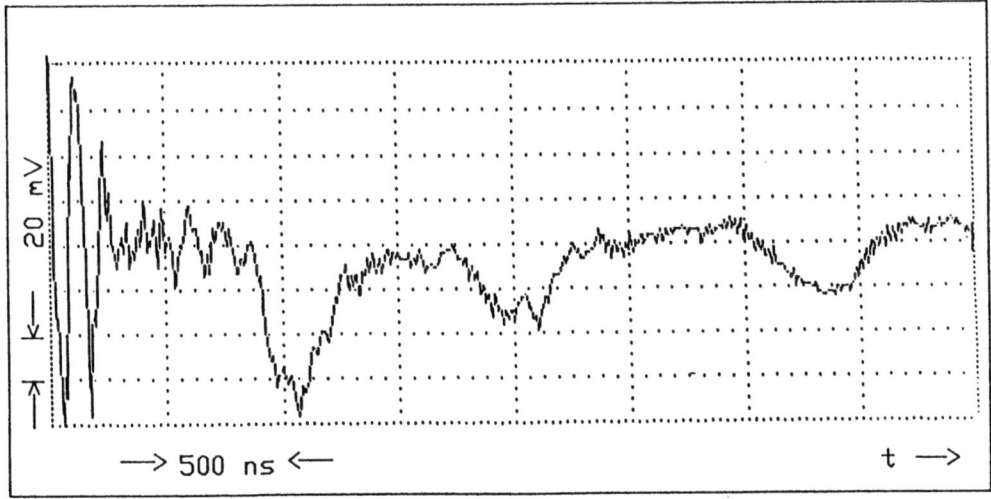

Fig. 5. Same as Fig. 4., but with pulsed dye laser (stone sample not identical with that of Fig. 4.! Distance d was 5 mm)

record a clear shockwave some mm inside the stone (Fig. 4.). However, with the dye laser the signal looks quite different (Fig. 5.). In this case a leading pulse is distinguishable with a pulse width comparable to that of the dye laser pulse, but this pulse is followed by two or more pulses which are in some cases partly overlapping. The origin of these secondary pulses is not yet clear.

Conclusion

We have shown that with a PVDF-foil transducer in 'strip geometry' shockwave signals can be measured in liquids and in stones. The recorded signals reflected the influence of different laser parameters (e.g. pulse length, risetime, wavelength etc.).
A systematic study with different lasers on different types of stones will help to find the optimal laser parameters for laser lithotripsy.

References

1) H. Schmidt-Kloiber, E. Reichel, H. Schöffmann
   Laserinduced Shock-Wave Lithotripsy (LISL)
   Biomed. Technik, 30, (1985), 173-181

2) N.S. Nishioka, P. Teng, Th. Deutsch, R.R. Anderson
   Mechanism of Laser-Induced Fragmentation of Urinary and Biliary Calculi
   Lasers in the Life Sciences, 1, (1987), 231-245

Laser Induced Shock Waves for Medical Applications

E. Steiger, W. Uebelacker
Dornier Medizintechnik GmbH, Applied Research, Germering/D

Abstract

Extracorporal shock wave lithotripsy (ESWL) is by now a well established method to fracture human kidney and gall bladder stones in vivo.
One method of generating shock waves in water is to focus a laser beam of short pulse width and high energy to a point.
We report on experiments with a Q-switched Nd:YAG laser causing an optical breakdown in the focal region of a lens. It was found that the shock wave formation and dynamic depends not only on the lens performance but also on the laser beam properties. Using a semi-elliptic reflector we measured the temporal and spatial behaviour of the reflected and focused shock wave and studied the pressure distribution at the second focal point of the reflector with an ultra-fast PVDF-transducer and time-resolved Schlieren photographs. First in vitro-experiments on kidney and gall bladder stones gave reasonable results.

Introduction

The application of shock waves produced by an electrical discharge in water and focused by an elliptical reflector is now an overall accepted method for the extracorporal destruction of human kidney stones (/1/). Another practicable method of generating these shock waves is to focus an intense light pulse in the nanosecond time scale by a Q-switched laser to a nearly pointlike source (/2/, /3/).
At sufficient intensity of the light pulse the electrical field-strength in the focal plane of the focusing lens causes plasma-production by multiphoton-ionization and inverse Bremsstrahlung. By further heating the plasma with the laser pulse a shock wave is emitted into the surrounding medium (/4/, /5/).

Methods and Results

Fig. 1 shows the experimental set-up for the laser induced generation of shock waves in a 3-D elliptic reflector attached to a tank with degassed water at room temperature. The Q-switched Nd:YAG laser (LASER 1) with a maximum pulse energy of 800 mJ at 1064 nm, a pulse duration of 8 nsec (FWHM), a beam divergence of 0.8 mrad and an unexpanded beam diameter of 8 mm is focused by a single moveable lens (L1) of variable shape and focal length at the first elliptic focal point F1. Besides the nearly spherically symmetric detonation wave of the optical breakdown at that point a cavitation bubble with a maximum diameter of 9 mm is produced by the laser pulse (/6/). The shock wave is then reflected by the brass ellipsoid and exits the reflector as a reinforced wave with increasing strength as it converges towards the second focal point F2. With an eccentricity of 0.828 F2 is 115 mm out of the mouth of the semi-elliptical reflector along the major axis. The sensitive element for measuring the pressure in the region around F2 consists of a thin film of poly-vinylidendifluorid (PVDF) with an active area of 1 mm in diameter. With a resonant frequency of about 55 MHz it delivers a pressure signal of approx. 8 mV/bar.

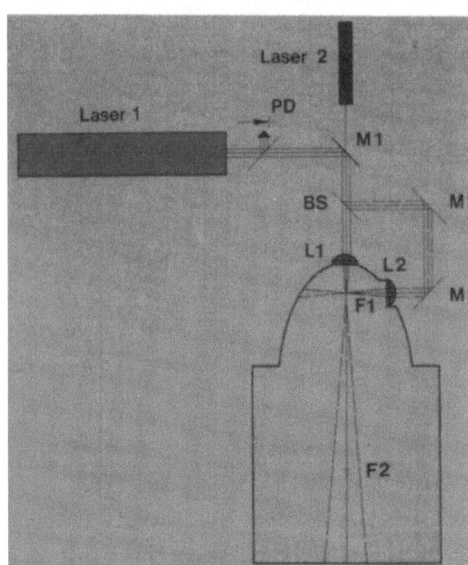

Fig. 1. Experimental set-up for laser induced shock wave generation

The sequence in Fig. 2 a-c shows the temporal response of this PVDF-transducer to a transient shock pulse in the second focal point at various time scales. The transducer is hereby oriented with the sensitive area normal to the wave front. The first pulse of the signal in Fig. 2a belongs to the laser induced shock wave, the second - separated by approx. 780 µsec - to the cavitation bubble collapse. The laser energy was focused by a lens with f = 20 mm in air. Fig. 2b shows the first pulse in more detail with a FWHM of 300 nsec and its tensile part. With the highest possible resolution of the oscilloscope Fig. 2c indicates a rise time of the shock pulse of about 50 nsec. By decreasing the laser energy the rise time, amplitude and shape of the pressure signal is changed considerably. Due to the smaller bubble diameter for lower laser energy the time to bubble collapse is also reduced. For a laser energy of 110 mJ this delay time reduces to about 460 µsec.

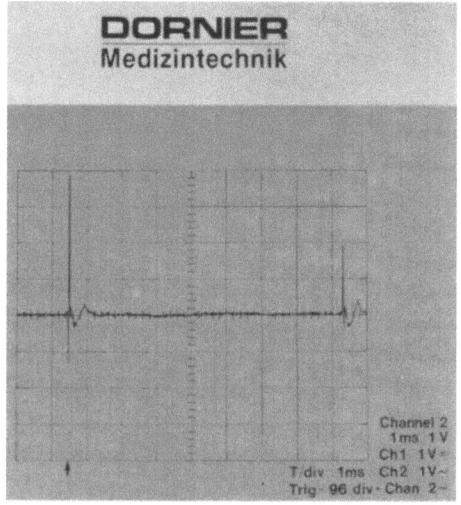

a

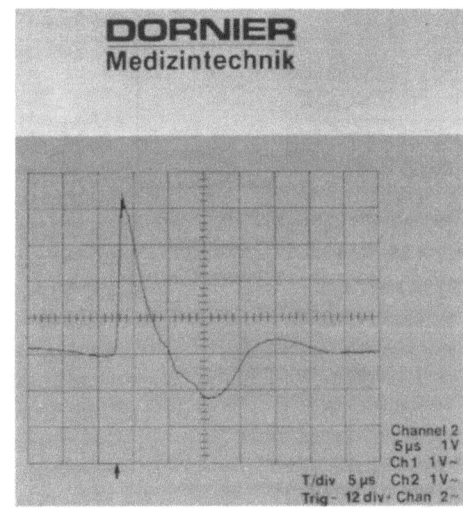

b

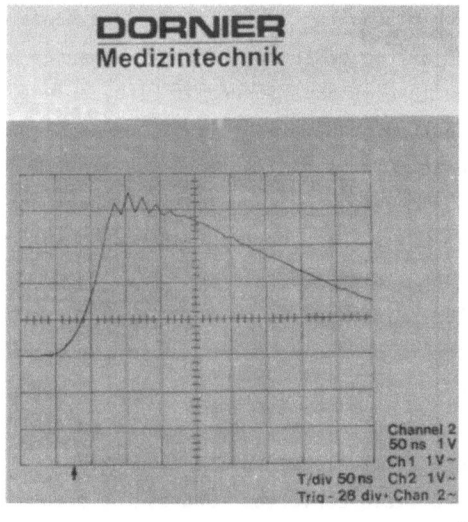

c

Fig. 2. PVDF-transducer response to a transient focused shock pulse (laser energy: 600 mJ)

a) 1 msec/div
b) 5 µsec/div
c) 50 nsec/div

If we consider only the shock wave pulse in the above pressure signals we can measure the pressure distribution of the reinforced wave in the region around the second focal point of the ellipsoid. This 2-D peak pressure distribution in the symmetry plane of the elliptic reflector is shown in Fig. 3. All the measured points are mean values of five laser pulses with the pressure transducer fixed at the same place. The laser pulse energy for this case is 600 mJ focused by a plano-convex lens with f = 20 mm in air. It is clearly visible that the pressure peak of the distribution corresponds exactly to the position of the second focal point F2 of the ellipsoid at z = 115 mm.

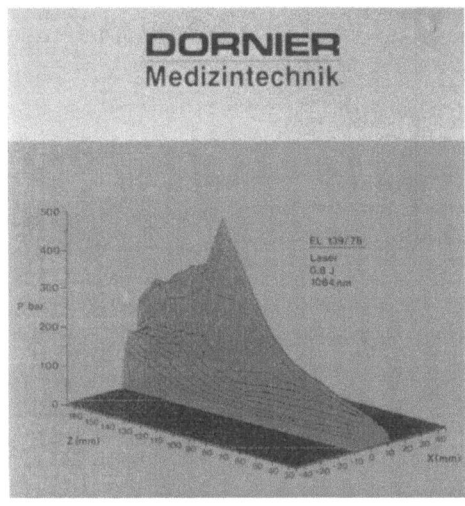

Fig. 3. 2-D peak pressure distribution of a laser induced shock wave in the second focal point of an ellipsoid

At that point all kidney and biliary stones were placed for destruction experiments. It is further interesting that the lateral FWHM of the distribution in F2 measures only 4 mm according to the conical shape of the laser plasma formed in F1 by a lens of short focal length. The shape of the distribution changed rapidly if the focal length of the lens is increased or the laser beam is expanded and focused with a nonspherical corrected lens of high aperture. In general the sphericity of the shock wave produced at the optical breakdown decreases as either the input energy or the focal length of the optics is increased. With the aid of a Schlieren-optical arrangement (/7/) we made the propagation of the reinforced laser induced shock wave in the water visible (Fig. 4 a-d). According to the recording technique the shock wave field appears dark against the undisturbed background. The photographs - made with the same optical configuration as for the pressure distribution - were taken with time delays of 394, 402, 408 and 422 μsec after the laser pulse respectively. Coming from the left side (Fig. 4a) the pressure field converges towards the second focal point F2 (Fig. 4c) and diverges very fast after its minimum extension of a few millimeters (Fig. 4d).

With this experimental set-up we shattered kidney and biliary stones in vitro. By applying some few thousand laser induced shock wave pulses with a laser repetition frequency of 10 Hz we reached stone destruction in the second focal point of the ellipsoid. It appears however that the stone - according to the small lateral extension of the reflected shock wave - had to be positioned very exactly to reach effective stone shattering.

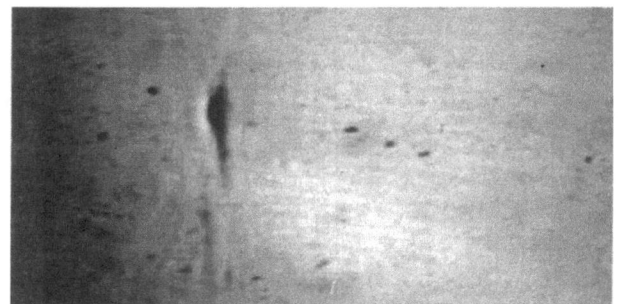

a)

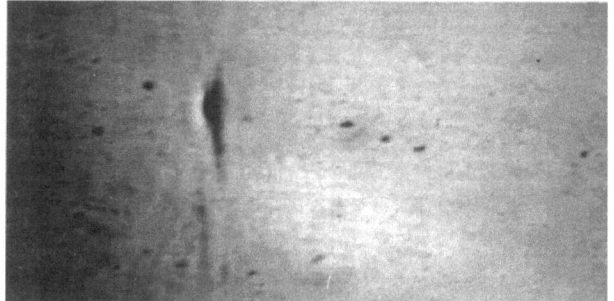

b)

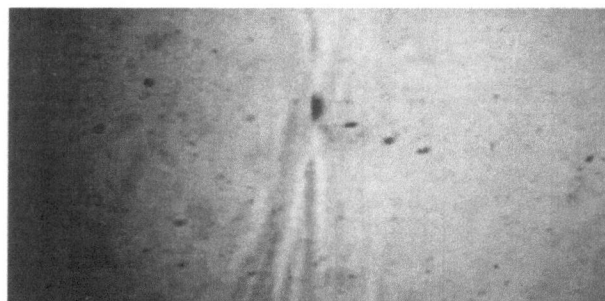

c)

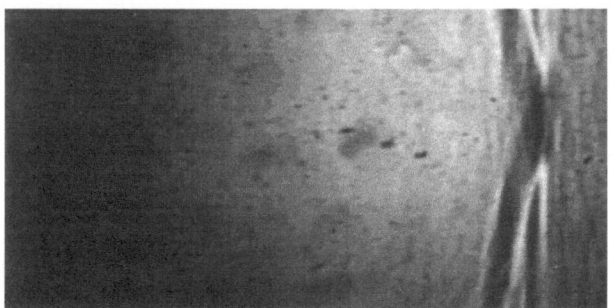

d)

Fig. 4.

Schlieren-optical photographs of a reflected laser induced shock wave field (laser energy: 600 mJ)

Time delay to the laser pulse:
a) 394 μsec
b) 402 μsec
c) 408 μsec
d) 422 μsec

Conclusion

Laser induced shock waves in water focused by a semi-elliptical reflector are a suitable means to shatter kidney and biliary stones in vitro. It turns out that the energy deposition efficiency of the laser pulses is very good and highly reproducible since no degradation can occur compared to the electric spark. Losses in the laser energy delivery system were attributable to reflection and/or absorbtion in the focusing optics and beam absorbtion in the intervening water. The shape and symmetry of the laser induced shock wave was found to be a function of the laser pulse energy, the spatial beam profile and the beam delivery optics of the complete system.

References

/1/ Chaussy, Ch. et al.
Extracorporeal Shock Wave Lithotripsy
Karger, Munich 1982

/2/ Charko, R.E.
Laser Shock Wave Lithotripsy
Master thesis of Science in Aeronautics and Astronautics
University of Washington, 1984

/3/ Russel, D.A.
Shock dynamics of noninvasive fracturing of kidney stones
Proceedings of the 15th International Symposium on Shock Waves and Shock Tubes, Standford University Press, 1986

/4/ Reichel, E. et al.
Interaction of intense ns-laserpulses with biological matter
2nd International ND:YAG Laser Conference, LASER 85, p. 285-289

/5/ Reichel E. et al.
Interaction of short laser pulses with biological structurs
Optics and Laser Technology 19 (1987) 1, p. 40-44

/6/ Lauterborn, W.
Kavitation durch Laserlicht
Acustica 31 (1974) 2, p. 51-78

/7/ Vogel, A. et al.
Cavitation bubble dynamics and acoustic transient generation in ocular surgery with pulsed Nd:YAG lasers
Third Physical Institute, University of Goettingen, FRG

Physical Foundations of the Laser-Induced Shockwave Lithotripsy (LISL)

E. Reichel[1], H. Schmidt-Kloiber[1], H. Schöffmann[1], G. Dohr[2], R. Hofmann[3], R. Hartung[3]
1) Institut für Experimentalphysik, 2) Institut für Histologie und Embryologie der Karl-Franzens-Universität Graz/ Austria
3) Urologische Klinik der Technischen Universität München/ FRG

1. INTRODUCTION

This paper describes the basic concepts of stone fragmentation by lasers and the possibilities of guiding laser-light through optical fibers. A section about the physics of the laser-induced breakdown (LIB) and the shockwaves produced thereby is followed. These shockwaves cause the stone fragmentation in the laser-induced shockwave lithotripsy (LISL) and the effectiveness of biliary and ureter stone destruction is dealt with in the last chapter.

2. METHODS OF LASER-INDUCED STONE FRAGMENTATION

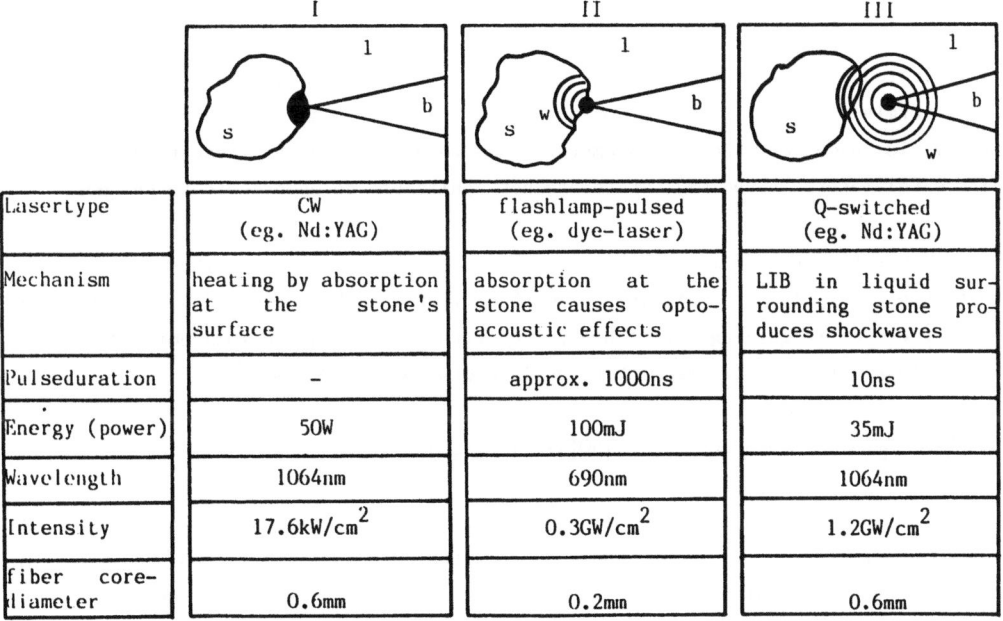

Lasertype	I CW (eg. Nd:YAG)	II flashlamp-pulsed (eg. dye-laser)	III Q-switched (eg. Nd:YAG)
Mechanism	heating by absorption at the stone's surface	absorption at the stone causes opto-acoustic effects	LIB in liquid surrounding stone produces shockwaves
Pulseduration	-	approx. 1000ns	10ns
Energy (power)	50W	100mJ	35mJ
Wavelength	1064nm	690nm	1064nm
Intensity	17.6kW/cm^2	0.3GW/cm^2	1.2GW/cm^2
fiber core-diameter	0.6mm	0.2mm	0.6mm

Fig.1. Survey of laser-induced stone fragmentation /1,2,3/.
(s...stone, l...liquid, b...laserbeam, w...shockwave)

Depending on the laser type there are three mechanisms for stone destruction, which are shown in Fig. 1.

Methods I and II use absorption of the laser-light at the stone's surface, producing strong thermal stresses or opto-acoustic released mechanical stresses respectively. Therefore method II depends on the selection of certain laser wavelengths (e.g. use of dye-lasers in II). Whereas for method I the use of high power CW-lasers is necessary (I), which leads to heating of the operation region. Method III ignites a laser-induced breakdown (LIB) in the liquid surrounding the stone and the stone composition is no longer decisive. Furthermore no thermic effects accompany the breakdown with the exception of plasma production in the focal region.

3. TRANSMISSION OF LASER-LIGHT THROUGH OPTICAL FIBERS

The second important aspect for the laser-induced lithotripsy is the possibility of transmitting the intensive laser-light through optical fibers. The limits for transmission are given by the intensity of the laser-light and the breakdown threshold of the particular fiber material:

$$\dot{I} = \frac{E}{T \cdot A} \leq 10 \ GW/cm^2$$

I ... intensity
E ... laserpulse energy
T ... laserpulse duration
A ... cross-section of the fiber-core

As indicated above this value should not exceed $10 GW/cm^2$ for silicone fibers. E and T are determined by the fragmentation mechanism, A depends on the fiber type. If more energy is necessary the core-diameters have to be made larger resulting in rigid fibers (diameters above 1mm), which are not applicable to endoscopic techniques.

The intensities needed for the three methods are given in Fig.1. These values show, that the laserpulse transmission for method III has to be performed very carefully. We succeeded in guiding Q-switched pulses with energies up to 70mJ emitted from a Nd:YAG-laser, through fibers with core-diameters down to 0.4mm.

4. THE LASER-INDUCED SHOCKWAVE LITHOTRIPSY (LISL)

One advantage of method III lies in the ignition of a laser-induced breakdown in the liquid surrounding the stone independent of the stone's surface, which makes this method independent of the stone's composition. A further aspect is the absence of thermal effects enabling application in narrow regions inside the body, such as ureter or bile-duct. These facts and the possibility of inserting the Q-switched Nd:YAG-laser, which is a very reliable and easy to operate laser-type, has caused us to develop a method based on this method.

4.1. THE LASER-INDUCED BREAKDOWN

On focussing the laserpulses of a Q-switched Nd:YAG-laser large photon flux densities can be reached, which are capable of producing free electrons by means of multiphoton ionization in matter. Inverse Bremsstrahlung caused by the then following photons of the same laserpulse accelerate the electrons until they are able to ionize matter by themselves. This results in an electron avalanche, which converts matter into the plasma state. The rapid expansion of the plasma at supersonic speed introduces shockwaves in the undisturbed matter- in our case in the liquid.

After emission of the shockwave the plasma expansion ceases and a cool, gas-filled void is left. This void collapses under the liquid pressure and leads to cavitation and emission of further shockwaves /4/.

4.2. LASER-INDUCED SHOCKWAVES

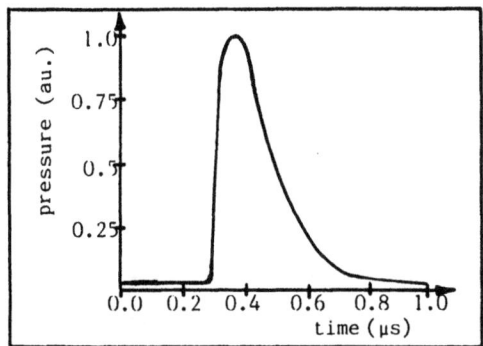

Fig.2. Time resolved shape of a laser-induced shockwave

Fig.2 shows the time resolved shape of a laser-induced shockwave. The rise of the pressure amplitude is less than 3ns and the overall duration is about 180ns. In the near-field of the LIB (approx. 3mm) the shockwave propagates with a supersonic velocity (2500m/s in water). The pressure amplitude at a distance of 1mm amounts to 1.5kbar given a laserpulse energy of 35mJ at the focal region.

Because of the plasma shape in the focal region the decrease of pressure with the distance from the plasma indicates a cylindrical waveform geometry, which is turning into spherical symmetry on leaving the near-field perpendicular to the optical axes (see Fig.3).

The shockwave pressure is connected to the laserpulse energy offered at the focal region by the following law:

$$p \sim (W)^{1/2}$$

p ... maximum pressure amplitude
W ... laserpulse energy at the focal region

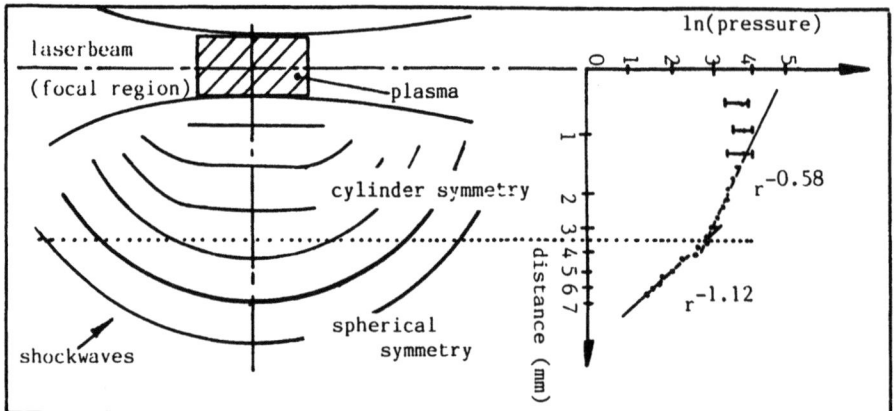

Fig.3. Shockwave pressure as a function of distance from the focal region

This means that doubling of the energy does not lead to a doubling in pressure. A typical value for the mechanical energy in the shockwave is about 1mJ for W=30mJ.

4.3. STONE FRAGMENTATION BY MEANS OF LASER-INDUCED SHOCKWAVES

The size of the stone particles and the effectiveness are determined by the mechanical energy, the peak pressure and the duration of the shockwave. The values from section 4.2. for the shockwaves indicate dimensions of the shattered particles in the order of 1mm.

In addition to the shockwave parameters the pulse repetition rate of the laser plays an important role, because it influences the duration of the destruction.

Experiments have shown that renal stones and biliary stones of any composition can be destroyed with the laser-induced shockwaves. Thereby the stones are shattered into tiny particles with dimensions of less than 1mm, which enables the irrigation of these particles out of the patient's body through a channel in the endoscope during operation.

5. SUMMARY

We have solved the problems of the transmission of laserpulses emitted by a Q-switched Nd:YAG-laser and realized a method for the in-vivo destruction of ureter and biliary calculi by means of a laser-induced breakdown. The shockwaves thereby produced are able to shatter stones of various compositions into tiny particles. These particles can be irrigated out of the patient's body through an endoscope simultaneously.

After pre-clinical tests examining side-effects of the laser-light and the shock-waves on tissue, the procedure is now under clinical testing. First results have shown that this method is very succesful in the destruction of ureter stones /5/.

6. REFERENCES

/1/ Tamahashi,Y., Orikasa,S., Numata,I., et al.
    Jap. J. Urol. 71 (1980)/ p 28
/2/ Teng,P., Nishioka,N.S., Rox Anderson,R., Deutsch,T.F.
    Appl. Phys. B 42 (1987)/ p 73
/3/ Schmidt- Kloiber,H., Reichel,E., Schöffmann,H.
    Biomed. Technik 30 (1985)/ p 173
/4/ Vogel,A., Hentschel,W., Holzfuss,J., Lauterborn,W.
    Klin. Mbl. Augenheilk. 189 (1986)/ p 308
/5/ Hofmann,R., Hartung,R., Schmidt-Kloiber,H., Reichel,E., et al.
    Urologia Internationalis (for publication accepted)

Laser Fragmentation of Urinary Calculi: In Vitro Studies

R. Friedrichs[1], R. Poprawe[2], R. Kohnemann[2], W. Schäfer[1], H. Rübben[1]
[1] Dept. of Urology RWTH Aachen, Pauwelsstr., D-5100 Aachen
[2] Fraunhofer Institute for Laser-Engineering and -Technology, Drosselweg 87, D-5100 Aachen

Abstract Parameters for effective in vitro laser fragmentation of urinary calculi by the neodymium-YAG (Nd:YAG) laser and the KrF-Excimer laser are examined. The results of reflection measurement of urinary calculi at wavelengths of different laser systems are presented. From $\lambda=1046$ nm (Nd:YAG laser) to $\lambda=249$ nm (KrF-Excimer laser) a continuous decline of reflection is found. The reflection at $\lambda=1046$ nm is above 90% whereas a complete absorption is found in the ultraviolet range. Furthermore a tube which contains as essential parts a water pump and a Nd:YAG laser system is presented. This tube allows by determination of its entrance size and by sucking off the urinary calculi fragmentation to particles which are not larger in diameter than the entrance size. Following these results experimental data with the KrF-Excimer laser are presented.

Introduction Although treatment of urinary calculi by different laser systems has been already introduced in clinical practice (1), many interactions between laser radiation and urinary calculi have not yet been examined. The purpose of this paper is the evaluation of some relevant parameters for effective calculi disintigration in vitro. The points discussed here are: What is the reflection of urinary calculi at wavelengths of different laser systems ? Is it possible to destroy urinary calculi by the Nd:YAG laser and to have as result fragments of a uniform and selected size ? What are specific effects of the KrF-Excimer laser upon urinary calculi ?

Materials and Methods Light of different wavelengths is dispersed by a prisma. The light of different wave lengths enters a sphere. Within this sphere the diffuse reflection is determined by a detector. The direct reflection is not considered because it can be neglected.(fig. 1) Urinary calculi of different composition are disintigrated by a Q-switched Nd:YAG laser (pulse duration $\tau=15$ ns, intensity $I=10^9$ W/cm^2, pulse energy E=25 mJ, focal radius $2r_F=500$ µm and laser frequency $\nu=20$ Hz). Urinary calculi are then disintigrated under the same conditions, using a tube shown in fig. 2. The calculi are sucked off by a water pump, thus being in direct contact with the tube in 90% of the

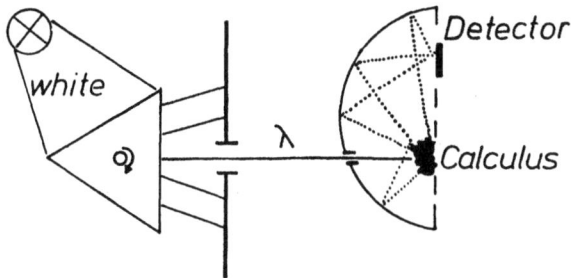

fig. 1. Schematic set up for reflection measurement

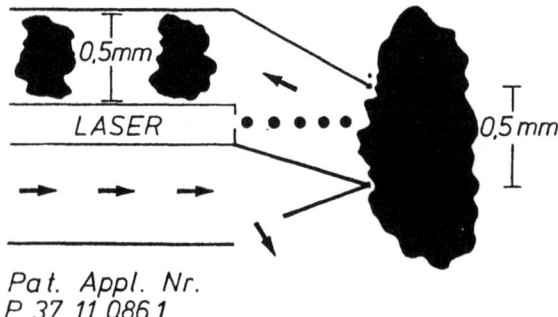

Pat. Appl. Nr.
P 37 11 086.1

fig. 2. Schematic set up of a tube which is developed
for limitation and selection of particle size

time. By selection of the entrance size the fragment size is determined. Urinary calculi of different composition are disintigrated by a KrF-Excimer laser ($\lambda=249$ nm, focal radius $2r_F=0,7$ mm x 3,5 mm, intensity $I=10^8$ W/cm^2, pulse energy E=30 mJ, pulse duration $\tau=15$ ns). The areas treated are examined by a scanning electron microscope.
Results The reflection of urinary calculi depends on the wavelength. From $\lambda=1046$ nm (Nd:YAG) to 249 nm (KrF-Excimer laser) a continuous decline in reflection is found. The reflection at $\lambda=1046$ nm is above 90% whereas a complete absorption is found in the ultraviolet range(fig.3).

The destruction of urinary calculi by the Nd:YAG laser results in fragments of different sizes. It is possible to select and to limit by application of the described tube mechanism (fig. 2) the fragment size using the Nd:YAG laser with all other parameters unchanged.- The KrF-Excimer laser allows effective destruction of urinary calculi. Stone disintigration was even achieved by a large focal radius and only 100 pulses. In contrast to the Nd:YAG laser a photoablative effect is

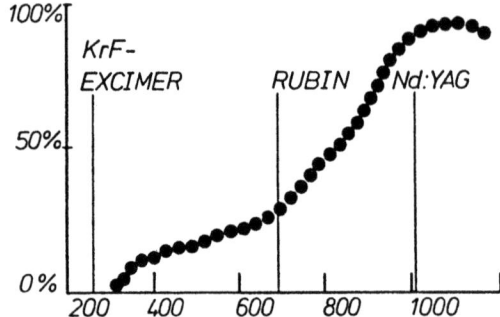

fig. 3. Reflection of a urinary calculus (calcium-oxalate) at wavelengths of different laser systems (axis of x=reflection in %, axis of y=wavelength λ (nm)

found after use of the KrF-Excimer laser. No areas of melting effects are detected by scanning electron microscopy.

Discussion Effective urinary stone disintigration can be performed in vitro by pulsed laser systems of different wave lengths (2-5). The technical principle of pulsed laser systems is that the absorption of a laser pulse by the calculus causes a plasma to form at the surface of the stone. This plasma is a rapidly expanding cavity of ions and electrons which collapses rapidly after the laser pulse. Thus a mechanical shockwave is produced (6-8). In most investigations carried out so far the technical application of laser systems of different wavelengths on urinary stone disintigration in general has been mainly studied. Neither the factors intensity, wavelength, pulse duration, pulse energy, focal radius, influence of the chemical stone composition on the disintigration, or particle size after laser treatment nor the influence between these factors have been intensely studied. Reviewing the literature it is found that from the technical point of view the results often can hardly be compared with each other, because important technical data like focal radius or intensity are not described (1,3,5). Some data are based on empiricism: it is suggested that particles after laser treatment are smaller than after ultrasound treatment (5). It is presumed that at 504 nm a complete absorption is found (1), but what is not the case as shown by our reflection measurements. The use of the Nd:YAG laser in combination with the tube system first described by us may lead to the introduction in clinical practice, because limitation of fragment size offers several advantages over existing methods. On the other hand the KrF-Excimer laser is most effective in destruction, the disadvantage is the difficult transport in fibres. Furthermore the biological effects are not yet completely known. - There seem to be only a few indications for invasive treatment of urinary calculi with laser energy. The treatment of choice for most urinary calculi is at present the non-invasive, non-contact ESWL. Therefore the definition of special cases of superiority of laser treatment compared to conventional methods will be necessary.

Literature
1. Dretler SP, Watson G, Parrish JA, Murray S: J Urol 137: 386-389 (1987)
2. Fair HD: Med Instrum J 12: 100-105 (1978)
3. Frank F, Hofstetter A, Keiditsch E, Wondrazek F: Eur Urol 12: suppl 1, 54-57 (1986)
4. Hofmann R, Schütz W: Urologe A 23: 181-184 (1984)
5. Watson GM, Wickham JEA, Mills TN, Bown SG, Swain P, Salmon PR: Br J Urol 55: 613-616 (1983)
6. Poprawe R, Beier E, Herziger G: Inst Phys Conf Series 72: 67-72 (1984)
7. Raizer YuP: Soviet Physics JETP 21: 1009 (1965)
8. Schmidt-Kloiber H, Reichel E, Schöffmann H: Biomed Technik 30: 173-181 (1985)

Laser-Induced Shock Wave Lithotripsy (LISL)

N. Schmeller(+), A. Hofstetter(+),
J. Pensel(*), F.Frank($), F.Wondrazek($)

(+) Klinik für Urologie, Medizinische Universität zu Lübeck,
(*) Medizinisches Laserzentrum Lübeck,
($) MBB Medizintechnik GmbH,
Ratzeburger Allee 160, 2400 Lübeck 1, F.R.G.

By continous Nd: YAG LASER it is possible to vaporize urinary calculi using high power. Because of tissue laceration due to the resulting heat, this is not possible in vivo.
Using suitable resonators, so called Q-switched mode, very short LASER pulses can be generated with high peak intensity. Thereby energy densities can be reached causing optical breakdown of gaseous, liquid and solid media. In this process shockwaves are generated. The difficult problem of coupling LASER pulses of 60 - 80 mJ and pulse duration of 13 ns into a quarz glas fiber could be solved reliably.
Thereafter a focussing device was developed to ensure optical break-down at a fixed point close to the distal tip of the fiber. With this device urinary calculi of every chemical composition could be fragmented in-vitro. Puls frequency was increased to 25 Hz to speed up fragmentation. The concretions were desintegrated into sandlike particles up the size of 2 - 3 mm.

Approximation of a finger to the tip of the probe causes sensations like small needle pricks without erythema or laceration.
To examine the effect on biological tissue the probe was inserted into the bladder of 5 rabbits by suprapubic cystotomy. Two points of the bladder wall were treated for 1 min. and for 3 min. at 10 Hz and 60 - 80 mJ/pulse at 1 mm distance between the tip of the probe and the bladder wall. Perforations were not observed. Only in one of the ten treatments a small petechial hemorrhage resulted in the bladder wall.
On histology only superficial lacerations of the mucosa were observed that healed within one week without scar formation.

The first prototype of the focussing device did not permit treatment of ureteral calculi due to its diameter (4.5 mm). Therefore its stone destruction ability and effects on human tissue were tested clinically during percutaneous nephrolithotomy in 3 patients. Tiny fragments were broken out of the stone under visual control. The sand was flushed out by continuous irrigation. Larger residual fragments were removed by forceps. Touching a papilla or the renal pelvis wall with the activated laser probe did not cause perforation, but only small hemorrhages, which stopped bleeding spontaneously in short time. No extravasations were observed. Kidney function was unchanged.

The succeeding prototype was used in the ureter in 16 patients (diameter: 2.2 mm, length: 6 mm). To check upon stone destruction and tissue effects it was used during rigid ureterorenoscopy by exchanging the telescope and the laser probe every 300 shocks. Concentric irrigation around the probe flushed out the stone fragments during desintegration. Confirming the animal experiments no perforations were observed and endoscopically only minor tissue lacerations were seen, less than by the ureteroscopy itself.

Generation of shockwaves by Q-switched Nd: YAG LASER pulses at energies between 60 and 80 mJ leads to fine fragmentation of urinary calculi and is harmless for surrounding tissue.
It may become an alternative to existing techniques during percutaneous nephrolithotomy, if the speed of stone destruction can be further increased.
In the treatment of ureteral calculi LISL is a promising new method, because these concretions of small mass can be desintegrated to sand-like particles by this flexible energy transducer, that is harmless for biological tissue. By further reducing the size of the focussing tip it should be possible to use this device under local anesthesia by fluoroscopic supervision.

Laser Lithotripsy of Gallstones by Means of Pulsed Nd: YAG Lasers

Ch. Ell, J. Hochberger, D. Müller, G. Lux, L. Demling
Medizinische Universitätsklinik Erlangen
Krankenhausstraße 12, D-8520 Erlangen, W-Germany

Method: Laser lithotripsy was performed with a flashlamp pulsed Nd: YAG laser (wave length 1064 nm) (by LASAG, Thun, Switzerland). The following parameters are freely adjustable: pulse frequency (1-20 Hz), pulse energy (0.1-4 Joule), and pulse duration (0.1-10 msec). The laser energy is transmitted via a highly flexible quartz fibre with a diameter of 0.2 mm.

Patients: Up to now we have treated 9 patients with one or several bile duct stones via laser lithotripsy.

Laser lithotripsy was only performed when the use of the other endoscopic techniques (removal with the basket, mechanical lithotripsy) was not possible or had failed.

Depending on the anatomic situation, laser lithotripsy was done under direct endoscopic vision (2 pat.) or under X-ray control with a specially developed laser lithotriptor basket (5 pat.) or a balloon catheter (2 pat.)

Results: Laser lithotripsy was successful in 6 of the 9 patients, i.e. the concrements could be destroyed and removed endoscopically from the bile duct. In 2 patients only a partial success could be achieved: The stones could be destroyed, but the fragments could not be removed as they were impacted in the bile duct. Therefore, patient no. 5 had surgery without complications, patient no. 4, who was in a really bad general state, was given internal bile drainage. In one patient lithotripsy was unsuccessful, although an adequate amount of energy was applied. For religious reasons the patient denied blood transfusions.

Therefore extracorporeal shock wave lithotripsy was performed that resulted in fragmenting the stone partially.

In every case between 40 and 150 pulses (80-300 Joule) were necessary for lithotripsy. A repetition frequency of 4 Hz, an impulse duration of 1-2 msec and an impulse energy of 1.5 (0.5-2.5) Joule per pulse have proved to be favourable working parameters. No complications or pathological changes in connection with the laser lithotripsy were observed neither during the acute follow-up nor during the long-term follow-up period now lasting 3-9 months.

Discussion: With a flashlamp-pulsed Nd:YAG laser (see methods) we were able to fragment gallstones in vitro reliably and reproducibly The fragmentation process is of thermal nature and can be explained by a high vaporisation pressure in the stone centre. For the in vivo use via the endoscope a sufficiently flexible transmission system is necessary, which is available in the form of a highly flexible, 0.2 mm thin quartz fibre. Mechanical damage of the fibre is not to be feared even in a radius of curvature down to 5 mm, transmission losses in extreme radii only amount to 15%. In acute animal experiments implanted human gallstones could be destroyed in 16 of 18 cases In chronic animal experiments in 8 dogs it could be shown by laboratory tests, X-rays and histological serial sections that even the direct pulsed laser irradiation of the bile duct wall does not cause any acute (cholangitis, peritonitis) or chronic (stenoses) complications (unpublished data).

No complications occurred in the first 9 applications in man. In 2 patients with choledochoduodenostomy lithotripsy was possible under direct endoscopic vision. Risks for the surrounding structures can be excluded in such a procedure. However, when the method is used under X-ray control only and not under direct vision, there certainly remains a risk, which cannot be totally excluded, that the bile duct is irradiated by mistake. In these cases a specially developed laser lithotriptor basket and its balloon modification contribute to the safety of the technique as the fibre is centrally guided in the catheter and the exact feed length of the fibre into the stone can be determined extracorporeally.

The first successful applications of endoscopic retrograde laserlithotripsy of bile duct stones in man described here mark the beginning of a new endoscopic technique. Further developments of the laser systems themselves and improvements in the endoscopy technique will open up the possibility for laser lithotripsy to become an economical, efficient and safe endoscopic technique and thus complement the non-surgical treatment methods of bile duct stones.

Gallstone-Lithotripsy by Pulsed Nd: YAG Laser

H.Wenk, V.Lange, K.O.Möller, F.W.Schildberg, A.Hofstetter
Department of Surgery and Medical Laser Center
University of Lübeck
Ratzeburger Allee 160, D-2400 Lübeck, West Germany

Nd:YAG-Laser are used in curative and palliative surgery. The development of a pulsed Nd:YAG Laser now also allows the desintegration of concrements. The presupposition for clinical use of such technique is a system that gives necessary energy in very short pulses and high repetition rate to avoid thermic lesion and a flexible transmission system that can be brought through the working channel of flexible endoscopes.

For our in vitro experiments we used as energy source a pulsed Nd:YAG laser with a wave length of 1.064 nm and a pulse duration of 12 nsec. The frequency was variable: for the examination was used pulse energy of 45 mJ and a frequency of 20 cycles/sec. The examinations were done with two different couples.

The first transmission system was a flexible quartz fibre with a diameter of 1.000 micrometer. At the distal end was put a lense system to focus laser emission directly in front of the frontal plane. The lense system used a diameter of 4.5 mm and was in this way not suitable for endoscopical application.

This was the reason for the development of a substantially smaller optomechanical couple. It's quartz guide has a diameter of 600 micrometer and is implanted concentrically into a rinsing tube. The optomechanical couple at the distal end has a diameter of 2.2 mm and can be used in modern flexible endoscopes.

Before destroyment all gallstones were measured in 3 planes and weighted. All stones could be destroyed in short time. Stones with a weight of up to 1/2 gramme were destroyed within 5 minutes. Only one stone used more than 15 minutes for total desintegration.

The duration of lithotripsy depended on size and weight and on the other hand on the hardness. The systems - lense system and optomechanical couple - showed no differences in quality of lithotripsy.

To examine the soft tissue reactions on the bile duct and the gall bladder we did experiments in 8 pigs with a weight of 30-40 kg. After laparotomy of the upper abdomen the main bile duct and the gall bladder were exposed. The bile duct and the gall bladder was opened between sutures over 2-3 cm. Different areas were exposed to the laser pulses over 5 and 15 minutes. The withdrawal of the areas was done immediately, after one hour, 3 days, 2 weeks, 4 weeks and 6 weeks. There were taken photos from the preparations, afterwards they were put into formalin and given to the histological processing.

The results: severe defects could not be recognized. There were no perforations by the treatment, neither coagulation of the tissure nor stenosis. The only residuum of treatment were foreign body cells in the regions of the suture markings.

Evident was an edema of the bile duct's wall and the gall bladder immediately after shock wave lithotripsy. After a treatment over 15 minutes petechial bleedings into the bile duct wall were recognized. They correspond to haematomas in the submucosa in the microscopical picture.

The tissue which was explanted one hour after laser exposition showed supplementary a leucocyt diapedisis.

The reactions of the bile duct wall were totally reversible and couldn't be recognized in the late explantated bile ducts.

The development of the pulsed Nd:YAG laser allows the destroyment of concrements in the bile tract by the use of thin transmission systems.

In our in vitro study all concrements could be destroyed to dust in relatively short time. Beneath the composition of the stone its consistence seems to be important. Hard stones can be destroyed better than soft stones. This phenomenon explains the exquisite lithotripsibility of stones in the urinary tract which are composed of inorganic salts in the majority.

Beneath the enodscopic application we see an indication for shock-wave-lithotripsy also in intraoprative situations, if it is possible to reduce the dimension of the operation. As an example we present a 40 year old female patient, who had pain in the stomach since her 17th birthday after holyday in a foreign country.

Diagnostic procedere in 1985 showed a chronic calcifying pancreatitis as the cause of pain. Endoscopic retrograde cholangiopancreatiocography showed an incarcerated concrement in the caput of the pancreas.

By acceleration of pain the operation was indicated and a pancreaticojejunostomy was planned. After incision of the pancreatic duct which was dilated, multiple concrements could be extracted. The big stone in the caput could neither be exposed nor be removed. Intraoperative endoscopy showed the concrement fixed in the small ducts. By endoscopical laser induced shock-wave-lithotripsy it was possible to destroy the concrement completely and to remove the fragments.

Afterwards the papilla of vater and the terminal bile duct could be inspected without difficulties.

The intervention could be finished as a pancreaticojejunostomy in favour of a duodenopancreatectomy.

On our opinion the 40 year old patient is better served by a draining operation, for resection of the pancreas is incriminated by endocrine insufficiency, diabetes and higher lethality in comparison to spontane progress.

The draining operation was made possible by laser lithotripsy of the impacted stone. Summarizing, we see indications for laser induced shock-wave-lithotripsy in impacted stones of the common bile and pancreatic duct that cannot be removed by any other methods. Beneath the endoscopical application intraoperative use can reduce the dimension of surgical intervention.

Literature

1. Hofstetter,A., Schmeller,N., Pensel,J., Arnholdt,H., Frank,F., Wondrazek, F. (1986): Harnstein-Lithotripsie mit laserinduzierten Stoßwellen.
Fortschr.Med. 104, 654.

2. Schildberg,F.W., Lange,V., Wenk,H., Schüller,J. (1987):
Die intraoperative, endoskopische Lithotripsie von Pankreasgangkonkrementen.
Chirurg 58, 239-242

3. Schmeller,N.T., Baumüller,A., Hofstetter,A.G. (1984):
Nichtoperative Behandlung von Harnleitersteinen mit Hilfe der Ureterorenoskopie.
Fortschr.Med. 102, 895

ENT

Laser Surgery – ENT (Upper Aero-Digestive Tract) – State of the Art

W. Steiner
ENT-Department, University of Göttingen
Geiststr. 5/10, 3400 Göttingen, FRG

The possibility of being able to use various laser systems (CO_2, Argon or Nd Yag) for endoscopic and microscopic surgery of benign and malignant lesions of the upper aero-digestive tract has opened up a new therapeutic dimension.

Lasers have proved of great advantage in improving precision in microsurgery and endoscopic surgery.

The addition of the CO_2 laser to the instrumentarium available to the laryngeal surgeon has improved the precision of traditional endolaryngeal procedures and has made the endolaryngeal approach available for procedures formerly requiring an external approach. The role of the CO_2 laser in the management of obstructive lesions of the pediatric airway is now firmly established. Its unique features, combined with the use of the surgical microscope, permit highly selective removal of tissue, and postoperative edema and scarring are minimal. The laser is recommended for the endoscopic and microscopic treatment of congenital abnormalities such as laryngoceles, cysts, webs, synechia or atresia, as well as hemangiomas and lymphangiomas.

Among the benign lesions of the larynx, such as vocal cord nodes, polyps and granulomas, the most important indications for endolaryngeal laser microsurgery are recurrent papillomatosis and laryngeal stenosis after endotracheal intubation.

The virus-induced papillomas are highly recurrent, whether treated conventionally or with the laser. Since there is a relative absence of bleeding during laser treatment, surgery can be performed with greater accuracy and safety. The definitive organic and functional results are better than after conventional surgery. Tracheotomy can usually be avoided.

Laryngeal stenosis caused by intubation is treated primarily endoscopically. Extensive circular stenosis usually requires a stent after endoscopic laser treatment. Severe stenosis in the cricoid region often requires classical surgical treatment.

The main indication for endoscopic and microscopic laser surgery is in my opinion, based on my experience, cancer of the upper aero-digestive tract. Since 1979 I have used laser surgery to treat more than 900 patients with cancer.

There can be no doubt about the progress made by the application of laser surgery in the symptomatic palliative treatment of far advanced, inoperable and/or incurable primaries and recurrent tumors or metastases deriving from other organs. The main aim of the procedure is to eliminate tumor-related stenosis, which is responsible for impairment of breathing and swallowing. Although, of course, this procedure will not cure the tumor, it can and does improve the patient's quality of life. This kind of surgery is not easy. If too much is resected in a functionally important region, the patient may have trouble with aspiration or other severe complications.

For treatment in the nasopharynx and the trachea, the argon or Nd Yag laser can be used under endoscopic control. For laser treatment in the oral cavity, in the oro-hypopharynx and the larynx, the CO_2 laser is employed together with the microscope.

In the early cancer stages enoral or transoral microsurgical resection using the CO_2 laser as curative monotherapy, is the method of choice. The great advantage of this procedure is its high, virtually bloodless precision in the removal of the tumor, which makes it oncologically reliable while permitting satisfactory functional results.

Laser surgery has become a practical means of removing not only small cancers of the vocal cords. It reduces the amount of normal tissue that has to be removed, since the procedure is done under binocular microscope in a bloodless field, allowing one clearly to differentiate between normal and cancerous tissues. In most cases the surgery can be carried out transorally, thus avoiding an external approach. Owing to the restoration capability of the tissue, even if almost the whole vocal cord is removed, a secondary vocal cord of scar tissue will develop and provide a functional vocal cord.

By not closing the defect after enoral or transoral laser resection of malignant tumors in the upper aero-digestive tract, excellent final results with largely preserved function may be obtained, even in the cases of large wound cavities.

The decisive advance of laser surgery is the possibility of being able to treat even advanced tumors transorally, alone or in combination with radiotherapy, while preserving functionally important organ structures-often without the need for tracheotomy.

We employ laser surgery as part of the combined modality treatment in which laser surgery is used for debulking prior to radiation therapy. Our experience with the CO_2 laser indicates that gross tumor ablation can be achieved with such minimal morbidity and rapid healing that potentially an ideal complementary relationship can be established between the surgeon and the radiotherapist in the combined treatment of patients with head and neck cancer.

In the cases of advanced laryngeal tumors we give preference to combined therapy rather than total laryngectomy.

It has been established that even extensive resections can often be performed without tracheotomy. Large areas of cartilage can be exposed or, when necessary, removed. Nevertheless, patients were able to receive irradiation considerably sooner than with conventional surgery, without having to fear such complications as edema or perichondritis.

The oncological and functional results so far achieved, justify further pursuance of the therapeutic concept.

Prerequisites for the successful application of endoscopic and microscopic laser surgery in the treatment of malignant tumors are :

Experience on the part of the therapist with conventional tumor surgery, endolaryngeal microsurgery and laser surgery. Optimal exposure of the region affected by the tumor. Close cooperation with an experienced pathologist. Intensive follow-up. Cooperation with the informed patient.

The conditions I have mentioned indicate that laser surgery is certainly not "surgery for everyman" and is not suitable for use in every patient. Our eight year experience with laser surgical removal of cancer of the upper aero-digestive tract have shown that it is a viable treatment modality.

The use of laser surgery means that the patient is often spared exposure to more invasive or mutilating surgery.

Long-term observations will show where the future possibilities and limitations of laser surgery lie, and what its final value will prove to be, within the framework of combined therapy procedures.

Endoscopic Therapy of Laryngeal Carcinomas with the CO_2 Laser

Dr. H. Rudert
E.N.T.-Department University of Kiel
Arnold-Heller-Str. 14, 2300 Kiel
Federal Republic of Germany

In many countries small vocal cord carcinomas are not treated primarily surgically, but radiologically because of voice impairment after surgery.
In Germany surgical treatment is a tradition of long standing. It is used in most hospitals as a first choice therapy of T1a- and T1b vocal cord carcinomas on account of the excellent cancerological results.
In 1983 we reported on 118 cases. After surgical treatment of 39 cases applying cordectomy and frontolateral partial resection we observed no recurrences, while after radiotherapy of 79 cases the amount of recurrences was equal to 30 %.

Since 1981, we have treated small vocal cord carcinomas also endoscopically with the CO_2-LASER.

The advantage of endoscopic CO_2-LASER therapy as compared with the therapy applying conventional micro-surgical instruments resides in the fact that a compact tissue block can be very accurately excised from the vocal cord with the LASER beam. The demands of carcinome surgery for an en bloc-resection are thus excellently fulfilled.

In 1981 we started with selected cases, old patients rejecting cordectomy or radiotherapy. In the past years we have cautiously expanded the indications. Until the end of 1986, we have treated 25 T1-vocal cord carcinomas and 10 T1-recurrences of irradiated vocal cord carcinomas with the CO_2-LASER.

Out of the 25 primarily treated vocal cord carcinomas the first 3 among them developed recurrences, probably due to insufficient resection (Fig.1). Two of these were controlled by the application of radiotherapy, while the third ultimately was controlled by laryngectomy. No patient died from his tumor. Two of them developed a secondary carcinoma. A small carcinoma of the palate was successfully treated with the LASER too. 23 of the cases are free from primary tumor.

CO_2-LASER-THERAPY OF VOCAL CORD CARCINOMAS

KIEL 1981 - 1986

Pat.	Rec.	Ther. of Rec.	2. Ca.	✝ from 1. Ca.	✝ from 2. Ca.	✝ indip. of tumor	N.E.D.
24 T1a	3	2 Rad.	2*	0	1	1	23
1 T1b		1 L.E.					

*2. Ca: 1 palatal Ca., treated by CO_2-LASER, N.E.D.
 1 bronchial Ca., ✝ died² by suicide

N.E.D: no evidence of disease
Rec. : Recurrence

Fig. 1.

The 10 recurrences after radiotherapy related to 6 unilateral and 4 bilateral vocal cord tumors (Fig.2).

CO_2-LASER-THERAPY OF RECURRENCES FOLLOWING RADIOTHERAPY

OF VOCAL CORD CARCINOMAS (KIEL 1981 - 1986)

Classif. before Rad.-Ther.	Classif. of the Rec.	2. Rec. after LASER	2. LASER-Therapy	L.E.	✝ from 1.Ca.	✝ from 2.Ca.	alive with 1.Ca.	alive with 2.Ca.	N.E.D.
6 T1a	5 T1a	1	1	0	0	0	1	2*	5
	1 T1b								
4 T1b	1 T1a	3	3	1**	0	1**	0	0	3
	3 T1b								

*2. Ca.: 1 Colon-Ca.
 1 Ca. of the mandibula
**2. Ca.: 1 malignant melanoma

N.E.D.: no evidence of disease
L.E. : laryngectomy

Fig. 2.

Four of them suffered a second recurrence being retreated with the LASER. One patient had to be laryngectomized because of a third recurrence. He died later from a secondary tumor, a malignant melanoma. Thus 8 of the patients live free of primary tumor with their larynx.

In these recurrent tumors formerly at least a hemilaryngectomy, as a rule however a total laryngectomy would have been carried out.

Depending on the size of the tumor, one can resect the entire vocal cord, including vocal cord muscles and perichondrium of the thyroid cartilage, thus achieving a big defect of the vocal cord with a minor voice quality. In case of superficial tumors, some muscles will remain. Anatomically and functionally the result obtained is considerably better.

We nowadays perform the LASER-resection of unilateral vocal cord carcinoma in all cases where the tumor has not reached the anterior commissure and the vocal process. The specimens are, of course, not vaporized but excised, fixed and histologically investigated. The intervention is implemented as an "incisional biopsy". Cases that could not be resected within tumorfree margins are subjected to one of the classical therapies.

While this treatment of small vocal cord carcinomas is still discussed controversely the palliative "debulking" of major airway obturating tumors is an uncontested indication for preventing or delaying a tracheostomy.

Ladies and gentlemen, I believe we thus can confirm the pioneer work of Dr. Geza Jako, our President, inasmuch as the CO_2-LASER is excellently suitable for the therapy of laryngeal carcinomas in certain indications. In order not to bring discredit upon the new instrument we should however emphasize that the CO_2-LASER represents a new tool, but not a new treatment principle for laryngeal carcinomas.

Vaporization of ORO-Pharyngeal Lymphoid Tissues – Indications, Techniques and Results in 40 Cases

M. Remacle, M. Hamoir, P. Van Heule, Y. Frederickx, B. Bertrand

University of Louvain, Department for ENT and Head and Neck Surgery

University Hospitals of Mont-Godinne and Woluwe, B-5180 Yvoir, Belgium

The role of the carbon dioxide laser has become established in the management of various congenital and acquired lesions of the airway. The method has proven to be efficient, safe, with minimal operative morbidity and bleeding. About 150 cases have been managed at our institution during the past 4 years.

We report our experience with 40 CO_2 laser procedures performed in patients with faucial or lingual tonsillitis.

A representative case report

A 17 year-old girl was referred for treatment of a major hypertrophic tonsillitis. In spite of a large antibiotic consumption, sore throat, fever, important dysphagie remains. The appetite is poor. The school is frequently missed. Her parents noted that she was a loud snorer who never really slept well at night. Her voice had a muffled quality. There was no need of a mirror to see huge cryptic lingual tonsils. Indirect laryngoscopy revealed that the valleculae and the epiglottis were totally masked. The patient was brought to the operating room and a lingual tonsillectomy performed with the CO_2 laser. She did well postoperatively, taking fluids by mouth the same day, and was discharged home the following day with minimal discomfort. Six months later, she remains asymptomatic.

Materials and methods

The group consists of 13 patients with faucial tonsillitis, 19 with lingual tonsillitis and 8 with both lingual and faucial tonsillitis. The faucial tonsillitis considered here are these coming from amygdalian stump or atrophic tonsils. The ages range from 6 to 71. The mean age is 34. There are 31 females and 9 males. The main symptoms are frequent sore throats, odynophagia and dysphagia, mild fever, feeling of lump in the throat, bad taste in the month. Otalgia is not uncommon.

The clinical examination shows redness of the oro-pharynx, enlargment of the faucial stump or of the lingual tonsils. The crypts are often enlarged and filled with exudate. Enlargement and tenderness of the anterior cervical lymph nodes are not rare. Usually, the faucial tonsils have been removed in the cases of lingual tonsilitis. When the clinical examination is not convincing, the pharyngitis inducing causes are investigated as rhino-sinusitis, with radio-tomograms, allergy with skin testing and rast on blood sample, as also a gastro-esophageal reflux with swallowing cineradiography and pHmetry. In some cases, however, the doubt can remains about a psychogenic or emotional origin (globus hystericus).

The patient is operated under general anesthesia with intubation. The safety rules for the CO_2 laser use are followed : the tube is wrapped with a aluminium sheet a wet towel is put on the face around the month. The lingual tonsil is approached much the same way as laryngeal lesions. A suspension laryngoscope is used to expose the lesions. The CO_2 surgical laser (Sharplan 1040) is coupled with a WILD operating microscope. Adequate resection of hypertrophic lingual tonsils requires special diligence on the part of the operative surgeon. Lingual tonsillar hypertrophy is diffuse and involves a majority of the bulk of the base of the tongue. Using the suspension laryngoscope directed at different portions of the tongue base, the hypertrophic tonsillar tissue is removed systematically. The hand-piece is used for the faucial stumps and the faucial atrophic tonsils. The lesions are viewed with a retractor as the same way as a standard tonsillectomy. The beam is used at an intensity of 10 to 15 watts, continuous with defocus so that one realizes a vaporization rather than a section. Should an artery of 0.5 mm or more in diameter be dammaged, haemostosis is effected by aspirator-coagulator. The patient is discharged from hospital after 48 hours.

Results
=======

The immediate courses are quite simple. The patients did well postoperatively, taking fluids by month the same day. There have been no cases of bleeding neither the days after the operation nor after the slough was Shed. The edema is trifling. The pain, though it is difficult to compare, seems to be really lesser, than with conventional technics. The follow-up ranges from 1 month to 36 months. The mean follow-up is 16 months. One case required a second procedure two months after the first, one for insufficiency of resection. Among the 40 patients, 28 are completely free of disease. 9 patients are improved, the symptoms are reduced but still remain. There is no improvement for 3 patients.

Discussion

Over the years, the procedure of lingual tonsillectomy as of faucial stumps resection has been avoided by most otolaryngologists because of the risk of serious hemorrhage and the difficulty of maintaining an airway both during and following the procedure.

Conventional methods have included cold knife, excision, electrocautery, and cryosurgery. Some patients required a tracheotomy. Based on our experience with 40 patients, we believe that the CO_2 laser is the method of choice for that still often neglected problem.

Benefit and Risks of Laser Surgery in Carcinomas of the Larynx and Pharynx

T. Lenarz, J. Haels
ENT Department, University of Heidelberg
Voss-Strasse 5-7, D-6900 Heidelberg, F.R.G.

Introduction

The incidence of laryngeal and pharyngeal cancer increased tremendously over the last 30 years in Europe (4). Several new concepts of therapy were developed in the last 10 years. Especially CO_2-laser surgery has gained much interest. The possibility of endoscopic surgery seems to be a major advantage over conventional surgery which requires a wide exposure of the operating field. However, the limited two dimensional view through the operating microscope can be deleterious as radical excision is required. Another objection was raised due to carbonization at the cutting borders which can hinder a true histological evaluation (2, 4, 5). In our present study we evaluated the benefits and risks of endolaryngeal and endopharyngeal CO_2-laser surgery in the management of carcinomas in these regions.

Material and Methods

A Coherent CO_2 laser unit modell 400 was used in combination with a Zeiss operating microscope. The tumors were excised with the laser beam focused and used as a cutting instrument. 25 patients entered the study. The site and the extend of the tumors are listed in table 1:

Table 1: Site and extent of tumor

	T_1	T_2	$T_{3/4}$	V.C.	F.V.C.	Epig.	B.T.	Hyp.	Tot.
n	10	5	10	10	3	5	2	5	25

V.C. = Vocal Cord; F.V.C. = False Vocal Cord; Epig. = Epiglottis
B.T. = Base of the Tongue; Hyp. = Hypopharynx;
Tot. = Total number of patients

The indication for T_1 tumors (vocal cord, epiglottis) was a radical excision, for $T_{3/4}$ tumors (n =10) a partial resection to restore swallowing or to avoid tracheostomy. The cutting borders were examined histologically to evaluate the surgical specimen. The follow up period lasted between 3 months and 5 years. Repeated lupe laryngoscopies were performed every 3 months to detect a relapse as soon as possible.

Results

By means of histological examination a complete excision of carcinoma was achieved in 9 out of 10 T_1 tumors, but only in 2 out of 5 T_2 tumors and in none of 10 $T_{3/4}$ tumors. The carbonization of the cutting borders was a severe limitation for histological analysis, especially in T_2 tumors. A recurrence of cancer could be observed in 2 T_1 tumors, one of the epiglottis and one of the lateral pharyngeal wall, but none in T_1 tumors of the vocal cord. Despite the high rate of relapse in partially resected $T_{3/4}$ carcinomas (8 out of 10 cases) the following benefits could be achieved. Swallowing was restored in 4 out of 6 cases, pain was markedly reduced in 7 out of 10 cases and tracheostomy could be prevented in 4 out of 4 cases. In 5 cases up to 4 palliative rescetions were repeated. During laser surgery bleeding was markedly reduced as compared with conventional endoscopic surgery. However, in 3 cases bleeding postoperative required a specific even surgical therapy. Other complications comprised a perforation of the recessus piriformis in one case and aspiration in 2 cases after resection of the epiglottis. All complications could be controlled after a short time.

Discussion

In accordance with reports in the literature (1, 2, 6, 7) our experience outlines CO_2-laser surgery as a safe and effective mode of therapy for laryngeal and pharyngeal carcinomas. Two groups of patients with different indications have to be distinguished. A radical and safe tumor excision can be achieved only in T_1 tumors of the middle part of the vocal cord and the upper part of the epiglottis. Tumors of other site or T_2 tumors should not be adopted to these technique because of the limited view in endoscopic surgery and the difficulties of histological evaluation of the cutting borders. In otherwise not curable extended tumors ($T_{3/4}$) endoscopic laser surgery is of special value. Palliative effects can be achieved and the health status of the patient is improved with low risk treatment. The endoscopic approach as limited surgery, the reduced bleeding and the precise cutting can be adopted as specific advantages of laser surgery over conventional surgery in this field (3, 4).

References

(1) ANDREWS AH (1974)
Experiences with the carbon dioxide laser in the larynx.
Ann. Otol. Rhinol. Laryngol. 83: 462.

(2) Burian K., Höfler H (1979)
Zur mikrochirurgischen Therapie von Stimmbandkarzinomen mit dem CO_2-Laser. Laryng Rhinol Otol 58: 551.

(3) GROSSENBACHER R (1985)
Laserchirurgie in der Oto-Rhino-Laryngologie.
Thieme, Stuttgart-New York.

(4) KLEINSASSER O (1983)
Bösartige Geschwülste des Kehlkopfes und des Hypopharynx.
in: Berendes, J., Link, R., Zöllner, F. (eds) Hals-Nasen-Ohren-Heilkunde in Praxis und Klinik, Vol 4, Part 2, 12.1 - 12.337

(5) MIEHLKE A, VOLLRATH M (1980)
Mikroskopische Laserchirurgie im Kehlkopfbereich.
Dtsch. Ärztebl. 74: 177

(6) RUDERT H (1983)
Erfahrungen mit dem CO_2-Laser unter besonderer Berücksichtigung der Therapie von Stimmbandkarzinomen. Laryng Rhinol Otol 62: 493

(7) STRONG MS (1975)
Laser excision of carcinoma of the larynx. Laryngoscope 85: 1286.

Laser Turbinectomy

Ronald Allen Kirschner
The Institute for Applied Laser Surgery
Suite IL-17
Two Bala Plaza
Bala Cynwyd, Pa. 19004, U.S.A.

The laser turbinectomy was popularized in the U.S. by Harry Mittelman and Stuart Selkin. At the International Society for Lasers in Medicine and Surgery Meeting that was held in Detroit, we presented a paper dealing with new instrumentation that facilitated the use of the carbon dioxide laser in intranasal surgery. To this instrumenation we have added the Nd:YAG laser as part of an FDA protocol that we have written for Cooper LaserSonics. This protocol covers a wide spectrum of Head and Neck Applications of the Nd:YAG laser.

In our original series, a carbon dioxide laser was used to ablate hypertrophic inferior turbinates. The nasal speculae that were utilized were designed with a right and a left handed model that were mirror images of one another. The longer blade served to protect the nasal septum from inadvertent laser damage. Utilizing this instrumentation, the surgeon is able to employ the speculum from a superior or an inferior vantage point.

In performing this procedure the patient's nose is packed with tetrahydalazine which provides a significant amount of hemostasis. The inferior turbinates are then swabbed with applicators impregnated with 10% cocaine. This affords adequate anesthesia. During the procedure with the carbon dioxide laser the patient's eyes are covered with sterile wet eyepads and the patient's face is covered with wet towels. The laser is set at between 5 and 10 watts and .5 seconds duration per pulse. The instrumentation incorporates a built in smoke channel to draw off the plume that is created by the laser tissue interaction. The instruments are especially fabricated for laser surgery. They are sandblasted with two different size glass beads and then ebonized. This combination allows the greatest reduction of reflection that the current state of the art provides.

Over the past six months we have additionally implemented the Nd:YAG laser for intranasal surgery. As opposed to the carbon dioxide laser, the Nd:YAG laser is an excellent coagulator and a rather poor cutting tool. The advent of the sapphire tip has further modified the effect that the Nd:YAG laser has on tissue.

The shape of the sapphire tip will effect the way in which the laser energy is transferred to the tissue. In performing a turbinectomy procedure with the Nd:YAG laser we are utilizing both a short scalpel tip and a chisel shaped sapphire tip. These tips are placed at the end of a fibre which is passed through a channel which is connected to the optics channel of the nasal telescope. There is a deflector at the end of the scope which creates a small angulation of the tip. This arrangement allows the Nd:YAG laser to be used on the turbinate tissue under direct observation. The ability of the tip to contact the tissue also facilitates the ablation of the excess turbinate tissue.

The ability of the surgeon to direct the laser energy in contact with the tissue removes the danger of distal laser damage and creates a procedure that is technically easier than the one that was previously utilized. The use of this wavelength also maximizes the coagulation abilities of the Nd:YAG laser. As bleeding is the greatest impediment to the proper performance of this procedure when it is done in a conventional fashion this is a definite plus.

The telescope is newly designed and will be available with a variety of lens angulations and lengths. There is a fibreoptic channel for viewing and a concentric one for providing illumination. A side channel provides both the ability to provide suction for removal of the plume and the ability to transmit the laser fibreoptic.

We follow all of our turbinectomy cases with intranasal beclamethasone for six to twelve weeks. The combination of the laser modalities and the postoperative medication have proven effective in our early work.

Advantages of the procedure are:
1. Office procedure
2. Less Bleeding
3. Better Vision and Control
4. Less Post-operative Pain
5. Less Invasive than conventional therapy

CO_2 Laser Microsurgery in Choanal Atresia – How to Protect the Alar Skin from Burning?

B.BERTRAND, PH.ELOY, M.REMACLE
ENT.DEPT. University of Louvain
Cliniques UNiversitaires UCL de Mont-Godinne
B. 5180 YVOIR – BELGIUM

The use of CO2 Laser beam combined with a surgical microscope has been, in our two years short experience, the best way for treating choanal atresia. The surgical tool is easy to move in the strenght field of the nasal fossa, there is less postsurgical pain for the young patient, and it is not necessary to leave in place a calibration tube for cicatrisation around. But some rules must absolutely be followed in order to avoid complications linked to the CO2 Laser microsurgery :
1) recurrence of the nasal stenosis, especially in case of a wide bony stenosis,
2) burning of alar skin that may lead to disaesthetic scars, and disfonctionnal stenosis.

The secondary nasal stenosis may be avoided in reducing the Laser power when working at the surgical border of the osseous atresia; so, the diathermic effect and the high temperatures in the next bony tissues become reduced at a minimal level.
Furthermore, in this kind of idea, it is important also to keep a sufficient lap of time between two CO2 Laser spots : the shorter the Laser-flashes and the longer the elapsed time between two flashes, the easier the blood flow and the air succion can be evacuating calories and so diminishing the depth of the diathermic effect.

The alar skin may be injured in different ways :
1) in missing to protect widely the face and the nose,
2) in misunderstanding the dangers from a too large Laser beam and from the parallax effect that sometimes is generated from the binocular view.

The solutions to avoid such problems are quiet simple, but must be employed all together at a time :
1) long focal distance lenses (400 mm) must be prefered to short focal distance lenses : the longer the distance, the shorter the diameter of the Laser beam at its point of entry in the nasal fossa;
2) the axis of the working Laser beam must be the same as the nasal fossa's one : if it is not, a parallax effect caused by a monocular view can induce a " touch " between the alar skin and the Laser beam;
3) a safe protection of the face and the nose must be provided : wet towels on the face, and aluminum tapes sticked around the narina before the operating speculum to be put into the nasal fossa.

Use of a Microspot Micromanipulator for CO_2 Laser Surgery in Otolaryncology

S.M. Shapshay, R. Wallace, J.F. Kveton, R. Hybels
R.K. Bohigian, S. Setzer

Lahey Clinic Medical Center, 41 Mall Rd., Burlington, Mass. 01805

A new microspot micromanipulator for the CO_2 laser has been developed and utilized in both laboratory setting and in clinical practice. Eight patients with various benign vocal cord pathologies and one patient with early dysplasia of the vocal cords were treated with the new microspot micromanipulator utilizing the operating microscope with a 400 mm lens. This new micromanipulator has the following unique features: a virtual image, utilizing a fiberoptic bundle with a green aiming light, and a spot size of .4 mm utilizing the 400 mm lens on the operating microscope. Elimination of a helium neon aiming laser obviates the problems with coincidence and a glaring effect of the laser upon the tissue. The spot size can be changed from .4 mm up to 3 mm in size.

Patients with bilateral vocal cord polypoid change were treated with this micromanipulator using a microflap technique. The vocal cord polypoid change was extracted after incision and raising of a microflap. After the excessive vocal cord lining was removed, the free edges of the incision were then coacted and "welded" with the use of a milliwatt setting on the laser at approximately 400 milliwatts. Due to the excellent cutting effect from the high power density and small impact size, only 1 watt of CO_2 laser energy was necessary for the incisions.

The microspot has also been used with a 250 mm lens on the microscope for experimental stapedotomy work on the cat model. Utilizing a 250 mm lens a 100 micron (.1 mm) spot size was achieved, allowing the otologic surgeon extreme precision in fenestration of the stapes footplate. Fenestration was achieved with one pulse of the CO_2 laser at 1/20th of a second with 900 milliwatts power. There was no thermal change in the perilymphatic fluid below the footplate as measured by thermocouple placement. This new microspot micromanipulator promises to refine present microlaryngeal and otologic techniques providing the laser microsurgeon greater precision than capable with standard micromanipulators.

Role of Laser Surgery in the Management of Recurrent Malignancies at the Base of Skull

N. Kunaratnam

Ear, Nose & Throat Dep., Singapore General Hospital, Singapore 0316

Laser has at present gained a foothold in the management of recurrent malignancies of the base of skull. Though this treatment modality is essentially palliative, it is gaining ground in many centres. In Singapore the use of laser is being increasingly used in the palliative management of recurrent Nasopharyngeal Carcinoma where other modes of treatment have gained, namely radiotherapy and chemotherapy. The incidence of new cases of NPC is in the region of 200 per year in Singapore hence there is increasing availability of such cases here.

The CO_2 laser can be delivered to the Nasopharynx through one or two of several approaches viz. Transnasal, the Transoral with retraction of palate and use of Silver Mirrors, the Transpalatal and the Lateral Rhinotomy' approaches. The transpalatal approach has good direct access to the tumour site for visualisation. The two way approach of beaming laser via transnasal and transpalatal approach gives adequate clearance of the growth. The palatal fenestration makes the postoperative follow up easy with possible repeat of laser at regular intervals if necessary. A dental palate is fitted to cover the fenestrated site to aid swallowing.

During the last three years we have tried this modality of treatment on twenty three cases of this clinical problem of recurrent nasopharyngeal carcinoma following radiation therapy. This has greatly benefited the patient's quality of life and even their quality of death with minimum perioperative morbidity. Lives of patients of these terminal cases have been prolonged for periods ranging from six to thirty months.

Reform of Traditional Treatment of Nasal Polyps by Using Laser

De Min Liu, Hong Deng, Pei Zhong Wang
83 Feng Yang Rd., Shanghai, PRC

This paper presents the use of laser for the treatment of nasal polyps instead of the traditional method. Traditionally, they are removed by snaring method. After operation, profused bleeding, possibility to recur, unsatisfactory result and so on may be the problems. Anterior nasal packing with gauze for hemostasis may make patient very distressing. To solve these problems, the authors used YAG Laser through optic fiber condition to treat 150 cases of nasal polyps recently with satisfactory results. This method might also be used in nasal polyp patients who are contradicted to the traditional treatment or complicated with blood and cardiovascular diseases.

Oral Surgery

Progress Report on Laser Therapy in Oral and Maxillo-Facial Surgery

H.-H. Horch, Herzog, M.
Clinic of Oral and Maxillo-Facial Surgery,
Klinikum rechts der Isar der Technischen
Universität München, Ismaningerstr. 22
D-8000 München 80

I. In oral and maxillo-facial surgery, the application of the Nd-YAG laser may be considered as a standard method in the treatment of patient suffering from hemorrhagic diathesis. ACKERMANN (1984) reportet his experiences of more than 1000 treatments in oral surgery during the last 10 years, executed in cooperation with the Munich Centre of Haemophilia. In his studies, the indication of laser-coagulation diseases (Haemophilia A and B), infirmity of thrombocytes (Thrombastenia, Thrombocytopenia, disorders of the function of thrombocytes) and the more exceptional vascular bleeding diseases. Postoperative bleeding was reported in 10% of the cases and therefore lies within the known limit. In most cases an ambulant treatment with local anaesthesia was possible. Only for patients with severe Haemophilia A with a remaining activity of factor VIII below 1% as well as in cases of inhibitors against factor VIII a stay in hospital for 1 or 2 days was necessary. Also the laser coagulation in anticoagulated patients has been successfully used. Ackermann's clinical studies show that the Nd-YAG-laser is a remarkable alternative to the classical methods of treatment, considering especially the possibility to avoid the problem of transferred plasma proteins during surgical treatment.

II. The application of CO_2-lasers in the treatment of multicentric premalignant oral dysplasia may be considered as another standard method. Clinical experiences of more than 10 years demonstrate the favorable use of the CO_2-laser especially in regions of the oral cavity where it is more difficult to operate in conventional manner (HORCH 1983, HORCH et al. 1986). After histological examination, the multicentric dysplasias are removed by the defocussed laser beam with a light dose of 15-20 W. In general, the patients can be treated in local anaesthesia without hospitalisation. This kind of laser surgery is characterised by a simple technique and little discomfort for the patients. Hardly any bleeding can be seen during the treatment.

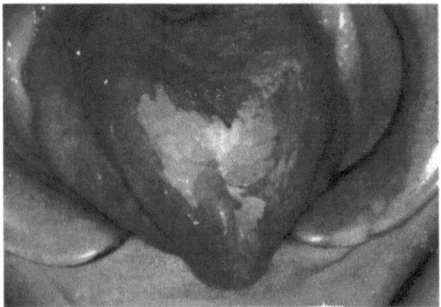
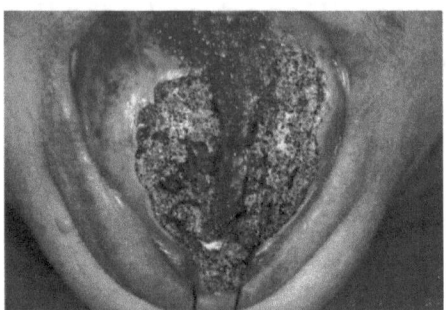
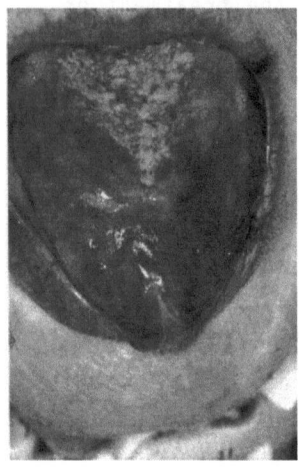

Fig. 1. Leukoplakia erosiva of the tongue (severe grade of dysplasia).
a. before CO_2 laser treatment; b. immediately post-operatively with carbonization of the superficial epithelium; c. 3 years post-operatively, still without any local recurrence

After 2 or 3 weeks, wounds of the oral mucosa are completely epithelized without any contractions. Therefore plastic reconstructive surgery is not necessary. Even large dysplasias of the lips, the angle and the floor of the mouth, and of the tongue can be treated without any loss of function. (Fig.1)
In comparison to the conventional-surgical or cryosurgical methods, the recurrence rate lies between 9 and 18% (HORCH et al. 1983, ROODENBURG 1985). Contrasting this with a recurrence rate of between 40 and 45% using conservative treatment with vitamine A and its derivatives and a recurrence rate of 33% after surgery,

the application of the CO_2-laser can be classified as superior to
the methods aforesaid. Also when compared to cryosurgery
(recurrence rate about 30%), the laser-method can be seen as a
favorable therapeutic alternative. Up to now more than 220
patients had been treated with the laser method (HORCH 1985,
ROODENBURG 1985).

III. Operative treatment of the cleft palate in small children may be
another indication to the clinical use of the CO_2-laser. Operating
the children (average age at time of operation: 23.6 months) the
blood loss using conventional operative technique was 13.4% whereas
using the CO_2-laser the blood loss was only 8.6% (PIEL and HORCH
1981, HORCH 1983). Considering that a blood loss of more than 10
or 15% in small children already indicates blood transfusions,
this blood loss could be reduced by 36% when executing the para-
marginal incisions of the bridge flap and pedicle flap method at
the palate by the CO_2-laser. Regarding also a blood loss of
10% caused by shock, the application of the CO_2-laser results in
a significant reduction of blood loss and blood transfusions.

IV. Therapeutic facilities in high risk patients with a poor general
condition, cardiac, pulmonary or other severe diseases may be improved, if parenchymatous or capillary bleeding could be reduced
by the Nd-YAG-laser or the CO_2-laser. Even if laser surgery may
not replace conventional surgery in the treatment of malignancies
in the maxillo-facial region , clinical experiences of more than
10 years suggest an enlargement and improvement of therapeutic
facilities in treating benign tumors and malignancies. (Fig. 2)

V. In the facial region, the application of argon lasers in treating
vascular diseases (Naevi flammei) or removing tatoos is well
established. The treatment of Naevi flammei with argon lasers in
adults show in 70% of the cases good results, which means a
significant clearing up or diminution. In the removing of
tatoos in regions where dermabrasions are not possible, the argon
laser enlarges the therapeutic facilities.

VI. In the field of the oral and maxillo-facial surgery it would be
convenient, after experimental and clinical trial, to treat malignancies with the photodynamic therapy, a combination of laser
therapy and chemotherapy. The effect of this therapy is based on
the concentration of special substances in malignancies. These
substances develop under the influence of light cytotoxic effects.

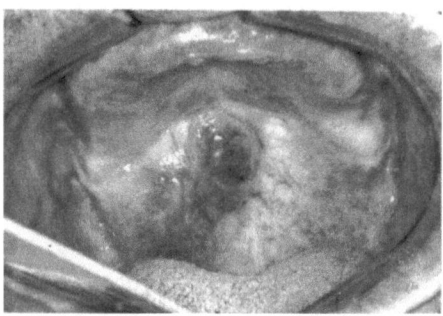
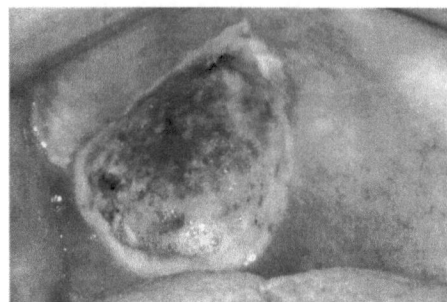
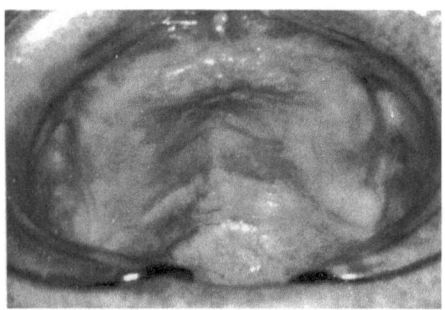

Fig. 2. Pleomorphic adenoma of the hard palate of a 84-years old patient:
a. before CO_2 laser excision; b. 14 days after laser excision without any reconstructive surgery; c. 3 years postoperatively, still without any local recurrence

The experimental and clinical tests to prove the efficiency of this method in the treatment of oral cancer are not finished yet (HERZOG et al. 1987). In Germany the mortality statistics show that 6 men and 2 women out of 100.000 inhabitants suffer from oral cancer (NEUMANN 1981). Despite the fact that the direct access to the oral cavity makes an early diagnosis and therapy possible, cancer of the oral mucosa is a dominant factor in these statistics. At this point the development of photodynamic therapy is necessary to improve the survival rate of 5 years from 30% to 40%. Therefore an early diagnosis and the enlargement of conventional therapy methods are the main points on which the research should concentrate.

REFERENCES:

Ackermann, K.: Neodym-YAG-Laser in der Zahnmedizin. Münch.Med.Wschr. 126: 1119-1121 (1984)

Apfelberg, D.B., R.A. Greene, M.R. Maser, H. Lash, J.L. Rivers, D.R. Laub: Results of Argon laser exposure of capillary hemangiomas of infancy-preliminary report. Plast.Reconstr.Surg. 67: 188-193 (1981)

Herzog, M., H.-H. Horch, R. Senekowitsch, E. Schröder: Experimentelle Untersuchungen zur Laser-Diagnostik und -therapie des Mundhöhlenkarzinoms nach tumorselektiver Photosensibilisierung mit Hämatoporphyrin-Derivat (HpD) - Vorläufige Mitteilung. Dtsch. Z Mund-Kiefer-Gesichtschir. 11: 18-22 (1987)

Horch, H.-H.: Laser-Osteotomie und Anwendungsmöglichkeiten des Lasers in der oralen Weichteilchirurgie. Eine tierexperimentelle und klinische Studie. Quintessenz, Berlin 1983

Horch, H.-H., K. Gerlach, H.E. Schaefer, H.-D. Pape: Erfahrungen mit der Laserbehandlung oberflächlicher Mundschleimhauterkrankungen. Dtsch. Z Mund-Kiefer-Gesichtschir. 7: 31-35 (1983)

Horch, H.-H.: Die Laser-Chirurgie im Mund-Kiefer-Gesichtsbereich. Zahnärztl. Mitt. 75: 2554-2568 (1985)

Horch, H.-H., K.L. Gerlach, H.-E. Schaefer: CO_2-laser surgery of oral premalignant lesions. Int. J. oral maxillofac.Surg. 15: 19-24 (1986)

Landthaler, M., D. Haina, R. Brunner, W. Waidelich, O. Braun-Falco: Laser in der Dermatologie und plastischen Chirurgie. In: E. Keiditsch, P.W. Ascher, F. Frank - Verhandlungsber. Dtsch.Ges.Lasermed. 2: 47-52 (1985)

Neumann, G.: Häufigkeit bösartiger Neubildungen. Dtsch.Ärztebl. 21: 1039 ff. (1981)

Piel, H.E., H.-H. Horch: Tierexperimentelle und klinische Untersuchungen zur Anwendung des Lasers bei Gaumenspaltplastiken. Dtsch. zahnärztl.Z. 36: 175-178 (1981)

Roodenburg, J.L.N.: CO_2-Laserchirurgie von Leukoplakie van het mondslijmvlies. Van Denderen, Groningen 1985

Seipp, W., D. Haina, V. Seipp, W. Waidelich: Argon- oder CO_2-Laser bei Tätowierungen und exophytischen Hautläsionen? In: E. Keiditsch, P.W. Ascher, F. Frank - Verhandlungsber. Dtsch.Ges.Lasermed. 2: 57-62 (1985)

Author's address:
Prof. Dr. Dr. Hans-Henning Horch, Dr. Dr. Michael Herzog.
Clinic of oral and maxillo-facial Surgery, Klinikum rechts der Isar, Technical University of Munich
Ismaningerstraße 22

D-8000 München 80
FRG

The Carbon Dioxide Laser in Oral Surgery

S. Barak, I. Kaplan, I. Rosenblum
Maccabi Sick Fund
Balfour 10, Tel Aviv, Israel. and Tel Aviv University

The CO_2 laser has a definite advantage in surgery of the oral cavity. This is related to the ability to perform accurate hemostatic surgery, while at the same time, sterilizing the operative area. Lesions of various kinds can be treated either by excision or vaporization. In the latter case, anesthesia can be avoided by using the pulsed mode. Minimal postoperative pain and edema with rapid healing results in speedy recovery without significant discomfort. We are presenting some demonstrative cases to support this assertion. Gingival Hyperplasia: In the treatment of gingival hyperplasia, the laser has an advantage because of its hemostatic potential and sterilizing capability. We also noted, in these cases, that postoperative discomfort is minimal, and the use of peripack after the operation is unnecessary. Epulis of the Gingiva: A case of epulis of the gingiva treated by vaporization without local anesthesia. Leukoplakia of the Residual Ridges and Palate: A case of a 64-year-old female with leukoplakia of the lower residual ridges and the palate. Treatment was by vaporization of the lesions with pulsed mode without anesthesia. Leukoplakia of the Tongue: The ability to treat lesions of the tongue occupying extensive surfaces without anesthesia and without bleeding while leaving the patient free of postoperative pain, is an impressive application of the CO_2 laser. A case of leukoplakia of the tongue in a 28-year-old male is presented. Lingual Tonsil: Another advantage of laser surgery in the oral cavity is the ability to gain access to the posterior portion of the tongue. A case of lingual tonsil, vaporized without anesthesia. Fibroma of the Tongue: A case of a reactive fibroma of the left side of the tongue vaporized without anesthesia and without bleeding. Fibroma of the Cheek Advantage of the CO_2 laser lies in the ability to vaporize tumors of the buccal mucosa without anesthesia and without bleeding. The following is an example of a 10-year-old child with a reactive fibroma of the left cheek. Fibroma of the Lip: Similar condition of the lower lip, treated as in fibroma of the cheek. Squamous Cell Carcinoma of the Lower Lip: A malignant tumor, squamous cell carcinoma of the   lower lip in a

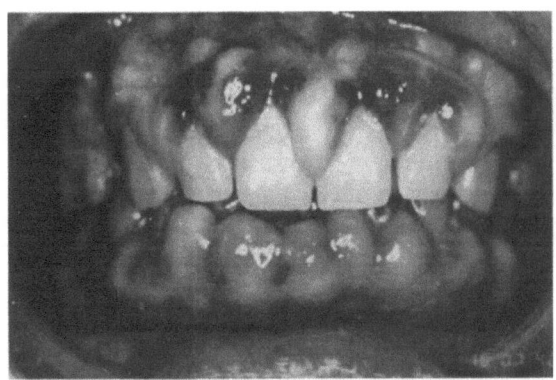

1. A 45-year-old male with nifedipine gingival hyperplasia

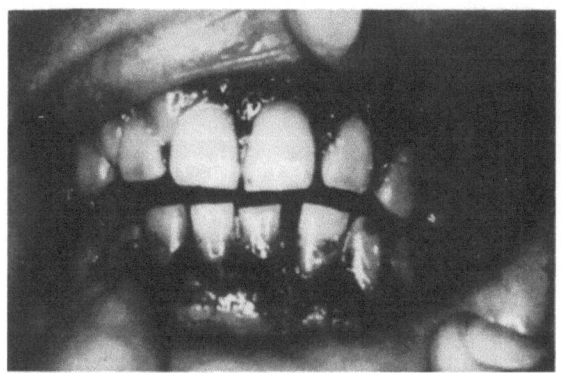

2. View of the same patient immediately after operation

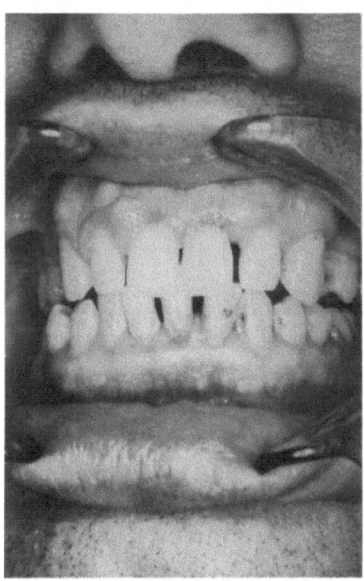

3. The same patient, four weeks after the operation

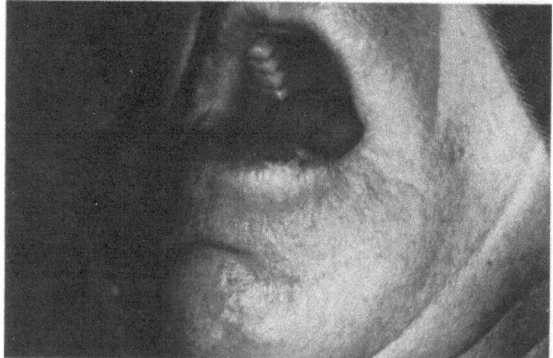

4. Squamous cell carcinoma in the lower lip

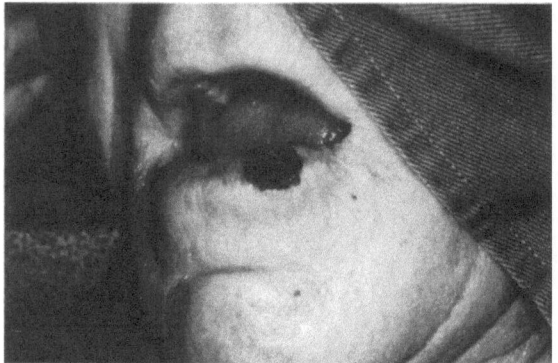

5. Laser ablation of the lesion

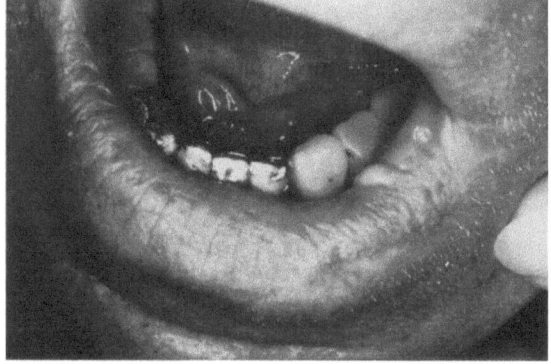

6. The same patient, five weeks later

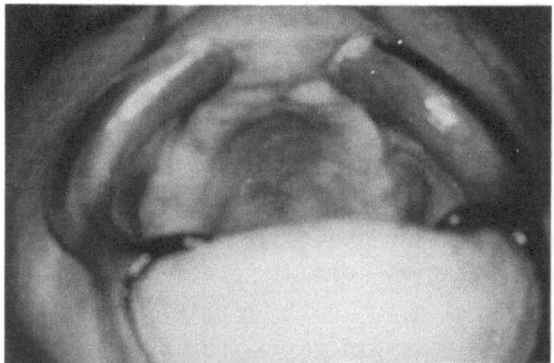

7. Reactive inflammatory papillary hyperplasia of the palate

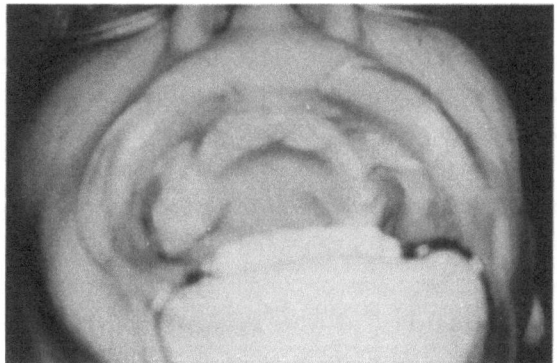

8. Four weeks after laser vaporization

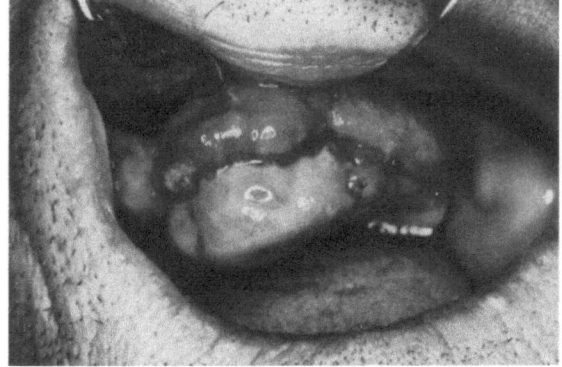

9. Peripheral giant cell tumor in the anterior region of the maxilla

72-year-old male. The tumor was excised; histology revealed adequate excision of the tumor. Reactive Inflammatory Papillary Hyperplasia of the Palate: Reactive inflammatory papillary hyperplasia of the palate is commonly associated with prolonged wearing of an ill-fitting maxillary full denture. A case of the above mentioned diagnosis was treated with vaporization. The depth of the penetration of the laser is to the submucosa, no bleeding was noted after the procedure, the denture was dressed with coe-comfort, no postoperative pain was claimed. Peripheral Giant Cell Tumor: A case of peripheral giant cell tumor with a residual cyst of the anterior maxilla in a 67-year-old male. Performing the biopsy with a scalpel, bleeding was almost uncontrollable. The tumor was excised and the cyst was vaporized with the CO_2 laser. One week later complete healing was observed. Two months after the operation, a full denture was fitted, demonstrating the preservation of the buccal sulcus which usually does not occur with conventional surgery. Hemangioma of the Oral Cavity: The ability to vaporize hemangioma of the oral cavity hemostatically is the main advantage of the CO_2 laser. A case of a 38-year-old female with a hemangioma of the lower lip and buccal sulcus. The lesion was vaporized with minimal bleeding. Hemangioma of the Lower Lip: It is well known that the treatment of strawberry nevi in infancy should be avoided, since they have a tendency to resorb spontaneously. When they occur in the vicinity of the eyes or mouth, however, one is obliged to resect them as they may comprise a functional disturbance, aside from the possibility of hemorrhage. The following case is an example of an 8-month-old baby with a hemangioma of the lower lip.

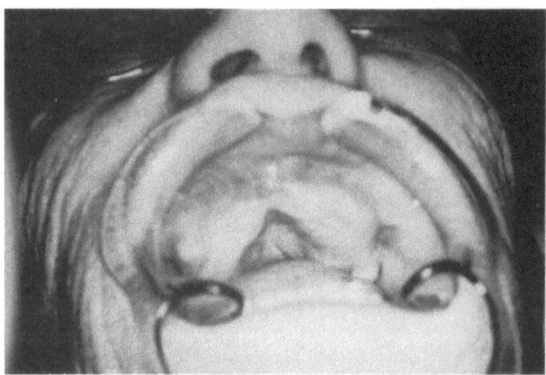

10. The same patient, six weeks after the operation. Note the buccal sulcus

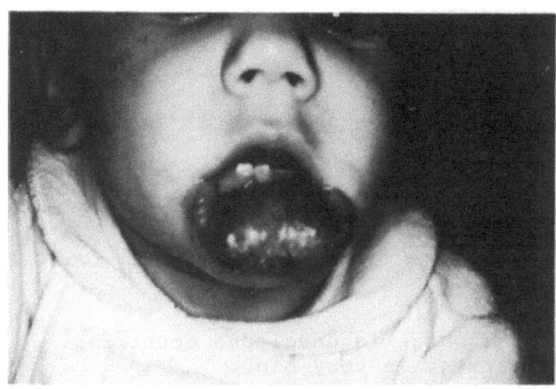

11. Haemangioma of lower lip in an infant

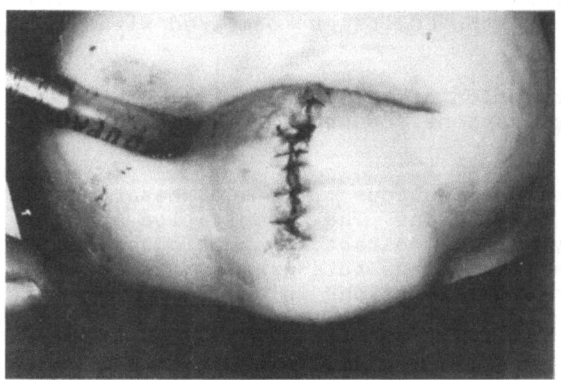

12. Immediate postoperative condition

References

1. Melcer J, Chaumette MT, Melcer F, Dejardin J, Hasson R, Merard R, Pinaudeau Y, Weill R: Treatment of dental decay by CO_2 laser beam: Preliminary results. Lasers Surg Med 4:311-321, 1984.
2. Pecaro BC, Garehime WJ: The CO_2 laser in oral and maxillofacial surgery. J Oral Maxillofac Surg 41:725-728, 1983.
3. Pick RM, Pecaro BC, Silberman CJ: The laser gingivectomy. The use of the CO_2 laser for the removal of phenytoin hyperplasia. J Periodontol 56:492-496, 1985.
4. Sachs SA, Borden GE: The utilization of the carbon dioxide laser in the treatment of recurrent papillomatosis: Report of a case. J Oral Surg 39:299, 1981.
5. Kaplan I, Giler s: CO_2 Laser Surgery. Springer-Verlag 1984.

Socio-Economic Appraisal of Dental Treatment Using CO_2 Laser

F.MELCER, J.MELCER, J.DEJARDIN.   Faculté   de   Chirurgie-Dentaire
Paris-V, O.R.S.T.O.M. (FRANCE)

INTRODUCTION
Dental decay is the third minor scourge in developed countries.
The cost of curative dental treatment is very high.
In France, 49 % of extractions result from decay and its
complications. The different kinds of treatment are complex and
haphazard, and iatrogenic pathology represents 40 % of our acts.
The role of prevention no longer has to be discussed. A socio-
economic appraisal of CO2-laser treatment in dentistry has been
carried out in order to locate the CO2-Laser compared with the
three forms of prevention.
- primary (lesions prevention)
- secondary (immediate interception of lesions)
- thirdly (treatment of complications resulting from lesions)

PRIMARY PREVENTION
It may be said that on the buccal mucous, the CO2-Laser beam
performs a role of primary prevention. The vaporization of the
fraenum and bridle (surgery without contact, atraumatic, and free
from postoperative complications) leads to a greater mastery of
dental hygiene and eliminates parafunctions which are important
etiological factors in pathology encountered in
- conservative odontology
- periodontology
- orthodontic
- speech therapy

SECONDARY PREVENTION
On the hard tissues of the vital tooth, the CO2-Laser performs a
secondary preventive role.
The local effects of the C02-Laser are beneficial in stopping
decay on the vital tooth.
The zone of sterile structural conversion is an obstacle to the
bacterial invasion and to the metabolic products and so fights
against the progression and recurrence of decay.
The further effects fight against the complications resulting
from decay.
The pulpal cells are activated. A dentin repair will permit the
pulpal healing and prevent pulpal complications of decay.

TERTIARY PREVENTION
As far as infective and periapical complications of decay are
concerned, the CO2-Laser beam will permit a periapical
sterilization and will induce a rapid periapical bone repair of
high quality.

ECONOMIC EVALUATION
In order to demonstrate this action and to make an economic
appraisal of the consequences of laser treatment, a computerized

analysis of clinical data, gathered in 7 french locations, has enabled us to compare the cost of conventional treatment with that of laser treatment.

It is based on more than 2000 cases and 912 have been checked at one week, three months and one year.
An economic evaluation of laser treatment has been carried out, and the problem has not been presented only from point of view of the practitioner who treats a relatively small number of illnesses and is only concern with technical efficiency.
It has also been presented from the point of view of health economists who want to know if the CO_2 laser beam is a good therapeutic to reduce the cost of curative dentistry.
It has been possible to calculate that the treatment of the vital tooth, completed with the laser effect, permitted a reduction of 24.8 % in the number of acts.
The therapeutic of infections complications caused by decay, permetted a reduction of 22.5 % in the number of acts, if we only include the surgical treatment, or else 68 % if we include both surgical treatment and prosthetic restauration of the extracted teeth.
It has been demonstrated that the use of the CO_2 laser beam would induce reduction in the rate of recurrence of decay, as well as a reduction in the endodontic treatment and a reduction in the iatrogenic pathology.
In the absolute, for one unit of hospital or private care, more patients may be treated, and over all dental health may be improved.

CONCLUSIONS
It may be stated that the CO_2 laser acts on the hard tissues of the tooth
- a SECONDARY PREVENTIVE role, intercepting immediately the lesions with a pulpal, apical, and periapical action on the tissue.
- a TERTIARY PREVENTIVE role figthing against general complications, local, in situ and further away in the case of diseases of the mouth and the teeth.
Technical progress in cardiac, vascular, renal, bone, or articular surgery increases considerably the number of patients wearing protheses.
The patients are receptive to infections of dental origin.
The responsability of focal infection of dental origin is greater in the case of failures of these surgical threrapies.
It is therefore reasonnable to reconsider the main objective of dental treatment and no longer to be satisfied to remain conservative but rather to be conservative in the area of healthy pulpal and periapical organs.
- On the buccal mucous the CO_2 laser beam performs a role of PRIMARY PREVENTION.

Finally, the CO_2 laser beam may be considered as an investiment in productivity since, by increasing the efficiency of the treatment of dental decay, it allows us to treat a greater number of patients. So that its contribution, in terms of PUBLIC HEALTH may be put into practice, it is imperative that access to the laser technique be as wide as possible.

This french work has been financed by PUBLIC FUNDS FROM THE MINISTRY OF INDUSTRY AND RESEARCH and the PUBLIC ESTABLISHMENTS : ANVAR and CNEH.

The Advantages of the CO_2 Laser Beam in Intentional Replantation, Implantation

MELCER,J.,MELCER F.,TARDIEU Ph. and BRUN J.P.
Faculté de Chirurgie-Dentaire PARIS-V.

INTRODUCTION

Since 1981 we have pointed out the benefits of the CO2 laser beam in Dentistry.
In TOKYO, we showed the structural changes, fusion and recrystallisation, on the surface of the dentinal tissue.
In DETROIT, we proved the biological repair of the dentino-pulpal tissue after laser treatment.
In ORLANDO (Florida),we gave the laser doses needed to obtain the sterilization of the infected apex.
In 1985 in JERUSALEM,these three principal results -structural changes,biological repair and sterilization -suggested a classification of the uses of CO2 laser in dental therapeutics.

Today,in 1987,we are giving another clinical use of the CO2 laser in Dentistry,namely in order to obtain the sterilization of the infected roots in the intentional replantation or implantation therapeutic.

DEFINITION

Intentional replantation or implantation of the infected tooth consists of the deliberate removal of a tooth and its reinsertion into the socket after obturation ,resection and sterilization of the root. This operation, limited to posterior teeth as the ultimate procedure, could be extended to other teeth.In this way the CO2 laser beam could be useful to improve the conservative dentistry with the object of sterilizing at 100 % the radicular infected areas while the tooth is out of its socket.
From our histological study on the bone repair,following apical surgery on Beagle dogs, we have shown that a young fibrous bone is formed against the surface of the root sterilized at 100 % by CO2 laser.

INDICATIONS

Intentional replantation and implantation of infected teeth are only indicated if the treatment completely removes the infection. CO2 laser surgery can only sterilize the infected dental structure.
1. Intentional replantation by means of CO2 laser is indicated in relatively few instances. The operation should be limited to posterior teeth,where resection is not feasible for anatomic reasons,risk of paresthesia, or inaccessibility.
2.Intentional implantation by means of CO2 laser is indicated when a portion of the alveolar crest is toothless, but the alveolar bone is dense and voluminous.

3. The contraindications to intentional replantation are periodontal involvement with extensive mobility of the tooth;a labial or buccal plate that has been destroyed or is missing;a septal bone destroyed at the bifurcation .
The tooth which is to be intentionally replanted should have a crown strong enough to resist the mechanical forces necessary to extract it. Whenever possible, the root canals should be filled the day before the operation.

TECHNIQUE

Intentional replantation by means of CO_2 laser should preferably be carried out by a two-man team. One person should be given the responsibility of extraction and curettement of the socket,the other of carrying out the necessary endodontic laser treatment and replacing the tooth in its socket.
The tooth is then carefully extracted; the wound is packed with sterile gauze, and the patient is asked to close his teeth together to immobilize the pack.
As soon as the tooth is removed from its socket, it is given to the person who is reponsible for the endodontic laser procedure. The tooth is immediately wrapped in sterile gauze saturated with the saline solution in such a manner that only the root tips protrude from the gauze. The operator then cuts about 2 or 3mm from the root apices with a bur.
A cavity is prepared in each of the resected roots and sterilized using the CO_2 laser beam .
Laser parameters are :
- focused beam
- minimal diameter spot
- minimal duration during shot (hundredth of a second)
- repetition
- power from 5 to 10 watts

The cavities are then filled with sterile gutta percha and again sterilized with a defocused laser spot.
The purpose of this is to keep the ligament viable and both volatilize the necrosed cement and sterilize the toxic dentinal areas . This method seems basically impossible, for it must both destroy the microbial germs impregnated into dentinal tubules and keep the viability of the ligament on the surface of the radicular root so as to reattach it to the alveolar wall of the socket. This can be done successfully in clinic if the external radicular wall is precooled by spraying chlorethyl for 30 seconds just before the laser application and if the energy doses are sufficient to sterilize the dentin. This clinical method reduces the extent of the thermal damage on the adjacent vital alveolo-dental ligament.
Then the tooth is returned to its socket.
A splint is then attached using at least two adjacent teeth for anchorage and removed one month later. By that time the tooth should be firm in its socket and the appearance of the gingiva should be normal.

CLINICAL CASES

1/ Intentional replantation.
Mr P. Michel comes for a consultation in May 1985 for an abscess in the third left maxillar molar.This pathology is due to fracture of the disto-buccal root.There is a deep and large

socket around the two buccal roots and the mobility IV is noted. This tooth,the posterior abutment of a bridge of three teeth, is functioning alone, the first abutment being detached.We recommend an intentional replantation after curettage of the socket and sterilization of the roots.

The dental prothesis and the third molar are extracted.The alveolar is curetted.The laser exposure treats the internal roots of the last molar with energy densities about 8.3×10 w/cm2,as well as the radicular necrosed surfaces contiguous with the periodontal abscess.Retrograde cement fillings are placed extraorally and the bridge is replanted.

The post- operative surgery was absolutely painless and the normal function was possible after a week.

After two years, there is no particular sign ,no aleolysis on X Ray and the mobility is reduced from IV to II.

2/Intentional implantation : in other words transplanting and submerging a root from another part of the same mouth.

Mr A.Robert comes for a consultation to restore his maxillary. He has lost his three left molars,all his other teeth are perfect except the first left premolar. A transplantation is recommended to place the first premolar in the position of the second molar.

The radicular bears a granuloma. After extraction, curettage, resection of the apex and laser treatment, an incision is made in the periosteum.A mucoperiosteal flap is raised and a surgical socket is made for the transplant. The premolar root is placed in the position of the second molar. The flap is repositioned and stitched.

The mucosa covering the transplanted tooth is removed after healing and a restoration is made from the canine to the second molar.

The clinical healing is maintained after two years.

DISCUSSION

In traditional techniques, some resorption occurs within one or two years; in other cases, the resorption is slow in developing. NINE CO2 laser intentional replantations and TWO CO2 laser intentional implantations were performed from 1985 to this year. All the eleven teeth are functional and the resorption seems static according to the X Rays.

Generally homotransplantation of teeth is not as successful as intentional replantation because of the immunological factor involved.Homograft rejection of teeth is similar to rejection of tissues elsewhere in the body and is mediated by cells which are derived from the reticulo-endothelial system. This new method using the CO2 laser beam can perhaps eliminate the antigenic factor and prevent ankylosis and root resorption.This possibility has still to be studied.

Conventional and Nd:YAG Laser Hyperthermia (Laserthermia): Effects on Rabbit Tongue Tissue

Y. Watanabe[1], H. Tsunekawa[1], K. Takeuchi[1], H. Okumura[1], K. Fujitsuka[1], S. Kitayama[2], T. Toyoda[2], Y. Kameyama[3], K. Hiranuma[4], C. Brünger[5]

1) Dept. of Dentistry and Oral Surgery, Meitetsu Hospital, Nagoya
2) Dept. of Oral Surgery, Japanese Red Cross Nagoya First Hospital, Nagoya
3) Dept. of Pathology, Aichi Gakuin University, Nagoya
4) Dept. of Prosthodontics, Aichi Gakuin University, Nagoya
5) Dept. of Internal Medicine, 2nd Teaching Hospital, Fujita-Gakuen Health University

Summary

To use laser hyperthermia (laserthermia) as a form of cancer therapy in the field of oral surgery, we have conducted several basic studies. Using rabbits, we recently investigated the differences between hyperthermia by laser light and by other means. More specifically, we experimentally compared the effects of the artificial sapphire probe commonly used for laserthermia and a new titanium probe of the same form which transmits heat but not laser light.

Results:
1) Ultrasonography showed that laserthermia penetrates deeper into the tissue than conventional hyperthermia.
2) Histo-pathological examination revealed that in identical conditions laserthermia has greater invasiveness in normal tissue than conventional hyperthermia.

Introduction

The development of medical lasers has been spectacular. Ever since we succeeded in developing an artificial sapphire probe for contact irradiation by Nd:YAG laser in 1984, we have reported on basic experiments using the contact-irradiation method.[1][2] In preference to high-output lasers which cause tissue vaporization, we have designed hyperthermia using low-power laser energy, and have produced a special high-divergence conic sapphire probe which combines stable power-output and high safety. We next designed a computer-controlled local laser hyperthermia system and attempted various clinical applications.[3] Recently, however, we detected degeneration of cancer tissue in sites where the temperature control during laser irradiation had been set to 40°C, suggesting that laserthermia is the synergistic effect of heat and laser light. To differentiate the two, we here compare laserthermia with traditional hyperthermia.

Materials and Methods

1. Experimental animals

For this experiment we used white Japanese domesticated rabbits weighing C. 2.0 kg, which were kept in our laboratory animal quarters at normal temperature ($23\pm1°C$) and normal humidity ($55\pm5\%$) and given solid chow (Oriental Re-5) and water ad libitum. The animals were observed under these conditions for at least four days prior to the experiment to determine that they were completely healthy.

2. Materials

As power source we used the 1064 nm Nd:YAG laser model CL-60 with attached computer-control (Fig. 1). This system's output is continuously adjustable from 1.0 - 60.0 W, and can be operated in both the continuous wave (CW) and pulse wave (PW) modes. To determine the irradiation site we used a He-Ne laser with axis parallel to the Nd:YAG laser. A water pump is attached to the laser system by which sterile water is transmitted to the irradiation site.

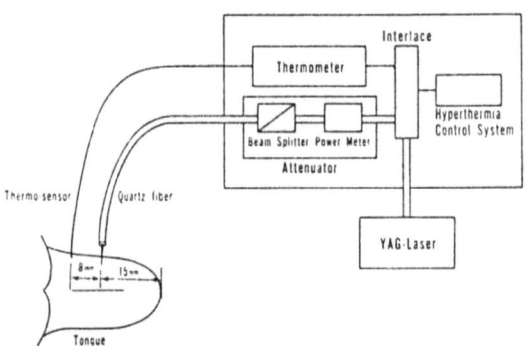

Fig. 1. Computer controled Laserthermia system

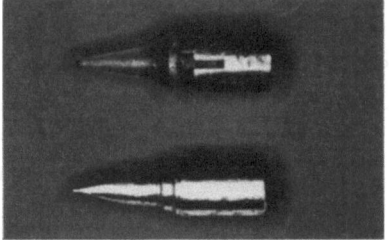

Fig. 2. Interstitial probes.
Above: Sapphire probe.
Below: Titanium (metal) probe

3. Interstitial probes (Fig. 2)

a. Artificial sapphire probe

To deliver uniformly dispersed laser energy to the tissue, we used our high-divergence conical probe (interstitial probe). This has good permeability for laser light, excellent heat stability, is made of one of the new ceramics, an aluminium oxide alloy, and has the advantage that tissue does not easily adhere to it.

b. Titanium (metal) probe

To block the laser light emitted from the power source and transmit heat only, we chose titanium, because it has superior heat conduction (0.20 W/cm x °C) and a high melting point (1680°C). This probe possesses the same form and size as the sapphire probe (2 x 1.5 mm). We performed computer-controlled hyperthermia with the power-generator as above.

4. Methods

Laserthermia was performed for 15 min according to the method of Tsunekawa et al.[4] The probe and thermosensor were 8 mm apart and the power output was 3 W.

a. Anaesthesia and fixation of the tongue

The animals were fixated in a lateral recumbent position under i.v. anaesthesia with sodium pentobarbital (0.4 mg/kg). The tongue was extended and held in place by tongue-clamps so that its total extended length was 25 mm. The clamps were so designed that the probe and sensor could be inserted at a right angle to the median line of the tongue. We inserted the probe 15 mm away from the apex of the tongue and the sensor a further 8 mm towards the radix.

b. Experimental groups

We used 40 rabbits in all which were divided into four groups of ten animals each. Group A was irradiated with the sapphire probe at 39-40°C for 15 min, group B likewise with the metal probe. Group C with the sapphire probe at 44-45°C for 15 min, and group D likewise with the metal probe.

The irradiation site was observed macroscopically one and seven days after irradiation and at each point half the animals were killed, the tongue removed and after fixation in a 10% phosphate buffer formalin solution embedded in paraffin and dyed with haematoxylin-eosin in the usual fashion. We also performed ultrasonography immediately after irradiation.

Results and Conclusions

1) As shown in Fig. 3, the heat distribution on the surface of the rabbit tongue was similar with the sapphire and the metal probe.

2) Ultrasonography immediately after treatment showed that laserthermia penetrates deeper into the tissue than hyperthermia with the metal probe (Fig.4).

3) Fig. 5 shows a macroscopic comparison between groups A and B one day after irradiation; namely in group A, treated with the sapphire probe, both the width and depth of the affected tissue are greater than in group B, treated with the metal probe. A comparison between groups C and D yielded similar results.

4) Histo-pathological examination one and seven days after irradiation (Fig. 6) showed greater invasiveness of irradiation in groups A and C (sapphire-probe treated) than in groups B and D (metal-probe treated).

All these findings demonstrate greater penetration into normal tissue of laserthermia and suggest that laser light has a cytocidal effect in addition to the thermic effect. We hope to apply our experimental findings of laserthermia effect in the clinical treatment of cancer in the field of oral surgery.

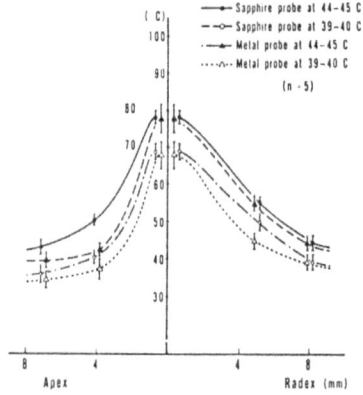
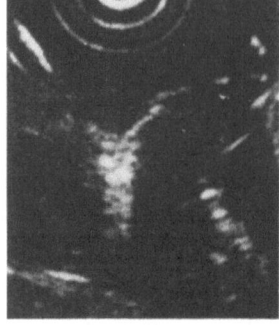
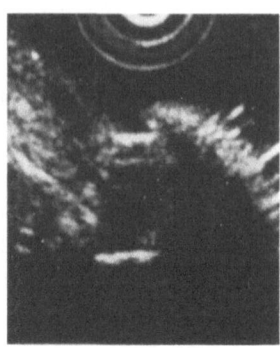

Fig 3. Temperature distribution on the surface of the tongue

Fig 4. Sapphire probe　　Metal probe
Ultrasonic changes immediately after irradiation

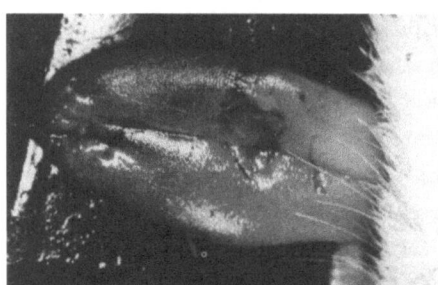
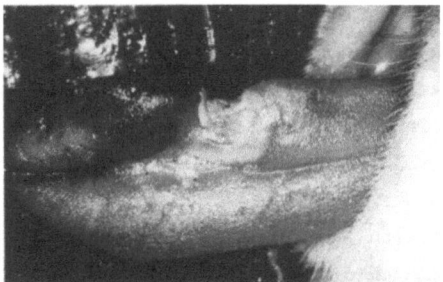

Fig 5. A group (Left)　　　　　　　B group (Right)
Rabbit tongue one day after laserthermia

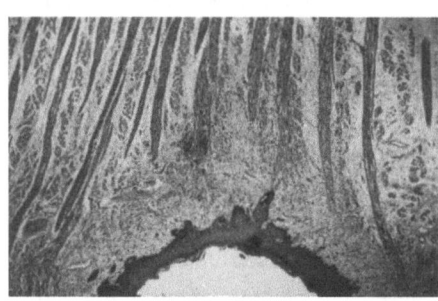
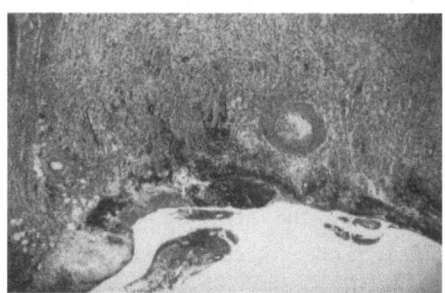

Fig 6. A group (Left)　　　　　　　B group (Right)
Histology one week after laserthermia

References

1) H. Tsunekawa et al.: Gastroenterological Endoscopy 1984, 26:1576
2) H. Tsunekawa et al.: Laser Optoelektronik in der Medizin, Springer-Verlag, Berlin, 1985, pp.360-366.
3) S. Suzuki et al.: Journal of the Japanese Society for Laser Medicine 1986, 6:347
4) H. Tsunekawa et al.: The 3rd International Nd:YAG Laser Symposium, PPS Tokyo, 1986, pp. 105

Nd: YAG Laser in Oral Cavity Cancer Report of 200 Cases – Minimum Follow up of one Year

DR. D. D. PATEL, M.S., F.R.C.S.
CHIEF SURGICAL SERVICE - I
GUJARAT CANCER AND RESEARCH INSTITUTE
ASARWA, AHMEDABAD - 380 016. INDIA

ORAL CANCER - Nd:YAG LASER

Abstract

Oral cavity cancers are one of the commonest cancers in our country. These cancers are treated by surgery, radiotherapy and chemotherapy either simultaneously or successively. Treatment of oral cancers by Nd:YAG Laser is an additional modality of treatment. Treatment by YAG Laser is simple, involves very little morbidity and no mortality and is cost effective. This treatment has special attraction for aged patients with cancers which otherwise need major ablative surgery and reconstructive procedures. It also permits adjuvant use of chemotherapy or radiotherapy if needed.

Introduction

Cancers of oropharyngolaryngeal region are the commonest cancers in our state. This group forms 45 % of the total cancers that we treat. Cancers of oral cavity form 30 % of these cancers. These cancers are treated by surgery, radiotherapy and chemotherapy either simultaneously or successively. Since February 1984, we have installed a mediLas Nd:YAG Laser at our Institute. All oral cancers admitted to our service are treated by Nd:YAG Laser. From February 1984 to March 1986 a total of 200 patients with oral cancers have been treated by YAG Laser.

Materials and Methods

This report gives out our experience of 200 patients with oral cancers treated by Nd:YAG Laser during the period February 1984 to July 1986. It thus gives follow up of one to three years for all the patients and allows to draw some conclusions about effectiveness of this modality of treatment.

All the patients had usual preoperative evaluation including biopsy of the lesion. They were all epidermoid cancers with variable degree of differentiation. There were 90 Females to 110 Males and age varied between 30 years and 85 years. All patients were admitted to the hospital and were scheduled for laser treatment on next day. The procedure was performed under general anaesthesia. The pulse frequency was 4 to 5 seconds of laser with power of 40 to 50 watts. The total joules received varied from 1000 to 12000 joules depending upon size of the lesion. The patients were then shifted to recovery beds. Most were allowed to go home next day but few were hospitalized for a further period of twenty-four hours. All were advised usual symptomatic treatment. Post operative period was free from pain but each patient complained of edema and swelling of the treated part, which subsided after four to five days.

These patients were seen in follow up clinic after three weeks. If the lesion had healed satisfactorily, further follow-up was advised. If not, re-biopsy was done and if the lesion was effective active laser was reapplied. The detailed anatomical location of the lesions as per Table I.

TABLE I. ANATOMICAL DISTRIBUTION OF ORAL CANCER PATIENTS

	SITE OF LESION	NO. OF CASES
1.	Hard Palate	30
2.	Soft Palate	40
3.	Buccal Mucosa	60
4.	Retromolar Region	15
5.	Tonsil	20
6.	Anterior Tongue	10
7.	Floor of mouth	10
8.	Lip	10
9.	Adenoid Cystic Carcinoma	5
	Buccal Mucosa	===
	Total	200

Results

From our experience of treatment of about 200 cases of oral cancers with Nd:YAG Laser, we believe that it offers an additional modality of treatment to conventional methods of surgery, radiotherapy and chemotherapy. It is observed that for T1-T2 and T2-T3 lesions it offers control with one treatment while T3-T4 lesions need more than one laser application. It has been our routine to use adjuvant radiation or chemotherapy for lesions which required more than two sittings. For T1-T2 lesions two years control rate was 80 % while for T2-T3 lesions, 2 years control rate was 70 %. Finer points of our observations are brought out in discussion.

Conclusions

1. In this paper we describe our experience of Nd:YAG Laser in the treatment of 200 patients with oral cavity cancers.

2. Treatment by Nd:YAG Laser offers attractive and equally effective additional modality of management for oral cavity cancers in comparision to surgery, radiotherapy and chemotherapy.

3. Short term tumor control up to 12 months to 24 months is quite promising. Longer follow up is necessary.

4. It offers simpler form of treatment, short hospitalization, minimum anaesthetic exposure and instrumentation, no blood transfusions, pain free recovery and resumption of oral feeding at the earliest.

5. There is no morbidity or disfigurement or modality. Vital functions of speech, mastication and deglutition are not disturbed.

6. Capital cost of equipment is high but there is tremendous saving in number of patient hospital days used if these patients are treated with Nd:YAG Laser. This modality is thus cost effective and strain on other hospital service is also minimal.

7. Nd:YAG Laser is very effective for tumor control for T1-T2 lesions of oral cavity. T2-T3 lesions need more than one sitting while T3 lesions need additional support in treatment by radiotherapy and chemotherapy. Treatment by Nd:YAG Laser for T3 lesions should be considered as cytoreductive surgery and has definite role in the management of such advanced lesions.

Acknowledgements

My thanks are due to Dr. T. B. Patel, Director of our Institute to give me permission to study this project. I am equally grateful to my patients for accepting this mode of treatment without hesitation.

Thermal Combination of Dental Alloys with a Commercial Nd: Glass Compact-Laser

A. Kasenbacher and E. Dielert
Klinik und Poliklinik für Zahn-, Mund- und
Kieferkrankheiten der Universität München
Lindwurmstraße 2a, D-8000 München 2

1. Introduction

In dental laboratories soldering is used almost exclusively for thermal combination in dental alloys. Despite careful techniques soldered joints always show low tensile strength with a wide range of values (1). The causes of this are: 1st) incomplete filling of soldering gap, 2nd) many partially connected shrinkholes, 3rd) small diffusion zones, 4th) oxide- and flux inclusions, 5th) microcracks in the connecting zone (2). These problems become apparent especially if alloys with extremely diverse expansion coefficients like, for instance, precious alloy Degulor^R M with non-precious alloy Wironium^R have to be soldered. Etched cross sections of this combination show that the edges of the Wironium^R sample do not differ from their original form. The bonding is achieved almost exclusively by adhesion, since diffusion of solder components hardly occurs and under the most favourable conditions only extends to a few micrometers. This is confirmed by distribution of the element gold recorded by wavelength dispersive x-ray spectroscopy (WDS). In order to obtain strong joints for clinical use, however, the connection planes have to be enlarged in dental laboratory and this hinders appearance, cleaning properties and parodontal hygiene.

2. Methods

In searching for more appropriate bonding techniques we have used microplasma-welding (3) since 1970 and laser-welding (4) since 1982 for dental alloys. Mechanical strength tests revealed that both welding methods are superior to soldering. Microplasma-welding is especially suited for thermal combination of non-precious alloys. Because of its low power density precious and non-precious alloys cannot be welded with this technique. We combined the previously mentioned alloys under argon protecting gas atmosphere without any additives with a commercial and easy to use pulsed Nd: glass laser which is obtainable at a reasonable cost.

3. Results and Discussion

In the ion-etched metal section (fig. 1a the cross section, fig. 1b the longitudinal section) the thermal bonding zone appears correct despite rather differing melting ranges of Wironium^R (left) and Degulor^R M (right).

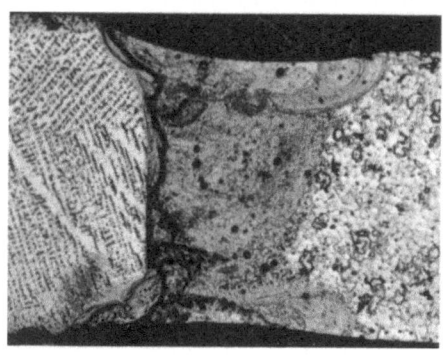
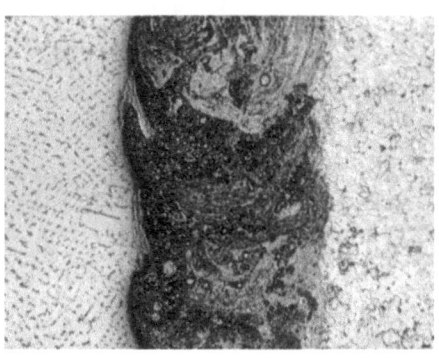

a
b

Fig. 1. Laser welded seam with base alloys Wironium^R (left), Degulor^R M (right) and fusion area (butt-configuration); a: ion-etched cross section, 50:1; b: ion-etched longitudinal section, 50:1

It measures only 0,5 mm in this 1 mm thick sample and consists of different eutectical phases, partially lamellar, partially globular with very fine distribution. Isolated pores in the welding seam are attributed to zinc evaporated from the precious alloy Degulor^R M. In fig. 1b round or oval structures are seen representing the Co-base alloy particles which did not melt completely during thermal bonding. Occasional microcracks are due to inherent tensions developing during the heating- or melting procedure. The length of these microcracks - 20 to 50 μm - and the fact that they are regularly filled with molten gold explain why the mechanical strength values are not affected very much. Since the thermal influence zone expands very little, there is only the slightest distortion with laser-welding. These advantages can be transfered to ordinary dental work. All Wironium^R - Degulor^R M combinations were obtained directly on the master stone cast with a very high degree of accuracy without the transfer work which for soldering is always necessary. Welding results could probably be improved by variation of the welding parameters and alloy components. Laser-welding increases the quality of the thermal bonding zone, reduces working time in dental laboratory (5,6) and is a great step forward if the demand for better weldable dental alloys could be realized.

References

1. E. Dielert: Werkstoffprüfungen an mikroplasmageschweißten und gelöteten Dentalgoldlegierungen. Dtsch. zahnärztl. Z. 34, 23 (1979).

2. E. Dielert: Mechanisch-technologische und metallographische Untersuchungen an Lötungen von Dentallegierungen. Dtsch. zahnärztl. Z. 33, 543 (1978).

3. E. Dielert: Zum Einsatz des gebündelten Lichtbogens beim Verbindungsschweißen von Gold- und Kobalt-Chrom-Molybdän-Legierungen. Dtsch. zahnärztl. Z. 33, 677 (1978).

4. E. Dielert and A. Kasenbacher: Lötungen, Mikroplasma- und Laserstrahlschweißungen an Dentallegierungen. Dtsch. zahnärztl. Z. 1987 (in press).

5. H. van Benthem, J. Vahl and B. Predel: Investigation of the grain structure of laser welded precious dental alloys. Proc. Europ. Prosthodontic Ass. 5, 40 (1982).

6. H. van Benthem and J. Vahl: The importance of the laser welding technique in prosthetic dentistry. Proc. ICALEO '83, E.A. Metzbower (Ed.), 38, 141 (1984).

Cardiology/Angiology

Applicability of 10 Watt Argon-Laser to Recanalisation of Obliterated Arterial Segments

C. Norden, F. Dähne, St. Müller, H. Heine, W. Ebert[*]

Central Institute of Cardiovascular Research and
[*]Physic-tecnical Institute Academy of Science, GDR

No. 50, Wiltbergstraße, Berlin, 1115, GDR

The aim of our study was to demonstrate the effect of Argon-Laser light on atherosclerotic obliterations of postmortal human vessels. The structure of the experiment was the following: 12 postmortal segments of the human A. femoralis with al length of 15 mm and atherosclerotic alterations were positioned in a basin containing physiological solution. The friction resistance between the vessel segment and the bottom of the basin was low. The distal fiber tip was directed into the obliterated vessel lumen. A steady velocity of 0.18 or 0.29 mm/s of the fiber was obtained by linear feeding. The proximal fiber tip was coupled to a 10-W-Argon-Laser. The initial distance between the distal fiber tip and the obliteration was 5 mm. With the beginning of irradiation the motor of the linear feeding was switched on. The laser process was observed through a stereo microscope and was interrupted either by the distal fiber tip appearing at the distal end of the vessel or the location of the vessel segment was changed. The diameter and depth of the channel and the level of fiber soiling were analysed.

The following parameters were measured:

n	12
initial power (fiber tip)	4.0 ± 0.2 W
decrease of power	49.3 ± 6.6 %
crater diameter	0.51 ± 0.07 mm
crater depth	2.1 ± 0.7 mm

In no case complete recanalization was achieved. After exposure a considerable power decrease of the axial light cone of 50 % was registered. The small crater depth of 1/5 of the total obliteration length is certainly associated with this fact. Furthermore it is of interest that the mean crater diameter corresponded to the diameter of the fiber. We classified the vessel segments used in the experiments into calcified and noncalcified segments. At nearly the same initial power of about 4 W only about half of the crater diameter was obtained in calcified vessels. The crater diameters reached both in calcified and in noncalcified obliterations are insufficient to develop a contactless laser therapy. Calcified areas are resistent against Argon laser light. However a sufficient crater diameter could be obtained when the fiber didn't get soiled. The axial direction of the laser beam from a clean distal fiber tip is demonstrated in figure 1a. Figure 1 b refers to the problem of fiber soiling in addition to parameters listed in the table. Please note the strong back radiation and the lateral diffraction of the laser beam.

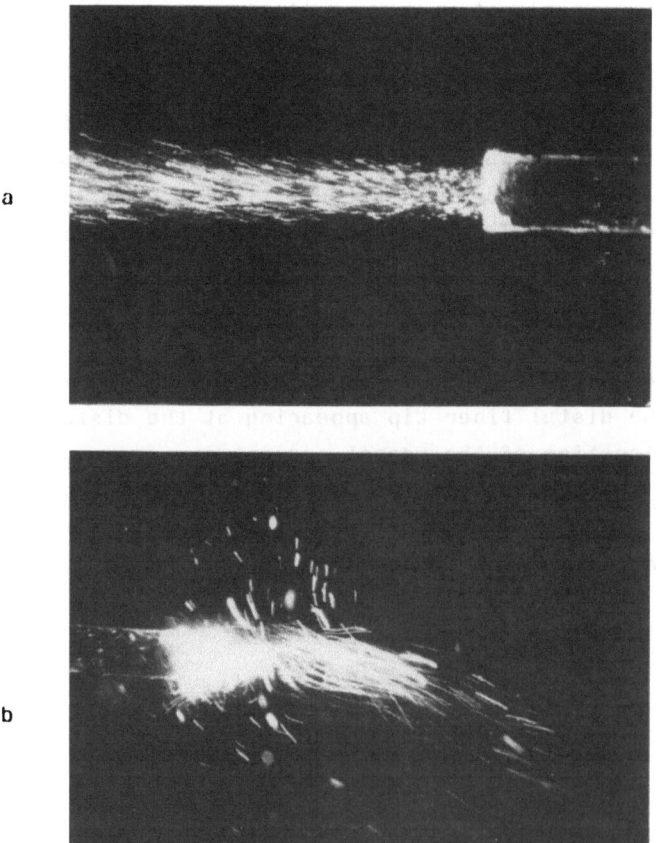

Fig. 1. Direction of laser beam before (a) and after (b) laser intervention

Besides the energy loss already reported and the decrease of effectivity connected with it there does appear the risk of a thermic vessel alteration. The laser beam leaves its axial direction. So, any directed exposure on the obliteration becomes impossible. Besides soiling of the distal fiber tip, scattering gas bubbles originating from vaporization cause a diffraction of straight direction, too. The light scattering is obviously determing also the crater configuration, which with increasing depth deviates more and more from a smooth walled cylinder. With increasing depth the relation of maximal to minimal crater diameter increases. The small penetration depth in calcified obliterations was previously shown in the table. During an exposure time of 1/2 minute the calcified area couldn't be destroyed. In contrast the adjoining tissue got heated up to such a level that it charred. Summing up all observations the negative result of Argon laser recanalization has revealed the following: We would divide the process of the laser ablation of the obliteration into 4 phases: The initial phase, the penetration phase, the soiling phase of the fiber tip and the contact phase. Up to and including the penetration phase the laser ablation plays the main role, the light induced component loses its importance in following due to growing fiber soiling. Subsequently the fiber penetrates the vessel segment in the contact phase as a "hot needle" without any possibility of control. As we advocate the concept of a contactless laser therapy, it is necessary to use pulsed high energy lasers. The stream of gas bubbles during exposure should be limited, a sufficient crater diameter must be achieved.

Cardiovascular Stability During Contact Nd:YAG Laser Surgery in the Abdominal Cavity

K. C. Moore, A Steger, N Hira
Oldham General Hospital
Oldham, England, U.K.

The introduction of contact tips and probes for use with low power Nd:YAG laser energy has been particularly beneficial to the specialty of General Surgery. The operative use of the Nd:YAG laser, formerly limited to endoscopic therapy, has now been extended to a wide range of open surgical procedures. The technological benefits of the low power contact method of applying laser energy have been well documented (1). For the patient, the operative advantages include reduced tissue trauma and greatly decreased blood loss. Postoperatively, reduced morbidity and improved recovery lead in many cases to early hospital discharge (2). The potential uses of low power contact Nd:YAG laser energy within the abdominal cavity have been detailed by Joffe (3).

Clinical Experience

Using the SLT range of contact probes we now have experience of some 200 cases, 25% being surgery within the abdominal cavity. These intra-abdominal cases were equally divided between upper and lower gastro-intestinal tract resections, cholecystectomy and solid organ surgery. Factors which affect operative cardio-vascular stability during these procedures include patient age and physical status, the degree of operative trauma and the amount of operative blood loss.

In this series of intra-abdominal surgery the age grouping of the patients was 50-90 years with an average of 74 years. The American Society of Anesthesiologist's (ASA) grading of physical status showed a range of Class 2 to Class 4 with an average of 3, in itself a further additional risk. To offset these disadvantages were the operative benefits of the Nd:YAG laser namely precision of use, reduced tissue trauma and minimal blood loss. It is known that increased age and poor physical status predispose a patient to cardiovascular instability during anaesthesia and abdominal surgery (4). Three examples are presented to support the contention that Nd:YAG laser surgery is, even in these high risk groups, associated with good cardiovascular stability.

Example 1. 58 year old female. ASA Class 2
    Diagnosis: Polycystic Disease of the Liver
    Operation: Partial resection of left lobe of liver.
    Operative time: 1½ hours   Operative blood loss: 80 ml
    CVS Stability: BP $\pm$ 15 mm Hg   Pulse $\pm$ 10 bpm

Example 2. 52 year old male. ASA Class 3
    Diagnosis: Carcinoma transverse colon
    Operation: Difficult resection of large necrotic tumour
    Operative time: 2 hours   Operative blood loss: 300 ml
    CVS Stability: BP $\pm$ 10 mm Hg   Pulse $\pm$ 10 bpm

Example 3. 86 year old female. ASA Class 4
    Diagnosis: Carcinoma of ascending colon
    Operation: Right hemicolectomy
    Operative time: 1½ hours   Operative blood loss 40 ml
    CVS Stability: BP $\pm$ 20 mm Hg   Pulse $\pm$ 5 bpm

Clinical Trial

In addition we have undertaken a prospective comparative trial of conventional versus laser surgery in cholecystectomy. A series of 20 consecutive patients were randomly allocated to either group. All patients underwent standardised operative and anaesthetic techniques (5). Non-invasive blood pressure and pulse rate measurements were taken every 5 minutes throughout operation. Preset monitoring parameters were $\pm$ 20 mm of Hg and $\pm$ 10 beats per minute for base line blood pressure and pulse rate respectively. There was no significant difference between the two groups in respect of age, sex, weight or physical status. The operating time and operative blood loss were similar in both groups.

However, the laser group of patients showed a significantly greater degree of cardiovascular stability throughout operation, only 20% demonstrating a variation in blood pressure and pulse rate which exceeded the preset monitoring parameters as compared with 100% of those undergoing conventional cholecystectomy.

Conclusion

Our experience to date suggests that in some aspects of intra-abdominal surgery the use of the low power contact Nd:YAG laser is superior to current conventional surgical techniques. Where large areas of dissection are required, particularly for necrotic or haemorrhagic lesions, the precise dissecting properties and excellent haemostasis provide the surgeon with a clear bloodless field. For solid organ surgery such as liver, spleen or pancreas resection, the superb small vessel haemostasis greatly reduces blood loss. As a consequence circulatory disturbance is minimised and blood transfusion is avoided in the majority of cases. The maintenance of good cardiovascular stability is of particular importance in the elderly and high risk patient.

References

1. Joffe S N, Daikuzono N: Multidisciplinary applications of contact Nd:YAG laser surgery. (Abstract 39) Lasers Surg. Med. 6:217 1986

2. Moore K C: Anaesthesia for Nd:YAG laser surgery. Today's Anaesthetist 1:6-7 1986.

3. Joffe S N: Contact Neodymium YAG Laser Surgery in gastroenterology: a preliminary report. Lasers Surg. Med. 6:155-157. 1986

4. Smith G, Aitkenhead A R: Textbook of Anaesthesia. Churchill Livingstone, Edinburgh 1985 pp 464-491.

5. Moore K C, Steger A, Hira N: The operative care of patients for Nd:YAG contact laser surgery. In: Oguro Y, Atsumi K, Joffe S N (Eds): Nd:YAG laser in Medicine and Surgery. Fundamental and Clinical Aspects. PPS Tokyo 1986. pp 124-127.

Fundamental Research in Laser Angioplasty (1): Effects of Nd:YAG, Argon-Ion and Excimer Lasers on Human Aortic Wall with or Without Atheromatous Plaque

Masaru Iwasaki, M.D., Kihachirou Kamiya, M.D.
Akira Ueno, M.D.
Second Department of Surgery
Yamanashi Medical College
1110 Shimogato, Tamaho-cho, Nakakoma-gun
Yamanashi, JAPAN 409-38

As the number of patients who have occlusive peripheral arterial disease grows, the clinical need of non-surgical treatments for this disorder is becoming stronger. In recent years, it has been reported that laser irradiation has the capability to vaporize and re-canalize occlusive lesions of a blood vessel [1-3]. Thus, angioplasty by laser has attracted considerable attention also in many countries, including ours.

We report here the results of our investigation on the effects of irradiation with several lasers on the human aortic walls with or without atherosclerotic change.

MATERIALS AND METHODS

For the purpose of this study, the authors selected, as continuous wave mode lasers, an Nd-YAG and an Argon-ion lasers (NIIC, Japan), and as a pulsed laser, an XeCl-excimer laser (Lumonics, Canada). Coupled to the Nd-YAG and Argon-ion lasers was a quartz fiber of 0.6 mm diameter so as to deliver the laser energy to the tissues. The output power of the Nd-YAG laser at the fiber tip was set at 50 and 80 watts, and that of the Argon-ion laser was 2.0, and 3.5 watts. The irradiation was sustained for 1, 2, 5, and 10 seconds. As for the xenon chloride excimer laser, pulse duration and repetition rate was set at 10 nanoseconds, and 40 Hz, respectively. A quartz fiber of 0.4 mm diameter was coupled to the excimer laser apparatus, and delivered 1 mJ per pulse. The duration of irradiation was varied from 1 to 5 minutes, that is 40 to 200 pulses.

Human aortas were obtained from seven cadavers. These aortas were dissected into 3 to 5 cm segments, 45 of them being selected for this study. The specimens, which were immersed in normal saline solution and positioned perpendicularly to the laser, were irradiated via the quartz fiber. The distance between the fiber tip and the specimen was maintained at 3 mm. Irradiated segments were examined by light microscopy, phase contrast microscopy and scanning electron microscopy.

RESULTS

Nd-YAG laser and Argon-ion laser:

The Nd-YAG laser was unable to ablate the aortic wall during a 1 or 2 seconds irradiation, with only whitening of the tissue being observed. For a 5 second irradiation or more, this laser produced a wide, ragged crater with extensive blast injury around it. With Argon-ion laser irradiation, crater formation was seen even at a 1 second irradiation. The margin of the crater was also irregular and carbonization was apparent. Figure 1 shows the typical histologic appearance of human aortic wall after irradiation with the Nd-YAG laser using 50 watts for 10 seconds. The aortic wall was ablated and a large irregular crater was observed. Surrounding the crater, carbonization and vacuolization of the tissue was evident throughout the whole length of the aortic wall. This thermal injury was laterally spread 4 mm from the margin of the laser crater. The shape of the crater formed by Argon-ion

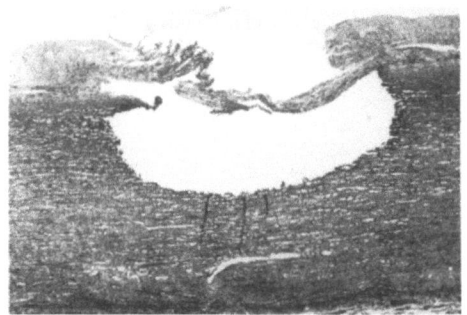

Fig. 1. Human aortic segment irradiated with Nd-YAG laser of 50 W for 10 sec. A large crater with extensive thermal injury is seen. (×40)

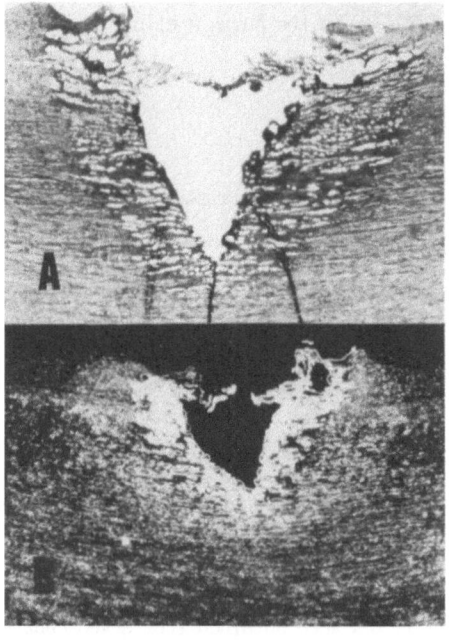

Fig. 2. Histology of an aortic wall irradiated with Argon-ion laser of 2 W for 10 sec. (A);Light microscopic view(×100), (B);Phase contrast microscopic view(×40)

laser irradiation of 2.0 watts for 10 seconds was somewhat sharper than that with the Nd-YAG laser (Fig. 2A), although, when examined with phase contrast microscopy, the zone of the thermal injury circumferentially extended 0.9 mm from the margin of crater, indicating lateral diffusion of laser energy (Fig. 2B).

Atheromatous plaques were also irradiated with these two lasers with both exhibiting the capability to vaporize these lesions. However, tissues irradiated by these two lasers demonstrated gross evidence of thermal injury, especially after Nd-YAG laser exposure (Fig. 3)

<u>XeCl-Excimer laser</u>: Aortic segments, which were irradiated with XeCl- excimer laser of 1 mJ, exhibited small craters with no gross evidence of thermal damage in adjacent tissues. By measuring the crater width and depth with micrometry, the relationship between the crater dimensions and duration of irradiation was examined. It was apparent that the depth of crater increased in a linear fashion with increasing duration of irradiation, while the width remained constant at about 0.3 mm

Fig. 4A shows scanning electron

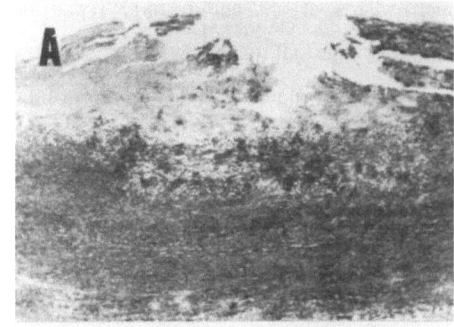

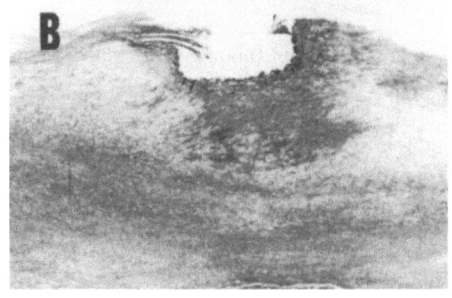

Fig. 3. Human aortic segments with atheromatous plaque irradiated with Nd-YAG laser (A), and Argon-ion laser (B). (×40)

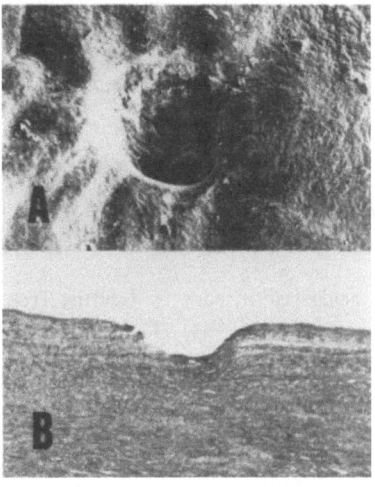

Fig. 4. An aortic wall irradiated with XeCl-excimer laser of 1 mJ for 3 min. (A) ;Scanning electron microscopic view (B) ;Light microscopic view

microscopic view of the aortic wall irradiated with the excimer laser using 1 mJ for 3 minutes. This examination revealed a smooth-walled crater with no recognizable evidence of thermal blast injury on adjacent tissues. Histologically, a clean incision was apparent with minimal thermal injury being restricted within very narrow limits (Fig. 4B). However, the capability of this system to vaporize the aortic wall was limited, and it was unable to penetrate the inner layer of the aortic wall, even after 5 minute radiation.

DISCUSSION

With regard to continuous wave mode lasers, the Argon-ion laser in this study was considered to be more suitable for angioplasty than the Nd-YAG laser. But even with the Argon-ion laser, the irradiated tissue exhibited a ragged and irregular central crater associated with a concentric thermal injured zone, which was probably due to the lateral diffusion of laser energy. Thus, by the photothermal effect caused by a laser of continous wave mode, it will be difficult to control the depth of ablation on the irradiated tissue. In contrast, the depth of crater produced by irradiation with an XeCl-excimer laser was proportional to the duration of irradiation, namely to the number of pulses, and thermal injury around the crater was negligible. From these results, it is suggested that by using excimer laser it will be possible to control the range of tissue ablation with minimal damage on adjacent tissues, and that this laser may be the most suitable for laser angioplasty. In our experiment, however, the excimer laser could only deliver 1 mJ/pulse energy through a quartz fiber of 0.4 mm diameter, and this power was not enough to vaporize and ablate long and hard occulusive lesions in the peripheral artery. Therefore, before excimer laser angioplasty is clinically adopted, effort shoud be made to develop a special fiber which can accomodate high pulses of energy.

This work was supported in part by funding from Mitsui Life Social Welfare Foundation.

References

1. Abela, G. S., Normann, S., et al. Effects of carbon dioxide, Nd-YAG and Argon laser radiation on coronary atheromatous plaques. Amer. J. Cardiol. 50;1199, 1982
2. Grundfest, W. S., Litvack, I. F., et al. Pulsed ultraviolet lasers and the potential for safe laser angioplasty. Amer. J. Surg. 150;220, 1985
3. Ginsburg, R., Wexler, L., et al. Percutaneous transluminal laser angioplasty for treatment of peripheral vascular disease. Radiology 156;619, 1985

Morphological Basis for Laser Isolation of the Ectopic Foci in Atria

V.A.Obelienius, A.J.Knèpa, E.J.Burneckis
Kaunas Medical Institute Central Research Laboratory
Kaunas, Lithuania, USSR

Surgical treatment of the supraventricular tachycardias caused by ectopic activity in the focus of the atrium is based on its excision, isolation or destruction applying electro- or cryotechnique (1, 2,3,4). If the localization of the focus is not precisely identified, surgical methods are proposed for the isolation of the right atrium, including the sinus node, complete electrical isolation of the left atrium etc. (5,6,7,8).

In previous works possibility of electrical isolation of the sinus node by Nd-YAG laser irradiation has been proved (9). Thus, experimental investigations of the morphological changes in the right atrial wall after their zone isolation by Nd-yag laser irradiation have been carried out in order to work out surgical methods for the treatment of the ectopic tachycardias.

Materials and Methods

The experiments were carried out on mongrel dogs weighing 10-20 kg under anesthesia of calypsol (5 mg/kg) and artifical lung ventilation. The heart was exposed through the right thoracotomy. Soviet Nd-YAG laser LTN-101 with a wavelenght of 1,064 mkm was used for the experiments. Irradiation at a power of 30 W with exposition lasting 40-60 s was used to formate circular coagulation strip around the sinus node zone, the right auricle or the part of a free wall of atrium. Coagulation was performed without burning-out or charring of the myocardium due to irradiation with simultaneous cooling (0,95 % saline solution 60 ml/min) of the irradiated surface (10,11). Irradiation and cooling were delivered through a special instrument containing 0,4 mm quartz fiber. A constant distance (1,5-2 mm) between the distal end of the fiber and irradiated surface was maintained.

Materials for histological investigations were obtained 24 hours after laser irradiation, after 7 and 25 days (3 experiments respectively) and were fixed in 10 % formaline solution and stained with hematoxylin-eosin.

Results

A brown strip of 2-3 mm width is observed in the area of laser destruction after 24 hours. No changes in colour or other macroscopical pathological findings were observed inside and outside of the isolated ring.

Histological examination of the irradiated zone revealed an expressed hemorrhagia and plasmorrhagia. The vessel walls in the subepicardial layer of atria are swollen with some ruptures in it. No signs of intravascular thrombosis are observed. The cardiomyocytes are stained inhomogenously, the form of the nuclei is altered, the part of cardiomyocytes are without nuclei. Swelling of the connective tissue with small foci of leucocyte infiltration are observed.

After 7 days in the area of laser destruction 3 zones are viewed: a central (necrotic) zone and the transient zones: outside and inside of it. Development of the granulation tissue is accomplished on the border of the central and transient zones. Thus, muscular fibers are found in the strip of damage in different stages of their desintegration: muscular fibers which turned into necrotic detritus and muscular fibers with a well-preserved anatomical integrity. In the transient zone myofibrils vanish and turn into basophilic. Obviously, during this stage the granulation tissue spreads out of the borders of the isolated ring to its center. On the periphery of the strip the connective tissue is collagenized in some places. Islets of the collagenized connective tissue appear around muscular stumps or close to the blood vessels. In the connective tissue there is a lot of thin-walled, dilated blood vessels of 0,2-0,3 mm in diameter. Microscopical changes of the atrial wall are insignificant.

Within 25 days a light isolation ring of 2 mm width is observed macroscopically. Definitively formed granulation tissue with its peculiar characteristics is microscopically viewed in the place of laser destruction. The zone of necrosis is formed from a rough connective tissue. Islets and bridges of the connective tissue are observed which seem to bind one border of the zone with another. On the margins of the connective scar we observe the stumps of muscular fibers gradually atrophing often splitting and branching. Thinned and splitted muscular stumps converge into the connective tissue of the transient zone. Majority of microvessels in the scar are patent, the walls are thickened and tracks of hemogenizate can be viewed in some of them.

Thus, the obtained results demonstrate that Nd-YAG laser irradiation can originate anatomical isolation of the atrial zone by forming a strip of the connective tissue in the place of laser destruction. No disintegration of the isolated zone or aneurysm formation is observed. The process of healing in the damaged zone is accomplished according to the analogous stages of organization in the foci of necrosis, but no marked leucocyte infiltration.

Discussion

The laser destruction may have many advantages as an ablative in the surgical treatment of intractable arrhythmias. The lesion has smooth borders, sharply demarcated from normal myocardium, no disrupts the anatomic continuity of heart wall (11). Laser beam destroying electrical activity in myocardium involves smaller amount of it as compared with cryotechnique. It is important that laser coagulation may be performed in transvenous operations combined with electrophysiological or endoscopical methods (10).

First clinical experience proves the laser beam to be effective in treatment of some cardiac arrhythmias (12,13). The laser coagulation technique seems to be very effective for electrical isolation of ectopic foci (9). It is necessary to emphasize that laser coagulation with simultaneous cooling of irradiated tissue induces neither charring nor defect of tissue.

Thus, we consider these morphological findings to be a background for the use of laser irradiation to isolate ectopic foci in surgical treatment of heart arrhythmias.

References

(1) Bredikis Yu., Bakschene D. et al.: Kardiologiia (Moskva), 5, 15 (1987).

(2) Revischvili A.: Kardiologiia (Moskva), 5, 9 (1987).

(3) Wyndham C., Arnsdorf M. et al.: Circulation, 63, 1365 (1980).

(4) Frank G., Baumgart D et al.: Thorac.Cardiovasc.Surgeon, 34, 398 (1986).

(5) Bokeria L., Revischvili A. et al.: Grudnaya Chirurgia (Moskva), 6, 28 (1981).

(6) Sealy W., Bache R. et al.: J.Thorac.Cardiovasc.Surg., 65, 841 (1973).

(7) Sealy W., Seaber A.: J.Thorac.Cardiovasc.Surg., 77, 436 (1979).

(8) Williams J., Ungerleider R. et al.: J.Thorac.Cardiovasc.Surg.,

50, 375 (1980).

(9) Bredikis J., Obelienius V. et al.:Laser Applications in Cardiovascular Diseases, Future Publ.Co., N.Y., in press (1987).

(10) Obelienius V., Knepa A. et al.:Lasers in Surgery and Medicine, 5, 469 (1985).

(11) Obelienius V., Knepa A. et al.:Lasers in Surgery and Medicine, 5, 479 (1985).

(12) Bredikis J., Obelienius V. et al.:In:Proceed. 2-nd Conference of Lithuanian cardiological society, Kaunas, 1984, p.77 (in Rus.).

(13) Obelienius V., Bredikis J. et al.:In:Proceed.2-nd International Nd-YAG Laser Conference, Springer-Verlag, Berlin, p.462 (1986).

Energy Threshold for Argon Laser Ablation of Arterial Plaque

Robert W. Gammon
Institute for Physical Science and Technology
University of Maryland, College Park, Maryland 20742

K.R. Fox
Atlantic Eye Center
2716 North Upshur Street, Arlington, Virginia 22207

A.A. Coster
Bradlee Medical Building
3451 West Braddock Road, Alexandria, Virginia 22302

Argon ion laser energy has been used for the removal of atheromatous plaque in vitro and in vivo and is a promising technique in recanalizing arterial channels for the surgical treatment of atherosclerotic cardiovascular disease.[1-4] It is important to understand the mechanism of tissue removal and laser tissue interaction to optimize the most efficient and safest method to deliver argon ion energy intravascularly, as well as the most appropriate wavelength, and dosage, optical geometry and methods to limit the laser activity to the intraluminal occlusion without damaging other tissues, including the vessel wall.

Kaminov, Wiesenfeld and Choy[5] described the first measurements to characterize plaque as an optical medium with scattering and absorption constants. More recently Sinofsky and Dumont[6] reported measurements of the scattering properties of plaque tissue. Welch[7] has reviewed the subject of laser induced thermal damage to tissues including the effects of scattering. The mechanisms are complicated and the modeling of multiple scattering or radiative diffusion in such strongly scattering systems does not appear to be adequate for optimizing the irradiation conditions for laser recanalization applications.

In this paper we present the measurements obtained from in vitro experiments in which plaque was removed from fresh human arterial samples recovered from autopsy (within 24 hours after death). These arterial specimens were from aorta, carotid and coronary arteries. Laser exposures were performed at the intimal surface of: (1) calcified fibrous plaques with necrosis and ulceration, (2) fibrous plaques with raised lesions or pearly plaques, and (3) fatty streaks with yellowish or white patches. We observed a constant minimal hole diameter of 500 ± 50 microns, no matter how tightly the laser was focused on the plaque. We believe this diameter is the result of anisotropic multiple-scattering and absorption in the plaque, but we know of no calculation which can predict this diameter. Given this diameter, there should be a well defined energy threshold for plaque removal: our measurements show a threshold of 200±50 mJ pulse for pulse lengths less than 60mS.

The measurements were made with a Spectra Physics Model 170 continuous argon ion laser, operating on all lines with powers to 9W. The laser output was focused with various lenses onto fresh arterial plaque mounted in air. The specimen saw the laser radiation as pulses of controlled length and number. The laser was controlled with a fast, mechanical shutter capable of opening and closing in 2mS. The focal diameter was varied from 50 to 500 microns and the pulse lengths were varied from 2 mS to 300 mS: anything longer than 300 mS was equivalent to continuous irradiation. The laser was pulsed at a slow rate of one pulse per second to allow conductive cooling between each pulse. After each set of laser pulses the sample was moved to a microscope with calibrated stage motion and dimensions of the hole in the tissue measured. Lenses of 40 cm and 9.4 cm focal length were used. With our particular laser and optical layout the calculated focal spot diameters are 100 microns and 50 microns. The focal spot diameters were checked by creating holes in black plastic targets: the measured holes were 100 microns in diameter. For either lens the holes made in plaque samples measured 500 microns in diameter. These results suggest that the minimum hole diameter is determined by scattering in the tissue and not the incident laser spot size: the hole diameter is set by a combination of strong, small-angle scattering and weak but finite absorption (owing to the presence of hemoglobin) in the plaque. The radiation is therefore spread over a larger volume than the focal region because of scattering. This enlarged illuminated volume leads to larger threshold for plaque removal. The minimum hole diameter dannot be controlled but the observed size is acceptable for laser recanalization procedures.

The idea of an ablation threshold energy (laser power x time) was checked and a value of 200 ± 60 mJ/pulse was consistent with our observations. We varied the incident power from 1.3 W to 7.5 W and the pulse lengths from 200 to 20 mS giving shot energies of 260 mJ to 150 mJ: tissue removal always occurred. The holes after ten shots were typically 500 microns in diameter at the surface and decreased in diameter towards the bottom by about 40%. The depth after ten shots was 230 ± 30 microns, giving an average cut depth of 23 microns/pulse. At 60 shots per minute this gives an ablation rate of 1.4 mm/minute, which seems acceptable for surgical recanalization procedures. Deep cuts of up to 80 microns/pulse were obtained in fatty plaque specimens, whereas the cuts in calcified plaques were as low as 4 microns/pulse. There was no evidence of charring noticed in the surface of these craters.

For comparison, continuous wave (CW) irradiation holes were produced using the same total energy dose, by delivering it in a single long exposure (For example, 7.5 W for 300 mS or 3.8 W for 600 mS.) The diameters of these craters were similar to those made with shorter pulses but the craters showed clear evidence of charring of the tissue on the edge and in the entire inner surface of the hole. Histology confirmed there is a marked difference in the extent and degree of thermal necrosis when the two types of craters were studied.

Other ivestigators have reported similar minimum hole diameters without comment. Fenech et al. used 500 micron fibers and saw 500 micron craters.[8] Eugene et al. used a 400 micron fiber and found 500 micron craters.[9] Gessman et al. used a 200 micron fibe and still found the minimum craters to be 500 microns.[10] Cothren et al. used a quartz shielded fiber, compression of the plaque samples by the shield tip, and long pulse exposures.[11] They found it possible to produces holes as small as 250 microns.

The threshold energy reported here is not completely accounted for by the simple model that ablation takes place predominantly by evaporation of the water in the tissue with resulting ablation of other tissue components in the steam jet. The calculated threshold energy is 10 mJ for a hole with 500 micron diameter and 23 micron depth. The thermal relaxation time for a 500 micron diameter cylinder is 175 mS. The measured threshold of 200 mJ is 20x larger than the calculated threshold. The laser pulse energy is probably absorbed in a larger volume of tissue, possibly to a depth of one millimeter, and out beyond the 500 micron hole diameter. It is also probable that the water is superheated in the evaporatd region, leading to other more energy consuming decompositions and leaving extra energy in the steam. There is strong jet and a modest localized shock wave to the tissue as the evaporated tissue rapidly leaves the hole following the laser pulse. Since optical scattering causes the energy absorption region to be enlarged radially to 500 microns diameter, it is reasonable to assume that a region at least 500 microns deep also absorbs energy during the laser pulse. If this region is superheated[12] to 305 C, then 111 mJ would be stored before explosive evaporation occurred. This description almost accounts for the measured threshold.

The findings, that there is a minimum spot size and an attendant energy threshold for adiabatic pulses roughly accounted for by evaporation and conduction, have important implications for laser vascular recanalization. If the pulse length and rate is controlled within the adiabatic regime, the thermal damage in surrounding tissue can be avoided and charring can be prevented.

We conclude that the argon ion laser operated in a suitable pulsed mode is able to thermally ablate all types of plaques and offers a safe, efficient, and effective approach to vascular recanalization.

REFERENCES

1. G. Lee, R.M. Ikeda, J. Kozina, D.T. Mason, "Laser-dissolution of coronary atherosclerotic obstruction," Am. Heart J. 102, 1074 (1981).
2. G.S. Abela, S. Normann, D. Cohen, R.L. Feldman, E.A. Geiser, C.R. Conti, "Effects of laser radiation to recanalize totally obstructed coronary arteries," Am. J. Cardiol. 50, 1199 (1982).
3. D.S. Choy, S.H. Stertzer, H.Z. Rotterdam, M.S. Bruno, "Laser coronary angioplasty: Experience with 9 cadaver hearts," Am. J. Cardiol. 50, 1209 (1982).
4. Geschwind, G. Boussignac, B. Teisseire, D. Laurent, N. Benaiem, A. Gaston, J.P. Becquemin, "Laser angioplasty: Effects in coronary artery stenosis," Lancet 2, 1134 (1983).
5. I.P. Kaminov, J.M. Wiesenfeld, and D.S. Choy, "Argon laser disintegration of thrombus and atherosclerotic plaque," Appl. Opt. 23, 1301 (1984).
6. Sinofsky and M. Dumont, "Measurement of Argon Laser Beam Spreading Through Arterial Plaque," Lasers in the Life Sciences, 1, 143 (1986).
7. A.J. Welch, "The Thermal Response of Laser Irradiated Tissue," IEEE J. Quantum Electron, QR-20, 1471 (1984).
8. A. French, G.S. Abela, F. Crea, W. Smith, R. Feldman, C.R. Conti, "A Comparative Study of Laser Beam Characteristics in Blood and Saline Media," Am. J. Cardiol. 55, 1389 (1985).

9. J. Eugene, S.J. McColgan, M. Hammer-Wilson, and M.W. Berns, "Laser Endarterectomy," Lasers Surg. Med., 5, 265 (1985).
10. L. Gessman, C. Reno, and V. Maranhao, "Transcatheter Laser Dissolution of Human Atherosclerotic Plaques," Cath. and Card. Diag. 10, 47 (1984).
11. R.M. Cothren, C. Kittrell, G.B. Hayes, R.L. Willett, B. Sacks, E.G. Malk, R.J. Ehmsen, C. Bott-Silverman, J.R. Kramer, and M.S. Feld, "Controlled Light Delivery for Laser Angiosurgery," IEE J. Quantum Electron. QE-22, 4 (1986).
12. J.D. Pendelton, "Water droplets irradiated by a pulsed CO_2 laser: comparison of computed temperature contours with explosive vaporization patterns," Appl. Opt. 24, 1631 (1985).

An Evaluation of Prostaglandin Activity and Pathologic Changes Following Carbon Dioxide Laser Endarterectomy

Francis W. Gamache, Jr., Babette Weksler, Daniel Alonso
Departments of Neurological Surgery, Hematology & Pathology
Cornell University Medical College
New York, New York, 10021 USA

Laser endarterectomy has been proposed as a method to recanalize narrowed or occluded arteries, especially coronaries. Since a substantial number of patients with anterior cerebral circulation ischemic symptoms have evidence of obstructive carotid lesions, laser angioplasty may perhaps be a useful technique for the treatment of cerebrovascular disease. Most of the endarterectomy studies performed to date have been performed using argon lasers (1). Alterations in clotting have been associated with argon laser angioplasty (2,3). Such alterations would have considerable impact on cerebro-vascular circulation where thrombosis and embolism are poorly tolerated. Very little basic science data has been published regarding carbon dioxide laser irradiation of vessel surfaces. CO_2 lasers generally induce more superficial lesions in tissue than argon or YAG so as to make them perhaps more useful in the performance of laser angioplasty. McVicker et al have recently published results from CO_2 laser treatments of canine carotid and femoral vessels studying the acute thrombotic consequences of laser irradiation (4). The current study set out to attempt to reproduce those data as well as to evaluate the delayed effects, observed after several hours of recirculation of CO_2 laser endarterectomy.

MATERIALS AND METHODS

Ten mongrel dogs (10-15 kg) were anesthetized with intravenous pentobarbital, intubated, and placed on a large animal ventilator (Harvard ventilator). Standard surgical tenchiques were employed to expose 20 common carotid arteries. A long segment of each artery was isolated between vascular clamps, and a 5 cm. linear arteriotomy was created. Using the operating microscope, each of 4 common carotid arteries underwent standard microsurgical endarterectomy. Two vessels were subjected to immediate pathologic examination and biochemical analysis of prostanoid formation (as an indicator of thrombotic potential) and two were allowed 3 hours of recirculation then subjected to pathologic and biochemical analysis. These four vessels served as standard micro-surgical endarterectomy technical controls against which the laser treated vessels were compared in the subsequent analysis.

Sixteen common carotid arteries underwent the same preparation and arteriotomies. Each vessel was divided into a proximal half which was not treated with laser irradiation and a distal half which was treated with laser irradiation. Eight vessels underwent immediate pathologic and thrombosis analysis; eight vessels were closed with 8/0 running prolene suture following endarterectomy and allowed 3 hours of recirculation and were then subjected to pathologic and thrombosis analysis.

Laser endarterectomy was performed utilizing a power setting of 2 watts of continuous laser energy in a maximally defocused mode (4mm diameter) through the use of a micro-slad attached to the operating microscope. Rapid scanning motions were made so as to provide a slow but gradual vaporization of endothelial intracellular water. All vessels were kept moist with heparinized saline. No frank char formation was allowed to form.

Harvested vessels were placed immediately in formalin for pathologic analysis, and iced Hepe's buffered saline for study of endothelial surface and whole vessel 6 Keto PGF1A and thromboxane B 2 activity as described elsewhere (5)

RESULTS

Light microscopic examination of surgically endarterectomized vessels revealed the same changes reported by McVicker et al: removal of the: Intima, elastic lamina, and part of the media (4). Following recirculation, a mild inflammatory infiltrate existed within the media of the blood vessel wall.

In the laser endarterectomized vessels, a smooth surface of coagulum was present with graded cellular injury extending from the intima through the full thickness of the media. In those vessels in which recirculation has been established, thrombi were detectable by carotid ultrasound within approximately 1.5 hrs. In those vessels allowed three complete hours of recirculation, when the vessels were re-opened, even greater degrees of thrombosis and in some cases frank occlusion were noted. Microscopically, clumps of platelets were documented.

Mean 6 keto PFG1A levels at the luminal surface for control vessels was 4131 pg/300 ul/10 min. compared to 918 pg/300/10 min.

for acutely laser treated vessels. For recirculated vessels, untreated vessel mean PGF1A was 3776 pg/300 ul/10 min. compared against 200 pg/300 ul/10 min for laser treated vessels. These were significantly different (p > .0 5). Mean thromboxane B2 at the luminal surface was 18 8 pg/300 ul/10 min. for acute controls compared to 20 6 pg/300 ul/10 min. for acutely lasered vessels. Mean thromboxane B 2 produced at the luminal surface in vessels exposed to three hours of recirculation demonstrated a mean value of 142 for untreated vessels and 608 pg/300 ul/10 min for laser irradiated tissue. These latter two values were significantly different (P > .02).

DISCUSSION

Our study confirms the results in a canine model recently described by McVicker et al (4) and extends those findings. CO_2 laser does, indeed, provide a greater degree of tissue injury than standard microsurgical endarterectomy. The greater degree of thrombus present on gross examination as well as microscopic examination is confirmed pathologically. While prostacyclin is clearly diminished by standard surgical endarterectomy, it is further diminished by laser irradiation. The laser coagulum and subsequent thrombus associated with platelet clumping together with the increase in luminal thromboxane encourages frank thrombosis. This in itself makes laser endarterectomy unattractive. In addition, however, inherent in the technique of laser angioplasty is the risk of vessel perforation or pseudo-aneurysm formation. Experiments employing antiplatelet substances and anticoagulants are currently underway to investigate the possible mitigating effects of these agents. Preliminary results are encouraging.

REFERENCES

1) Abela G, Normann S, Cohen D, et al: Effects of carbon dioxide, Nd-YAG, and argon laser radiation on coronary artheromatous plaques. Am J Cardiol 50:1199-1205, 1982.
2) Weichert W, Pauliks V, Breddin H: Laser induced thrombi in rat mesenteric vessels and antithrombotic drugs. Haemostasis 13: 61-71, 1983.
3) Treat M, Weld F, White J: Effect of CO_2 laser on the luminal surface of blood vessels in-vivo. Lasers Surg Med 31:247-254, 1983.
4) McVicker J, Day A, Savage D, et al: Laser endarterectomy: A comparison of thrombotic potential following CO_2 laser versus surgical endarterectomy. Stroke 17:266-270, 1986.
5) Weksler, B, Pett S, Alonso D, et al. Differential inhibition by aspirin of vascular & Platelet prostaglandin synthesis in atherosclerotic patients. N Engl J Med 308:800-805, 1983.

Laser Application in the Fields of Cardiovascular Surgery; Experimental and Clinical Studies

Masayoshi Okada, Yoshihiko Tsuji, Masato Yoshida, Kazuta Shimizu, Hiroshi Ikuta, Hiroyuki Horii and Kazuo Nakamura
Second Department of Surgery, Kobe University
School of Medicine, Kobe, Japan

A) **A new method of mycocardial revascularization by high energy laser**

Recently, several kinds of lasers have been widely employed in the fields of medicine and surgery. However, laser applications are very rare in the field of cardiovascular surgery throughout the world. By the way, surgical treatment for ischemic heart disease has been widely performed in Japan. Especially aortocoronary bypass (A-C bypass) for these patients has been down as a popular surgical intervention.

Among these patients there are a few cases for whom A-C bypass could not be carried out, because of diffuse stenosis and small caliber of coronary arteries. A new method of myocardial revascularization by high energy CO_2 laser was experimentally performed to save severely ill patients.

In this study a feasibility of myocardial revascularization from left ventricular cavity through artificially created channels by laser was precisely evaluated.   Anatomically, there are many channels between the coronary arteries and their veins or myocardial sinusoids in the myocardium (Fig. 1)[5,6]

1) Materials and methods

Thirty-six mongrel dogs weighing 7~16 kg were used in this study. Their chests were opened through the left fifth intercostal space under general anesthesia. Acute myocardial infarction was produced by multiple ligations of the left coronary artery. On the other hand myocardial punctures were created under beating heart or temporary ventricular fibrillation in the area of the infarcted myocardium by high energy CO_2 laser. Laser output was 60~90 W, and irradiation time was 0.12~0.25 sec. to make transventricular laser holes (Fig.2).

Transmyocardial punctures of 0.2 mm in diameter and 10 mm in depth were safely created by laser.[7,8]

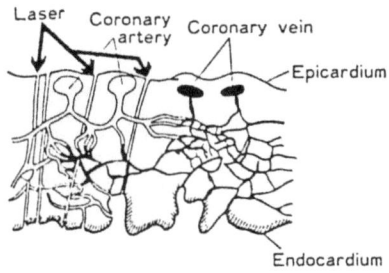

Fig. 1. Microcirculation in the myocardium

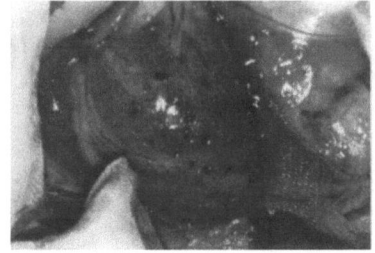

Fig. 2. Punctured laser channels

2) Results

a) Evaluation of the infarcted area produced by coronary ligations
Avascular area of the 30 ~55% of the free wall in the left ventricle was confirmed by postmortem coronary angiography and the staining of nitroblue tetrazolium.

b) Prognosis of acute myocardial infarction
Five out of 36 dogs were observed as control group, and were only subjected to coronary ligations. Four (80 %) out of 5 control dogs died of refractory arrhythmias to medication and low cardiac output syndrome within 1 hour after acute myocardial infarction. Thus, prognosis of acute myocardial infarction was very poor.
The remaining 31 dogs were studied as an experimental group. Four out of 18 dogs in initial group with laser holes which were followed up in the long-term period died of 2 of heart failure, 1 of respiratory failure and 1 of bleeding. Satisfactory results were obtained through laser myocardial revascularization by laser. The remaining 27 dogs were utilized for long-term follow-up, especially histological examinations. Follow-up period ranged from 3 years to 24 hours after surgery. [9)10)]

c) Microscopic findings of newly produced myocardial channels
Carbonization of the myocardium was found in the first layer and co-agulation necrosis was observed in the 2nd layer of the punctured laser channels. Figure 3a shows microscopic findings soon after creation of the myocardial channels. Fig. 3b shows histological findings in 1 week and in 1 month after laser surgery; in which tissue reaction in early stage disappeared. Recently, patency of the myocardial laser channels 3 years after surgery could be confirmed

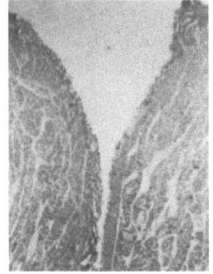 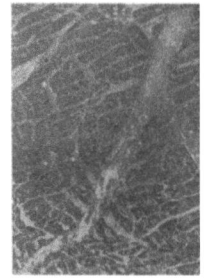 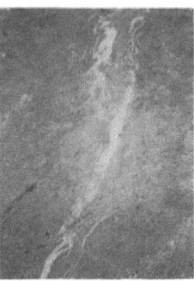 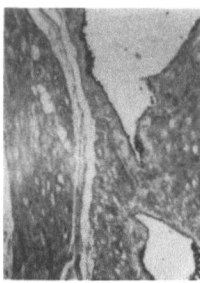

a) Soon after creation   b) 1 week and 1 month later   c) 3 years later

Fig. 3. Microscopic findings of the punctured laser channels

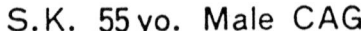
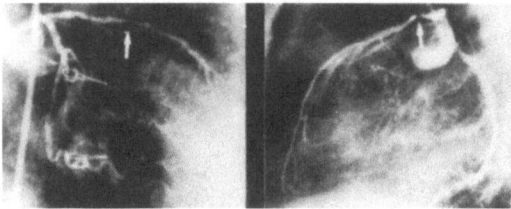

Fig. 4. Coronary angiogram

microscopically (Fig. 3c). These findings revealed a feasibility of the long-term patency of the newly created laser holes and clinical application.

3) Clinical application

On the basis of the satisfactory experimental results the new surgical method was employed for a 55 year-old male patient with constrictive pericarditis and anginal attack. Pericardiectomy was already done 7 years ago for severe constrictive pericarditis. At this time he was admitted to our hospital, because of severe anginal pain. His coronary angiogram disclosed 90 % of stenosis of the left anterior descending artery (LAD) (Fig. 4)[1]

Operation was planned in performing A-C bypass to the LAD on November 12, 1985. But the LAD could not be detected, because of a marked adhesion of the epicardium. Therefore, six myocardial punctures were made by laser (85 W, 0.2 sec) in the anterior wall of the left ventricle (Fig. 5). Postoperative course was uneventful, except for application of IABP during 3 days. No abnormal changes were noted in cardiac catheterization data and ECG findings before and after surgery. He is now doing well 1 year and 7 months after laser surgery.

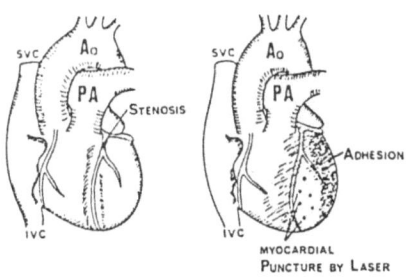
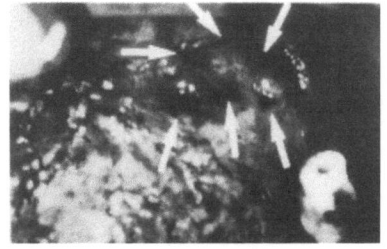

a) Schematic illustration   b) Punctured laser channels

Fig. 5. Operative findings

4) Discussion

A new method of myocardial revascularization was performed by CO_2 laser experimentally and clinically. Principle of this procedure is to apply additional arterial blood from the left ventricular cavity into the ischemic area of the myocardium. A minimal tissue reaction was microscopically observed in the created laser channels.[11] In experimental study, it could be clearly recognized that laser channels in the myocardium were patent even 3 years after surgery. Besides, endothelial cells surrounding insides of the laser channels were obviously confirmed histologically.[1] It was considered that tissue defects of fine transventricular punctures by high energy laser caused long-term patency of laser channels.[12,13] These findings revealed a possibility of long-term patency of the laser channels and clinical application. Until now, experimental procedures that supply arterial blood from the left ventricle into the ischemic myocardium have been reported since 1965.[14] However, there were no successful results in this field.[15] But recently, successful clinical report of myocardial revascularization by CO_2 laser was presented by Mirhoseini.[13] He created laser holes in the akinetic and dyskinetic area of the left ventricle and simultaneously performed A-C bypass in all clinical cases. Up to date combined procedures were carried out in 10 patients who had anginal attack and they were doing well postoperatively. Thus, myocardial revascularization by laser should be recommended for the patients for whom A-C bypass could not be done at all.

B) **Vascular anastomosis by low energy laser**

At present, in vascular surgery there are some problems to keep long-term patency after anastomosis of the conventional suture method,

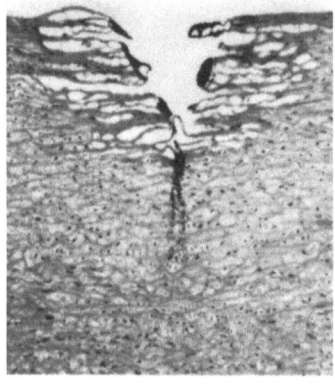 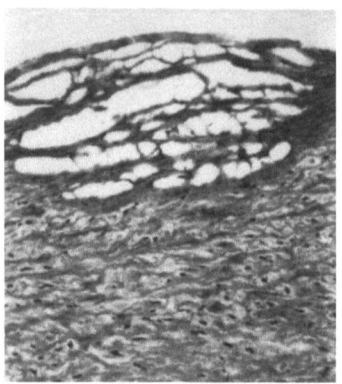

a) 100mW, 10 sec   b) 50mW, 10 sec

Fig. 6. Tissue reaction (aorta) by laser

especially for small caliber vessels. From these standpoints, a low energy CO_2 laser was employed experimentally in vascular anastomosis for small caliber vessels.[16)-20)]

1) Materials and methods

Sixty-five mongrel dogs were used in this study. First of all, the relationship between output and irradiation time of a CO_2 laser was analyzed as well as tissue reaction to the laser in a preliminary experiment (Fig. 6). From these preliminary experiments it could be concluded that the optimal laser output was 20 ∼40 mW and irradiation time 6 ∼12 sec/mm for vascular anastomosis of a small caliber vessel in the extremities. Thereafter, side-to-side, end-to-side, and end-to-end anastomosis at the sites of the femoral arteries and their veins or the carotid arteries and their veins were carefully performed using a low energy laser (Fig. 7). Diameter of these vessels ranged from 2 to 10 mm with a mean of 4 mm. Stay sutures of 5∼0 monofilamentous suture material were anchored at the incised ends of the vessels and were located to hold tightly the rim of the vessels. Recently, vascular anastomosis for small caliber vessels has been routinely made by CO_2 laser and just four stay sutures on the suture line.

On the other hand, vascular anastomosis between the internal mammary artery and the left anterior descending artery (LAD) could also be carried out by laser under beating heart (Fig. 8).

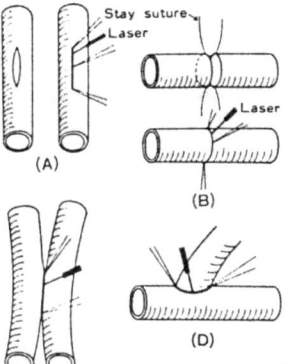

Fig. 7. Schema of vascular anastomosis

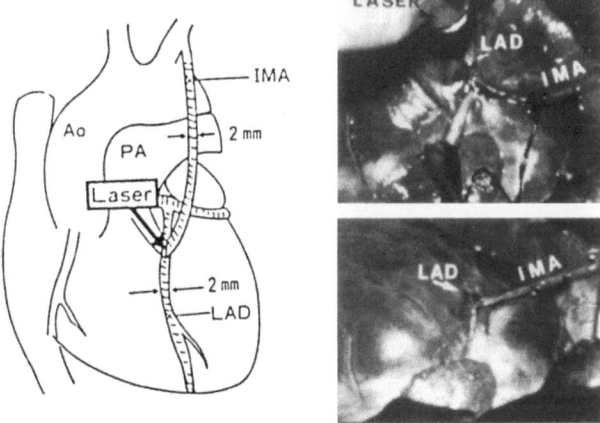

Fig. 8. Coronary artery bypass by laser

2) Results
The number of vascular anastomoses is shown in Table 1.
Bleeding from the anastomotic sites was seen at only 5 points among 137 anastomoses. Anastomotic sites were picked out for histological examinations which were patent at the time of exstirpation in several weeks after surgery.

a) Microscopic findings of the anastomotic sites
In microscopic findings 1 week after laser surgery, good adaptation and a marked proliferation of fibroblast can be seen in the adventitia and the media (Fig. 9a). In histological findings 2,5 months after surgery all layers of the vessels were adequately connected by welding of a lot of collagen fibers. Thus, excellent healing of the

Table 1. No. of Vascular Anastomosis by Laser

A) Experimental study

Method of anastomosis	No. of anastomosis
1) End-to-end (Artery 15, Vein 26)	41
2) Side-to-side (Arterio-Venous)	23
3) End-to-side	6
total	70

B) Clinical study

Method of anastomosis	No. of anastomosis
1) End-to-end (Artery 43, Vein 3)	46
2) End-to-side	21
total	67
Grand total	137

Fig. 9. Microscopic findings by laser anastomosis

(Upper: Laser method / Lower: Suture method)

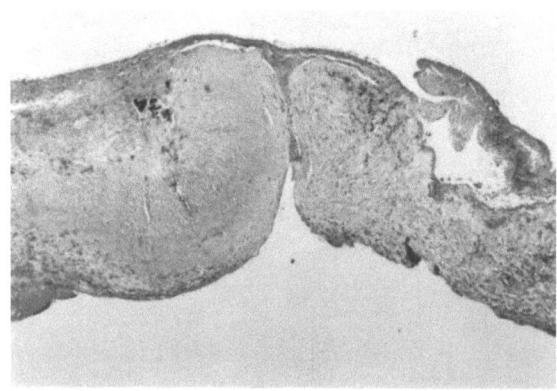
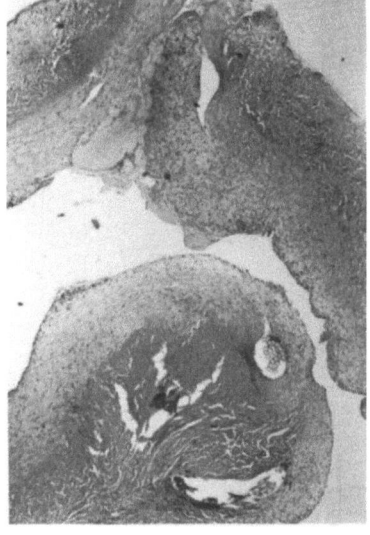

a) 1 week later   b) 2,5 months

anastomotic sites by laser were clearly confirmed histologically. On the other hand, anastomotic sites of the conventional suture method were also investigated microscopically (Fig. 9b). Subsequently, remarkable granulations in chronic stage were observed.[19]

b) Pressure tolerance test
Pressure tolerance tests were performed to evaluate intensity of the anastomotic sites. There were no hemorrhages from all sites of anastomoses even with a pressure of 300 mm Hg (Fig. 10).

c) Tensile strength test
Intensity of the sites of laser or conventional suture anastomosis was examined by weighing. Consequently, the anastomotic sites by

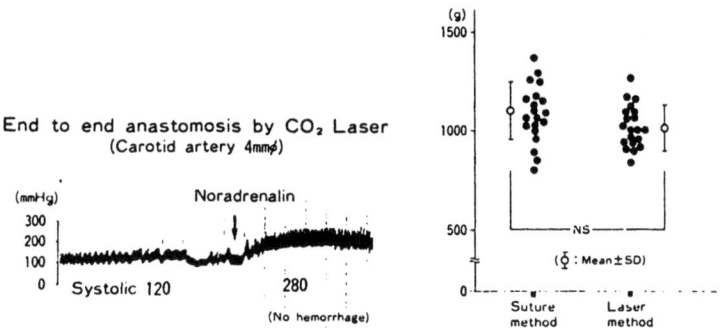

Fig. 10. Pressure tolerance test Fig. 11. Tensile strenght test

laser with only 4 stay sutures were separated in average weights 1034.2±103.9 g. On the other hand, sites of anastomoses sutured by 5-0 suture materials were also separated into weights in average 1103.7±144.8 g. Thus, there were no significant differences in the intensity of the sites of vascular anastomoses in either group (Fig.11). From these findings advantages of vascular anastomosis by laser were recognized and it could be recommended for clinical applications.[19)20)]

d) Clinical application

On the basis of our excellent experimental results a low energy of CO_2 laser was employed for vascular anastomoses of peripheral vessels in 56 patients (Table 2). There were 39 men and 17 women. Age ranged from 18 to 80 years old with a mean of 56. The first successful vascular anastomosis by laser was made in a 44 year-old female patient with severe renal failure on 21 February 1985 in the world.[20)]

End-to-end anastomoses of the femoral artery used for extracorporeal circulation were carried out in 46, and end-to-side anastomoses were performed in 21 sites of several vessels. In latter E-S anastomosis group, there were A-V shunt for hemodialysis and anastomosis of the femoral vein used for cardiopulmonary bypass in the patient who underwent re-mitral valve replacement, and anastomosis of the brachial artery after thrombectomy, arterial reconstructions consisting of femoro-popliteal bypass, or proximal popliteal and distal popliteal bypass. Arterial reconstructions were carefully performed, because of severe intermittent claudication due to chronik obstructive arterial disease. In these cases the great saphenous vein was used as bypass graft (Fig. 12). Recently, laser method was also applied in a 52 year-

Table 2. Clinical Experience of Vascular Anastomosis by Laser

No. of case : 56 cases (Male 39, Female 17)
Age : 18~80 year   (mean 56 Y)

Site of Anastomosis	No. of Anastomosis
Femoral artery (E-E)	42
Femoro-popliteal bypass (E-S anast. by SVG)	14
Radial artery-ceph. V. (E-S)	4
Femoral vein (E-E)	3
Pop.-popliteal bypass (E-S anast. by SVG)	2
Brachial artery (E-E)	1
LIMA-LAD (E-S)	1
Total	67

E-E : End-to-end anastomosis
E-S : End-to-side

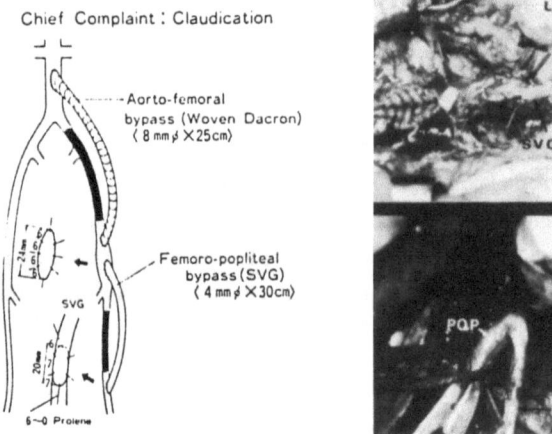

Fig. 12. Femoro-popliteal bypass (72Y, Male)

old male patient with severe anginal pain who underwent triple A-C bypass. Laser anastomosis was done beetween the left internal mammary artery and the LAD (Fig. 13).

All patients are doing well postoperatively without any complications. From these clinical experiences, vascular anastomosis by laser might be safely and faster performed and therefore recommended for small caliber vessels.

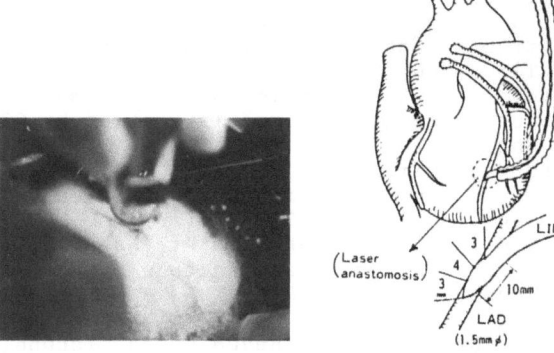

Fig. 13. A-C (LIMA-LAD) bypass (52Y, Male)

CONCLUSIONS

1) Transventricular punctures by laser could be created even under beating heart.
2) Minimal tissue reactions to myocardium were observed microscopically.
3) A long-term patency of the newly created myocardial punctures was clearly recognized even 3 years after surgery.
4) Laser application was available in a clinical case.
5) Vascular anastomosis could be safely performed by low energy laser.
6) Optimal conditions of vascular anastomoses for small caliber vessels were 20-40 mW in output and 6-12 sec/mm in irradiation time.
7) Good healings of the anastomotic sites were observed microscopically.
8) Excellent results of vascular anastomosis by laser were obtained in our clinical cases.

REFERENCES

1) Okada M: Modern trends of surgical treatment for coronary heart disease. (English abstract). Jap. Ann. Thorac. Surg. 6: 207, 1986.
2) Okada M, Shimizu K, Horii H, Matsuda S., Nakamura K.: Current problems in coronary artery surgery: New methods for myocardial revascularization and vascular anastomosis. (English abstract) J. Jap. Surg. Soc. 86: 1203, 1985.
3) Mirhoseini M., Cayton M.M.: Revascularization of the heart by laser. J. Microsurgery 2: 253, 1969.
4) Mirhoseini, M., Mucherheide M., Cayton M.M.: Transventricular revascularization by laser. Lasers in Surgery Medicine 2: 187,1982.

5) Beck C.S.: The development of a new blood supply to the heart by operation. Ann. Surg. 102: 801, 1985.
6) Vineberg A.M.: Development of an anastomosis between the coronary vessels and a transplanted internal mammary artery. Can. Med. Assoc. J. 55: 117, 1946.
7) Okada M.: Horii H., Ikuta H., Shimizu K., Nakamura K.: Experimental studies on myocardial revascularization by CO_2 laser. J. Jap. Coll. Angiology 23: 627, 1983.
8) Okada M.: Ikuta H., Shimizu K., Horii H., Nakamura K.: An alternative procedure of myocardial revascularization by CO_2 laser. Jap. J. Laser Medicine 4: 201, 1984.
9) Okada M.: Horii H., Ikuta H., Shimizu K., Nakamura K.: Application of fibringlue for transmyocardial puncture by CO_2 laser. Medical Postgraduates Suppl. p. 15. 1983.
10) Okada M., Ikuta H., Shimizu K., Horii H., Nakamura K.: Myocardial revascularization by CO_2 laser. Revue Europ. Technol. Biomed. 7: 100, 1985.
11) Goldman L., Rockwell R.J.: Laser action at the cellular level. JAMA 198: 641, 1966.
12) Mirhoseini M., Fisher J.C., Cayton M.M.: Myocardial revascularization by laser: A clinical report. Lasers in Surgery Medicine 3: 241, 1983.
13) Personal Communication: At the 6th American Society for Laser Medicine and Surgery. Boston, May 1986.
14) Sen P.K., Udwadia T.E., Kinare S.G., Parulkar G.B.: Transmyocardial acupuncture. J. Thorac. Cardiovasc. Surg. 50: 181, 1965.
15) Pifarre R., Jasuja M.L., Lynch R.D., Neville W.E.: Myocardial revascularization by transmyocardial acupuncture. J. Thorac. Cardiovasc. Surg. 58: 424, 1969.
16) Okada M., Ikuta H., Horii H., Shimizu K., Nakamura K.: A new method of vascular anastomosis by low power CO_2 laser. J. Jap. Soc. for Laser 5: 209, 1985.
17) Jain K.K.: Sutureless microvascular anastomosis using a Neodoymium - YAG laser. J. Microsurg. 1: 436, 1980.
18) Kurokawa Y., Taguchi Y. Ohara I., Kasei M.: Optimal condition of laser power for microsurgical vascular anastomosis with CO_2 laser. J. Jap. Soc. Laser Med. 5: 203, 1985.
19) Choy D.S.J.: Lasers in Cardiovascular disease - The International Textbook of Cardiology, P664 - 673, 1986.
20) Okada M., Shimizu K., Ikuta H., Horii H., Nakamura K.: A new method of vascular anastomosis by laser, Experimental and clinical studies. IGAKUNO AYUMI 139: 411, 1986.

Laser Angioplasty by Means of Sapphire Contract Probe

J. Lammer, E. Pilger, H. Schreyer, P.W. Ascher
Karl-Franzens-University and Medical School
Departments of Radiology, Internal Medicine and Neurosurgery
A-8036 Graz, Austria

Univ.-Doz. Dr. Johannes Lammer
Department of Radiology
Auenbruggerplatz 9
A-8036 Graz, Austria

The first experimental studies on the ablation of thrombi and atheromatous plaques by laser energy have been done in the early 1980s (1, 2). The feasibility of percutaneous transluminal laser angioplasty (PTLA) in men in peripheral (3, 4), coronary (5), and carotid arteries (6) were demonstrated by clinical pilot studies. At the Department of Radiology of the Karl-Franzens-University Graz, Austria, a research program on PTLA is underway since 1984. In the present study we report our clinical experience with PTLA of peripheral arterial occlusions.

MATERIAL AND METHODS

In 45 patients (33 males, 12 females) with a mean age of 64 years PTLA was carried out with a sapphire contact probe. The indications were femoro-popliteal occlusions with a mean length of 8 cm (range 2 - 24 cm) causing limiting claudication, rest pain or gangrene.
As energy source a Neodym: YAG laser with the wave length of 1064 nm (type C160, Surgical Laser Technologies) was used. The laser was coupled to a silica fiber with an internal diameter of 600 µ and a length of 1.5 m. For contact irradiation a sapphire probe (Surgical Laser Technologies) was used. The synthetically hardened sapphire crystal (Fig. 1) was attached to the silica fiber by means of an universal metal connector. This sapphire 2.2 mm in diameter has the melting point at 2030 ° C, a 90 % transmittance and a refraction index of 1.77. Due to the spherical configuration of the sapphire the laser beam will be focused. The focal area is about 0.5 mm from the surface of the sapphire.

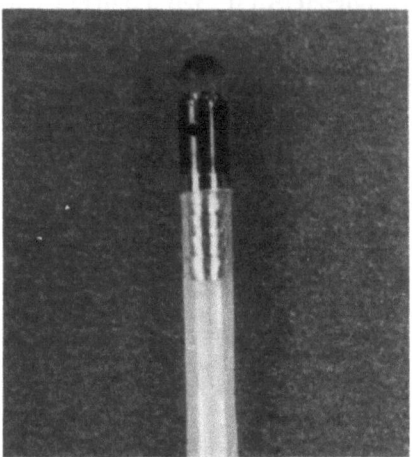

Figure 1. Sapphire probe attached to silica fiber

All recanalization procedures of femoral popliteal arteries were done under fluoroscopic visualization. The ipsilateral femoral artery was punctured antegradely under local anesthesia using the Seldinger technique. After insertion of a 7 French catheter introducer sheath a base-line angiogram of the occluded arterial segment was performed. Under fluoroscopic control the laser catheter with the 2.2 mm sapphire probe was advanced to the proximal end of the occlusion. The power setting for PTLA was 10 - 20 W in bursts of 1 sec ever 2 - 2.5 sec. During laser treatment the sapphire was in direct tissue contact at the side of the vessel occlusion. After successful recanalization balloon angioplasty was carried out in the majority of the patients. On the day before PTLA acetyl-salicylic acid 330 mg and dipyradimole 75 mg were given 3 times daily. During PTLA anticoagulation was carried out by an initial dose of 5000 units heparin intraarterially followed by continuous intravenous infusion of 1000 units heparin per hour. Three days after the procedure patients were switched to an oral anticoagulation or platelet inhibition therapy. Peripheral circulation was assessed by determination of the Doppler Index before and after PTLA.

RESULTS

Experimental results revealed a tissue crater due to photothermal ablation at temperatures of more than 250 °C. This tissue defect was surrounded by a zone of thermal necrosis. Corresponding to the heat distribution a superficial zone of carbonization followed by a zone of cell rupture and dehydration with pycnotic nuclei could be observed (Fig. 2). The depth of the thermal necrosis around the laser crater was between 50 - 200 µm.

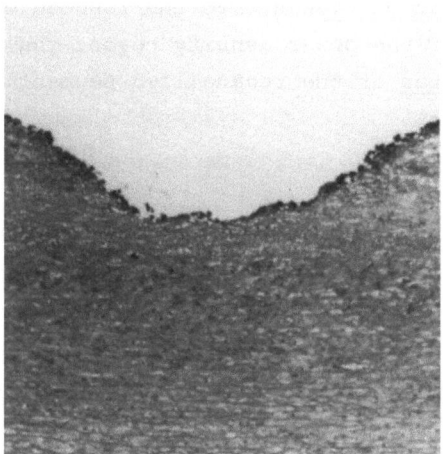

Figure 2. Histologic specimen of an aortic plaque demonstrating a laser crater and surrounding thermal necrosis

Clinical results: Initial recanalization of the femoro-popliteal occlusions was achieved in 36 out of 45 patients (80 %). The diameter of the recanalized channel prior to angioplasty was 2 - 3 mm (Fig. 2). Additional dilatation with a balloon catheter was necessary in 30 out of 36 patients. The total energy required for laser recanalization ranged between 137 - 2897 Joule. Perforation of the vessel wall occurred in 5 patients (11 %). After perforation further attempt to recanalize the obstructed segment were obmitted and the non-perfused perforation underwent rethrombosis without sequilae. Reocclusion within 48 hours after PTLA and balloon dilatation occurred in 2 patients. In 1 patient within the first 3 months and into within 6 months. Therefore after 9 months the reocclusion rate was 17 %.

DISCUSSION

Neodym: YAG laser recanalization of occluded arteries is based on photothermal principles. Vaporization of obstructing thrombi and plaques occurs after absorption of the photons of the laser light on contact with the target tissue. Prior experimental series with increasing laser energies on plaques and normal vessel wall revealed an almost linear relation between the irradiation dose and the volume

of the ablated tissue (7). A comparison between the bare fiber and
the sapphire probe revealed that larger volumes of tissue could be
ablated with the same dose of laser energy by using the sapphire probe.
Additional advantages of the sapphire probe for PTLA are:
1. A decreased perforation risk due to the rounded configuration and
   a rapid decrease of the power density beyond the focal spot.
2. An increased diameter of the recanalized segment up to 3 mm.

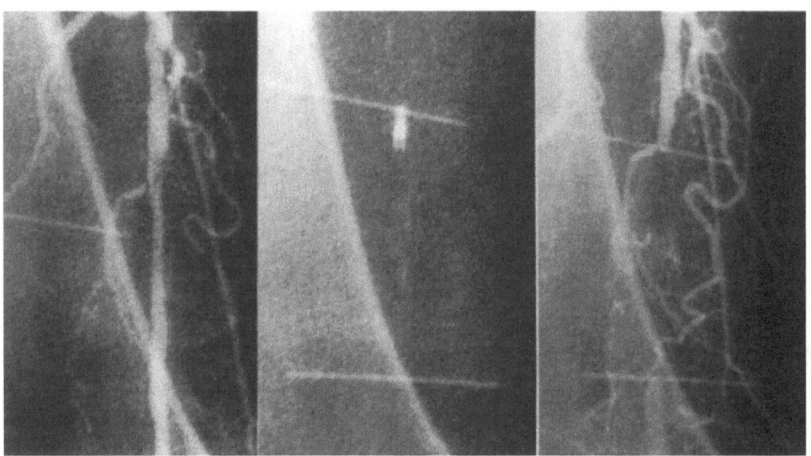

Figure 3. Femoral artery occlusion before and after PTLA

The initial clinical experience resulted in a successful recanalization of obstructing thrombi and fibrofatty plaques in 80 % of 45 patients. A high calcium content of the occluding plaque has proven
to be a serious limitation of PTLA because photothermal elimination
of calcium salts require temperatures in excess of 1000 ° C.
Nevertheless PTLA by Neodym: YAG irradiation through a sapphire contact probe has proven to be a safe and successful method for recanalization of peripheral arterial occlusions.

REFERENCES

1. Lee G, Ikeda RM, Kozina J, Mason DT: Laser dissolution of coronary atherosclerotic obstruction. Am Heart J 102: 1074-1075, 1981

2. Choy DSJ, Sterzer SH, Rotterdam HZ, Sharrock N, Kaminow IP: Transluminal laser catheter angioplasty. Am J Cardiol 50: 1206-1208, 1982

3. Geschwind H, Boussignac G, Teisseire B, et al: Percutaneous transluminal laser angioplasty in man (letter). Lancet 7: 844, 1984

4. Ginsburg R, Kim DS, Guthaner D, Toth J, Mitchell RS: Salvage of an ischemic limb by laser angioplasty: description of a new technique. Clin Cardiol 7: 54-58, 1984

5. Choy DSJ, Sterzer SH, Myler RK, Marco J, Fournial G: Human coronary laser recanalization. Clin Cardiol 7: 377-381, 1984

6. Lammer J, Ascher PW, Choy DSJ: Transfemorale Katheter-Laser-Thrombendarterektomie (TEA) der A. carotis. Dtsch med Wschr 11: 607-610, 1986

7. Lammer J, Pilger E, Kleinert R, Ascher PW: Laserangioplastie peripherer arterieller Verschlüsse. Experimentelle und klinische Ergebnisse. Fortschr Röntgenstr 147: 1-5, 1987

Ophthalmology

The Use of Nd: YAG Laser in the Treatment of Hyperplastic Persistent Pupillary Membrane

Charles Chia Lee Lin, J.K. Wu,& J.H. Liu
Department of Ophthalmology
Veterans General Hospital
Yang Ming Medical College
Taipei, Taiwan. R.O.C.

INTRODUCTION

Hyperplastic persistence of the pupillary membrane is a rare but devastating congenital anomaly. Extensive and thick membrane arised from the collarette of iris covering the whole or most of the pupil and sometimes adhering to the anterior surface of the lens forming anterior capsular cataract. Victims of this anomaly often suffered from clinical significant intractable organic amblyopia. Few early medical or surgical management to prevent visual disturbance were reported in the literature [1,2,3,4]. However, only certain cases with less extensive persistent pupillary membrane and at least pupillary aperture of 1.5mm in diameter could achieve successful medical treatment by mydriatics and occlusion therapy[2]. Available surgical methods such as sector iridectomy & coreoplasty[1] are often complicated with severe iritis, hyphema and cataract. Using the Nd-YAG laser as a new therapeutic tool, we have successfully treated 7 patients of persistent pupillary membrane. The detached membranes were easily removed from pupillary margin with only limited complications.

MATERIALS & METHODS

Seven consecutive patients, 9 eyes, suffered from congenital hyperplastic persistent pupillary membrane received Nd-YAG laser memebranectomy. They were 3 males and 4 females. The mean age at the time of treatment, was 20.28 years old. Our average follow up period was 22 months. Prior to and after treatment, they had received complete eye examinations including visual acuity, slit lamp biomicroscopy, tonometry, tonography, gonioscopy and Kodachrome slit lamp photography.
LASAG (Microruptor II), Q-switch Nd-YAG laser, with the power of 4-7 mJ, was used as the choice of fundamental mode. During the

treatment, patients' pupil were maximally dilated. The laser focus were directly on the iris strands and cut across the anchorage of the pupillary membrane. Most of the patients could stand the procedure well, and only topic anesthesia was necessary. Multiple sessions were occasionally used for dense pupillary membrane.

Postmembranectomy, steroid eye drop and cycloplegic agent were given to each of patients for one week. Antiglaucoma medications such as 0.5% Timolol, 2% pilocarpin, or carbonic anhydrase inhibitor, were occasionally used if patient suffered temporary IOP elevation.

RESULTS

55% of patients showed improved visual acuity and that of the rest 45% remained the same due to amblyopia, retinal abnormality or cataract (Table 1). Transient elevation of intraocular pressure and decreased outflow facility could be easily controlled by antiglaucomatous agents (Table 2 & 3). Gonioscopy of the patients revealed mild to moderate pigment deposition at the anterior chamber angle, especially on lower portion. However, it did not influence the final aqueous outflow function. Minor complications and anterior chamber reactions, such as mild iritis, 100%; pigment dispersion, 100%; hemorrhage from iris strands during operation, 77%; transient IOP elevation, 44% and transient corneal edema, 77% were easy to handle(Table 4).

DISCUSSION

Persistent pupillary membrane is the most common congenital anomaly of iris. The incidence is 30-95% in normal individuals. It follows as autosomal dominant trait with family inheritance[5]. Embryologically, the presence of this persistent membrane is due to the failure of normal sequence of complete atrophy or absorption of the infantile mesodermal connective tissues and blood vessels of the iris from the stage of 5-month gestation[6]. They are usually of no clinical significance. However, the extensive membrane which covers the whole or most of the pupil was suggested the term of hyperplastic persistent pupillary membrane by Merin[3]. It is rare and sporadic, often associated with other ocular abnormalities, such as cataract, microcornea, megalocornea, nystagmus and aniridia. Early therapeutic neglect may result in organic amblyopia.

There are three ways to approach the treatment. First, spontaneous atrophy or absorption of the less thick persistent membrane during the first year of life might be expected[6]. Second, medical management should be considered, on such condition that patients suffered extensive membrane with still a clear central pupillary aperture larger than 1.5mm in diameter. Mydriatic agents and occlusive therapy might help to get effective diffraction and retinal illumination in preventing amblyopia[2]. Third, early surgical removal of [1,4] the dense extensive opaque pupillary membrane is indicated if the above two alternatives are ineffective. Skillful microsurgical technique could minimize the operative complications. Yet, iritis, hyphema, and cataract can not be totally avoided.

We have used the Nd-YAG laser to successfully treat 7 patients of hyperplastic persistent pupillary membrane with only minor temporary complications. Technically, after pupil dilated, the membrane-iris adhesion became thin and tense. The laser focus was easily on the iris strands and cut across the anchorage of the membrane. During the procedure, little hemorrhage was occasionally seen from the vessel in the iris strands and subsequently stopped itself. Mild to moderate iritis and pigment dispersion in chamber angle were observed after laser. They were easily controlled by steroid eye drops and cycloplegic agents. Transient elevation of IOP and decrease of outflow facility revealed no clinical significance and most of the time, the treatment was not even necessary. Among two of our cases, the membranes firmly adhered to the anterior surface of lens. After the membrane stands were totally cut off by the laser microdisruption, we made a 2mm limbal incision from 11 o'clock position. Healon was injected to reform the anterior chamber. A Kelman-McPherson forcep was introduced into anterior chamber and the membrane was easily peeled off without lens damage.

To the best of our knowledge, this is the first report in the world by using the Nd-YAG laser in the treatment of hyperplastic persistent pupillary membrane. The advantage is to minimize the complications of surgery and hold the progression of amblyopia. However, the difficulty in performing the Nd-YAG on young children is the only technical shortcoming.

REFERENCE
1. Levy WJ:Congenital iris lesion.Brit J Ophthalmol 41:120,1957
2. Miller SD, Judisch GF: Persistent pupillary membrane:successful medical management.Arch Ophthalmol 97:1911,1979
3. Merlin S, Crawford JS, Cardarelli J: Hyperplastic persistent pupillary membrane. Am J Ophthalmol 72:717,1971
4. James D. Reynolds, David A. Hilles: Hyperplastic persistent pupillary membrane-Surgical management.J Pediatr Ophthalmol & Strabismus 4(20):149,1983
5. Cassady JR, Light A: Familial persistent pupillary membrane. Arch Ophthalmol 58:438,1957
6. Duke-Elder S: Normal and Abnormal Development. Congenital Deformities. In Duke-Elder S(ed):System of Ophthalmology, vol.3, pt.2, St.Louis, CV Mosby,1964,pp.752-782.

Table 1 VISUAL ACUITY

Case	Age	Sex	Eye	VA Initial	VA Final
1	12	F	OD	6/12 cc	• 6/10 cc
2	20	M	OD	6/30	6/7.5
			OS	6/6	6/6
3	25	M	OD	6/60	• 6/30
4	16	M	OD	2/60 cc	• 6/60 cc
5	15	F	OS	6/15 cc	6/10 cc
6	8	F	OS	6/20 cc	• 6/20 cc
7	16	F	OD	6/20 cc	6/20 cc
			OS	6/20 cc	6/20 cc

Table 2 INTRAOCULAR PRESSURE

Case	Eye	I.O.P. Initial	1hr	2hr	1 D	3 M
1	OD	12	24	20	16	13
2	OD	18	20	20	18	10
	OS	18	20	20	18	10
3	OD	16	26	24	14	16
4	OD	14	16	16	14	16
5	OS	18	52	40	16	18
6	OS	14	16	16	14	14
7	OD	14	16	14	15	11
	OS	12	15	11	13	10

Table 3 TONOGRAPHY

Case	Eye	Outflow Facility (ul/min/mmHG) Initial	Immediate	Final
1	OD	0.24	0.08	0.18
2	OD	0.28	0.12	0.20
	OS	0.22	0.14	0.20
3	OD	0.26	0.12	0.20
4	OD	0.24	0.16	0.26
5	OS	0.16	0.07	0.16
6	OS	0.20	0.18	0.14
7	OD	0.20	0.10	0.16
	OS	0.18	0.12	0.12
Mean		0.22	<0.121	0.18

Table 4 COMPLICATIONS

1) Iritis	9/9 (100%)
2) Pigment dispersion	9/9 (100%)
3) Hemorrhage from iris strain	7/9 (77%)
4) Transient IOP elevation	4/9 (44%)
5) Transient corneal edema	7/9 (77%)

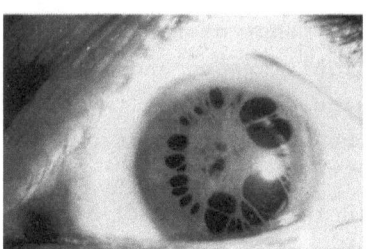

Fig 1. BEFORE LASER

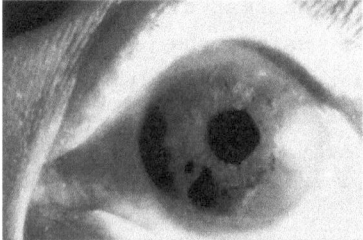

Fig 2. AFTER LASER

Intraocular Microsurgery by Short Pulsed Nd:YAG Laser Effects Clinical Application and its Microsurgical Alternatives

V.-P. Gabel, R.Birngruber
Augenklinik der Universität München
8000 München 2, Mathildenstr.8

INTRODUCTION

Advocates and sceptics stand opposite sides of the fence at the beginning regarding almost every new procedure which is introduced in medicine. While the one side accepts a new procedure opens up previously unattainable possibilities. The situation is not different regarding the use of short-pulsed lasers on the eye. Inasmuch as comparative prospective studies of this laser application and the microsurgical methods alternative to it are still lacking today, 5 years after the first clinical use, we wish in the following to juxtapose contrary aspects of laser application and microsurgery in some clinically common operations - especially those in which we ourselves have practical experience of both methods.

IRIDOTOMY

Photodisruption iridotomy is a quick and uncomplicated methode which has proved useful especially in prophylactic iridotomy, in cases of iris bombé and following acute attacks of glaucoma (Fankhauser et al.1981). A likewise frequent indication is the opportunity of deepening the chamber angle by such an iridotomy prior to laser trabeculoplasty. Surgical iridectomy on the other hand (done in only about 25% of all iridectomies in our hospital), is unavoidable when conservative measures fail to lower pressure in an acute glaucoma attack. A further indication for microsurgery is also present when the anterior chamber is very shallow, that is, in many instances of iris bombé, since laser damage to the endothelium would otherwise be extensive (Gabel et al.1985). There is no question that laser iridotomy is psychologically and physically less burdensome for
the patient - especially the elderly patient - than an operative procedure which, even when brief, requires a stay in the hospital. In the case of outpatient Neodymium:YAG iridotomy a subsequent monitoring must be guaranted for at least 3 hours following the operation to

detect any secondary pressure rise. Such rises in pressure, which were in our experience in a series of 192 iridectomies to be found in 20% higher than i.o.p. 30 mm Hg (Gabel et al.1987), can be arrested with conservative medication as pilocarpin, beta blockers or carbonic anhydrase inhibitors in practically all patient. Preoperatively the prophylactic use of 250 mg of Diamox orally and pilocarpine drops is to be recommended. Wether the proposed prior treatment with prostaglandine inhibitors actually reduces the risk of a rise in pressure appears not yet fully established (Schrems 1985, Pappas et al.1985, Gabel et al.1987).

ANTERIOR CAPSULOTOMY

Anterior capsulotomy was one of the main reasons a few years ago for promoting the developement of a short-pulsed laser (Aron Rosa et al.1981). There is no question that the anterior lens capsule can be opened elegantly with this methode and without mechanical stress on the zonular fibres; the technique, however, was not successful in winning general acceptance. The reasons for this are both the frequent high rises in pressure due to flow-off of tumescent lens material and organisational problems which can arise from the necessity of transporting premedicated patients from the Nd:YAG-Laser instrument to the operating room when capsulotomy is to be done immediately before cataract extraction. Wether it is sensible to evade this by installing a ceiling mounted laser in the operating room seems questionable.

Noteworthy among alternative microsurgical techniques is the stamp technique using a Sato knife, a bent needle or the Magnetron; in particular, however, also the capsulorhexis mentioned by Neuhann (1987). The latter moreover permits a complitely smooth capsulotomy border with no danger of slight tears in the capsule toward the periphery like those occurring in other penetrating techniques.

POSTERIOR CAPSULOTOMY WITH I.O.L.

Posterior capsulotomy with lens implant is clearly the domain of the short-pulsed laser (Deutsch 1985, Bath 1986 a), which can be used to create exactly central capsule openings even in the presence of post cataract membrane elements of different thickness. Precisely in such a case the use of a Sato knife, for instancee, would tend to lead to unpredictable tears along mechanically stabile structures, whereas in treatment with the Nd:YAG laser the incisions can be positioned exactly at the points dictated by optical considerations. Posterior capsulotomy also has the advantage that it can practically always be done on an outpatient basis. Here, too, postoperative pressure checks are necessary for the first three hours, since pressure rises after this technique are to be expected, e.g. we found in a series of 108 posterior capsulotomies in 10% the i.o.p. higher than 30 mmHg. A further complication, which, however, causes few problems, is possible damage to the posterior chamber lens implant. This may consist either of small lens defects (pitting) on the posterior lens surface or larger cracks in the lens; regarding the first it has been shown (Bath 1986 b) that different lens materials possess different degrees of mechanical restistance; the second results above all from inadvertend focusing at a point within the lens. While this damage must be avoided at all costs and can be avoided by care and practice, the first type is apparently not always completely avoidable, since the material to be cut rests against the posterior lens surface. The frequency of such lens damage clearly depends on the aiming beam system and the surgeon's skill. The small lens lesions have astonishingly little effect on visual acuity but should become evident upon a test of the patient's glare sensitivity.

POSTERIOR CAPSULOTOMY WITHOUT I.O.L.

Similar in principle to postcataractmembranotomy in the presence of intraocular lens is also the situation of post cataract membranes without intraocular lenses, where pupillary membranes may also appear (for example in chronic uveitis). The optical pathway is easily freed with the Nd:YAG laser. The danger of endothelial damage is comparatively slight due to the relatively large distance between the postcatarct membrane and the cornea; problems with postoperativ pressure rises are also few. When, however, a pronouncedly thickened postcataract membrane (possibly with lens remnants, pupillary distortion and/or synechias) is present, e.g. after trauma, it appears necessary to reflect whether numerous therapeutic sessions with laser are not better avoided in favor of a once only microsurgical cleanup, where the pars plana access in particular is suitable. In this manner all lens remnants can be removed, synechias eliminated and an anterior vitrectomy performed.

ND:YAG APPLICATION IN THE VITREOUS

The indications for use of the Neodymium:YAG laser in the vitreous are appreciably less common than those for the anterior segment, even though here in particular both possibilities for non-absorbing structures, that is, vitreous strands or vitreous membranes, are more than likely. The problem lies in the fact that the vitreous strands are not always so distinct and distinguishable from one another that they can be severed with a few pulsed; rather they are often diffuse and unclearly defined, so that a very large number of exposures is required, leading in turn to relatively pronounced endothelial damage. The vitreous strands best suited for laser application appear to be those which pass anteriorly through the pupillary opening, e.g. to a cataract incision. In such cases an already existing Irvine-Gass syndrome may regress, as reported by Little (1986). Another good but also rare indication is the vitreolysis in order to open the anterior hyaloid surface in cases of malignant glaucoma, as observerd by Epstein (1984). Severing vitreous strands in the posterior eye segment is in our experience an extremely rare indication for the short-pulsed Neodymium:YAG laser, since whether a traction on the flap of a retinal tear nor a traction detachment itself can be permanently solved in this manner only in scattered cases (Aron-Rosa 1985, Kreissig 1986). In such cases episcleral measures or complete posterior vitrectomy is often preferable, if need be with use of silicone oil as well.

Individual, relatively thick strands, such as those observed following double perforating injuries, do not necessarily require therapy in many cases when scarring to the sclera has appeared. Since they are often also very thick and rigid, they can be cut by laser only with the greatest exertion and with a large number of single exposures or salvos. It is our experience that using a Neodymium:YAG laser to prepare for a vitrectomy as proposed by Fankhauser (1985 a,b) is not to be viewed as an indication.

In contrast, subhyaloidal hemorrhages or hemhorrhages extending under the internal limiting membrane, are an excellent indication for the short-pulsed Nd:YAG laser in the vitreous. Such hemorrhages may be spontaneous after physical stress or accompany diabetic retinopathy or other vascular diseases. They can be opened with a few single shots at the bottom edge of the bubble; the blood enters the vitreous and resorbs in a few days, and vitrectomy can thus be avoided (Gabel 1987).

References from the authors.

Infrared Versus Visible Laser Photocoagulation in the Treatment of Specific Eye Diseases

B.Lorenz, R.Birngruber
Hermann Wacker Laboratory for Laser Applications in Medicine.
University Eye Clinic, LMU München (Head: Prof.Dr.O.-E.Lund), FRG

In the visible and near infrared wavelength region melanin is the main absorbing chromophore of the fundus. As melanin absorption decreases with increasing wavelength (8), an increased penetration depth into the choroid can be expected for longer wavelengths (10,15,21), and is indicated by some experimental results (1,3,13,17), though quantification is still lacking.

Photocoagulation therapy of various chorioretinal diseases should be as selective as possible. In diabetic retinopathy, localised destruction of part of the photoreceptor cells would be responsible for the therapeutic effect of photocoagulation (18,19), but there is also experimental evidence that photocoagulation of deeper choroidal layers could be beneficial (16). In aging related macular degeneration, sealing of the subretinal neovascularisations is attempted, the high recurrence rate (2,20) indicating the need for further optimization of this treatment modality. In the treatment of choroidal melanomas, therapy has been much improved by the use of ruthenium applicators with preservation of the globes (11), one of the problems being the still considerable incidence of radiation retinopathy and optic neuropathy (4). Therefore, further reduction of the irradiation dosage is desirable. Increased reliability of the cutting-off of the choroidal blood supply to the tumor by encircling photocoagulation might be helpful (5).

Experimental set-up

Experiments in chinchilla gray rabbits and in the rhesus monkey (macaca mulatta) aimed at quantifying the choroidal effects in depth as a pure function of wavelength, and with respect to the actual geometry of the choroid that shows intra- as well as interspecies variation as to its pigmentation (6) and to its thickness (14). To visualize maximal wavelength dependent differences, an argon green laser ($\lambda=514nm$) and a CW-Nd:YAG-laser ($\lambda=1064nm$) were used. 2 criteria of dosage were applied: [1] Comparable degrees of retinal blanching. Single lesions of different intensity were compared histologically in rabbits (13). [2] Closure of all choroidal vessels at the site of coagulation as visualized by fluorescein angiography and plastic corrosion casts. Overlapping lesions forming a ring 5 to 10mm below the optic disc (rabbit eyes) or within the region of the big arcade (monkey eyes) allowed to study the functional effects in a closed system with special consideration of the actual choroidal geometry (14).

Fig.1. Micrograph of histological sections through the center of ophthalmoscopically similar lesions in the rabbit with constant exposure time (t=200ms) and constant retinal spot size (diameter 330µm). Top: argon laser lesion, bottom: Nd:YAG laser lesion. Note deeper choroidal damage for similar retinal damage in the Nd:YAG laser lesion ➡

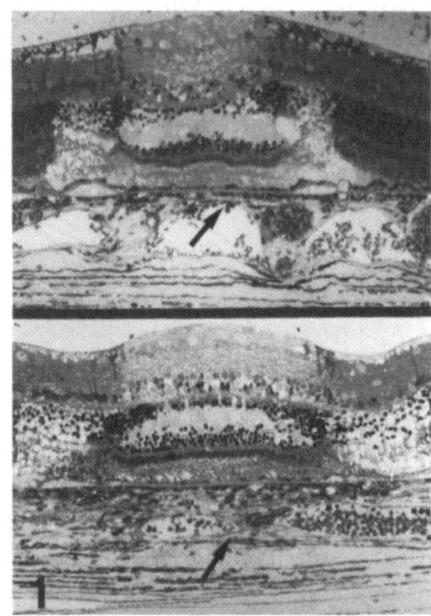

Fig.2. Fundus photograph of retinal lesions with complete closure of the underlying choroidal vessels. Left: in the rabbit, ophthalmoscopically comparably heavy lesions were necessary for both wavelengths at an exposure time of 200ms. Right: in the rhesus monkey, much heavier retinal lesions with undesirable bleeding from the retinal vessels were necessary than in the rabbit, when an argon laser was used

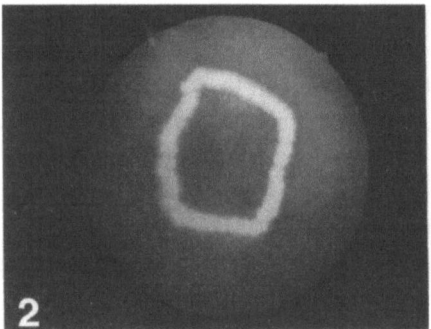
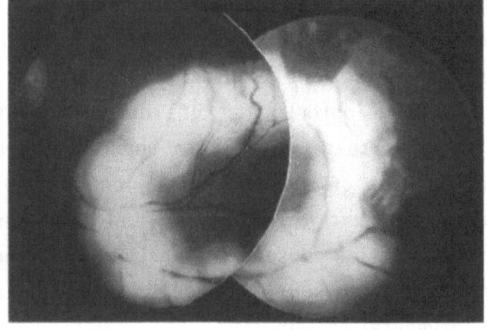

Fig.3. Comparison of choroidal thicknesses after identical mode of enucleation and fixation. Center: human choroid, left rabbit, right rhesus monkey. The human choroid is at least 3 times thicker than the rabbit choroid. Note also heavier pigmentation of the monkey choroid

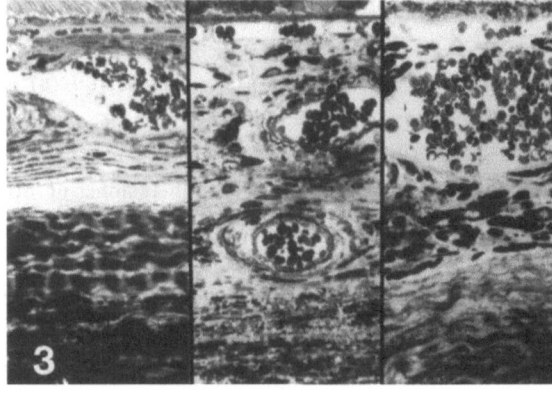

Results

[1] Threshold criterion = retinal blanching.

Single lesions that were ophthalmoscopically gray = weak or gray-whitish = moderate disclosed a deeper damage into the choroid for the Nd:YAG-laser than for the argon laser (fig.1) indicating the greater penetration depth of longer wavelengths.

[2] Threshold criterion = closure of all choroidal vessels at the site of coagulation.

In the rabbit, for both wavelengths, ophthalmoscopically very white = heavy lesions were needed when an exposure time of 200 ms was used (fig.2). Reducing the exposure time to 20 ms allowed to get the same circulatory stop but with less retinal damage with the ND:YAG-laser than with the argon laser. Apparently, for exposure times of 200 ms (and more), the wavelength dependence of the choroidal effects is smeared out in heavy lesions in the rabbit.

In the rhesus monkey, only the argon laser was used. Because of the different pigmentation (6), no experiments were carried out with a CW Nd:YAG-laser: differences in pigmentation become increasingly important with the use of longer wavelengths because of the decreasing melanin absorption. Hence no valid conclusions would have been possible from experiments in monkeys at 1064 nm in view of the clinical situation. With the argon laser, much heavier exposures were needed in the monkey than in the rabbit to induce closure of all choroidal vessels at the site of coagulation with unacceptable bleeding from the overlying retinal vessels (fig.2).

Discussion

The rabbit choroid is relatively thin i.e. 80 to 100 μm at maximum, whereas the monkey choroid is about twice as thick, and the human choroid 3 to 4 times thicker than the rabbit choroid (fig.3). Closure of vessels that are no more than 100 μm from the retinal pigment epithelium i.e. the thickness of the rabbit choroid, can be achieved with clinically acceptable exposure parameters with either wavelength. When, in the rabbit, heavy effects i.e. coagulative closure of all choroidal vessels at the site of coagulation are produced which are much above threshold for retinal blanching, wavelength dependent differences in penetration depth can be visualized only when reducing the exposure time such that heat conduction from the main absorbing layer i.e. the retinal pigment epithelium is not yet predominant. Thicker choroids i.e. the human choroid should, however, show an increasing wavelength dependence of the depth of the laser induced choroidal damage. This is already indicated by the limited efficiency of the argon laser in the monkey when heavy choroidal effects are aimed at. As animal models with a choroidal geometry similar to the human situation are lacking, a rabbit model has been developed where the exposure parameters are reduced to scale in such a way that similar spatial temperature profiles will result in similar relative depths of the human choroid and of the rabbit choroid (Birngruber and Lorenz, in preparation). According to that model, there is a linear dependence of the spot size and the power from the choroidal thickness, and a dependence to the square from the exposure time. In the rabbit, choroidal vessel closure could be achieved with less retinal damage with a Nd:YAG-laser than with an argon laser for a spot size of 250μm and an exposure time of 20 ms. That means that it should be possible to get similar effects within the human choroid with clinically acceptable parameters at the condition that the rabbit choroid is a true reduction to scale of the human choroid. Variations in the degree and spatial distribution of the melanin in the human choroid (9) point out the limitations of the model.

Clinical consequences from the experimental results

Near ophthalmoscopical visibility threshold lesions show a net wavelength dependence even within thin layers. If such moderate choroidal lesions can induce different far effects onto the retinal vasculature (16), a wavelength dependence of the therapeutical potential of photocoagulation in diabetic retinopathy should result. Because of the very complex pathology, the clinical value of possible wavelength dependences is hard to establish. If heavy effects close to the retinal pigment epithelium are aimed at e.g. closure of subretinal neovascularisations in aging related macular degeneration, no wavelength dependence should act if other factors such as scatter through preretinal opacities or xanthophyll absorption (7) are left out of consideration. Cutting-off of the choroidal blood supply to choroidal tumors i.e. very heavy choroidal effects should be achieved more easily and with less adverse vitreoretinal effects with the ND:YAG-laser than with shorter wavelengths. However, variations in the choroidal geometry could prove to be critical. Hence the potential of the Nd:YAG-laser in tumor photocoagulation should be considered with precaution, and cannot be recommended, at the actual stage of the experiments, for a clinical trial of a life-threatening disease.

References
1) Brown G.C. et al. (1984) Ophthalmology 91:1397
2) Coscas G., Soubrane G., Koenig F. (1986) Lasers in Ophthalmology 1:107
3) Fankhauser F., Kwasniewska S., van der Zypen E. (1985) Arch.Ophthalmol. 103:1406
4) Foerster M.H. et al. (1983): Intraocular Tumors. Academie Verlag, Berlin pp.316
5) Foulds W.S. and Damato B.E. (1986) Graefe's Arch.Clin.Exp.Ophthalmol. 224:26
6) Gabel V.-P., Birngruber R., Hillenkamp F. (1976) GSF-Bericht A55.
7) Gabel V.-P., Birngruber R. (1979) Ber.Dtsch.Ophthal.Ges. 76:475
8) Gabel V.-P. (1980) Lasers in Biology and Medicine. Plenum Publ. Coop., NY pp.383
9) Geeraets W.J., Ghosh M., Guerry DuP. III (1962) A.J.O. 59:277
10) Lachenmayer B., Birngruber R., Gabel V.-P. (1984) Docum.Ophthal.Proc.Series 36:3
11) Lommatzsch P. (1979) Klin.Mbl.Augenheilk. 174:948
12) Lorenz B. et al. (1982) Fortschr.Ophthalmol. 79:159
13) Lorenz B. et al. (1986) Fortschr.Ophthalmol. 83:436
14) Lorenz B., Birngruber R.: Proc. DOG-Symposium Laser in Ophthalmology, Berlin 1987
15) Mainster M.A. (1986) Ophthalmology 93:952
16) Marshall J., Clover G., Rothery St. (1984) Docum.Ophthal.Proc.Series 36:21
17) Peyman G.A., Larson B. (1984) Ophthalmology 91:1034
18) Welter J.J., Zuckerman R. (1980) Ophthalmology 87:1133
19) Wolbarsht M.L., Landers III M.B. (1980) Ophthalmic Surgery 11:235
20) Yannuzzi L.A., Shakin J.L. (1982) Retina 2:1
21) Yannuzzi L.A. (1982) Retina 2:29

The Role of Heat Dissipation in Living Tissue During and After Laser Exposure

R. Birngruber, V.-P. Gabel, B. Lorenz

H. Wacker Lab for Medical Laser Applications Eye Clinic of the University Munich
Mathildenstr. 8, 8000 Munich 2, Fed. Republic of Germany

Heat convection and heat conduction are the two types for the spread of heat in tissue. Heat convection means transport of heat due to mass transport whereas heat conduction is characterized by heat diffusion without mass transport. In tissue with dense vascularity, e.g. parenchymal tissue or the choroid of the eye, heat convection should contribute essentially to heat dissipation.

Blood flow in the choroid has at least a ten times higher perfusion rate and a much less arteriovenous oxygen loss than other systems or organs in the body. Every second about 50 % of the choroidal blood volume is exchanged by this fast circulation. Therefore we undertook measurements as well as calculations of the temperature-time dependance in the retina (directly adjacent to the choroid) during laser exposure. The measurements were done with and without choroidal circulation, that means before and after the animal was sacrified. All other conditions and parameters like the position of the thermal probe, the exposed retinal area, the exposure time, the delivered energy etc. were identical during each series of exposures (1). Figure 1 presents a typical series of temperature curves and shows no measurable cooling effect due to blood circulation.

In order to prove our experimental results and to compare the case of photocoagulation with the conditions during normal life situations where the temperature stabilisation should work well we also performed theramal calculations using a newly developed heat conduction and heat convection model (2). With a perfusion rate of 50% per second only a minor temperature reduction due to the blood circulation can be calculated in the case of Argon laser photocoagulation as shown in Figure 2. However the influence of blood flow increases with larger spot sizes and longer exposure times. As an example the situation of a large exposed field of 7.5 mm in diameter for about one hour shows a very high cooling effect even with perfusion rates of a few % per second (Fig. 3).

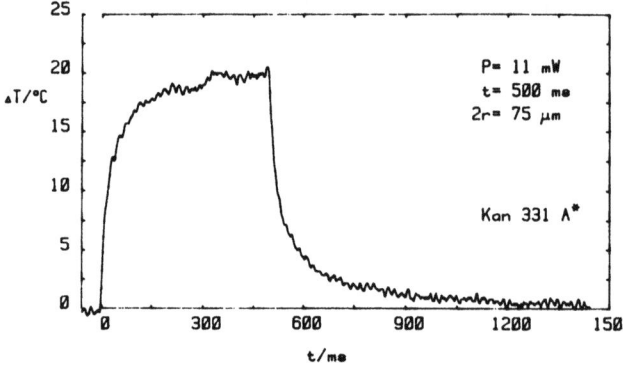
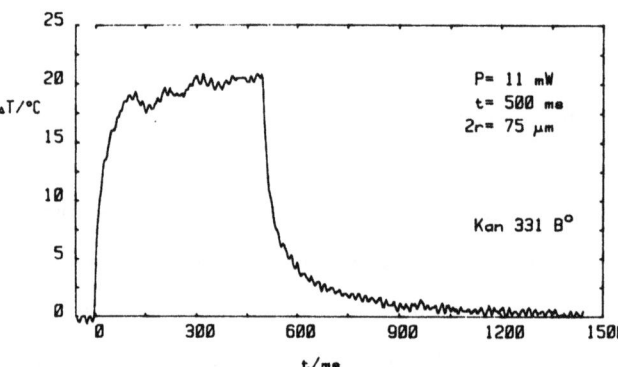

Fig.1. Time course of measured temperature increases T in the center of the exposed area during Argon laser exposure of the retina in a rabbit eye. The upper graph shows the situation with choroidal blood circulation (living animal), the lower graph shows the situation without blood flow (dead animal). (P: Laserpower t: Exposure time, 2r: Spot size diameter)

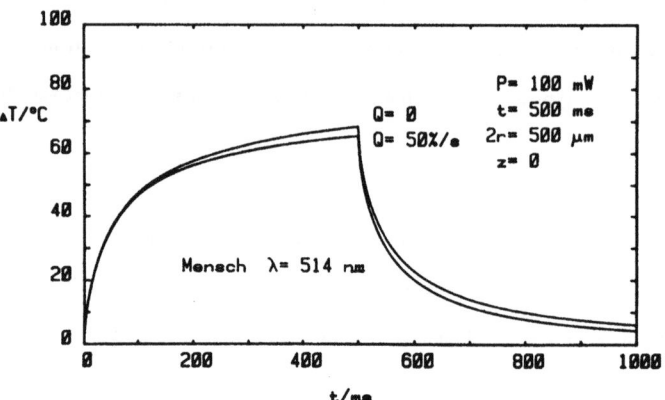

Fig.2. Calculated temperature increases during Argon laser photocoalgulation without (Q = 0 and with Q = 50%/s) perfusion

In conclusion one can state that even in cases where the temperature stabilisation effect for long lasting and large extended thermal influences (e.g. environmental temperature changes) is very effective(e.g. retina or skin), the cooling effect due to blood circulation can be neglected for highly localized and short-term thermal loads like the extremely artificial situation of laser photocoagulation.

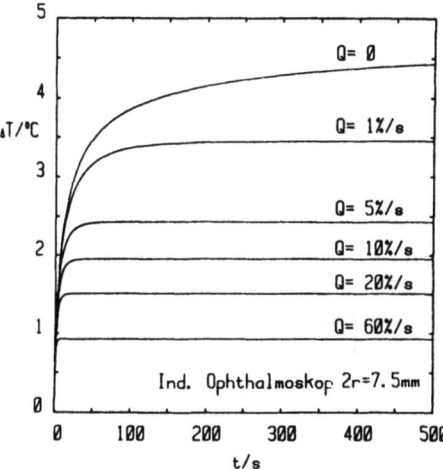

Fig.3. Temperature increases due to long lasting (500 s) light exposure of the retina with a large illuminated area of 7.5 mm in diameter calculated for perfusionrates between 0 and 60% /s.

References

(1): R.Birngruber, B.Lorenz, V.P.Gabel, Fortschr.Ophthalmol.84, 92-95, 1987

(2): A.J.Welch, E.H.Wissler, L.A.Priebe, IEEE Trans. Act.Birmed.Eng., 27, 164, 1980

Our Clinical Experience with the new Scanning Laser Ophthalmoscope – A Preliminary Report

M. Mertz, E. Fabian, Chr. Foos
Dept. of Ophthalmology, Technical University of Munich
Ismaninger Str. 22, D-8000 München 80, F.R.G.

Introduction

Since the days of Helmholtz (2) in the middle of the last century, the inner surface of the living eye can be observed: by ophthalmoscopy. The hand hold ophthalmoscope therefore is the instrument most frequently used by the ophthalmologist, whereas for documentation with film or video bigger and stationary equipments are necessary, called "fundus cameras". Due to their high technical standard the pictures gained with the aid of modern fundus cameras are of the utmost quality. On the other hand, there are some limitations of the method. Pupils must be widened artefically (by eye drops), and even small opacifications of the transparent media of the eye (localized in cornea, aqueous humour, lens or vitreous body) can disturb the image by glare.

In order to minimize these effects, the illuminating source has been reduced from the broad illumination of the fundus cameras to only one single laser beam which reaches the fundus even through a very narrow pupil. However, with this aid, the retinal surface cannot simultaneously be illuminated as a total, naturally, and a scanning procedure becomes neccessary.

Based on the technical experience of two teams of investigators headed by Bille in Heidelberg (1) and Webb in Boston (4), Rodenstock recently has realized a new scanning laser ophthalmoscope (SLO). Since we had a first opportunity to investigate our patients in the Rodenstock laboratories in Munich we thankfully can demonstrate our first clinical results.

The technical features of the instrument such as wave length, light energy etc. are given elsewhere (3). As a main fact it should just be noticed that the spatial resolution of the SLO is in the range of that of the fundus cameras.

Our demonstration concerns clinical features to be observed at the ocular fundus and in its regions of main interest:

- the papilla (optic nerve head),
- the vessels of the retina and the underlying choreoid, and
- the macula (central retinal region responsible for the visual acuity)

Results

1) Optic nerve head
In laser scanning ophthalmoscopy, the papilla of the optic nerve has a quite different aspect as compared to the well known picture gained by usual ophthalmoscopy (Fig.1). Due to the elimination of glare, the inner wall of the cupshaped nerve head remains dark, reflecting a lower amount of laser light, and thus giving an impression of the three dimensional arrangement of the tissue. Moreover, the thickness of this neuro-retinal rim can be estimated more easily. This is very important in various eye diseases e.g. in glaucoma.

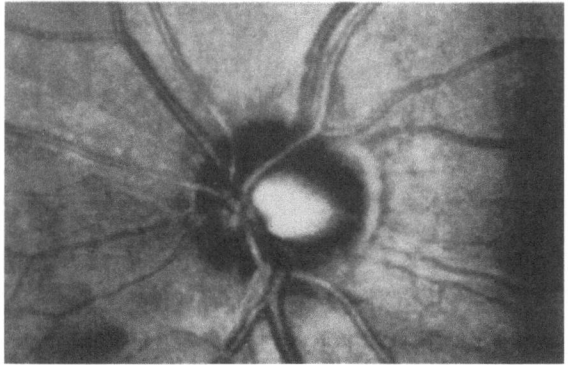

Fig.1. The papilla of the optic nerve as shown by scanning laser ophthalmoscopy. Note the well contrasted delineation of the (black looking) rim corresponding to the thickness of the optic nerve fiber layer leaving the globe in this region on its way towards the brain (Picture quality being reduced here by double step recording via videotape and monitor screen photography)

With the aid of a special optical arrangement in the SLO, not only changes of the surface, but even abnormalities inside the tissue can be visualized. This is done by excluding the central reflected laser beam from measurement and instead gathering the scattered light only. As demonstrated recently (3), pathological inclusions in the tissue like cysts (the so called Drusen) can be observed very clearly, and their three dimensional localization in the Papilla can be demonstrated easily by only small changes of the SLO observation angle.

2) Vascular pattern
The architecture of retinal and underlying choreoidal blood vessel systems is of extreme importance for the estimation of pathological changes caused by most common diseases - such as hypertonus and diabetes. The SLO proves feasable for this kind of examination of the fundus. The intraretinal scatter being suppressed, the retina virtually becomes more transparent, thus enabling a better view of the vessels and their possible abnormalities. E.g. in myopia, the chorioidal vessel sheet in the surrounding of the optic nerve often has vanished due to a progressing atrophy. This fact can be recognized prior to and more distinctly delineated than with usual ophthalmoscopy.

Clinically, it is well known that vessel abnormalities often become apparent at crossing points. SLO reveals details of those regions more informative, too.

3) Macula
In severe macular degeneration, pathological subretinal vessels cause the central detachment of the retina - one of the most commen reasons for blindness. Normally, they can only be visualized by fluorescence angiography. With the aid of SLO, the newformation of this vessel layer can be imaged by a non-invasive method (Fig.2, arrows). Thus scanning laser ophthalmoscopy will be of great advance in fundus angiology.

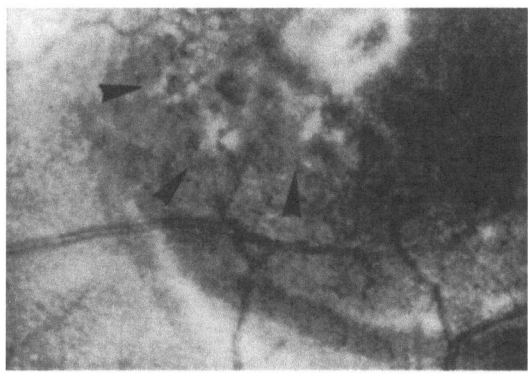

Fig.2. Lower part of the macula in a case of severe degeneration. Note subretinal edema and pathological vessel layer (arrows) as visualized by mere scanning laser ophthalmoscopy without intravenous fluoresceine application.
(For rather poor picture print quality see legend of fig.1)

Discussion

The SLO-prototype as used in the Rodenstock laboratories for this study, is just designed for mere fundus observation purposes. But there is no doubt that this is only the beginning of a great carreer of this type of instrumentation in ophthalmology. Once a picture being scanned - and the SLO pictures are scanned from the very beginning - all advantages of modern image analysis can be utilized rather easily. This concerns e.g. contrast and contour enhancement, shading correction, and automated artifact elimination. Moreover, SLO could be the basic tool of a new eye investigation system presenting a broad variety of tasks, such as quantitative fundus morphometry and angiology, low dose fluoresceine angiography, micronized fundus perimetry, refractometry, and image controlled laser koagulation therapy.

Nevertheless, a lot of technical inventive capacity has still to be stressed on the prototype, for there is still a remarkable gap between the imaging quality as primarily seen at the monitor during the investigation, and that gained for documentation purposes with the aid of videotape or monitor screen photography.

Summary

Clinical pictures are demonstrated illuminating some of the great expectations that we are focussing on scanning laser ophthalmoscopy. At the moment, SLO is just a special observation tool, enabling more accurate examination of the fundus morphology. Examples are given for fine structures of the papilla, the macula, and the vascular pattern hardly to be visualized by usual ophthalmoscopy. Future experience hopefully will reveal a lot of additional advantages and will probably prove the scanning laser ophthalmoscope one of the instruments most frequently used in ophthalmology.

References

(1) Klingbeil U., Rauh H., Bille J., Käfer O.: Ein hochauflösendes optisch- elektronisches Verfahren zur Darstellung des Augenhintergrundes. Ber.Dtsch.Ophthalm.Ges. 77 , 337-339 (1980)
(2) Helmholtz H.v.: Beschreibung eines Augenspiegels zur Untersuchung der Netzhaut im lebenden Auge. Berlin 1851, cit. Heydenreich A.: Untersuchungsmethoden. In: Velhagen K.: Der Augenarzt, Vol 1, p 604, Leipzig: VEB Thieme 1969
(3) Mertz M., Fabian E., Foos Chr.: Erste klinische Untersuchungen mit dem Rodenstock Laser Scanning Ophthalmoskop. Münchn. Ophthalm. Ges. 31.1.87, Klin. Mbl. Augenheilk. (in press)
(4) Webb R.H., Hughes G.W.: Scanning Laser Opthalmoscope. IEEE Trans. Biomed. Engin. (1981) BME-28:488-492

Interaction of Q-Switched and Mode-Locked Nd:YAG Laser Pulsed with Ocular Media: An Experimental Analysis

C.A. Sacchi, F. Docchio
Istituto de Fisica del Politecnico
Piazza Leonardo da Vinci 32, 20133 Milano, Italy

We report on a wide series of experiments performed with the aim of clarifying basic aspects of the interaction between short and ultrashort laser pulses and ocular media which occur in the photodisruption of ocular membranes. We performed, on a simple eye model

i) the determination of the threshold intensities required for optical breakdown, and their dependence on pulse duration and geometrical conditions, with pulses ranging from the nanosecond to the picosecond regine;

ii) measurements on the shielding properties of single pulses, to evaluate the intrapulse shielding, and of plasma lifetime as a means of determining possible inter-pulse shielding effect;

iii) experiments to investigate the occurrence of non-linear effects like Brillouin scattering in the nanosecond regime.

We found that the breakdown threshold intensities increase substantially by decreasing the pulse duration, and by increasing the power of the focusing lens. The shielding effect appears more pronounced with single ps pulses than with ns pulses. The lifetime of the plasma generated by single ps pulses results of the order of one nanosecond. This excludes a direct interpulse shielding in the case of a train of ps pulses generated by commercial mode-locked photodisruptors. The implications for the clinical use of this procedure are discussed.

Intraocular Pressure Changes After Nd:YAG Laser Capsulotomy

Kang-Sun Wang, Ling Wang
Dept. of Ophthalmology, Rui Jin Hospital
197, 2nd Rui Jin Rd., Shangai, PRC

3 mJ Q-Switched Nd:YAG laser anterior capsulotomies with 30 burns in circular arrangement were performed on 10 rabbits 20 eyes. Intraocular pressure measurements, anterior segment fluorescent angiography, aqueous humour protein amount determination, optic microscopy and electron microscopy observation were examined at different intervals after operation. Discussion on the relationship between intraoccular pressure and other measurement and observation mentioned above were presented.

Corneal Laser Trauma

E. Fabian

Augenklinik und -poliklinik der Technischen Universität, München
(Direktor: Professor Dr.med. H.J.Merté)

In ophthalmology laser surgery is a well established method of therapy. It had been one of the first laser applications in medicine which has been introduced into routinly used clinical therapy. Nowadays in ophthalmology a variety of different lasers are used for:

    photo-coagulation

- argon laser (blue, green),
- krypton laser (yellow, red),
- dye laser (blue, green, yellow, orange, red),
- CO_2-laser

    photo-disruption

- Nd:YAG-laser (Q-switched, mode-locked).

Other laserapplications are under investigation :

    photo-ablation

    UV-laser (ArF excimer)
- Infrared (HF, Er:YAG).

The clinically used lasers - which I want to concentrate on - are applied to different parts of the eye. Photocoagulation is used on the iris, in the angle of the anterior chamber and on the retina. Photodisruption is used on the iris and at the posterior capsule after cataract extraction.

All these lasers are based on the supposition of transparent media of the eyeball. One of them is the cornea, the first and most powerful refracting surface of the optical system of the eye.

The cornea is composed of six layers:

- epithelium
- basement membrane
- Bowman's membrane
- stroma or substantia propria
- Descemet's membrane
- endothelium.

Specific morphological organisations and physiological functions of the corneal layers are important for the transparency of the cornea. All laser energy, applied to structures of the eyeball has to pass the cornea. That is why the examination, the knowledge, and the judgement of possible trauma to the cornea is important.

Ophthalmologists treating with laser energy should be aware of wo different types of corneal trauma that can occure:

- thermal injury by an undesired amount of absorption in the cornea, corneal burns (epithelium, stroma endothelium),
- mechanical injury by an acustic wave or shock wave (endothelium).

Corneal burns can occure during argon laser coagulation of the iris (laser iridectomy) or of the angle of the anterior chamber (laser trabeculoplasty). One example of corneal epithelial burns can be seen after argon-laser trabeculoplasty. Small white dots are caused by absorption of energy in the corneal epithelium in the presence of opacifications. These dots are located near the center of the cornea where the laser beam is passing the cornea. They will disapear some hours later.

Injury of the corneal endothelium can occure during Nd:YAG-laser iridectomy. This iridectomy is a noninvasive surgical therapy of narrow angle or anlge closure glaucoma. The energy of this laser is used to disrupt mechanically tissue thus creating an incision or a hole into the iris. Doing this in the far periphery of the anterior chamber in the eyeball, space between the iris and the inner layer of the cornea, the corneal endothelium, is very narrow.

Controlling the corneal endothelium on the oposite of the iridectomy will detect small changes of the corneal cells. The homogenious specular reflex of the corneal endothelial cells is disturbed. Multiple, tiny, well defined, dark areas - that are regions with no specular reflex - can be documented as the region of injury of some endothelial cells. The edges of these dark areas do not correspond to the borders of the corneal cells thus indicating that the peripheral cells of this area are not completely distroyed. These cell defects had been quantitated by image analysis of the corneal endothelium, indicating that nearly 100 endothelial cells disrupted during the Nd:YAG-laser iridectomy using 10 - 20 mJ.

Different mechanisms of injury had been discussed:

- absorption of energy of the laser beam when passing the cornea,
- mechanical energy of the shockwave come from the spot of photodisruption,
- small air bubbles, produced from the optical breakdown,
- particles of iristissue flining in the anterior chamber after photodisruption.

To differenciate between these supposed mechanisms we injected a visco-elastic material into the anterior chamber of a rabbit eye and performed Nd:YAG-laser iridectomies. In the presence of this vicoelastic material between the iris and the corneal endothelium no injury of the endothelial cells could be recorded. Less or even no injury of the corneal endothelial cells occurred with greater distance between the cornea and the iris performing the irdectomies more centrally. Thus we think the mechanism of injury is mechanically caused by the shockwave arsing from the plasmaformation at the spot of photodisruption.

Using different types of Nd:YAG-lasers different typs and different areas of injuries are created. Small individual areas of injury are caused by the original mode-locked laser. When the same laser-system had been changed into a q-switched Nd:YAG-laser (using monomode for both lasers and the same slitlamp) a great coherent area of destroyed endothelial cells could be documentated. An other laser-system with a low order mode and a diverent slit lamp created a very big area of destroyed cells and even disrupted the cells from Descemet´s membrane.

Argon-laser- and Nd:YAG-laser-systems are routinly used in ophthalmology. Potential side effects should be well known to avoid them. If the corneal endothalial cell count of a certain eye is already very low these side effects could become hazardous. Usually the injury of the corneal endothelial cell layer is often of no or of low clinical importance and will disappeared without special treatment within hours.

Literatur
1. Schubert,D., St.Trokel: Endo-thelial repair following Nd:YAG laser injury. Invest.Ophthalmol.Vis.Sci. 25 (1984) 971.
2. Khodadoust,A.A., D.F.Arkfeld, F. Caprioli, M.L.Sears: Ocular effect of neodymium-YAG laser. Am.J. Ophthalmol. 98 (1984) 144.
3. Neubauer,L., V.P.Gabel, R. Birngruber: Hornhautendothelveränderungen bei vorderer Kapsulotomie und Nachstardiszision mit dem Neodym: YAG-Laser. Fortschr.Ophthalmol. 82 (1985) 80.
4. Kerr Muir,M.G., E.S.Sherrard: Damage to the corneal endothelium during Nd/YAG photodisruption. Br.J. Ophthalmol. 69 (1985) 77.
5. Fabian,E., H.v.Denffer: Nd:YAG- Laser-Iridektomie und Hornhautendothelzellveränderungen. Laser 1 (1985) 68.

Dermatology

Laser Dermatology – State of the Art

Toshio Ohshiro, M.D., R.Glen Calderhead, M.A.
Japan Medical Laser Laboratory
TBR Bldg. #607, 5-7 Kojimachi, Chiyoda-ku, Tokyo 102, JAPAN

ABSTRACT

The use of the laser in dermatology has one of the longest histories in the medical application of the laser. Despite a period where dermatologists moved away from the use of the laser because of unwanted side effects such as scarring and hyperpigmentation, the past three years have seen a resurgence of interest in the use of this still-new modality. A better understanding of basic laser physics, biophysics, laser-tissue interaction and beam manipulation has led to good results, consistently achieved. The emergence of new wavelengths with highly specific tissue interactions has added to this growth phenomenon. Basic scientific studies and solid clinical data on photobiostimulation have added Low Level Laser Therapy (LLLT) to the growing list of both new and tried and tested High Level Laser (HLL) modalities which form the armamentarium of the laser dermatologist. This paper will examine the basics of HLLT and LLLT, and look at the state-of-the-art applications of the laser in dermatology from both a theoretical and practical standpoint. It will become clear that, as Professor Leon Goldman has long said; "If you don't need the laser, don't use it". However, if you *have* need of it, then *do* use it, always provided the user has the multidisciplinary background so necessary for successful application of the laser in any of the medical specialties, especially dermatology.

INTRODUCTION

Doctor Theodore Maiman's development of the ruby laser in 1960 opened up the flood gates of laser medium discovery, but only five "medical" lasers emerged from the thousands developed in the first four years from 1960 to 1964: the argon, helium neon (HeNe), ruby, neodymium yttrium aluminium garnet (Nd:YAG) and carbon dioxide (CO_2) lasers. First the ruby then the argon found applications in dermatology with the pioneering work of Francis L'Esperance Jr. and others. Professor Leon Goldman pioneered the use of the ruby laser in dermatology, followed by the Lash group in Palo Alto, including David Apfelberg, presenting the dermatological applications of the argon laser, particularly for the removal of pigmented skin lesions. The addition of the Nd:YAG and CO laser wavelengths, using the visible red HeNe beam as an aiming beam for the invisible infrared energy, broadened the use of the laser in medicine, and soon all major specialties were using the laser to supplement, and even to take the place of, conventional incisional, vaporisational and coagulative techniques.

To the existing wavelengths with real medical utility have been added the "superpulsed" or quasicontinuous CO beam, consisting of thousands of high peak power pulses per second, the superpulsed frequency-doubled green YAG beam, the copper vapour laser with its twin lines of green and yellow (also superpulsed in some systems), and the rainbow of wavelengths from dye lasers. Not too far away is the eximer laser, with a "cool", nonthermal tissue reaction from an ultraviolet beam, and other exciting systems. The "dial-a-wavelength" idea is no longer a mere pipe dream. However, with all these wavelengths comes some confusion for the clinician: "Which one should I use?" Without careful clinical evaluation and really substantial biophysical knowledge on the surgeon's part, the creation of more and more wavelengths is like filling a Pandora's Box, waiting then to be opened by some unsuspecting person. The final choice of wavelength or wavelengths must be goverened by firstly the basic desired laser-tissue interaction, then the desired surgical effect.

LASERS IN DERMATOLOGY

The first application, and subsequent main applications, of lasers in dermatology was the removal of pigmented cutaneous lesions, or naevi. These birthmarks were of two main groups: the blood vessel anomaly group, such as haemangioma simplex (port wine stain) and telangiectasia; and the melanin anomaly group, such as naevus spilus or naevus cell naevus. Other applications, such as tattoo removal, have been added to the original applications. In order to remove the excess pigment from the skin, the laser has traditionally been used to create heat in the target tissue: this photothermal reaction has by necessity been destructive in nature, causing irreversible changes in irradiated tissue. We would like to refer to this as High Level Laser Therapy (HLLT). We define the word "Level" as the damage level of the skin or tissue, based on a completely reversible reaction following laser irradiation: thus HLLT denotes laser-tissue interactions producing heat in the tissue above 40°C. From around that temperature, protein denaturation occurs, up to about 60°C. However, the higher the temperature, the greater the irreversible changes in the target tissue. Normal body temperature is around 36.5°C. Tissue temperature changes from 36.5°C to 40°C produce completely reversible changes in the target tissue: we refer to this as Mid Level Laser Therapy (MLLT). A laser-tisue reaction eliciting no temperature change we classify as Low Level Laser Therapy (LLLT). LLLT and MLLT therefore form a photoactivation zone, while those reactions occurring over 40°C form a photodestructive zone.

HLLT: In traditional HLLT, various phothermal reactions are targeted, depending on the biological result required. From around 40°C, protein denaturation occurs, with irreversible changes in the collagen matrix increasing as the temperature rises. From around 68°C, tissue coagulation and haemocoagulation occur. Temperatures of around 95°C produce small vacuoles in the tissue as the intra- and extracellular fluids expand, and from 100°C frank vaporisation occurs as the fluids boil, causing disruption of overlying tissue components. When temperatures are in the region of 110°c, due to boiling under pressure, a sudden rapid rise in temperature occurs, accompanied by burning off of the dessicated tissue, resulting in carbonisation of the irradiated area (figure 1).

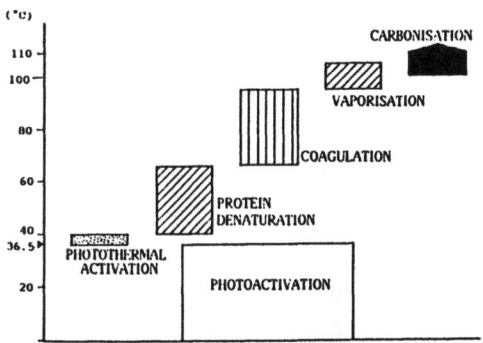

Fig 1. Biothermal ranges & surgical effects

The basic tissue reaction is primarily wavelength dependent, as the wavelength of a laser beam determines the absorption mechanism and the depth of penetration. The visible light lasers are all pigment-absorbed, the particular pigment depending on the colour of the laser beam. Near infrared energy, such as the Nd:YAG at 1064nm, is mostly absorbed in protein, with little pigment specificity, while the 10,600nm beam of the CO laser is almost totally absorbed in water. Biological tissue contains pigments, protein and water, and so provides an excellent target for these laser groups. In addition to the wavelength, however, the beam parameters play a very important part in determining the final surgical result.

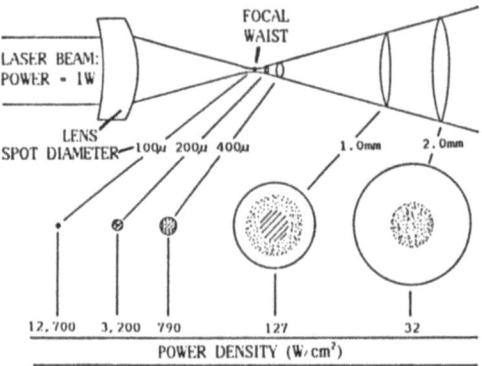

Fig 2. Spot size/power density relationship

Greatest control over the power density is achieved using a lens system to bring the beam to a focal waist. Figure 2 shows how dramatically defocusing or focusing a beam can alter the power density. By using a focused beam we can create pinholes, or a fine linear incision: by using a defocused beam, discrete spots of coagulation and protein denaturation are produced, or discrete lines with similar characteristics using the linear technique. With a defocused beam, large areas can be treated in the area technique. This is seen in figure 3.

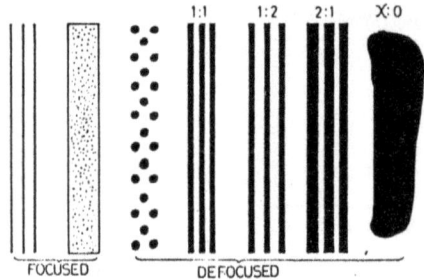

Fig 3. Focused and unfocused linear, spot and area techniques

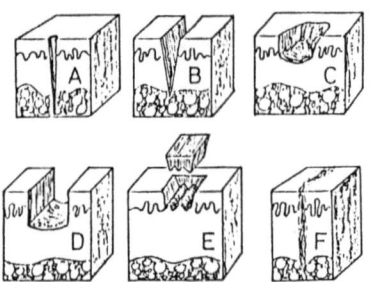

Fig 4. Spot, linear and area techniques illustrated diagrammatically

Figure 4 demonstrates clinical application of the spot, linear and area techniques. A focused beam used in the spot technique creates a pinhole in tissue (4A). This can be used in treating acne foci. By moving the focused beam steadily across tissue in the linear technique, a laser incision is created (4B). Slightly defocusing the beam gives power densities capable of vaporising raised lesions or producing laser abrasion (4C, 4D). Further defocussing lowers the power density to achieve laser detachment (4E). In the linear technique, using various ratios of treated to untreated skin as seen in figure 3, pigment removal on large lesions is achieved: we call this the "Zebra" method. Scarring is prevented by leaving the untreated areas to assist in the reepithelialisation of the treated areas. Further defocusing with short irradiation times produces protein denaturation, which enables tissue welding.

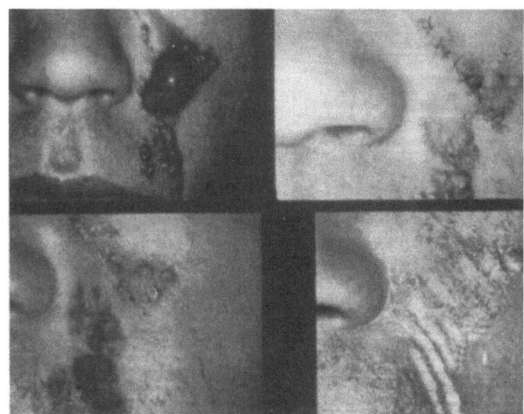

Fig 5. Clinical applications of linear, spot and area technique

In practical clinical terms, this is seen in figure 5. This 36-year-old male presented with haemangioma simplex of the left cheek, accompanied with one large and several small soft tumours (5A). Using a focused CO laser beam in linear technique, the large tumour was excised with blood loss of less than 10ml (5B). The ruby laser was then indicated at 35J/cm^2 to coagulate the larger, more superficial blood vessels (areas marked "R"), and the argon was used to vaporise the smaller tumorous growths (marked "A" in 5C). Next, the argon was used with a more defocused beam in the "zebra" technique to treat the deeper-lying blood vessels. Configurational abnormalities are usually dealt with first in this way, and then the colour is removed in layered stages. Naturally it takes a little longer, but the results show much less visible scarring with maximum colour removal. Comprehensive patient education is a most important part of the process too, so that they know firstly how long the process will take, and secondly, have a _realistic_ expectation of the final result.

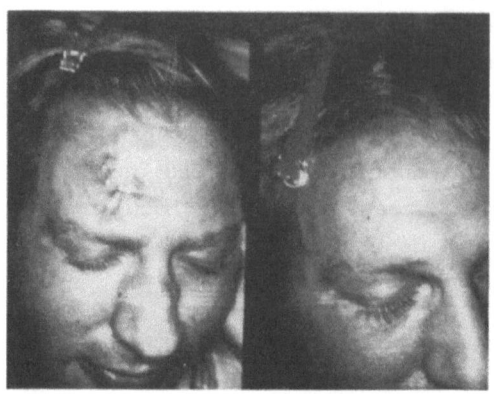

Fig 6. Ruby laser in caucasian skin

Another consideration which affects laser parameters is the race of the patient. In general, the oriental skin is much more prone to scarring than the caucasian skin, and thus lower power densities are needed for the former. Figure 6 above shows haemangioma simplex on the forehead of a 33-year-old caucasian male. The ruby laser was used at 90J/cm², and 6B shows the result 4 weeks after treatment, with no visible scarring and good skin texture. In the case of the oriental,- 90J/cm² would be certain to produce hypertrophic scarring and secondary hyperpigmentation. The oriental skin is usually treated within the range of 30-40J/cm². These considerations apply equally to tattoo lesions and lesions in the melanin anomaly group, as to naevi in the blood vessel anomaly group.

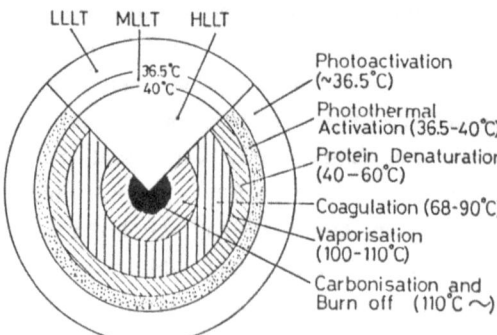

Fig 7. Plane schematic of laser imprint in tissue, showing biological reaction zones

LLLT: Low level laser (LLL) reactions have always existed, even when using HLLT. Consider figure 7: this shows the schematic imprint pattern of a beam set to vaporise tissue. At the centre of the beam is an area of carbonisation, surrounded by areas of vaporisation, coagulation, protein denaturation and thermal and nonthermal activation, all in outward-radiating concentric circles. As light travels at 3 x 10 - metres per second, all these effects occur virtually simultaneously with the radiant heat produced as the absorbed light energy is transformed. This concurrent photobiostimulative effect is only now being realised.

The law of Arndt-Schultz states that, in biologic tissue, mild stimuli excite the organism, moderately strong ones sustain activity, strong stimuli inhibit it, and very strong ones completely retard it.

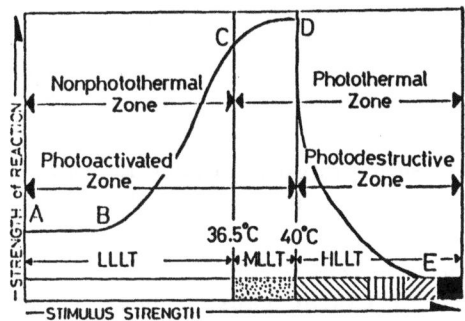

Fig 8. Ohshiro's Arndt-Schultz laser tissue reaction curve

Figure 8 shows Ohshiro's Arndt-Schultz curve for photothermal and non-photothermal reactions. Area AB is the normal activity level for the organism. From B to C the stimulation activity exhibits a sharp rise, levelling off from C to D. Thus area AD is the activated zone, composed of the nonthermal LLLT and the nondestructive photothermal MLLT areas, AC and CD. From point D where the tissue temperature reaches 40°C, the photodestructive HLLT zone begins, and the activity level of the organism shows a sharp decrease, gradually declining with increased stimulus level until death occurs at point E. Accordingly, for the maximum biostimulative effect, tissue temperature should never be-raised above normal, and must certainly never exceed 40°C.

The late Professor Endre Mester of Budapest is the father of LLLT, and his tremendous volume of clinical and experimental data is being constantly expanded and updated by his sons, Drs. Adam and Andrew-Mester. He demonstrated the increased vascularisation of LLLT-treated tissue. His work prompted further experimentation in our laboratory into the use of LLLT to improve the take of failing grafts and flaps.

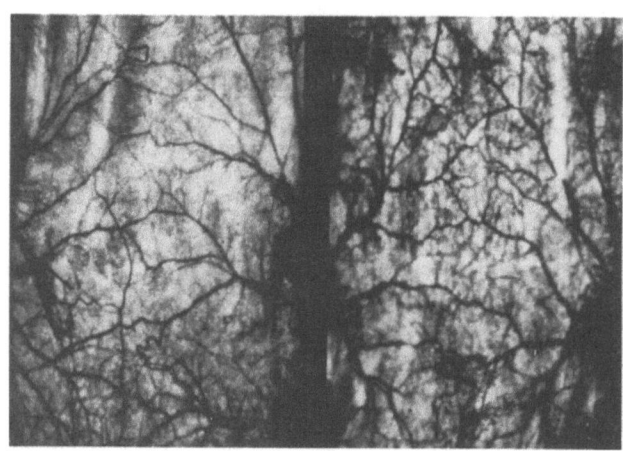

Fig 9: Control (left) and LLLT-treated (right) flaps on Wistar rat dorsum, one hour post irradiation, flourescein angiography. (Print courtesy of J. Kubota, M.D.)

Figure 9 shows the result of an experiment using the LLLT diode laser on flaps raised on the backs of Wistar rats, 1 hour after irradiation. The increased vascularisation of the treated flap on the right is clearly visible when compared with the control specimen on the left. Even shortly after irradiation, increased blood flow with reactive vasodilation could be seen around the irradiated points. In addition to the vascular system reaction, Professor and Drs Mester found a local cellular response of a photoenzymatic nature. Recent research has shown that these photoproducts regulate a number of biologic reactions: collagen synthesis and lysis are regulated; haemolytic activity is stimulated; excess seral mucopolysaccharides are reabsorbed; local endorphin synthesis is stimulated; and prostoglandin production is affected, elevating the levels of some and decreasing that of others. Because of this, the low level laser has found increasing acceptance in dermatologic applications for pigment removal or stimulation; for scarring control; for accelerated wound healing; for pain therapy; and for the augumentation of failing grafts and flaps.

Naturally, further research is necessary to establish in exact scientific detail how LLLT really works: only the basic "bones" of its mechanisms and pathways are known at present. However, good, solid double-blind trials are proving the effeciveness of this latest additon to the laser surgeon's arsenal, and the growing number of experimental and clinical papers presented on LLLT at national and international symposia reflect the growing awareness that LLLT is part of the art and science of dermatologic surgery.

CONCLUSIONS

The state-of-the-art in dermatologic surgery today can be summed up in one word: combination. The modern dermatologist has to be able to combine the knowledge and skills of medicine, physics and chemistry; and must have the ability to combine the different treatment techniques of HLLT, LLLT and conventional medicine and surgery. Given this ability to combine, we can look ahead at an even brighter future for the laser in the field of dermatology, helping to achieve the best results for every patient on a truly individual basis.

Argon Laser Treatment of Portwine Stain, its Application and Limitations

T. Matsumoto, M.D., T. Ohura, M.D.
Department of Plastic Surgery, School of
Medicine, Hokkaido University, Sapporo, Japan

1. Introduction

Application of argon laser (Ar) treatment to portwine stain (PS) and other superficial lesions of the skin was studied for an 8-year period in about 800 cases. Results of the treatment and some of its limitations were reported.

2. Method and Materials

The equipment, 770 Ar laser photocoagulator, by Spectra Physics Co., was used. It was adjusted to irradiate about 6 J/cm^2 on the skin surface. The single spot irradiation method was used for areas smaller than 20x10 cm^2 and the multispots method for areas larger than that. (1,2,3). Zebra method was applied for poorly healed lesions.

After irradiation, ointment therapy was administered so that a new epidermis would be formed within about 10 days. Once the epidermis was formed, pigmentation by ultraviolet light was prevented by applying a screen gauze for 2 months and cosmetics for 4 months.

The subjects were 364 cases of PS, who were followed-up for over 6 months after laser treatment. The histological types and therapeutic evaluations according to various sites were summarized in Table 1. There were two main histological types: the superficially located type (SLT), in which PS was observed mainly in the upper dermis ; and the deeply located type (DLT), in which PS appeared mainly in the deeper dermis (Fig.1, Fig.2).

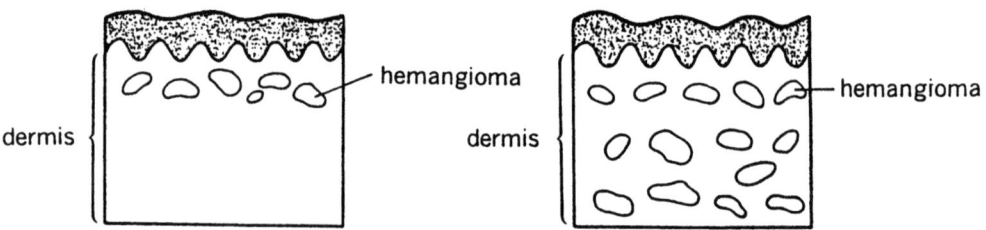

Fig.1. Histological schema of superficially located type of PS

Fig.2. Histological schema of deeply located type of PS

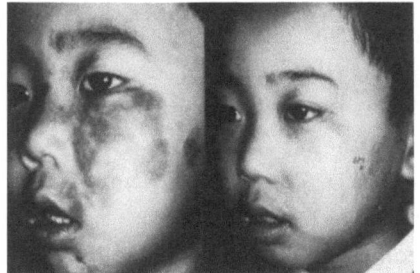

Fig.3. A 6-year-old boy with superficially located type PS.
b; 7 months after the last treatment. showing Good result

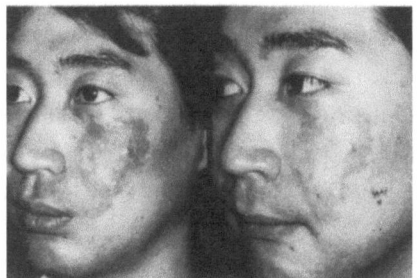

Fig.4. A 24-year-old man with deeply located type PS.
b; 6 months after the last treatment. showing Fair result

Evaluation was made according to the degree of blanching of the lesion: Good denotes remarkable blanching (Fig.3); Fair indicates still existing reddish coloring of the skin (Fig.4); and Poor means that there is almost no change in the PS.

3. Results (Table 1)

Of the 364 cases examined, there were 114 cases (31%) of SLT - PS. The lesion significantly reduced the degree of coloration in this type of stain (Fig.3). This type was observed mostly on the face and neck, and rarely on the trunk or the upper and lower extremities. The DLT -PS accounted for 250 cases (69%) and was mainly on the extremities. The lesion, which was deeply located in the lower layer of dermis, did not blanch satisfactory (Fig.4).

The evaluation of good was made in 108 cases (30%) , who showed mainly face and neck lesions. However, the effectiveness of laser treatment on deeply located lesions of the extremities and trunk was considered as 11-24%.

Table 1. Histological type and Therapeutic evaluation according to sites of portwine stain

Sites	No. of cases	Histological type		Therapeutic evaluation		
		superficial	deep	Good	Fair	Poor
Face	180	59(33%)	121(67%)	58(32%)	86(48%)	36(20%)
Neck	51	24(47%)	27(53%)	24(47%)	19(37%)	8(16%)
Trunk	31	8(26%)	23(74%)	7(23%)	18(58%)	6(19%)
Upper Limbs	58	15(26%)	43(74%)	14(24%)	28(48%)	16(28%)
Lower Limbs	44	8(18%)	36(82%)	5(11%)	21(48%)	18(41%)
Total	364	114(31%)	250(69%)	108(30%)	172(47%)	84(23%)

4. Procedures of Laser Treatment of PS (Table 2)

Treatment was decided according to histological types and sites of lesions as shown in Table 2. The superficially located type, which was demonstrated in 30% of the 364 cases, was remarkably improved by laser treatment, indicating optimal effectiveness for this type. As for hairly lesions on the face (eyebrows, mustache, hair lines and so on) and vermillions, of which the anatomical structure may be damaged by surgery, laser treatment was considered the first choice. In most of the cases, incomplete regression of PS was considered clinically acceptable. In the cases of deeply located type, which accounted for 70% of cases, 45% of the cases were evaluated as partially effective when they demonstrated regression of PS in the upper dermis with color lightening. The cases of this type showing small area lesions, which could also be treated by local flap, were treated first by laser irradiation, and remained lesion was then excised and sutured. Medium sized lesions, which are treated by skin graft, were irradiated by laser and covered with cosmetics at the appropriate interval. Indications of skin graft vary according to the age, sex and site of PS. However, skin graft is not recommended before the age of 30, when good skin tension is expected. Good results are achieved by skin grafts made after the age of 40. Laser treatment proved to be effective for wide spread PS in which skin graft could

Table 2. Guidelines for Argon Laser Treatment of Portwine Stain

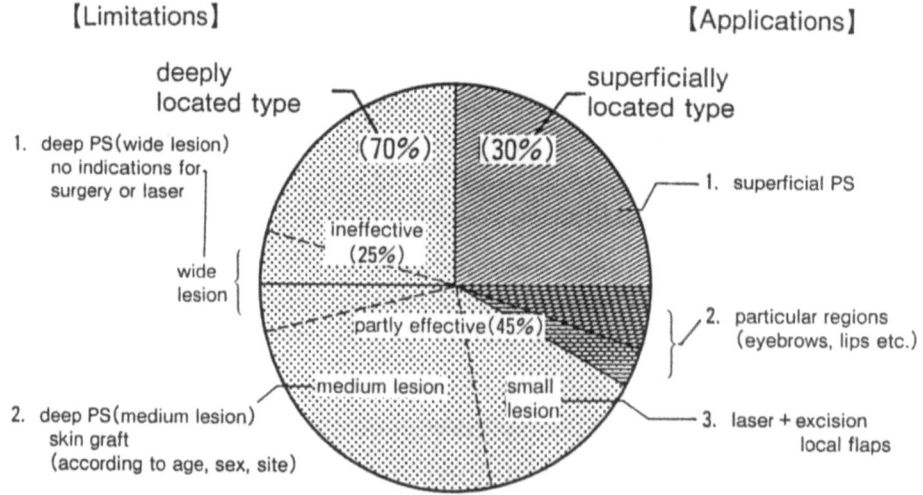

be applied. However, most wide lesions belonged to the deeply located type of PS and were considerably resistant to laser treatment. The search for improved methods to treat this type is a subject for future research.

The side effects of Ar laser, that is pigmentation and hypertrophic scarring, are recognized drawbacks, but they are outweighed by the advantages of easy maintenance and operation of the laser device, as well as the effectiveness of the whole treatment. Careful consideration of the type of lesion and the suitable irradiation dose should lead to enhanced effectiveness of Ar laser treatment for PS.

References
1. Matsumoto,T.,Ohura,T.,Fujii,H.,et al.: Argon laser treatment of portwine stains using fiber bundle scanner. Transaction of The 4th Congress of the International Society for Laser Surgery, edited by Atsumi,K., 1, 17-20, Lap.Soc. Laser Medicine, Tokyo, 1981.
2. Matsumoto,T.,Ohura,T.,Saikawa,M.,et al.: Argon laser treatment of Portwine stains using fiber bundle scanner. J.Japan Soc.Plast.Reconstr.Surg. 3: 1-15, 1983.
3. Matsumoto,T.,Ohura,T.,Sugihara,T.,et al.: Argon laser treatment of cutaneous lesions —— A new device for the mode of laser irradiation in each cutaneous lesion and its problem. J.Japan Soc. Laser Medicine 5: 137-142, 1985.

Laser Treatment of Cutan and Deep Vessel Anomalies

H.-P. Berlien, J. Waldschmidt, G. Müller
Laser-Medizin-Zentrum and Pediatric surgical Dep.
Klinikum Steglitz, Freie Universität Berlin
Krahmerstr. 6-10, D-1000 Berlin 45

Haemangioms are the most often occuring malformations in childhood and their treatment is controversial. Most haemangioms heal spontaneously before the age of 8, and it is advisable to wait till then. If located at an exposed position, e.g. on the face or on functionally important structures, further growth can result in significant functional disorders or disfigurations. This requires early treatment in infancy and childhood. Until now all treatment methods have been radical and have caused further injury. One prominent example is X-ray therapy. Treatment can result after a period of 20-30 years can result in a development of malignomas (Fig. 1 + 2).

Angiomatosis	Ar+	Ar+-Dye	Nd:YAG non contact	Nd:YAG contact	CO_2
spider naevi	+		(+)		
port wine stain	+		(+)		
cutaneous hemangiomas					
strawberry hemangioma	++		++		
cavernous			++		
combined	+		++		
angioma (cavernoma)					
resection			++	+	
volume reduction			++	++	
vascular hamartia			++	+	
hemangioendothelioma			++	+	
venectasia				++	
teleangiectasia	+		+		
varices					(+)

Fig. 1. Types of angiomatous and the laser types which we prefer for the therapy

Indications for the laser therapy at angiomas

- rapid growth with spreading on mucosa membrane and conjunctiva
- functional disorders with occlusion of luminas and destructions of organs (pharynx, larnyx, trachea and bronchia)
- exulceration, superinfection and bleeding
- gastrointestinal bleeding
- AV shunts with cardiac disease or steal effect
- preoperative volume reduction
- angiomas of parenchymatous organs
- cosmetic correction

Fig. 2. Due to the spontaneous heeling of sometimes of angiomatosous the indications for laser therapy is very strong. Only these indications need early laser therapy

The initial hopes in using the laser were not always satisfying, especially the cosmetic results in children. Treatment was carried out almost entirely in using the Argon laser. This radiation has a high absorption in hemoglobin, permitting selective treatment of vessel anomalies.

Since 1983 we have used the Argon laser. At former laser instruments relatively low power of 2-3 W output with long pulse duration of 0,1 s have been possible. Thermal skin damage was not always to avoid. Further development of the instrument technique allowed to increase the selectivity for the haemoglobin with an output of 5-6 W and exposition times of 0,02 s and a minimizing at the same time of the heat conduct effect caused by the short exposition time. With this technique you can treat successful plane and strawberry haemangiomas, spider naevi, port wine stains naevus flammeus. Because of good experiences of the high selectivity and a minimum of wound ache caused by short exposition time we start with the treatment already in childhood. This is very important as children themselves will suffer of the anomalies during the play and in the kindergarten. Very seldom a general anesthesia was necessary. Normally a sedation and a local anesthesia were sufficient. In order to avoid scares it is important not to get a coagulation of the radiated area during the treatment, but to induce the so-called thermodynamic reaction (Katalinic). Within 3-4 weeks it will come to due to the following vasculitis to an increasing blanching of the lesion. Therefore the following sessions shouldn't occur within the next 4-6 weeks. Normally we wait 8-12 weeks (Fig. 3).

Treatment of superficial lesions
argon laser 0.48/0.51 um

    power : 5 watts
    spot size : 0.5 mm
    pulse duration : 0.02 sec
    rep. rate : 6/sec

Remark: prevent surfacecoagulation
late thermodynamic sequelae,
period of treatment 8 weeks

Fig. 3. Therapeutical procedure using the Argon laser

Treatment of combined vessel anomalies
Nd:YAG laser 1.06 um

For the intradermal parts
    power : 20 watts
    spot size : 1.5 mm
    pulse duration : 0.05 sec
    rep. rate : 6/sec

Remark: prevent visual surfacecoagulation
thermodynamic late sequelae,
period of 8 weeks

Fig. 4. Treatment of the intradermal parts of combined angiomas with the Nd:YAG laser

Because of the high selectivity with absorption in the haemoglobin the Argon laser is not useful for the treatment of larger vessel anomalies. For the treatment of these larger respectively deeper situated anomalies the Nd:YAG laser is predestinates due to its relatively high penetration depths. Conventional application still caused skin burns, therefore these treatments have been left. In literature mentioned procedures for skin cooling with chlorethyl or saline solution couldn't achieve sufficient protecting effect.

Because the transmission of the near infrared of the Nd:YAG laser in water is quite high an efficient surface cooling can be obtain also by icecubes. Conventionally produced icecubes have substantial air occlusions, which can lead to a diffusion of the irradiation because of their opaque structure. These icecubes could not be used for application. Icecubes made by ice machines which are produced at nearly 0° C and under high pressure, air occlusions were nearly missing. These icecubes nearly show a crystal-clear structure. Because of the still remaining rest absorption and deviation an output of ca. 50 W has to be applied. Furthermore you have to consider, that the cube has good contact with the skin. Otherwise you will have skin burns. Another important effect is the compression of the haemangioma caused by the icecube, so that first the blood can be pressed out partially causing a better irradiation of the vessel walls, and second irradiation can penetrate deeper into the tissue. With this procedure large haemangiomas could be treated and brought regression. At part-remissions it was possible to resected inoperable angiomas before, without any problem (Fig. 5).

Treatment of combined vessel anomalies
Nd:YAG laser 1.06 um

For the subcutaneous parts
    power : 50 watts
    spot size : 1.5 mm
    pulse duration : cw

Remark O sufficient cooling of the surface is necessary
    O water or chlorethyl is not enough
    O cooling procedure: ice-cubes without air pockets
    O good skin contact with the ice-cube; otherwise burning wounds are possible
    O compression of angiomas

Fig. 5. Treatment of the subcutaneous parts of combined anomalies with the YAG laser to induce the vasculitis with following vessel occlusion of the deeper parts, sufficient cooling of the skin is necessary. Here we use icecubes with great advantage

Treatment of ectatic veins:
percutaneous intraluminal irradiation
with the −bare fiber−
Nd:YAG laser 1.06 μm

    power : 10 − 20 watts
    pulse duration : 1 − 5 sec
    speed : 0.2 − 1 mm/sec

Remark: fiber tip always in saline solution

Fig. 6. Treatment of ectatic veines and varices. after puncture of the ectatic veines it is possible to irradiate intraluminal with following shrinking and occlusion of the ectatic veines

Another application form is the percutan intraluminal irradiation of larger cavernomas by bare fiber. After puncture of the angioma with a special canula it follows the introducing into the vascular lumen. With an output of 10-20 W and slowly withdrawing of the fiber the vessel will irradiated with an expedition time of 0,2 - 1 mm/s. Continuous rinsing of the fiber tip with NaCl-solution prevents on one hand a destroying of the fiber caused by the adhered blood and a thrombus formation on the other, so that radiation can reach the vessel wall with following vasculitis and obliteration. Even with this procedure a volume reduction can be achieved, so primarily inoperable angiomas can be resected. Also for resection of angioma the Nd:YAG laser proved effective (Fig. 6). Using a focus handpiece with a focus of 0,5 mm and an output of about 50 W a clean preparing of the angiomas in the surrounding can occur in order to prepare cavernous haemangiomas respectively lymph-angiomas from the soft tissue. In order to avoid a thermal slack in the tissue with following uncontrolable coagulation, pulse duration don't have to be over 0,3-0,5 s. If necessary it is always helpful to spread the tissue with an instrument apart so larger vessels can be coagulated with the defocussed beam respectively can be cut after ligature. Further you can achieve the radicality of the resection with protection of functional important sturctures at the same time. Hereby eventually existing rests of angioma can be coagulated homogenously with the defocussed beam. For this reason the formation of rezidives will be extremely reduced.

For treatment of angiomas of parenchymatous organs like liver, lung and spleen the Nd:YAG laser is of important surgical help. With an output of 100-120 W and by using a focus handpiece with a beam diameter of 0,5 mm, resections of these parenchymatous organs can be made without essential intraoperatively bleeding from the resection surface. But it is important that the cutting speed is just about 1 mm/s. Otherwise not sufficient high power densities for carbonisation and vaporisation of the tissue are produced. Eventually extravasating blood out of the parenchym should be removed by intermittent rinsing and suction, because the Nd:YAG radiation will be absorbed in the haemoglobin and doesn't lead to a cutting effect.

Through the well-calculated use of the laser to treat vessel anomalies depending on the indication, either the Argon or the Nd:YAG laser, then children can be treated intime without a high risk. This is important for these particular psycholical problems and especially at angiomas of parenchymatous organs, vital risk of bleeding.

But nevertheless all angiomas in the face and at functional important parts should be treated in time, as despite of the tendency towards spontaneous remission the meanwhile occuring growing can lead to enormous anomalies in children.

Preparation, resection
Nd:YAG laser 1.06 μm

power   : 50 watts
spot size   : 0.5 mm
pulse duration : 0.2 – 0.3 sec

Remark: spreading of tissue, defocussed coagulation of bigger vessels, or ligature

Fig. 7. Preparation of cavernous angiomas by the YAG laser with short pulse duration and small focus it is possible to prepare the angiomas from the healthy tissue with good success and without bleeding and damage of the healthy tissue

Resection
tumors, parenchymatous organs
Nd:YAG laser 1.06 μm

power   : 100–120 watts
spot size by focussing handpiece   : 0.5 mm
pulse duration   : cw
speed   : 1 mm/sec

Remark: continuously aspiration and intermittent rising with high–pressure saline solution during the resection

Fig. 8. For intrahepatic angiomas and angiomas in other parenchymatous organs it is possible to resected these with great advantage and bloodless by the Nd:YAG laser

Argon Laser Photodermoabration for Cicatrical Acne Sequella Treatment

Trelles M.A.*, Martínez Morillo M.**, Mayayo E.***, Rigau J.*, Sánchez J.****, Sala Francino P.*****

* Instituto Médico Vilafortuny, Cambrils/Tarragona -E
** Cátedra de Radiología y Medicina Física, Fctad. de Medicina Univ. de Málaga -E
*** Serv. de Anatomía Patológica del Hosp. Juan XXIII de Tarragona y Dpto. de Histología de la Fctad. de Medicina de Reus, Univ. de Barcelona -E.
**** Serv. de Cirugía del Hosp. Gral. de San Pablo y Sta. Tecla, Tarragona -E
***** Serv. de Anestesiología y Reanimación del Hosp. Gral. de San Pablo y Sta. Tecla, Tarragona -E

INTRODUCTION

Scarring constitutes one of the most frequent unaesthetic acne complications (1). For its correction there have been several methods of treatment proposed of which chemical peeling (2), which produces destruction of first cutaneous layers, is the most common. Nevertheless, this method doesn't always achieve satisfactory results, especially if lesion is too deep or when peeling complicates with haemorrhages (3), infections (4), etc.

Argon laser can be used as an efficient tool for elimination of cutaneous lesions, because of the particular absortion of its wave length by the pigments of the skin. When Argon laser is used in continous waves, at 4 to 5 W output with a focalized beam of 0,5 mm, elimination of the first layers of skin can be obtained by previously painting the epidermis with mercurochrome.

MATERIAL AND METHOD

Previous to surgical procedure, the phototype of patients should be carefully evaluated as well as their psycological equilibrium with the aim of knowing their expectations regarding the results of treatment.

It is necessary to use an analgesic medication (Paracetamol for example) accompained by 10 mgrs Valium (R). Both should be given approximately thirty minutes before Argon-dermoabration. Afterwards, the areas that are going to be treated are marked, paying special attention to the natural orifices and capilar lines. In order to have some aditional information of the vascularization of the involved area termographic control should be recorded (5). After this control, vascularization can be stimulated by using He/Ne laser irradiation at 1 J/cm2 (6). We then painted the area with mercurochrome taking into account that the dermoabration would overlap the limits of the lesion. In order to protect the neighbouring skin it is covered with a transparent plastic, strong enough to stop Argon beams. Dermoabration is then programmed with the assistence of a computer which makes the Argon laser scan the whole area selected for dermoabration. The scan technique is performed point by point with an irradiation of 1 sec. per point and 0,1 sec. relapsing time between pulses. Particular attention should be taken so that any point in which the scanner irradiation occurs should be located at a maximum distance of 0,5 mm from the next point.

When using Argon-dermoabration a frank haemorrhage of the tissue should not occur, but just a mild bleeding. After dermoabration has being performed we proceed to irradiate the lesion with He/Ne laser in order to decrease inflammation and pain (7) and, at the same time, to activate cicatrization. Afterwards, we cover the lesion with a cream which in our experience, constitutes a good aid for rapid recovery of the dermoabradeted area (Table I).

***T A B L E   I.* CICATRIZIAL   POMADE**

- Blue Camomile..................... 2%
- Glucosamin Glicano Precursor.... 3%
- Equinacea Extract................ 2%
- Centella Extract................. 3%
- Steril Greese component, up to.. 100

We continue controling the lesion every 24 hours after dermoabration, using the same cream each time. No other local or general medication is needed. The patient must avoid exposure of the lesion to sun for four months after treatment.

CLINICAL CASE

Female, 26 years old, has been suffering from a depressed scar on the left side of the face for the last 4 years (Fig. 1). The pathological cicatrization arose after surgical elimination of a cystic acne lesion. Argon-dermoabration was practised under the previously described parameters. The different pictures taken during the procedure and 4 months after dermoabration showed the cosmetic results obtained which can be classified as excellent (Fig. 2-8).

COMMENTS

1) We don't possess experience of Argon laser dermoabration of extensive areas but, nevertheless, we have used this method to correct cutaneous strech-marks on areas of abdomen and thighs of approximately 20 x 25 cm in size. The results obtained were fairly satisfactory, and directly related to the age of the lesion (e.g. when they are too old, brown coloured or too deep, results are less impressive).

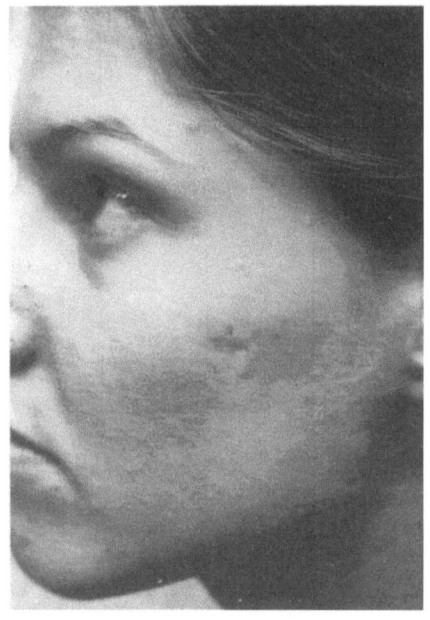
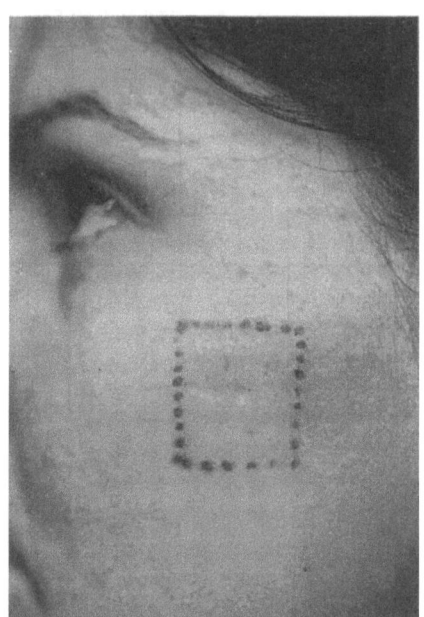

Fig. 1.- Acne sequella. 26 year-old female

Fig. 2.- Marking of the area to be dermoabraded

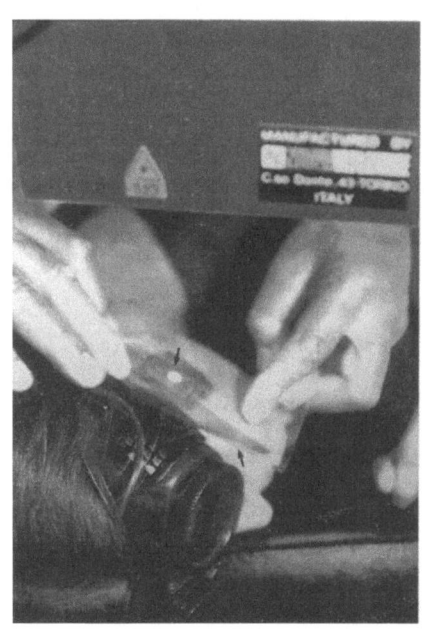
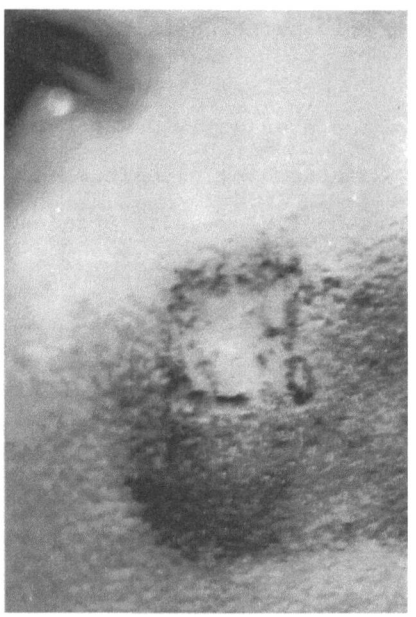

Fig. 3.- The patient is positioned for laser dermoabration. Note the laser-guide-light at the center of the lesion and the plastic sheet to protect the surrounding tissues

Fig. 4.- Immediately after Argon-laser-dermoabration

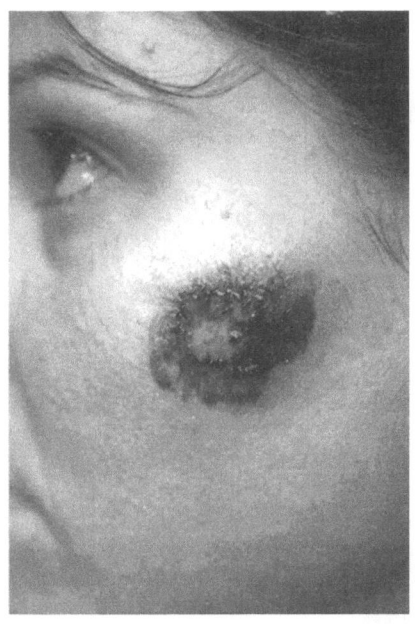 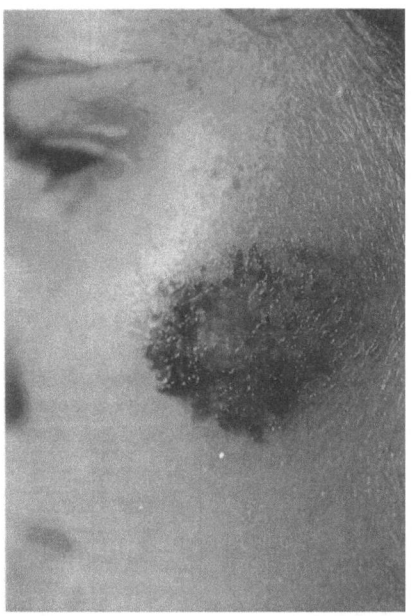

Fig. 5.- Twenty-four hours after dermoabration. Observe that there is no inflamation. Rest of the cream used to cover the lesion (Table I) can be observed

Fig. 6.- Four days after Argon-dermoabration

2) Our casuistic is formed by 37 patients. Obviously this is not large but results obtained in all these cases are promising.

3) Since we started to used low power He/Ne laser irradiation to improve cicatrization quality of dermoabraded areas, cosmetic results were better and we have not witnessed scarring problems (8). At the same time, He/Ne laser irradiation significantly decreases pain and inflammation after dermoabration.

4) To activate cicatrization and to improve its quality we also rely on the composition of the cream used. Its components are well-known because of the benefits they produce on cicatrization.

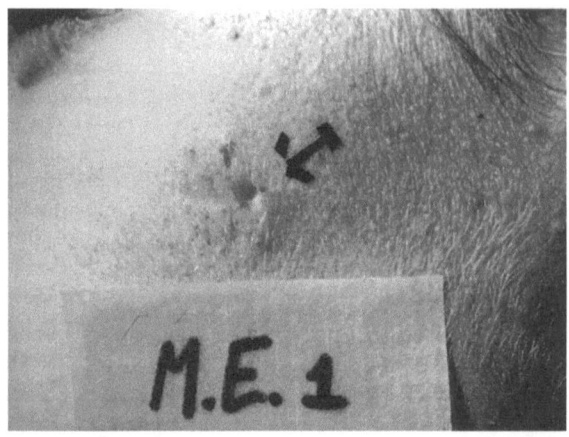

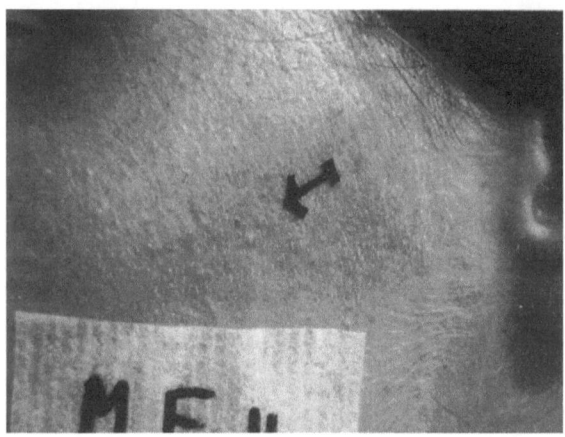

Fig. 7 and 8.- Comparative photographies prior to and 4 months after Argon-dermoabration

5) When the lesion to repair is too deep we previously inject collagen and after two to three weeks, photodermoabration can be performed. If the depth of scarring tissue is too important, correction can be tried by surgery using the so-called punch-technique (see graph A), before dermoabration.

6) Argon dermoabration practiced under computer programme allows the use of standarized parameters which contributes to better the quality of results.

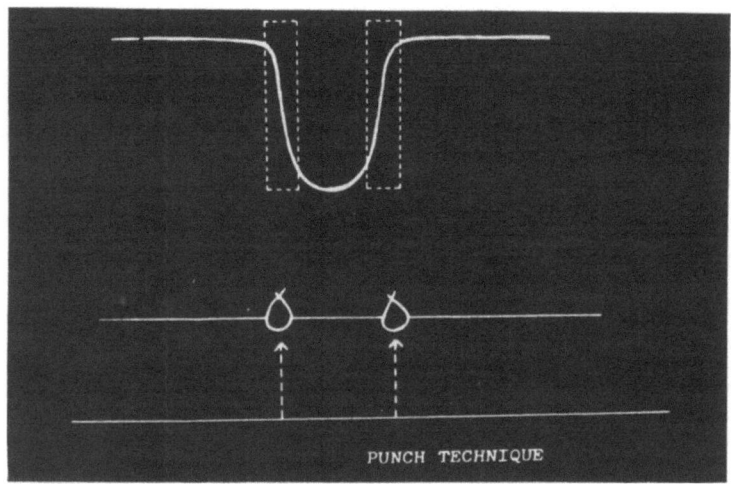

Graph A. <u>Surgical punch Technique</u>, for depressed scar reparation

7) Comparison of Argon-dermoabration with common peeling techniques favours the former especially regarding the risk of haemorrhages, infections or reactive eczema when chemical products are used for dermoabration.

8) In order to avoid the risk of hiper or hipochromia and to evaluate the risk of scarring, the old scars of the patient should be evaluated to consider their colour and aspect. We beleive that, in order to improve the prognosis and results of dermoabration, He/Ne laser, as a stimulatory radiation, should be considered as an important aid (9).

9) It seems that the 4 W is the most suitable laser output for dermoabration. This parameter we have found after experimentation on animals (Fig. 9). By histological analysis of the tissue submitted to Argon-dermoabration we observed destruction of the epidermis, superficial dermis and almost all of the deep dermis (Fig. 10).

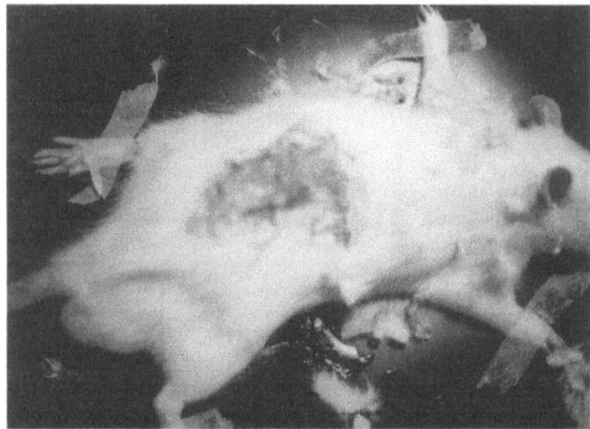

Fig. 9.- Protocol of experiment of Argon dermoabration on a Swiss lab mouse

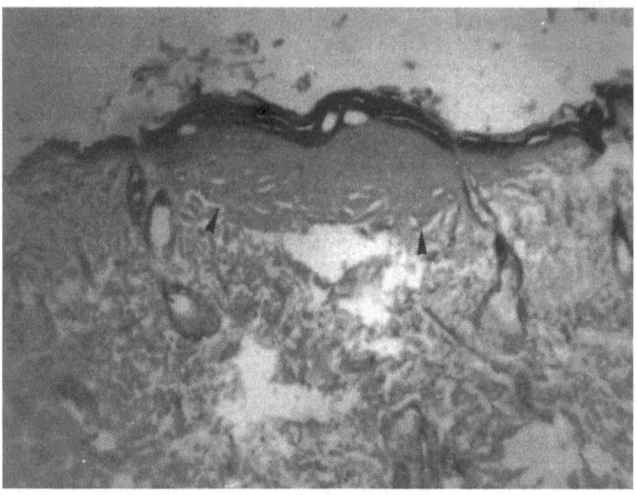

Fig. 10.- Histological sample of Argon-dermoabraded tissue (Swiss lab mouse). Observe that the lesion has been produced at the epidermis and at superficial dermis level (arrows). Note the necrosis effect

10) By studying the characteristics of laser impacts on the skin of the laboratory-mouse, we conclude that some parameters, which are constant, should be taken into account, as for example the depth of the laser action which is related to

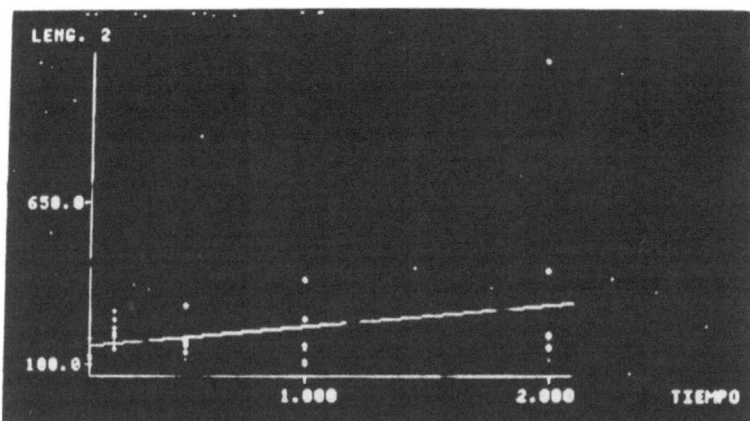

Graph B. <u>Photodermoabration for Laser of Argon.</u>
Deepth and time

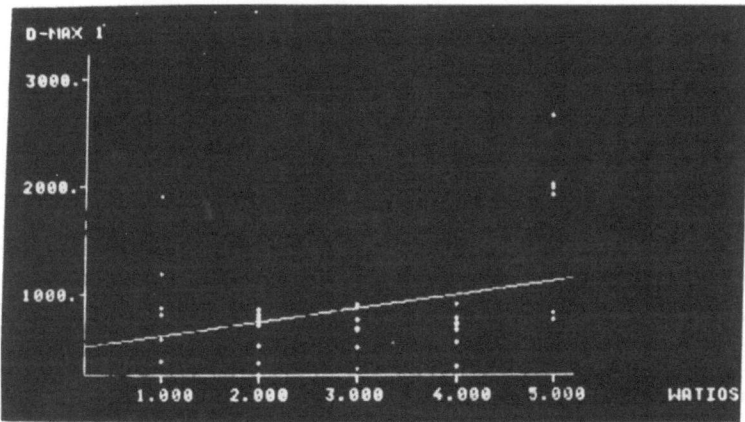

Graph C. <u>Photodermoabration for Laser of Argon.</u>
Maximum Diameter and power

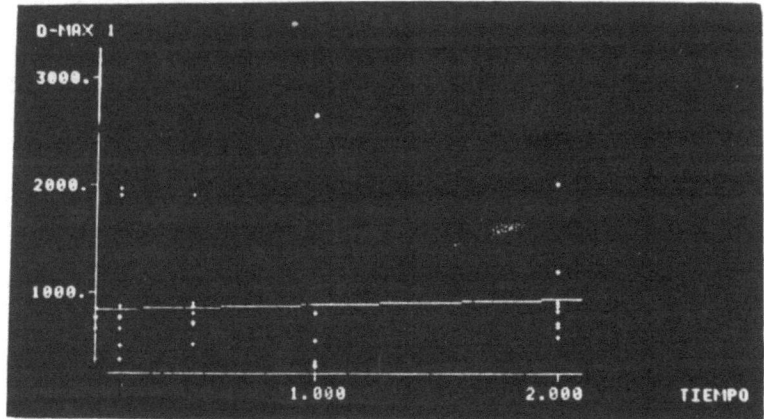

Graph D. <u>Photodermoabrarion for Laser of Argon.</u>
Maximum diameter and time

power (Graph B). By the same token the lesion diameter progressively increases by augmentates the laser power (Graph C). In the same way the lesion diameter remains constant at a fixt laser power without influence of the laser time work (Graph D).

Argon-laser-dermoabration appears as a promising technique, but nevertheless more clinical long term controls and extensive casuistic are necessary to explore its potencial possibilities.

REFERENCES

1.- T.B. Fitzpatrick, M.K. Polano, D. Surmond (1985) Atlas de Dermatologia clinica. Ed. Doyma, Barcelona.

2.- R. Amar (1981) ABC de Chirurgie plastique et esthètique. Ed. Masson, barcelona.

3.- J. Quetglas (1971) Breve manual de Cirugia Plàstica y Estètica de la Cara. Publicaciones Controladas S.A., Madrid

4.- J. Marquis Converse (1964) Reconstructive Plastic Surgery. Ed. Saunders Company

5.- J.A.S. Carruth, P. Shakespeare (1986) Toward the Ideal Treatment for the Port Wine Stain with the Argon Laser: Better Prediction and an "Optimal" Technique. Lasers in Surgery and Medicine, 6, pp2:4

6.- L. Miro, M. Coupe, C. Charras, C. Jambon, J.M. Chevalier (1984) Estudio capilaroscópico de la acción de un láser AsGa sobre la microcirculación. Inv. y Clínica Láser, vol.I n.2, pp9:14

7.- J.L. Cisneros, M.A. Trelles (1987) Láser y terapéutica en Medicina y Cirugia Cutánea. Ed. Centro Documentación Láser, S.A. Barcelona.

8.- M.A. Trelles, E. Mayayo, C. Schmidt, J.M. Iglesias, J.I. Barber (1983) Láser para la salud y la estética. Ed. Etecnes, Barcelona.

9.- S. Fuertes Lanzuela (1986) Láser de baja potencia y bioestimulación. Inv. y Clínica Láser, vol.III n.1, pp21:26

Possibilities for the Increase of the Coagulation Depth in Skin with the Argonlaser

D. Haina, M. Landthaler, W. Waidelich

H: GSF, Inst. f. Angewandte Optik
   Ingoldstädter Landstr.1, D-8042 Neuherberg, FRG
L: Dermatol. Klinik und Poliklinik, Univ. München
W: GSF und Inst. f. Medizinische Optik, Univ. München

The depth, to which tissue will be coagulated by irradiation with laser light of defined wavelength, cannot be increased arbitrarily by simply raising the laser power. The surface of the tissue carbonizes and evaporates above a certain power density. Therefore, the optical absorption becomes larger and the laser beam now is absorbed to a higher amount on the surface and the depth of coagulation decreases. For every type of laser there exists a maximum coagulation depth (MCD), which cannot be exceeded by increasing the laser power /1/.

But this MCD is not a constant. Due to heat conduction in tissue, toward long irradiation times the deeper layers of the skin are heated up not only by absorption of radiation but also by heat transfer from the upper hotter layers. Consequently MCD has to increase with longer irradiation times. Heat conduction also is the cause for the increase of MCD with increasing diameter of the laser beam. A further drastic increase of MCD can be achieved by cooling the skin surface. If the latter is moistened with floating water, the heat, which is created in the upper skin layers, is partially removed by the water. The surface carbonizes at a higher laser power and therefore MCD increases.

For the argonlaser the MCD has been measured in vitro in full thickness human skin samples at beam diameters of 1 mm and 2 mm (fig.1). The exposure time was varied between 0.1 sec and 10 sec. The maximum coagulation depth raises from 0.3 mm at 0.1 sec exposure time up to 1.2 mm for a 10 sec irradiation and 1 mm diameter. The increase of MCD with the diameter of the laser beam is evident. At 10 sec irradiation time MCD increases from 1.2 mm to 1.7 mm, if a beam diameter of 2 mm is used instead of 1 mm. In fig.2 the necessary irradiation dose is specified.

This effect can be used in clinical application of the argonlaser for deeper coagulation of tissue, for example for treatment of dermal

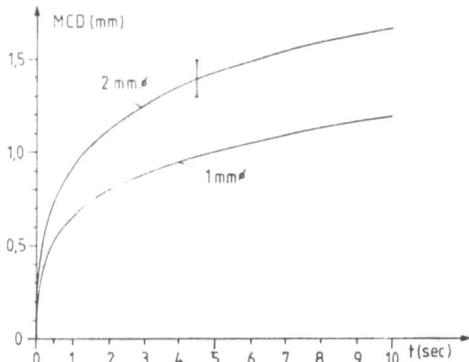

Fig.1. MCD in human skin samples, achieved with the argon-laser for different beam diameters

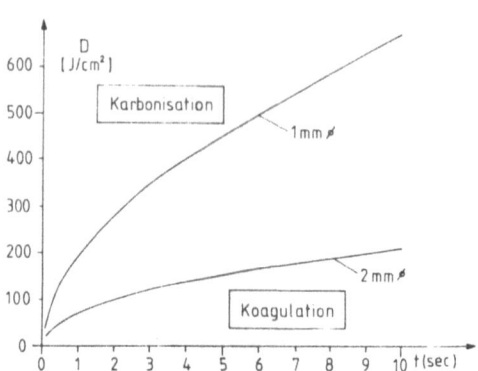

Fig.2. Irradiation dose which is necessary to reach MCD. At higher doses the skin surface will carbonize

fibroma, hypertrophic scars, hemangioma or in special cases for port wine stains. Of course one has to consider, that damage of the skin surface is more intense and more extended and scar formation may occur.

For cooling respectively protection of the skin surface during treatment with the argonlaser we have developed two different equipments which work by a similar principle /2/. One of them is a spoon like equipment, consisting of an aluminum frame covered with 1 mm thick slide of glas. Between this glas and the skin destillated water flow from a dropper bath. In the other case instead of the spacer a cooling equipment is mounted on the light pencil of the fiber optic (fig.3). After contact with the skin surface water is sucked through the gap between

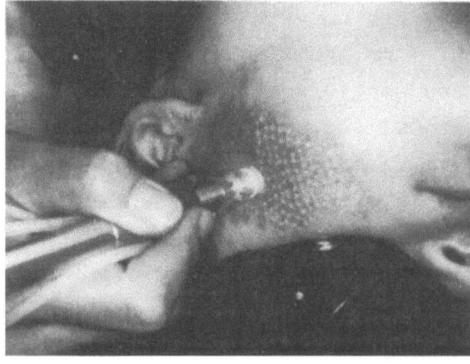

Fig.3. Cooling equipment at the end of the light pencil

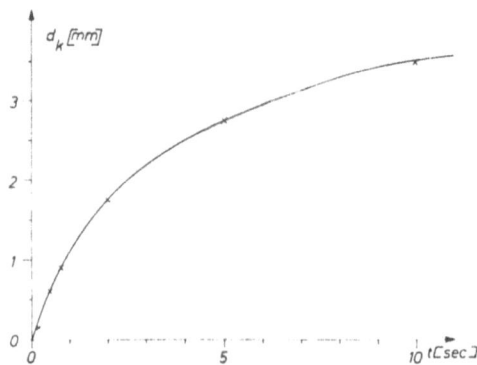

Fig.4. Coagulation depth in human skin, achieved with water cooling and a laser power of 5.1 W

glas slide and skin. By this way the heat, which is generated in the upper skin layers during laser exposure, is partially removed by the water.

In human connective tissue the coagulation depth has been measured for an argonlaser beam diameter of 2 mm and water protection of the skin surface (fig.4). The laser power has been kept constant, irradiation time has been varied between 0.2 sec and 10 sec. Only at this long exposure time the MCD has been achieved for this laser power. The connective tissue is coagulated to a depth of 3.5 mm.

Our investigations have shown that it is possible to increase the coagulation depth in dermal connective tissue
from 0.5 mm at common argonlaser treatment parameters
   to 1.2 mm by increasing the exposure time to 10 sec,
   to 1.7 mm by increasing the beam diameter from 1 mm to 2 mm and
   to 3.5 mm by an additional protection of the skin surface by floating
water.

For treatment of vascular birthmarks /3,4,/, which in our experience is the main indication for dermatological laser application, the absorbtion of the laser light in hemoglobin is of great importance. In blood the blue and green light of the argonlaser is stronger absorbed

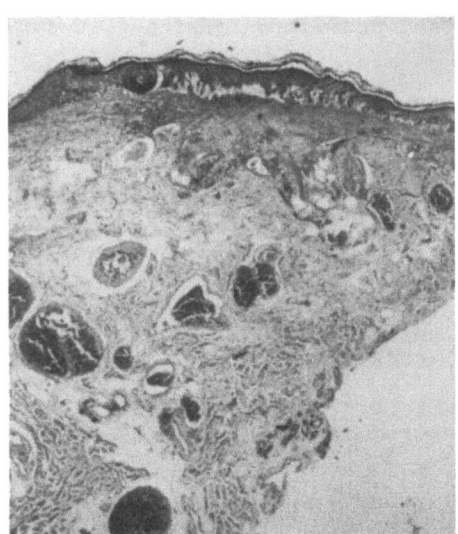 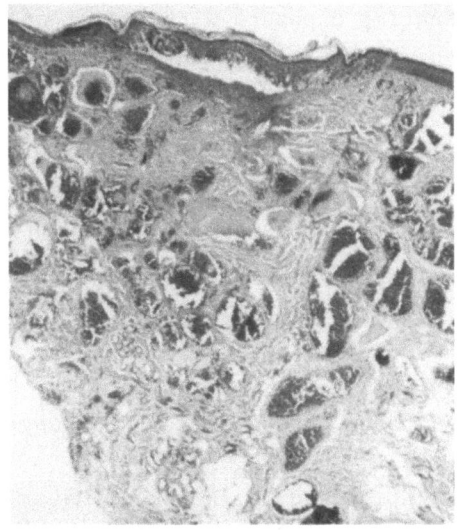

a)   b)

Fig.5. Coagulation necrosis in a port wine stain. a) Without cooling, 18 J/cm^2. b) With water protection of the skin surface, 96 J/cm^2

than in connective tissue and therefore blood vessels are coagulated in deeper layers of skin than connective tissue. Let me recall to your mind that under normal treatment conditions vessels are coagulated to a depth of 1 mm, connective tissue to 0.5 mm /5,6/.

It was not possible to determinate the MCD for blood vessels systematically because such investigations should be done in patients with port wine stains. Shurely towards long exposure times, where heat conduction is of importance the differences between coagulation depth of blood vessels and connective tissue will decrease and disappear.

From some biopsies taken from patients with port wine stains we saw, that without cooling, 2 mm beam diameter, 0.3 sec exposure time and an irradiation dose of 18 J/cm^2, the common values of 0.5 mm and 1 mm are achieved. With additional cooling of the skin surface, 0.8 sec exposure time and 48 J/cm^2 irradiation dose, the blood vessels have been coagulated to a depth of 1.8 mm and connective tissue to 1.0 mm. At the twofold irradiation time (96 J/cm^2) blood vessels are coagulated to a depth of 2.2 mm and connective tissue to 1.7 mm. Histologically (fig.5) the damage of the skin surface seems to be equal for normal treatment conditions and longtime exposure under water protection. In both cases dermis and epidermis are separated by a blister, basal membrane seems undamaged.

Longtime exposure with the argonlaser and protection of the skin surface with floating water is a very good possibility to improve the therapy results in treatment of PWS with deep lying blood vessels.

Literature
/1/ Haina D, Landthaler M, Braun-Falco O, Waidelich W: Comparison of the maximum coagulation depth in human skin for differnt types of medical lasers. Lasers Surg Med 7: in print, 1987.
/2/ Haina D, Landthaler M, Braun-Falco O, Waidelich W: Kühlung der Haut bei der Laserbehandlung von Gefäßmälern. In Waidelich W, Kiefhaber P (eds): "Laser 85 Optoelektronik in der Medizin." Berlin-Heidelberg-New York-Tokyo: Springer, 1985, pp 86-94.
/3/ Seipp W, Haina D, Justen V, Waidelich W: Erfahrungen mit dem Argonlaser. Akt Derm 7:85-124, 1981.
/4/ Noe JM, Barsky SH, Geer DE, Rosen S: Port wine stains and the response to argon laser therapy:Successful treatment and the predictive role of colour, age and biopsy. J Plast Reconstr Surg 65: 130-136, 1980.
/5/ Apfelberg DB, Kosek J, Maser MR, Lash H: Histology of port wine stains following argon laser treatment. Br J Plast Surg 32:232-237, 1979.
/6/ Falco O: Morphologische Untersuchungen zu Behandlung von Naevi flammei mit dem Argonlaser. Hautarzt 34:548-554, 1983.

Improvement of Therapy Results in Treatment of Port Wine Stains with the Argonlaser

D. Haina, W. Seipp, M. Landthaler, W. Waidelich

H.: GSF, Institut für Angewandte Optik
    Ingolstädter Landstr. 1, D-8042 Neuherberg, FRG
S.: Dermatologische Gemeinschaftspraxis, D-6100 Darmstadt, FRG
L.: Dermatologische Klinik und Poliklinik, Univ. München,
W.: GSF und Inst. f. Medizinische Optik, Univ. München

The report in "Possibilities for the increase of the coagulation depth in skin with the argonlaser" by D. Haina, M. Landthaler, W. Waidelich describes the technical and physical means of water cooling which helps to improve the results in treatment of Portwine stains with the argonlaser /1/.

Our report describes the clinical application of the water cooling method. The reported results were obtained from treatment of 109 patients (W1 and W2). Fig. 1 shows the distribution of age of the patients. Most of them are between 16 and 20 years old.

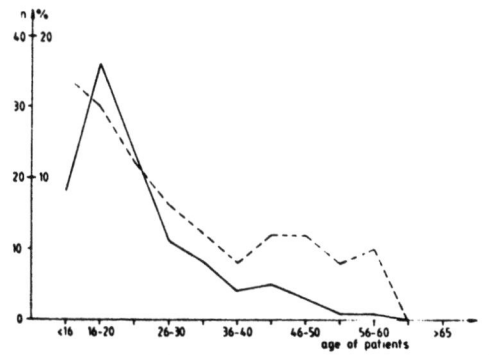

Fig. 1. Distribution of age of port wine stain patients treated under water cooling. Solid line represents number of patients. Dotted line represents percentage of patients

The experimental studies suggested to apply cooling of the skin during treatment with the argonlaser for two different purposes:

<u>The water cooling method W1</u> (Clue "Careful treatment")

In this method the usual and accepted radiation parameters (i.e. 2 mm beam diameter, 0.3 sec pulse duration, laser power 2 - 2.5 watts) remain largely unchanged. Possibly the laser power could be slightly increased to offset the reflection loss at the glass plate.

This method of cooling the skin has the effect of a protection of epidermis and upper dermis. The time required for the treatment is doubled, however, the danger of scar formation after healing is clearly reduced.

The W1 method will be applied in sensitive areas (e.g. breast, shoulder, uper arms) when the test radiation indicates increased risks (fig. 2).

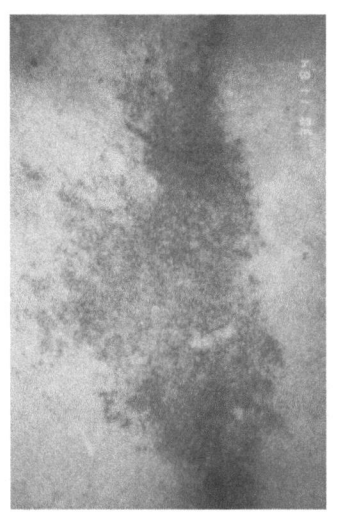 

a) b)

Fig. 2. Vascular birthmark in a 27 years old female patient,
a) before treatment, b) Scarless blanching after 7 treatments with the argonlaser under the "Careful treatment" of water cooling W1

Clinical results

In all 25 patients where this method has been applied the bleaching effect was the same like without cooling and scarring has been totally avoided. The only disadvantage in the W1 method is the doubled time of treatment.

The water cooling method W2 (Clue "Deeper coagulation")

In treatment of port wine stains with deep lying blood vessels after some treatments with the argonlaser no further blanching of the lesion can be achieved because under normal treatment conditions blood vessels are coagulated only to a depth of 1 mm. With this result, a remaining redness, the treatment has to be terminated.

In the W2 method the laser dosis will be increased by means of longer pulse duration and simultaneous power increase (1.5 sec pulse duration, 2.8 watts). Without water cooling, treatment with these parameters would lead to a destruction of the upper skin layers. With water cooling, this destruction will be avoided; at the same time the higher laser dosis leads to an increase in coagulation depth for the blood vessels from 1 mm to over 2 mm. This allows the possibility of blanching stains in a deeper skin layer, which up to now had to be left as remaining redness. The possibility of a deeper coagulation therefore leads to a considerable improvement of the treatment results (fig. 3).

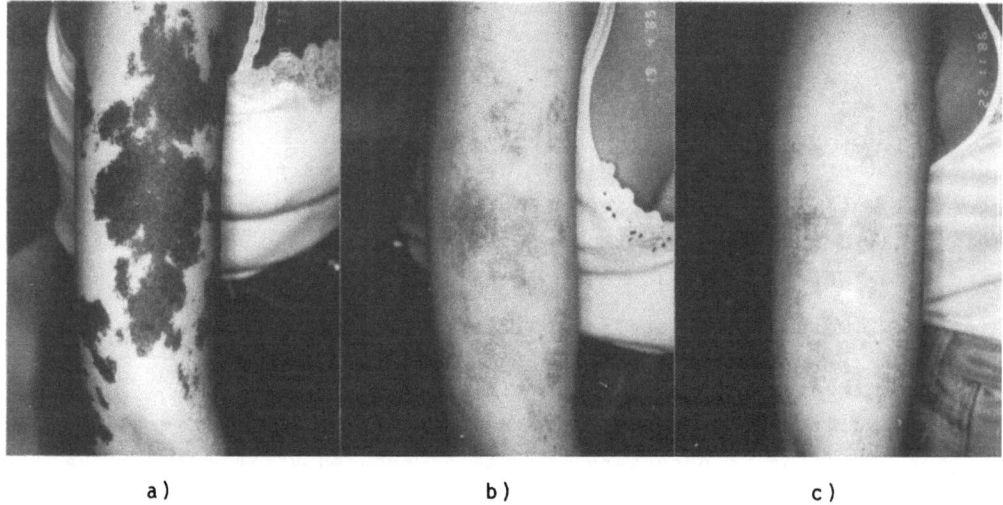

a)   b)   c)

Fig. 3. Dark blue-red port wine stain in a 19 years old patient.
a) Before treatment. b) Rest redness after 8 treatments with the argonlaser without water cooling. c) Optimum blanching after further 4 irradiations under W2 conditions (Deeper coagulation)

Clinical results

So far we have 65 W2 cases from which we can draw final conclusions. The diagram shows that in 69% of the cases a favourable result was obtained (fig. 4). The criteria for the judgement are as follow:

Additional lightening	> 60 % :	excellent
Additional lightening	30-60 % :	good
Additional lightening	< 30 % :	moderate
No additional lightening:		poor

When grouping the treatment results of these 65 W2 cases by age, it can be seen that the rate of fair results is much higher for younger patients (fig. 5).

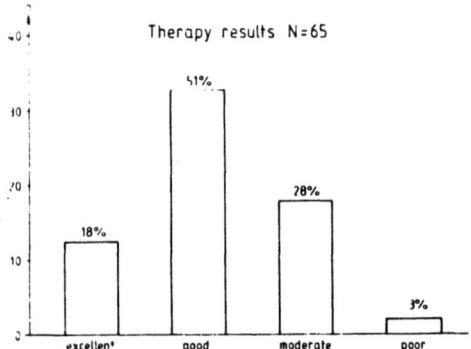

Fig. 4. Therapy results of 65 W2 cases

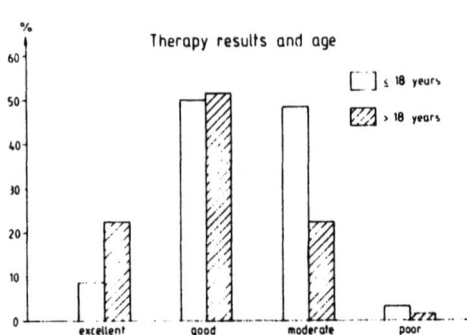

Fig. 5. Grouping by age of the therapy results shown in fig. 4

On the other hand there is higher necessity of water cooling for younger patients. This can be seen from the dotted line in fig. 1, which gives the percentage of port wine stain patients who have been treated under water cooling.

In the W2 method there are several disadvantages:

Time for treatment is about 6 times longer.
The healing time of epidermis damge is longer by the factor 1.5.
Higher attention is necessary because of reduced visibility of the aiming beam.
Intervals of treatment have to be at least 3 months because of the stronger wound redness.

Our clinical results have shown that protection of the skin surface with floating water during argonlaser irradiation is helpful to avoid scar formation ("Careful treatment" W1) and to improve therapy results in treatment of port wine stains with deep lying blood vessels ("Deeper coagulation" W2).

Literatur

/1/ Haina D, Landthaler M, Waidelich W (1987) Possibilities for the increase of the coagulation depth in skin with the argonlaser. In: Waidelich W .....(eds.)......, Springer, Berlin-Heidelberg-New York-Tokyo

New Light Guide with a Sapphire Tip for the Argon Laser

Michael Landthaler[1], Diether Haina[2], Erich Weimel[3],
Wilhelm Waidelich[2,4] and Otto Braun-Falco[1]

1. Dermatologische Klinik und Poliklinik der LMU München
   (Direktor: Prof.Dr.Dr.h.c.O.Braun-Falco)
2. Gesellschaft für Strahlen- und Umweltforschung, Institut für
   Angewandte Optik; Neuherberg
3. Meditec, R. Thyzel GmbH, 8501 Heroldsberg
4. Institut für Medizinische Optik der LMU München (Direktor:
   Prof.Dr.W.Waidelich)

The argon laser is well established for treatment of vascular lesions like port wine stains (3). But the argon laser does not work vessel specific since coagulation of epidermis and superficial dermis occurs. With the usually used parameters of irradiation depth of coagulation is limited to about 1 mm (1, 2, 4).

Aim of the present study was to examine whether it is possible to avoid thermal damage of epidermis and superficial dermis by means of a thin light guide, that can be sticked in the skin and be placed near, or even in the vessel that should be coagulated.

Material and methods

For this purpose a light guide of Meditec Company was used. This light guide ends in a conically shaped 0.2 mm thick sapphire tip. By turning a ring on the hand piece the tip can be extended up to 3 mm. The target of the experimental study were small venous vessels of guinea pig ears. These animal model has proved to be effective in a previous study about the effects of different lasers on epidermis, dermis, and venous vessels (5).

The light guide was sticked in the skin over these vessels and 24 hours after laser exposures of different power an exposure tile (Table 1) lasered tissue was excised and prepared according to routine histological techniques. Controls were irradiations without sticking in the light guide and without laser irradiations. Epidermal damage was measured histometrically, dermal damage judged histologically.

Table 1. Parameters of irradiations

Power	exposure times (s)				
3.0 W	0.8	0.5	0.3	0.2	0.1
1.5 W	0.8	0.5	0.3	0.2	0.1

Controls: irradiation without sticking in (3.0 W/0.8 s); sticking in without irradiation

Results

Exposures of 3 watts output power and an exposure time of 0.8 seconds resulted in broad epidermal damage (1.1 mm), coagulation of dermal tissue and thrombosis of the vessel. Reduction of exposure time to 0.3 and 0.1 seconds respectively led to less dermal and epidermal damage (0.7 and 0.4 mm respectively). A reduction of epidermal damage (0.7 to 0.4 mm) and dermal damage could also be observed with the 1.5 watts series.

Without sticking in the tip of the light guide broad coagulation of epidermis and dermis could be observed, much broader compared to the epidermal damage after sticking in the light guide. Sticking in the tip without irradiation resulted in mechanical disruption of tissue.

Conclusions

The results of this study indicate that it may be possible to reduce epidermal and dermal damage by this new procedure. It remains to be tested whether this light guide is suitable for the treatment of superficial varices and of special deeply located vascular lesions.

Literature

1. Apfelberg DB, Kosek J, Maser MR, Lash H (1979) Histology of port wine stains following argon laser treatment. Br J Plast Surg 32: 232-237

2. Finley JL, Arndt KA, Noe J, Rosen S (1984) Argon laser - port-wine stain interaction. Immediate effects. Arch Dermatol 120:613-619

3. Landthaler M, Haina D, Waidelich W, Braun-Falco O (1984) A three-years experience with the argon laser in dermatotherapy. J Dermatol Surg Oncol 10:456-461

4. Landthaler M, Dorn M, Haina D, Klepzig K, Waidelich W, Braun-Falco O (1983) Morphologische Untersuchungen zur Behandlung von Naevi flammei mit dem Argon-Laser. Hautarzt 34:548-554

5. Landthaler M, Haina D, Brunner R, Waidelich W, Braun-Falco O (1986) Effects of argon, dye, and Nd:YAG lasers on epidermis, dermis, and venous vessels. Lasers Surg Med 6:87-93

A Comparative Study of the Wavelength Dependent Effect of the Argon, Nd: YAG and CO_2 Lasers in ddY Mouse Skin

Toshio Ohshiro, M.D.
Japan Medical Laser Laboratory
TBR Bldg. #607, 5-7 Kojimachi, Chiyoda-ku, Tokyo 102, JAPAN

ABSTRACT

The argon, Nd:YAG and CO_2 lasers are the lasers used most in medicine and surgery. The biological tissue reaction to each laser is primarily wavelength dependent, but basically similar early histologic changes can be achieved by all three laser types despite their wavelength difference. This study was designed to find the irradiation time needed to achieve a similar repeatable biologic reaction for each laser type, and to correlate the findings. Positive Evans blue exudation (EBE) from the laser-irradiated dorsum skin of the ddY mouse was used as the indicator. The correlation of the irradiation times to achieve EBE with the argon laser standardised at 1 was 47.5 for the Nd:YAG and 0.1 for the CO_2. The possible use of these figures in the medical application of the laser is explored.

INTRODUCTION

There have been a number of excellent studies on the wavelength-dependent tissue reactions of each of the main medical lasers, however no study has yet been made of the irradiation time required for each of the lasers to achieve a similar biological effect, given equal spot size and output power, i.e., power density. We felt this might be an interesting parameter to study, since, knowing the correlation factor, one type of laser could in theory be used to replace another.

Accordingly a study was designed using the dorsal skin of the ddY mouse as a target. Since this is a genetically purebred laboratory animal, the data for each result must hold true and be repeatable for all such target subjects.

MATERIALS & METHODS

The argon system used was a Lexell model 295, the Nd:YAG was a Control Systems system, and the CO_2 laser was a NIIC (Nippon Infrared Industries Company) Lasery 30Z system. Both the argon and the YAG systems employ a flexible fibreoptic light guide terminating in a pencil-type handpiece with a 10mm focal length lens, while the CO_2 system uses an articulated arm terminating in a handpiece incorporating a 30mm focal length lens. A HeNe laser provides the aiming beam for both the Nd:YAG and the CO_2 lasers.

Six white male ddY mice, each 25g, were used as a group for each laser. The hair was shaved to 0.7mm in length, and 2ml of 1% Evans blue (Merck Co., Ltd.) in saline solution was injected intraperitoneally into each animal. The mice were then anaesthetised with ether.

5 exposures were duplicated bilaterally on each mouse dorsum, with an output power of 3W, and a spot size of 2mm in diameter, maintained by means of a distancing probe. This is shown in figure 1. 40 minutes postirradiation, the subjects were checked for Evans blue exudation, and the doses at which EBE ocurred were noted for each laser system, from which the energy densities could then be calculated. The irradiated areas were then routinely processed and were evaluated with haematoxylin eosin, Van-Geison's and Mallory's staining. Histological changes in the irradiated skin were recorded by 3 layers. The data were tested statistically using χ^2 and U tests, with the significant difference set at a p value less than 0.05.

RESULTS

The results are summarised in tables 1,2 and 3 (argon, Nd:YAG and CO_2 repectively) for the macroscopic appearance of EBE as seen in figures 2, 3, and 4. EBE appeared at 0.4s for the argon laser, 19.0s for the Nd:YAG and 0.04s for the CO_2. Figures 5, 6 and 7 show EBE histology for the argon, YAG and CO_2 lasers respectively, and the histological data are tabulated in tables 4, 5 and 6.

DISCUSSION

When the dermal capillary walls receive exogenous stimulation of a thermal nature, such as occurs following laser irradiation, protein denaturation occurs in the vessel walls, and the permeability of the walls is affected. Progressively larger particles in the blood stream are then passed through the vessel wall into the surrounding dermal collagen matrix. This process is staged, so the size of particles allowed through is precisely limited. Evans blue particles are consis-

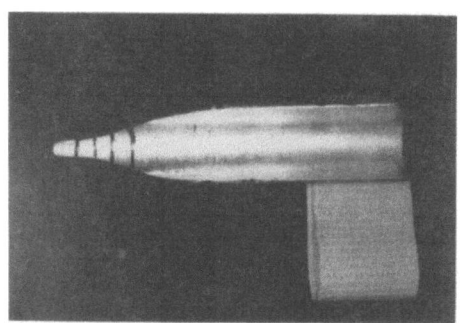

Fig 1. Probe distancing piece. Note Velcro strap to hold piece to probe.

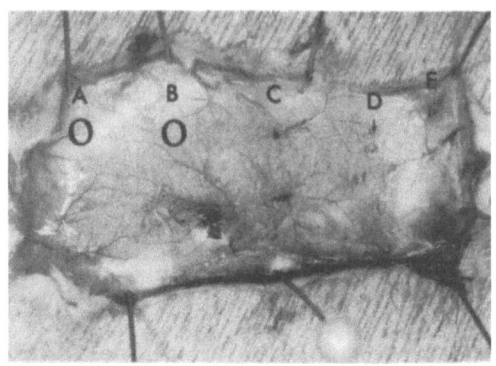

Fig 2. EBE in mouse skin, argon laser at 3W, 2mm dia. spot. Note sharp points.

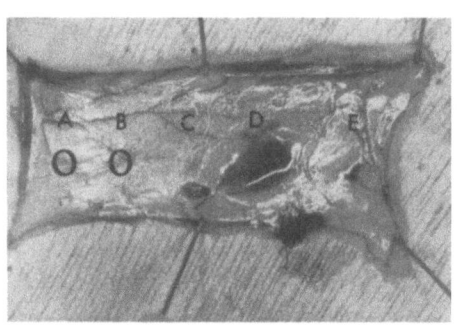

Fig 3. EBE, mouse kin, Nd:YAG laser, 3W, 2mm dia. spot. Note large diffuse spots.

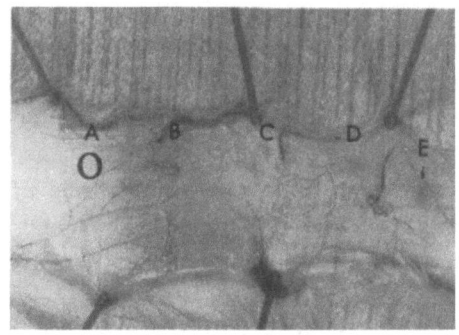

Fig 4. EBE in mouse skin, CO_2 laser, 3W, 2mm dia. Very sharp points.

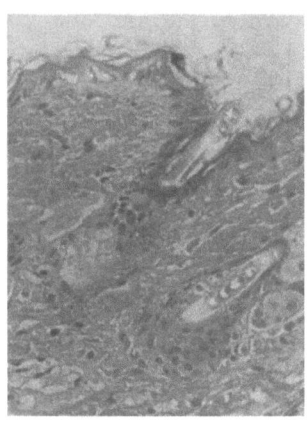

Fig. 5.
ddY mouse skin, argon laser.
H-E stain, x400.

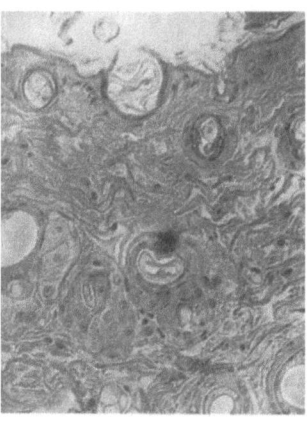

Fig. 6.
ddY mouse skin, CO_2 laser.
H-E stain, x400.

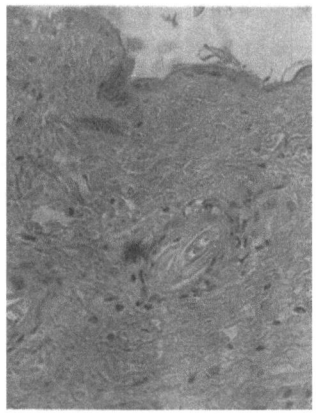

Fig. 7.
ddY mouse skin, Nd:YAG laser.
H-E stain, x400

Table I.
Macroscopic evaluation of visible EBE
with argon laser

Irradiation Time (s)	−	+	x^2 test
0.2	12	0	
0.3	10	2	10.7
0.4	1	11	[p 0.01]
0.5	0	12	
0.6	0	12	

Table II.
Macroscopic evaluation of visible EBE
with Nd:YAG laser

Irradiation Time (s)	−	+	x^2 test
17	12	0	
18	10	2	8.2
19	2	10	[p 0.01]
20	0	12	
21	0	12	

Table III.
Macroscopic evaluation of visible EBE
with CO laser

Irradiation Time (s)	−	+	x^2 test
0.03	10	2	8.2
0.04	2	10	[p 0.01]
0.05	0	12	
0.06	0	12	
0.07	0	12	

Table IV.
Histological evaluation of tissue damage depth
with argon laser

Irradiation time (s)	Epidermis	Upper Dermis	Mid Dermis	U test
0.2	11	1	0	
0.3	9	3	0	3.08
0.4	0	11	1	[p 0.01]
0.5	0	7	5	
0.6	0	1	11	

Table V.
Histological evaluation of tissue damage depth
with Nd:YAG laser

Irradiation time (s)	Epidermis	Upper Dermis	Mid Dermis	U test
17	11	1	0	
18	9	3	0	2.84
19	2	9	1	p [0.01]
20	0	4	8	
21	0	0	12	

Table VI.
Histological evaluation of tissue damage depth
with CO laser

Irradiation time (s)	Epidermis	Upper Dermis	Mid Dermis	U test
0.03	12	0	0	3.4
0.04	4	8	0	[p 0.001]
0.05	0	12	0	
0.06	0	4	8	
0.07	0	0	12	

tently sized (0.5nm0.6nm), thus Evans blue particles in the blood stream will pass through the affected capillary walls into the superficial dermis at a precise stage of the reaction, and will become macroscopically visible as a blue stain in the skin. The appearance of this blue stain is therefore a positive and reliable indication that Evans blue exudation (EBE) is occurring, and for genetically similar tissue types will be easily repeatable with the same laser doses.

Basic laser/tissue reactions are wavelength dependent. The visible blue/green argon laser light is absorbed preferentially in pigment, especially the red pigment of haemoglobin. The energy density required to achieve EBE with the argon laser was approximately $38.2J/cm^2$. The YAG wavelength on the other hand is absorbed mainly in protein. Accordingly the YAG energy penetrates and scatters well in tissue. The energy density necessary to achieve EBE with the YAG laser was approximately $1814J/cm^2$. The CO laser energy at 10600nm is absorbed almost 100% by water molecules. Its heating effect is thus very quick and local. The energy density required to achieve EBE for the CO laser was $3.8J/cm^2$.

The fact that the argon laser is so well absorbed by haemoglobin would indicate that it should cause EBE more efficiently than the CO laser. However, because of the refractive, diffusive effect of the skin and its appendages, the actual energy required to elicit EBE was ten times greater than the CO laser beam. The YAG laser has more of a volume effect, due to its scattering and penetration. The greater the volume, the more energy is required to heat it to any given temperature. The YAG laser required 475 times the CO laser energy to achieve a similar EBE.

With the argon standardised at 1, the correlation factors for the Nd:YAG and CO were 47.5 and 0.1 respectively. These correlations could therefore allow a clinician to use the YAG or CO laser in place of the argon, for example.

Effects of Laserlight of Low Power Density on Sebaceous Glands

Michael Landthaler[1], Diether Haina[2], Christoph Ohngemach[1], Wilhelm Waidelich[3] and Otto Braun-Falco[1]

1. Dermatologische Klinik der LMU München (Direktor: Prof.Dr.Dr.h.c. O.Braun-Falco)
2. Gesellschaft für Strahlen- und Umweltforschung, Institut für Angewandte Optik, Neuherberg
3. Institut für Medizinische Optik der LMU München (Direktor. Prof.Dr. W. Waidelich)

In contrast to laserlight of high power density therapeutical application of laserlight of low power density remains still questionable (1, 2). At least in Europe the so called soft lasers and MID lasers are recommended for treatment of various conditions and in dermatology especially for the treatment of acne vulgaris. But up to now no scientific data are available. We therefore decided to examine the effect of laserlight of low power density on sebaceous glands, since these glands play an important role in the pathogenesis of acne vulgaris. Sebum output is an absolute prerequisite of acne and all measures which reduce sebum production improve the disease (3).

Material and methods

We have used the animal model of Syrian hamsters, which is well established in sebaceous gland research (4). The study was performed in adult male hamsters with a bodyweight of about 100 g. The earlobes are richly endowed with sebaceous glands, which are rather similar to human sebaceous follicle (4).

The following light sources and physical parameters of irradiation were used (Table 1).

Five groups of animals were irradiated, in each of the groups 5 hamsters (Table 2).

The left ear was irradiated, the right ear was the individual control. After at least 20 daily irradiations the animals were sacrificed and the ears prepared according to routine histological techniques. At

Table 1   Physical parameters of irradiations

	(nm)	PD (mW/cm²)	t	number of irrad.	total dose (J/cm²)
Incoherent red light source (irls)	633	9.7	72 s	20	14
Biolas (MBB-AT)	633	0.75	5 min	22	5
Model 124a (Spectra Physics)	633	9.7	72 s	20	14

Table 2   Irradiation of hamster ears

Group	n	light source	irradiated side
A	5	irls	dorsal
B	5	Biolas	dorsal
C	5	m 124a	ventral
D	5	m 124a	dorsal
E	5		controls

least 50 dorsal and 50 ventral glands of each ear were measured histometrically by means of a Contron IBAS 2000.

Results

In no one of the groups differences between the irradiated and non-irradiated sebaceus glands could be found (Fig. 1).

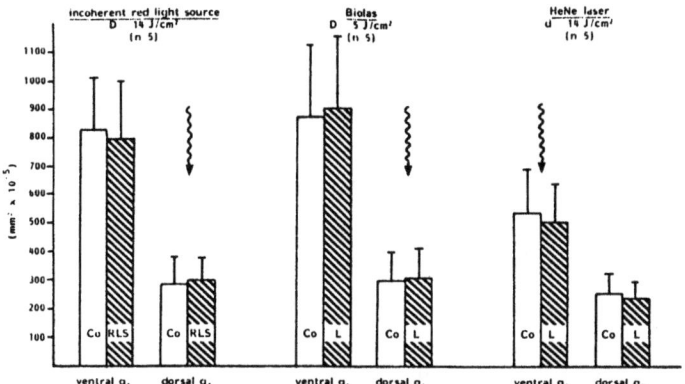

Fig. 1. Effects of irradiations with different red light sources on sebaceous glands

Conclusion

These data clearly demonstrate that laser light of low power density of the used wavelength had no effect on size of the sebaceous glands in Syrian hamsters. A beneficial effect on sebum production, the major pathogenetic factor of acne, could be excluded by the study.

Literature

1. Brunner , Haina D, Landthaler M, Waidelich W, Braun-Falco O (1986) Appplication of laser light of low power density. Experimental and clinical investigations. In: Hönigsmann H, Stingl G (eds) Therapeutic photomedicine. Curr Prbl Dermatol 15. Karger, Basel, pp 111-116

2. Greguss P (1984) Low-level laser therapy - reality or myth? Optics Laser Technol IV:81-85

3. Plewig G, Kligman A (1975) Acne. Morphogenesis and treatment. Springer, Berlin-Heidelberg-New York

4. Plewig G, Luderschmidt C (1977) Hamster ear model for sebaceous glands. J Invest Dermatol 68:171-176

Large Scale Treatment of Dermatoses Using He Ne- and IR-Laser Radiation

S. Chlebarov

Abteilung fuer Dermatologie und Allergologie
der Klinik Borkum Riff der BfA
Hindenburgstr. 126, D-2972 Borkum

Materials, methods and results

The apparatus [1] used by us has been developed for external treatment of large size skin areas. It is equipped with a He-Ne-Laser (632.8 nm wavelength, 10 mW peak power) and a GaAs-Laserdiode (904 nm wavelength in the infra red) emitting pulses with a peak power of 72 W, 200 ns pulse duration and 600- 1400 Hz repetition frequency. The visible He-Ne laser beam also provides a guiding aid for the infrared application. The area of irradiation can be varied at different oscillation frequencies by means of a vibrating electrodynamical scanner.

In addition an UV-source (275 nm wavelength, 8 W power) is also provided and can be applied if necessary. As regard to the depth effect both lasers (He-Ne and IR) influence the therapeutic results favourably.

88 patients exhibiting dermatological findings were treated with the apparatus. The irradiation was carried out without any other treatment. The distance of the laser head was adjusted according to the appropriate area of treatment. On the average the distance was 50 cm. Duration of irradiation was set at 15 min once a day. Care was taken such that the laser beam hits the skin being treated perpendicularly. Energy dose and duration can be adjusted individually by a built-in timer. This combined irradation was very compatible to all patients; it did not cause any kind of unpleasant sensations. There were no undesirable side-effects observed.

---

1) Felas Medical Laser MED 10

Table 1. Results

Kind of Diseases	Number of treatment	completely healed	changed for better	unchanged	total
ulcus cruris and others	25	5	5	1	11
zoster	8	12	5	-	17
scars, keloides	18	-	9	5	14
verrucae, plantares	19	1	-	4	5
acne	23	2	6	3	11
vitiligo	12	-	2	1	3
loss of hair	20	-	-	3	3
herpes simpl. recid.	7	2	-	-	2
prurigo	12	-	2	2	4
facial wrinkles	15	-	1	2	3
granuloma anulare	15	-	1	-	1
eczema chronicum	8	-	1	1	2
prerioral dermatitis	5	-	1	-	1
pruritus vulvae	12	1	1	-	2
pain	6	1	3	-	4
arthralgia	12	1	2	2	5
		2 (28%)	3 (45%)	2 (27%)	88 (100%)

The types of dermatoses which were treated, the number of irradiations applied and the therapeutic results are listed in the table below.

Comment on the results

To begin with it must be noted that out of a total of 88 dermatoses treated 25 of them healed completely and in 39 cases have been improved significantly. Together there are 73 % of finding influenced favourably. Only 24 (27%) of the cases remained unchanged.

The effects of the treatment of ulcus cruris and of other ulcerations resistent to other therapies were very favourable. Spontaneous cleansing of the ulcus took place, fresh granulation has formed, significant vascularisation and subsequent epithelization and pain relief were achieved. An average of 25 irradiations were carried out. The ulcus was already completely closed at the end of 16 irradiation treatments on one women patient. Another patient had two small ulcers on the outside of her right ankle of which only one was treated. This one healed completely about six weeks later. The one which received no radiation remained almost unchanged.

All those patients suffering from zoster were completely healed or improved significantly after 8 irradiations on the average. One has to emphasize that laser irradiation is not a miracle cure for zoster which would heal completely anyway but it is established that the process of healing proceeds more quickly in comparison to the application of other methods and that the unpleasant pain is soothed and above all very quickly soothed.

9 out of the 14 hypertrophic scars and scar keloids respectively, have improved noticably. 5 remained unchanged after an average of 18 irradiations. It was also noticed that the scar became flatter and the scar tissue became softer and smoother on keloids which had been in existence longer.

We experienced a marked improvement on 8 out of 11 patients being treated for acne. Two of them were free of symtoms after 23 irradiations. Acute inflamation, infiltrates and erythema disappeared slowly and the infected skin was calmed and no forming of efflorences typical of acne took place.

On two vitiligo patients we observed a repigmentation of the skin in small patches which was unfortunately only temopary after concluding the average 12 irradiations which were carried out.

Only on one patient with <u>verrucae plantares</u> did these disappear after 17 irradiations. The remaining 4 continued to exist during the period of observation.

The <u>diffuse loss of hair</u> on three patients could not be influenced favourably after an average of 20 irradiations.

Both patients suffering from <u>chronic recidivating herpes simplex,</u> accompanied by unpleasant pain, itching and taughtness could be discharged after a very short time free of symtoms and ailments.

On two patients the <u>prurigo knot</u> became flatter and the irritation was lessened; two remained unchanged.

A lady's <u>facial wrinkles</u> have also been clearly improved after the application of this combined irradiation. After about 15 irradiations of the face the tissue of the skin was tightend and the wrinkles flatter. The application of this method on subjective sensations such as pruritus vulvae, postzoster neuralgae and arthralgia in the case of arthropathies were influenced favourably in 9 cases out of a total 11 patients treated. In 3 of the patients the symtoms disappeared completely.

Discussion

The majority of work done in this field is concerned with the combined application of the He-Ne-laser plus the IR laser on ulcerations, the treatment of scars and keloids and pain conditions of varying genesis.

Clearly positive results and effective therapy were observed during treatment of these symtoms. We also suppose that an acceleration of the blood circulation by widening of capillaries and subsequent stimulation of cellular metabolism which causes in turn accelerated formation of granulation tissue and rapid epithelization to be responsible for these findings (Haas et al 1986).

The recession of oedema swellings could be explained by the

change in the hydrostatic intracapillary pressure causing larger absorption of tissue liquid within intercellular fissures.

It might be suggested that the threshold of perception of the algotrophic nerve endings is raised which results in a pain killing action. As a secondary action an electrolyte exchange , due to influences on the ionic charge reversal at the cell membrane, is obtained which stimulates the metabolism.

A certain stimulation of the immune system and an increase in antibody formation is also observed .

The quantum energy transferable is perhaps sufficient in order to induce conformation changes e.g. in proteins. We presume the laser irradiation causes photochemical changes so that the mitochondrial transport system of the orithine membrane is "damaged". (Pratzel and Chlebarov 1982,1984; Chlebarov 1983, 1984, 1985,1986). This system reacts extremely sensitively to UV radiation (Pratzel and Geiger 1977). Therefore one might call this effect biostimulation. The failure of mitochondriae is quite a normal process in epidermal differentiation (Pratzel 1985).

The action mechanism of laser radiation has still to be investigated in order to prove the clear biological effects.

Literature is available from the author .

Tunable Lasers in Dermatology: Determination of Action Spectra

A. Anders, M. Knälmann, E.-G. Niemann, H. Tronnier[x]
Inst. für Biophysik Universität Hannover
Hautklinik, Städt. Kliniken Dortmund[x]/ FRG

Tunable lasers are ideal light sources for photodermatological research because of their monochromaticity, high spectral intensity and tunability of the wavelength. Thus action spectra e.g. of erythema and pigmentation can be determined with high accuracy. An improved knowledge of erythema and pigmentation reactions is of great interest concerning the photo- and photochemotherapy of special skin diseases like psoriasis with UV light or the use of intense UVA irradiation for cosmetic tanning.

Action spectra

The following action spectra in the UV are of photomedical interest:
- erythema effectiveness curve
- melagonesis spectrum
- these curves after administration of photosensitizers (e.g. 8-methoxy-psoralen)
- action spectra for photo- and photochemotherapy of skin diseases (e.g. psoriasis)

Most of these action spectra are not yet exactly determined. Also, contradictory results are found in the literature. Up till now, lamps

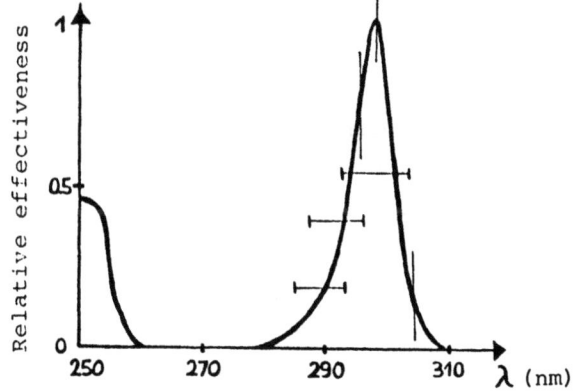

Fig. 1. Example of an action spectrum - erythema effectiveness curve - (effect versus irradiation wavelength); vertical line (|): indication of the laser bandwidth; horizontal line (⊢⊣): typical spectral bandwidth of lamps with monochromators

and monochromators were nearly always used for the determination of
action spectra. Such irradiation systems normally have to be operated
with spectral bandwidths of 5-2o nm to get enough intensity. Fig. 1
shows that spectral bandwidths of lamps and monochromators are often in
the order of magnitude of the halfbandwidths of the curves to be determined.
On the contrary action spectra can be determined with high accuracy
using tunable lasers. These lasers have spectral bandwidths smaller
than o,1 nm and the wavelength can be tuned over the whole spectrum.

Experimental

For our experiments we used pulsed laser systems in the UV: 25o-37o nm.
- Flashlamp-pumped dye laser
- Excimer laser pumped dye laser

The action spectra were determined as follows:
- Selection of suitable probands (Caucasians)
- Irradiation of small skin areas
- Variation of the irradiation intensity and -wavelength
- Observation of the skin reaction (erythema, pigmentation)

Examples

1. Erythema effectiveness curve

This action spectrum was very often measured in the wavelength range
25o-31o nm (UVC,UVB). The spectrum investigated with dye lasers is more
narrow-banded than the ones which were determined with lamps and monochromators.
The halfbandwidth of the erythema effectiveness curve around
the maximum at 297 nm is in the order of magnitude of 1o nm. The reaction
of the skin is strongly dependent on the irradiation wavelength as
this result shows (1). This dependency was also shown in theoretical
calculations in which irradiation sources with different bandwidths for
the determination of an action spectrum were presumed (1).

2. Action spectrum of 8-methoxypsoralen in the UVA

The information about the efficiency of 8-methoxypsoralen in the UVA are
contradictorily in the literature (3), e.g. two different maxima of
this photosensitizer were postulated. By our dye laser measurements it
was shown that these contradictions exist no longer. We found a maximum
at 355 nm confirming earlier findings in the literature and a hint
that there is another maximum at about 33o nm (2). Some more experiments
will be done to clarify further discrepancies.

3. Erythema and pigmentation reactions

Determining the minimal erythema and pigmentation doses we observed discrepancies with values in the literature known so far. Our erythema curve, found by laser irradiation, e.g. decreases much stronger than the curve of Parrish et al. (4) (Fig. 2). Furthermore, our preliminary results concerning a persistent (delayed) pigmentation in the UVA are inconsistent with the experiments carried out by Parrish et al.. For example we need much more intensity (J/cm^2) about 360 nm for producing a minimal pigmentation. As, besides, the curve of Parrish et al. was investigated with broad spectral bandwidths (up to 20 nm) and great steps of measurements (up to 30 nm) in the UVA a further re-evaluation and completion should be performed.

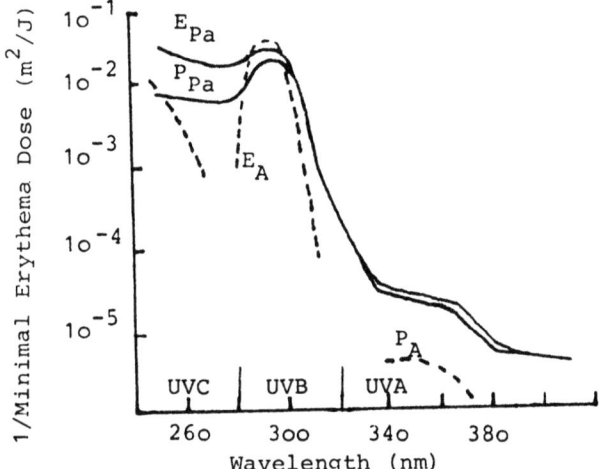

Fig. 2. Minimal erythema and pigmentation doses (reciprocal values) in dependence on the irradiation wavelength.

Solid line E_{Pa}: erythema (Parrish et al. (4) - read after 24 h
Solid line P_{Pa}: pigmentation (Parrish et al.(4)- read after 7 days
Dotted line E_A: erythema (Anders et al. (1); to be published) - read after 24 h
Dotted line P_A: pigmentation (Anders et al., to be published) - read after 3 days

References

1. A. Anders, A. Aufmuth, E.-M. Böttger, H. Tronnier:
   Investigation of the erythema effectiveness curve with tunable lasers: Dermatosen: 32, 166 (1984)
2. A. Anders, M. Knälmann, H. Tronnier:
   The UVA action spectrum of 8-methoxypsoralen in human skin investigated with dye lasers: Dermatosen, in press
3. D.J. Cripps, N.J. Lowe, A.B. Lerner:
   Action spectrum of topical psoralens: a re-evaluation. Brit. J. Dermatol. 107, 77 (1982)
4. J.A. Parrish, K.F. Jaenicke, R.R. Anderson:
   Erythema and melagonesis spectra of normal human skin. Photochem. Photobiol.: 36, 187 (1982)

Morphologic Effects of Short Argon and Dye Laser Pulses

K. Klepzig[1], M. Landthaler[1], D. Haina[2], W. Waidelich[2,3], O. Braun-Falco[1]

1. Department of Dermatology, University of Munich (Chairman: Prof.Dr.Dr.h.c.O.Braun-Falco), Frauenlobstraße 9-11, D-8000 Munich 2, Federal Republic of Germany
2. GSF, Inst. für Angewendete Optik, Neuherberg
3. Inst. für Medizinische Optik, Universität München

The goal of the present study was to characterize the effect of different durations of dye laser pulses in comparison to the changes following short argon laser pulses.

MATERIALS AND METHODS

The study was performed at the dorsal aspects of male white guinea pigs. Argon and dye lasers were used as described elsewhere (4).

Following irradiation series were performed:

1) Dye laser spot size 0,5 mm, output power (N) 0,7 W, pulse duration (t) 0.02 s, power density (PD) 356 W/cm^2 dose (D) 7,1 J/cm^2.
2) Dye laser spot size 0,5 mm, N=0.7 W, t=0,05 s, PD=356 W/cm^2, D=17.8 J/cm^2.
3) Argon laser spot size 0,5 mm, N=1,5 W, t=0,02 s, PD=746 W/cm^2, D=15.3 J/cm^2.

Laser defects were excized 24 hours following irradiation and prepared for routine histological technique using hemalaun and eosin staining. For electron microscopy pieces of tissue were fixed with osmium tetroxide and epon embedded. Electron microscop Philips 300.

RESULTS

Dye laser pulses of 0.02 s induced a specific injury of blood vessels beneath an intact epidermis as could be seen lightmicroscopically. Ultrastructural examination of the epidermis revealed the presence of some small cytoplasmatic vacuoles in the basal keratinocytes although organelles including nuclei, mitochondria, endoplasmatic reticulum and basement membrane zone remained intact, as did the adjacent dermal collagen. Blood vessels showed marked endothelial swelling and narrowed vascular lumen with aggregation of platelets and abnormal shaped and abnormal electron dense red blood cells. On higher magnification swelling of mitochondria, perinuclear edema and myelinoid artificial membrane structures were obvious (Fig 1.).

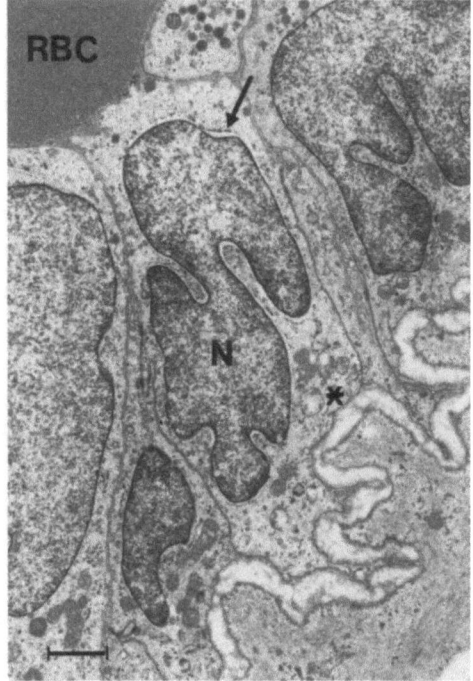

Fig 1. (left side) Dye laser - 7.1 J/cm^2. Anoxic injury of endothelial cells with perinuclear edema (↑), swelling of mitochondria (*); intraluminal red blood cells (RBC). (⊢ 1μm)

In surrounding smooth muscle cells marked and more severe cytoplasmatic vacuolisation was found. There was a slight perivascular edema but perivascular collagen seemed to be intact.

Application of dye laser pulses of 0.05 s resulted - as could be seen lightmicroscopically - in a necrosis of keratinocytes throughout all epidermal layers, a widerspread cleft formation through the basal layer and edematous injury of adjacent dermal collagen. Electronmicroscopically the cellular outlines of basal keratinocytes could hardly be discerned. The basement membrane, however, was intact and followed every part of the contour in the upper dermis. The adjacent collagen revealed focal loss of periodic structure of collagen fibrils and well defined foci of flocculent material between the fibrils. Blood vessels showed marked transmural necrosis with destruction and disintegration of endothelial cells, smooth muscle cells and pericytes (Fig 2.). Intraluminally they contained large masses of agglutinated red blood cells and platelets. Changes of perivascular collagen were equal to those of upper dermal collagen.

Argon laser pulses of 0.02 s duration but with a comparable dose (15.3 J/cm^2) induced injuries similar to those of 0.05 s dye laser pulses (17.8 J/cm^2). Keratinocytes were necrotic throughout all epidermal layers, intrabasal cleft formation was prominent, adjacent dermal and perivascular collagen showed foci of denaturation and blood vessels revealed transmural necrosis and intraluminal thrombusformation.

DISCUSSION

The results of this study confirm the findings which recently had been reported that specific vessel injury could be achieved by application of short dye laser pulses. Dye laser pulses at 577nm are selectively absorbed by oxyhemoglobin and lead when laser exposure is short enough to a selective coagulation of red blood cells.

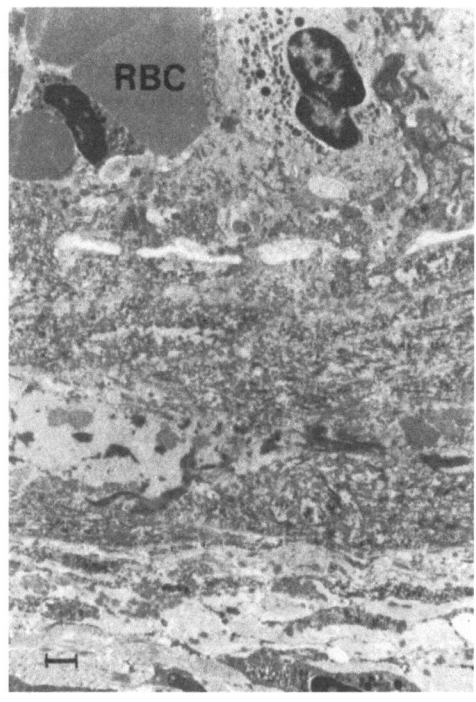

Fig 2. (right side) Dye laser - 17.8 J/cm². Transmural necrosis of blood vessels. (⊢ 1µm)

This results in a intravascular thrombusformation. Vascular occlusion and ischemia causes metabolic stress due to hypoxemia and anoxia to endothelial cells, pericytes and smooth muscle cells. Ultrastructural effects of pronounced anoxic injury are generalized edema, edematous swelling of perinuclear sac, endoplasmatic reticulum (RER) and mitochondria leading in some cases to total rupture of their outer envelope. As further anoxia takes part, myelinoid "artificial membrane" structures from the reassembly of the phospholipid and cholesterol break down products of disintegrated unit membranes develop (2).
Our findings confirm the observations of Tong AKF et al. (7). The fact that smooth muscle cells are more susceptible to anoxic injury may explain the more severe intracytoplasmatic vacuolisation in smooth muscle cells in comparison to those seen in endothelial cells despite being ana-

tomically in greater distance from the blood vessel lumen than endothelial cells. This fact had been documented by Nakagawa et al. (5) too. Prolongation of dye laser pulse duration - in our irradiation series from 0.02 s to 0,05 s - leads to a thermal diffusion from the target tissue (red blood cells) to the other nearby structures in heating these to denaturating or vaporizing temperatures (7). The tissue destruction following dye laser pulses of 0.05 s (D 17.8 J/cm^2) equally to the injuries following argon laser pulses of 0.02 s (D 15.3 J/cm^2) are comparable to those induced by acute burn (1). Although there could hardly be detected a quantitative difference by electronmicroscopy qualitative changes were almost the same.

REFERENCES

1. Cuppage FE, Leape LL, Tate A: Morphologic changes in rhesus monkey skin after acute burn. Arch Pathol 95:402-406, 1973.
2. Constantinides P: Ultrastructural Pathobiology. Elsevier Amsterdam, New York, Oxford, 1984.
3. Greenwald J, Rosen S, Anderson SS, Harrist T, MacFarland F, Noe J, Parrish JA: Comparable histological studies of the tunable dye (at 577nm) and argon laser: The specific vascular effects of dye laser. J Invest Dermatol 77:305-310, 1981.
4. Landthaler M, Haina D, Brunner R, Waidelich W, Braun-Falco O: Effects of Argon, Dye and ND: YAG lasers on epidermis, dermis, and veneous vessels. Lasers Surg Med 6:87-93, 1986.
5. Nakagawa H, Tan OT, Parrish JA: Ultrastructural changes in human skin after exposure to a pulsed laser. J Invest Dermatol 84:396-400, 1985.
6. Tan OT, Carney JM, Margolis R, Seki Y, Boll J, Anderson RR, Parrish JA: Histologic responses of port wine stains treated by argon, carbon dioxide, and tunable dye laser. Arch Dermatol 122:1018-1022, 1986.
7. Tong AWF, Tan OT, Boll J, Parrish JA, Murphy GF: Ultrastucture: Effects of melanin pigment on target specificity using a pulsed dye laser (577nm). J Invest Dermatol 88:747-752, 1987.

CO_2 Laser Microsurgery for Skin Lesions

G.BANDIERAMONTE, O.SANTORO, P.LEPERA, G.FAVA, G.DE PALO

National Tumor Institute
Via G. Venezian 1, 20133 - Milano, Italy

Abstract
A series of 52 malignant and 310 benign skin lesions was selected for laser microsurgery from Jan. 1982 to Dec. 1985. Epithelial (13.3%), pigmented (17.2%) soft tissue (32.1%), pseudotumoral (33.1%) and inflammatory lesions (4.4%) were located on the face (58%), scalp (5%), extremities (10.2%), trunk or limbs (16%) and perianal area (10.5%). CO_2 laser models used were Valfivre LSS 25, Coherent 450, and Cooper 250 Z coupled with the ZEISS OPMI-6 operating microscope (focal lens 200 mm). Laser systems were used at 10 to 15 W, CW and superpulsed emission spot size was 0.5 to 1.5 mm. Resection was used in 58% of cases, vaporization or combined procedure were used in the remaining cases. Of the 52 malignant lesions, 4 (7.7%) had unevaluable radicality for thermal damage, 7 (13.5%) persisted, and 1 (1.9%) recurred in a follow up ranging from 6 to 36 months. Of the 310 benign lesions, 96.4% had good to excellent cosmetic results without complications, 3 cases (1%) had prolonged pain and edema, 5 cases (1.6%) had hyperplastic scars and 8 cases (2.6%) recurred. CO_2 laser microsurgery appears to be a precise and effective alternative treatment modality especially for benign exophytic and critically located lesions.

Introduction
A compact platform of multidisciplinary collaboration has enabled us to use the CO_2 laser in many different surgical fields. CO_2 laser was recognized particularly suitable for a wide range of surgical requirements, being precise incision, istantaneous sealing of small blood and lymphatic vessels and absorption independent from the tissue surface color the main characteristcs of this type of laser (1). The progressive insertion of this new technique for skin surgery have made it possible the routine use for selected malignant and benign lesions (2-4). In this study our experience is reviewed in order to check the indications, the technique, used and the clinical results of CO_2 laser microsurgical treatment for skin lesions.

Materials and Methods
Study population
From Jan. 1982 to Dec. 1985, a total of 362 patients affected with benign or malignant skin lesions were selected for CO2 laser microsurgery. 178 were male and 184 were female. Median age was 46 years (range 8-84). Selection of the case was based on the following criteria: 1) presumable diameter of vessels less than 1 mm, within the lesion area, 2) minimal depth of infiltration (not reaching the fat dermal layer), 3) questionable result obtainable with conventional surgery, especially for anatomic location. Anatomic location of the selected skin lesions was: 211 of the face (58%), 18 lesions of the scalp (5%), 17 of hand and foot areas (4.7%), 20 of the fingers (5.5%), 58 of the trunk and limbs (16%), 38 perianal lesions (10.5%). Of the 211 lesions of the face, 38 were located on the

surface of the cheeks, chin and forehead (18%), 24 on the eyelids (11.4%), 23 on the ear surface (10.9%), 34 on the nose (16.1%) and 92 on the cutaneous portion of the lips (43.6%).

Except for 3 lesions of about 70 mm maximum diameter, the range of lesion diameter varied from 3 to 30 mm. The distribution of the 362 cases by histology was: 1) benign epithelial (1.4%), 2) malignant epithelial (11.9%), 3) benign pigmented (17.2%), 4) benign soft tissue lesions (29.6%), 5 malignant soft tissue lesions (2.5%), 6) pseudotumoral (33.1%), 7) inflammatory (4.4%). Benign lesions were evaluated monthly for the first 3 months after surgery and quarterly thereafter. Malignant lesions were followed monthly for the first three months postoperatively and bimonthly thereafter.

Instruments and techniques

Three CO_2 laser instruments were used for skin microsurgery: 1) the Valfivre LSS 25 reaches 25 W maximum output power. Its beam mode is combined between TEM 00 and TEM 11, 2) the Coherent 450 has a maximum output power of 20 W with a doughnut-shaped transverse beam mode (TEM 01 *), 3) the Cooper 250 Z model reaches 35 W, CW, with a TEM 00 beam mode. It has pulsed emission of the beam, repetition rate available up to 999 HZ. All lasers were used in association with the Zeiss OPMI-6 operating microscope at 200 mm focal distance. Beam spot diameter varied from 0.5 to 2 mm. Average irradiance was 2×10^3 W/cm^2

Training of the surgeon, nursing staff education and safety measures were applied. Particular attention was given to the surgical expertise in order to minimize the tissue thermal damage and to optimize the recognition of the anatomic land-marks, while operating under microscopic magnification, thus having an exact control over the depth of penetration during laser procedure. Under local anesthesia, for the removal of the 362 skin lesions the following procedures were used: 1) excisional technique without subsequent suturing of the wound, in 209 cases (57.8%), 2) Excision plus sutures in 11 cases (3%), 3) vaporization in 103 benign lesions (28.4%) and 4) combined technique (5) (resection plus peripheral vaporization of the outer margins of the lesion) in 39 cases (10.8%). Wet gauze sponges were always used to cool the tissue and to remove carbonized particles after laser removal. Hydrogen peroxide was used to surface medication and dressing was used for 1 to 3 days postoperatively.

Results

Of the 52 malignant lesions treated by laser microsurgery 12 (19.4%) had unfavorable clinical results. Four of the 12 had unvaluable radicality of the surgical specimen, because of the thermal damage at the lesion borders (1 case of basal cell ca., 1 squamous cell ca., 1 sebaceous ca., and 1 leiomyosarcoma). This led to the need of further radicalization which was performed by external radiation therapy (3 cases) and cold knife excision (1 case). Seven cases revealed persistent disease within 3 months after laser microsurgery, confirmed by positive histologic examination, (3 cases of basal cell ca., 2 cases of squamous cell ca., 1 malignant fibrous histiocytoma and 1 Kaposi' sarcoma) which required further surgery (6 cases) and external beam radiation (Kaposi' sa.).

Its is noteworthy that 3 of the persistent disease (2 basal cell ca. of the facial area and 1 squamous cell of the lower right eyelid) were recurrences after radiation therapy).

After all these combined treatments, only 1 case recurred (basal cell carcinoma of the left cheek) in a follow-up period ranging from 6 to 36 months.

No other complications were observed as regards to the postoperative course and the cosmetic result for the cured cases was good.

Of the 310 benign lesions treated by laser microsurgery a very low incidence of unfavourabale results were observed. Small hemangiomas (36 cases) had a rate of complications of 4/36 since 1 case had prolonged pain and edema, 1 case had hyperplastic scar, and 2 out of the 8 retreated cases have recurred (5.5%); one case of warts of the fingers had prolonged pain and edema, whereas 6/69 cases of wart of the sole and perianal area recurred after primary treatment. The other three unfavourable results were 1 case of prolonged pain and edema which was noted after wide resection for an inflammatory lesion of the left leg, and 2 cases of hyperplastic scar after laser vaporization for keratosis of the hand and after resection of a pyogenic granuloma of the auricular region.

Discussion and conclusion

The rationale for using the carbon dioxide laser to treat the cited lesion was the removal of the entire area of the lesion under microscopic magnification to a desired depth so that minimizing the intraoperative bleeding, the postoperative complications and that rapid healing would occur from the underlying tissue at the base of the wound. Intraoperative microscopic detection and laser removal was important both for malignant and benign lesions, thus the width and depth of tissue removal were related to the type and site of the lesion. Nonetheless irregular spreading patterns of cancer cells led to an amount persistent disease (6). For these reason laser microsurgery for malignant skin lesions should be selectively indicated when very conservative management is requested especially for critical sites or poorly accesible anatomic location, i.e. eyelid margins or ears. Here, careful attention and the highest magnification power of the surgical field should be used to avoid poor cosmetic results and treatment failure. For critical sites, improved result may be obtained when using a combination procedure (sub-total excision + peripheral vaporization with radicalization or modelling purpose). Benign exophytic lesions were considered the most suitable indications for CO_2 laser microsurgery. The lack of the need for surgical sutures led usually good or excellent cosmetic result, with a negligible amount of complications. Healing by secondary intention is considered of choice when a special conservative management of superficial lesions is required, owing to the possibility of avoiding suture disfigurement while simplifying the surgical procedure.

References

1. Fuller T.A. Foundamentals of lasers in surgery and medicine. In: Dixon J.A. (Ed.): Surgical applications of lasers. Chicago Yearbook Med. Publ. 1983, pp. 11-28.
2. Goldman L. Laser surgery for skin cancer. New York State J. Med. 81 1897-1900, 1977.
3. Kirschner R.A. Cutaneous plastic surgery with CO_2 laser. Surg. Clin. North Am. 64: 871-883, 1984.
4. Oshiro T. The CO_2 laser as an ideal microsurgical tool. Lasers Surg. Med. 6: 29-37, 1986.
5. Bailin P.L. Use of CO_2 laser for Non-PWS cutaneous lesions. In "Cutaneous laser therapy: Principles and methods". K.A. Arndt, J.M. Noe and S. Rosen (Eds), John Wiley & Sons Ltd; 1983, pp 187-199.
6. Mohs F.E., Latrop T.G., Modes of spread of cancer of skin. Arch. Dermatol. Syph. 66: 427-432, 1952.

CO₂ Laser and Cavernous Haemangiomas

F. LAFFITTE, J.P. CHAVOIN, D. ROUGE, M. COSTAGLIOLA
Department of Plastic Surgery, Rangueil Hospital 31054 TOULOUSE - France

During our five year's experience of the CO_2 laser, we have been able to pick out a certain number of indications where this laser is particularly useful. Cavernous haemangiomas are among them.

The cutting and haemostatic qualities of the laser beam result in a distinct improvement in ease of operation for the surgeon, as bleeding is considerably reduced and the field of operation can be clearly seen.

According to the case, the CO_2 laser can be used on a focalised mode, to cut the skin facing the angioma, or on a defocalised mode to vaporise progressively the cavernous lesion. Cutting out the lesion, which was formerly the tricky part of the operation, is thus unnecessary. We always use a handpiece with a short focal distance of 50 mm, or less if possible. The output necessary at tissue level varies from 10 to 50 watts depending on the size of the lesion. The tissue is vaporised by successive scanning until healthy tissue is reached. The electric knife can be used occasionally if the CO_2 laser is not sufficient for haemostasis of a pedicle or a large blood lake (diameter between 0,5 mm and 1 mm).

Depending on tumour volume, the patient can be treated as an outpatient, with local anaesthetic, or loco-regional or general anaesthetic can be used during a short stay in hospital (3 days).

The patient always benefits from excellent post-operative comfort (no oedema or inflammation). Healing takes place in 10 days to 3 weeks, without fibrosis or scar retraction, particularly in mucous tissue (inside the mouth, for example). Contrary to conventional methods, there is no crust to fall later, so the danger of post-operative haemorrhage is removed.

Embolisation is not always necessary beforehand, especially with capillary cavernous haemangiomas, but it is indispensable with large diameter venous lakes. In our series, one patient presented with a cheek lesion which had previously been operated on somewhere else and various vessels had been ligated including the external carotid artery. Embolisation was thus impossible, and when we treated the lesion inside the cheek, the patient lost 2 litres of blood during the operation and transfusion was necessary in spite of the CO_2 laser. Nevertheless, the result was very satisfactory.

Where embolisation is not done, vasopressin must be injected locally at the correct dilution. This gives very effective vasoconstriction and it is easier to use the laser.

After our small series of 32 patients with lesions of varying size, form and location (face, mouth, fingers), we believe the CO_2 laser represents a considerable progress in the treatment of cavernous haemangiomas, both for the surgeon while operating and for the patient's comfort and post-operative course.

Dermabrasion Versus CO_2 Laser in the Removal of Tattoos – A Comparative Study

U. Hohenleutner[1], M. Landthaler[1], Diether Haina[2], W. Waidelich[2], and O. Braun-Falco[1]

1. Dermatologische Klinik und Poliklinik der LMU München (Direktor: Prof.Dr.Dr.h.c.O.Braun-Falco)
2. Abt. für angewandte Optik, Gesellschaft für Strahlen- und Umweltforschung, Neuherberg bei München

Since the first days of laser application in dermatology the removal of tattoos was of special intrest and different lasers have been employed (Ruby, Argon, CO_2, Nd:YAG) (3).

Nowadays the CO_2 laser is considered the laser of choice for tattoo removal. Most laser therapists state that it is superior compared to other lasers or other therapeutic modalities including dermabrasion, but no comparative studies are available.

We therefore decided to compare the removal of tattoos by means of CO_2 laser and dermabrasion inn one and the same patient with regard to amount of time needed, removal of pigment, time of wound healing and cosmetic result.

We report first results in three male patients aged 25, 30 and 33 years. Therapy was performed on an outpatients basis in local anaestesia.

In patient 1, tattoos on the right forearm were removed by dermabrasion, on the left by laser. In patients 2 and 3, half of a tattoo was removed by laser and the other half by dermabrasion.

If we summarize our preliminary results, we can state that the CO_2 laser has advantages as well as disadvantages compared to dermabrasion (2).

If we summarize our preliminary results, we can state that the CO_2 laser has advantages as well as disadvantages compared to dermabrasion (2).

With the laser pigment can always be removed completely and therapy is possible even in skin areas where dermabrasion cannot be performed (1). Additionally there is no risk of bleeding or infection and neither sterile conditions nor dressings are needed.

On the other side, the time needed for treatment and the length of the healing period are the main disadvantages of the laser.

Dermabrasion (DA) is at least three times faster than laser treatment (DA $\geq$ 3 cm²/min, CO_2 $\approx$ 1 cm²/min), and the time of wound healing is shorter (DA 2 - 3 weeks, CO_2 2 - 7 weeks).

Additionally, due to the checkerboard technique used in laser-removal, several treatments with intermissions of at least 4 weeks are needed for one tattoo. Overall treatment times of 6 to 12 months are not unusual for extensive tattoos.

With regard to the cosmetic results, we found no difference between the two therapeutic modalities.

Our conclusions are that dermabrasion is the method of choice for the removal of tattoos, but that the CO_2 laser is helpful in skin areas, where dermabrasion cannot be performed or where complete removal of pigment, especially in deep, non-professional tattoos, is important.

Literature

1. Grösser A, Konz B, Landthaler M (1982) Behandlungsmöglichkeiten von Tätowierungen. Fortschr Med 100:687-693

2. Landthaler M, Haina D, Waidelich W, Braun-Falco O (1987) Laser in der Dermatotherapie. In: Petres J (Hrsg) Fortschritte der operativen Dermatologie, Band 3:27-35

3. Seipp W, Landthaler M, Haina D, Justen V, Waidelich W (1981) Die Entfernung von Tätowierungen mit dem Argon-Laser. Dtsch Ärztebl 78:1809-1811

Nd: YAG Laser Ablation of Superficial Varices

Ronald Allen Kirschner

The Institute for Applied Laser Surgery

Suite IL-17

Two Bala Plaza

Bala Cynwyd, Pa. 19004, U.S.A.

Superficial Varices or spider veins comprise a long standing problem for a large number of women. A number of procedures have been utilized in the past for eradication of these vessels.

Sclerosis of superficial varices remains an excellent technique in the proper hands. Although infrequent, this procedure has been known to cause areas of gross discoloration and areas of slough. Electrocoagulation procedures have been used as well. This procedure has produced dissappointing results in the number of vessels that are ablated and in frequently causing areas of depigmentation.

The argon laser was the first laser that was utilized to ablate varices. This wavelength allowed very selective absorption by the hemoglobin in the vessels. In theory, at least, the surrounding tissue should have been spared the effects of the laser. In actual practice there were a number of changes that were noted in the surrounding skin.

The carbon dioxide laser was also utilized in an attempt to remove superficial varices. The available power was greater than the argon laser but the ability to coagulate was severely diminished.

Several years ago, we started to use the Nd:YAG laser in an attempt to ablate superficial varices. Before starting with this group we performed a considerable amount of work in the laboratory. This work consisted of ablating vessels in the nude mouse belly and in rabbit ears. For this purppose a focusing handpiece was utilized with the Cooper LaserSonics 4000 and with the MBB Nd:YAG lasers. Dosimetry evaluations were done and tissue effects were evaluated by serial H&E preps as well as scanning electronmicroscopy.

There were several problem associated with the use of this instrumentation: The HeNe aiming beam proved to be a problem in that the glare and the color that were produced were very distracting to the surgeon. The size of the aiming beam and the necessity to maintain it at a perpendicualr attitude to the skin made it difficult. The available focal length lenses also made their use cumbersome by some surgeons.

When the sapphire tip was introduced, we utilized it on several animal models. We found that a truncated conical tip was the ideal shape for use on superficial varices. We also noted that the diameter of the tip should ideally be slightly smaller than that of the size vessel we were ablating.

The procedure that we currently employ is as follows: The patient is brought to the out-patient O.R. without benefit of any preoperative medication. The area to be treated is photographed with a color bar. The area is then topically iced for about 10-12 minutes. This amount of cooling will usually provide sufficient anesthesia If necessary, a small amount of 1%

lidocaine is also injected. This has only been needed several times and this is presumably due to the fact that the operative site was insufficiently cooled. The area is then prepped with 70% alcohol. It is imperative that the alcohol be entirely removed from the operative area with sterile saline because alcohol will support combustion. The area is draped with sterile towels. The patient and everyone in the suite is then fitted with wavelength specific goggles. The varices are then ablated touching the superficial vessels every couple of millimeters with the contact tip. It is important that when the surgeon is treating a cluster, he must start at areas peripheral to the cluster. If he starts centrally, there will be diminution of the flow to the peripheral vessels and the surgeon wil be deceived as to what is and what is not ablated. The power settings are between 12-15 watts with the machine set to cut out at .5 seconds. At the end of the procedure the patient is instructed to keep the area clean and to avoid exposure to the sun.

The main difficulty with this procedure is that the sapphire tip tends to stick to tissue. The surgeon muast coordinate his application of power to the way in which he places the tip on the skin. The tips are also very expensive and will detereriorate after about ten treatments.

At the end of two weeks the treated vessels will appear dark as areas of coagulation are noted through the skin. These areas become light over the next four to six weeks as phagocytosis removes the coagulum. Any residual vessels in this area are then retreated. We find that it is necessarry to treat each area several imes to obtain the greatest effect.

This procedure shows promise for the future. We have not seen any objectionable scarring or other problems with the technique. Our main problem has been incomplete obliteration.

Possibility of Treating Hyperpigmented Skin Lesions Using the Nd: YAG Laser

Kenji Iwasaki, Medical Systems Division, Toshiba Corporation, 1-1 Shibaura 1-chome, Minato, Tokyo, Japan 105,
Susumu Shimizu, Toshiba Medical Engineering Co., Ltd.
Mitsuhiro Osada, Ryuzaburo Tanino, Muneo Miyasaka, Department of Plastic Surgery, Tokai University, Japan

1. Preface

The authors have developed a ruby laser system having a device to provide uniform output, the "Kaleidoscope" handpiece. This equipment can be used for the treatment of a hyperpigmented skin lesions, such as nevus spilus and nevus cell nevus. As a result, acceptable clinical results have been obtained[*]. However, the ruby laser was not effective for the treatment of deeply located intra-dermal hyper-melanoses.

The Nd-YAG laser with a wavelength of 1.06 micron has been considered unsuitable for the treatment of hyperpigmented skin lesions. However, it is expected that the use of this new technique will make possible the application of the Nd-YAG laser in the treatment of these lesions. This is because the "Kaleidoscope" can simply and accurately control the depth of the laser beam's penetration into human tissues. This report deals with the study from this point of view.

2. Principle of uniform intensity distribution

The laser beam generated by the resonator is focused by a lens and directed upon the end surface of an optical glass or quartz square pillar. The beam enters the square pillar at a predetermined incident angle, repeats total reflection on the inner walls of the pillar, and emerges from the surface of the opposite end (Fig. 1).

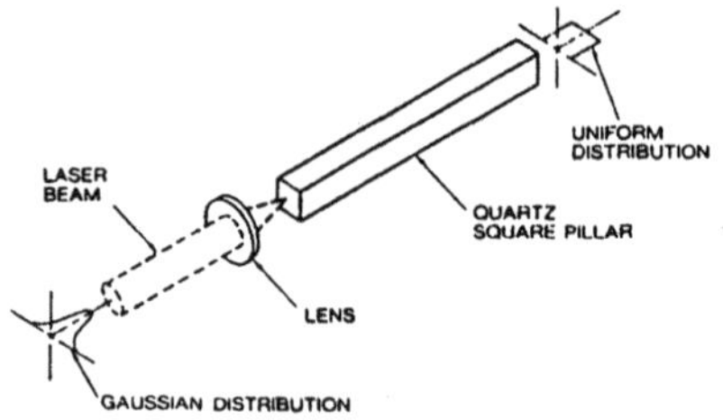

The intensity distribution of the output beam is made uniform and square by selecting the correct combination of

Fig. 1 Principle of "Kaleidoscope"

---

[*]K. Iwasaki et al.: "Development of new ruby laser system for treatment of nevus". The 6th Congress of the International Society for Laser Surgery and Medicine. (1985)

incident angle and size of square pillar (Fig. 2).

3. "Kaleidoscope" handpiece

The handpiece adpoting the method described in item 2 is called the "Kaleidoscope". When the laser beam passes through the "Kaleidoscope" handpiece, the output is converted from a Gaussian distribution to a uniform square distribution. Consequently, irradiation with predetermined intensity is possible. (Fig. 3.)

In order to test in the same condition, the Nd-glass rod was inserted to the laser oscillating cavity instead of the ruby rod. As a result, we obtained 1.06 micron laser beam.

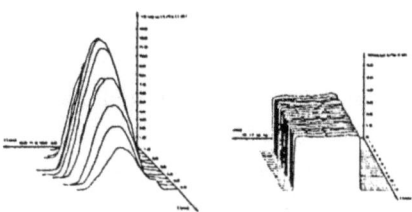

(a) Conventional   (b) New

Fig. 2. Output intensity distribution

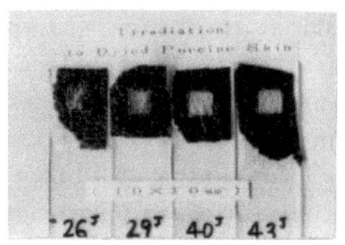

Fig. 3. Example of uniform irradiation

4. Consideration of Reflection characteristics

(1) Fig. 4 shows the reflection characteristics of the test materials, "Meipack" atellocollagen sheet, painted in yellow, red, brown, blue, purple and black, measured with the spectrophotometer manufactured by ourselves. Fig. 5 shows the results of irradiation on those test materials by the ruby laser (0.69 micron pulse) and Nd-glass laser (1.06 micron pulse) through "Kaleidoscope" handpiece at 30 J/cm^2, 2 ms. The Nd-glass laser breaches the material painted in black, but the other colors scarcely react to it. Though the degree of reaction differs depending on the color, the ruby laser breaches purple, blue, brown and red as well as black much more than the Nd-glass laser does. These facts correspond to the results of spectral analysis shown in Fig. 4.

(2) Fig. 6 shows light reflection and transmission by melanin and

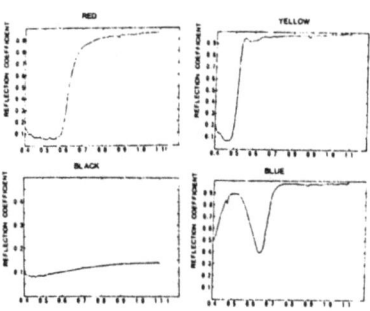

Fig. 4. Spectral reflection of the various colors

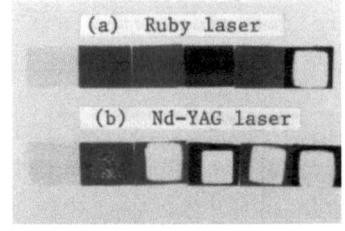

Fig. 5. Results of irradiation to the various colors

collagen*.

Tabel 1 shows the calculation of light absorption at wavelengthes of 1.06, 0.7. and 0.5 micron, almost corresponding to those of the Nd-YAG, ruby and argon lasers respectively. It clearly shows that, the difference and ratio of light absorption by melanin against collagen reach their maximum at 1.0 micron. It indicates the possibility of application to deeply located intra-dermal hyper-melanosis, which has never been applied before because of high transmission into the skin.

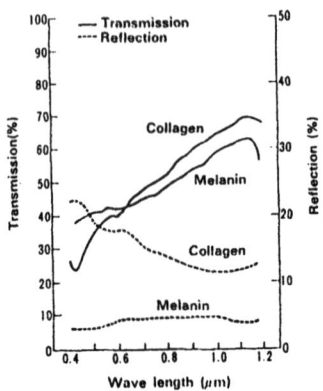

Fig. 6. Spectroscopic characteriestics of melanin and collagen

5. Examination of tissue effectiveness according to wavelength

(1) We measured the transmission ratio of human nevus cell nevus in vitro and obtained the results shown in Table 2. In our histological findings, considerable alteration was seen in the superficial region of the skin when the ruby laser was used. However, no such abnormality was detected when the Nd-glass laser was used, and only coagulation of red blood cells in the vein was seen.

Items Wavelength	Tissue	Reflection A	Penetration B	Transmission C	Absorption D	Whole absorptions B×D	Absorption by melanin against collagen (value m×B)	Ratio
1.0 μm	Melanin	0.05	0.95	0.60	0.40	0.38	0.12	1.46
	Collagen	0.12	0.88	0.70	0.30	0.26		
0.7 μm	Melanin	0.05	0.95	0.45	0.55	0.52	0.07	1.15
	Collagen	0.15	0.85	0.48	0.53	0.45		
0.5 μm	Melanin	0.05	0.95	0.40	0.60	0.57	0.05	1.10
	Collagen	0.20	0.80	0.35	0.65	0.52		

Table 1. Calculation of light absorption by melanin and collagen

(2) In the case of the artificial tattoo, clear hypertrophic scars were made after one year of the last treatment by ruby laser, while those were not made after six months of the last treatment by the Nd-glass laser.

6. Conclusion

In this study, we found that laser therapy for deeply located nevus cell nevus would be possible without giving much damage to the normal skin using a laser with the following characteristics:

Wave length Tissue	1.06 μm	0.964 μm
Normal human skin (t=0.4mm)	76~80%	37%
Nevus cell nevus (t=4mm)	10%	1.2%
Nevus cell nevus (t=9mm)	1%	not measured

Table 2. Light transmission rate of tissues in vitro

---

*M. Kikuchi et al.: "Clinical application to laser" (in Japanese), Medical Planning, p.61 (1981)

　　　　　Wave length:　1.06 micron (Nd-YAG)
　　　　　Irradiation time:　Approx. 2 m sec (pulse)
　　　　　Output intensity:　uniformed and predetermined by
　　　　　　　　　　　　　　"Kaleidoscope" handpiece.
We intend to continue this study to expand the application of our laser system.

Nd: YAG Laser Treatment of Tattoos

Ronald Allen Kirschner

THE INSTITUTE FOR APPLIED LASER SURGERY

Suite IL - 17

Two Bala Plaza

Bala Cynwyd, Pa. 19004, U.S.A.

There are a variety of techniques tht are currently employed for the eradication of tattoos. Each one of the techniques has its own distinctive advantages and disadvantages.

The earliest laser that was utilized for tattoo removal was the argon. The argon laser was selectively absorbed by the pigment of the tattoo and spared the non-pigmented tissue that surrounds the tattoo. This laser proved itself to be a major improvement over techniques such as salabrasion and over-tattooing. The laser did, however, frequently cause hypertrophic scarring.

The next laser to be widely employed for this purpose was the carbon dioxide laser. The carbon dioxide laser is an excellent cutter and a relatively poor coagulator. This laser was widely employed in the eradication of tattoos over the last five years. The results obtained with this wavelength covered the gamut from excellent to poor. The carbon dioxide laser was utilized to cut through the more superficial skin layers and then to debride the pigment from the deeper layers. The results were highly variable. In some cases, we might see excellent ablation in wide areas interspersed with small ares of hypertrophic scarring.

The more experienced laser surgeon would always do a small inobtrusive area with the carbon dioxide laser to see how the area healed. As with all of the laser wavelengths that have been employed for eradication of tattoos, the lighter the skin the better degree of healing experienced by the patient.

The Nd:YAG laser is an excellent coagulator and a poor cutter. This type of radiation is better absorbed by dark pigments such a melanin and hemaglobin than by lighter colored material. The absorption spectrum is not nearly as selective as argon. We have termed this facultative selectivity. We feel that this degree of selectivity, when combined with the relatively high power levels available with the Nd:YAG lase is responsible for the results that we have obtained.

Our preliminry study is comprised of a series of eighten patients. They are evenly divided as to sex. They range in age from the second to the fifth decade. Sixteen of these tattos were professionally done and of high quality. Two of the tattoos were amateurish and of very poor quality.

In our series, we treated a test spot on each individual. This test spot allowed the patient and the physician to evaluate the possible results. The test area would be followed for a three month period before any additional work would be done. In no instance did the patient not wish to continue treatment.

The procedure ensues with the skin area being prepped with 70% alcohol. The treatment site is then infiltrated with 1% lidocaine with 1/100,000 epinephrine. The Nd:YAG laser is set at

12-15 watts with a cut off point at .5 seconds. Each segment of the area is lased once and then a sponge that has been impregnated with hydrogen peroxide is used to remove the byproducts of the laser - tissue interaction. After this first pass with the laser the areas that contain the tattoo pigment will be much brighter than they were previously. The areas of brightened pigment will be surrounded by areas that have undergone some degree of oxidation from the hydrogen peroxide. They will be whitened and somewhat raggedy in appearance. The laser is then used to make one additional pass over the pigmented areas. An antibiotic ointment is then placed over the site with a light dressing.

The patient is instructed to wash the area twice daily with a textured washcloth. They will then clean it with hydrogen peroxide and reapply a thin film of ointment. After the first day they leave the operative site without a dressing. Most of the pigment is thusly removed by the patient in a mechanical fashion. The way in which the pigment is separated from the wound has been reported to either come off as speckles of pigment when the peroxide is applied or as a thin sheet of material which contains the pigment.

Most of the residual pigment that is left behind as the most superficial superficial layers of skin regenerate appears to fade slowly. This is probably due to phagocytic action.

After the first two to three weeks, the healing areas appear more injected, thinner, and shinier than the surrounding tissue. This effect diminishes over the next three to six weeks. We have not biopsied the reddened areas; however, they do blanche when a glass slide is placed over the area. This indicates that the redness is of a vascular nature. As the phagocytic action decreases, the capillary dilatation seems to ebb as well.

The post treatment areas differ from cases that have been treated with other laser modalities. The skin in all of our cases appears close in pigmentation to the surrounding tissue. We have experienced no permanent hyperpigmentation or hypopigmentation. All of our patients are instructed to avoid exposure to the sun. The younger individuals in our series usually ignore our instructions and the treated areas in these patients appear to undergo normal tanning. An additional difference in the result is in the way the resultant tissue feels. It is much closer to normal texture than tissue treated with other modalities. There may, indeed, be a place for this procedure in our plastic surgery armamentarium.

The Percutaneous and Subcutaneous Application of the Nd: YAG Laser for Animal Experiments

Dimtrije Katalinic, MD
Privatklinik, Am Plärrer 35, 8500 Nürnberg
West Germany

In the case of a percutaneous laser application the laser beam at first hits the superficial layers of the epidermis which are also the first to coagulate. The layers of the skin that follow, which are deeper are less and less hit by the laser coagulation cone. The tip of this cone marks the limit of the so-called depth of penetration (in the case of the CO 2 laser 0.1 mm, in the case of the Argon Laser 1-2 mm, in the case of the Nd-Yag-laser 3-5 mm).

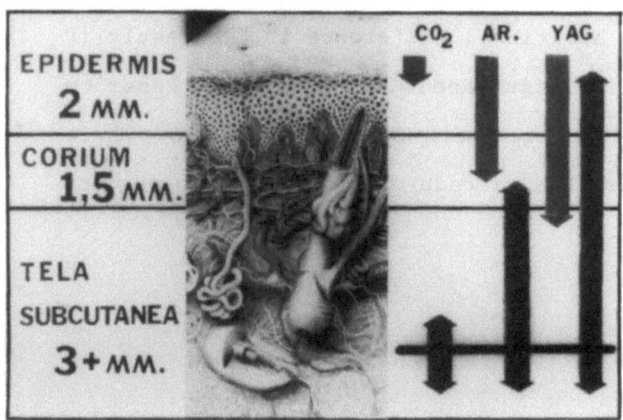

Fig. 1.   Penetration of different laser systems in the percutaneous application. Assumed penetration range in the subcutaneous application

Further layers are only then hit by the laser beam if the coagulated tissue is either mechanically removed or if it is vaporated by the laser. Through the percutaneous application different lesions can be treated more or less successfully which depends on the colour but decisively on the depth of the lesion. Some deep-seated anatomic skin regions are not accessible by the laser beam in the percutaneous way. The fact that in case of the percutaneous laser application the skin

surface is hurt either in a microscopic or macroscopic way and the
fact that the superficial skin layers do not represent a transparent
medium but a medium that absorbs the laser energy, all this causes
skin lesions in the surface which, consecutively causes a more or less
visible cicatrisation. The two disadvantageous points of the percutaneous laser therapy - insufficient depth and injure of the skin surface -
were impulsive to think about the problem of whether or not a subcutaneous application of the laser beam would be possible. Early in 1986
our team has made animal experiments in the department for experimental
surgery of the University of Ulm, in order to come closer to an answer
of this question. The basic question was to make a comparison between
the laser effect of the percutaneous and the subcutaneous application
and to find an answer to the question whether a sophisticated subcutaneous application is possible at all. We used a pulsed new Nd-Yag-Laser
system of the LASAG company of Thun/Switzerland. The parametra of the
unit was 0.2 to 10 ms and the energy was 1 - 20 joules. Tests were
made in 70 rats. 35 rats were destined for the percutaneous application
and 35 rats for the subcutaneous application. Each rat was exposed to
two tests:

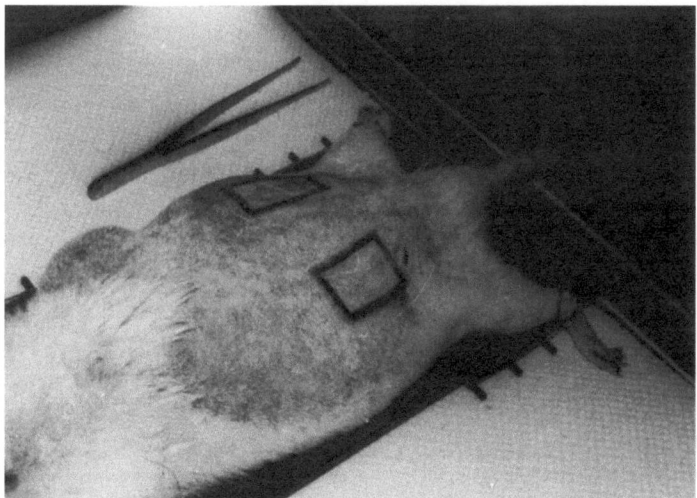

Fig. 2. Two tests, i.e. for the percutaneous as well
as for the subcutaneous application, were
made on the backs of rats

One on the left and one on the right side of the body, which means that
we carried out 140 tests. We chose suitable power and duration of exposition in order to be able to administer the lowest and highest laser impulses. We used among others identical parametra in the subcutaneous and percutaneous tests in order to register the differences.
The percutaneous application was made in the conventional way. Each
animal received 30 impulses in one line, one beside the other, left
and right within a marked region on the shaved animal skin. For the
subcutaneous application a technically and optically not uncomplicated
cannula was made to suit this purpose. By a cut of 1 cm of length the
skin was opened, well dissected, undermined, and then the cannula was
slid forward deeply below the skin (about 8 cm). In this way also 30
laser shots of the respective parametra were administered.

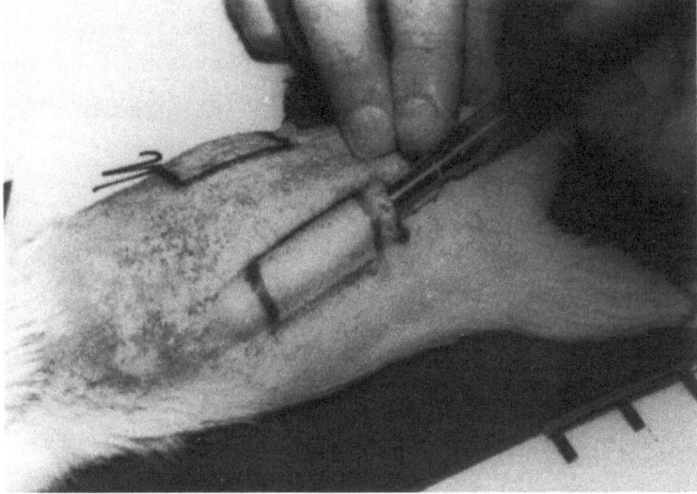

Fig. 3. The subcutaneous test was made with a newly
developped canula

The histological analysis was carried out on the first, third, fifth,
seventh,   twelfth and forteenth day in order to obtain an overview on the healing of the laser lesions. The tissue specimens were
analysed by the Pathological Institute of the University of Erlangen-
Nürnberg by Prof. Dr. Becker, pathologist. The histomorphometric evaluation was made with the MOP-Image-plan-Morphometric Program. With an
calibration grid and an Orthoplan microscope and a video camera the
histological pictures were taken over by a monitor and exact measure-

ments were made. We received the results in mm, with 2 digits behind
the decimal point, i.e. always on the depth and width of the coagulation or necrosis and its symptoms caused by the laser.

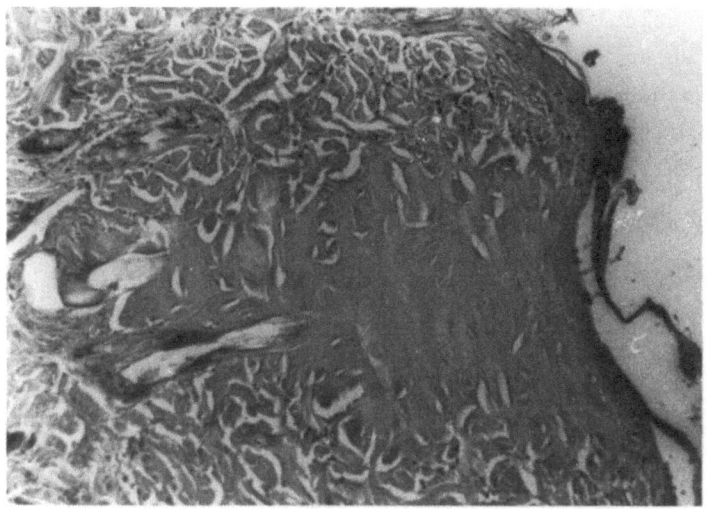

Fig. 4. A typical percutaneous Nd-Yag laser coagulation
cone. The epidermis on the surface is injured

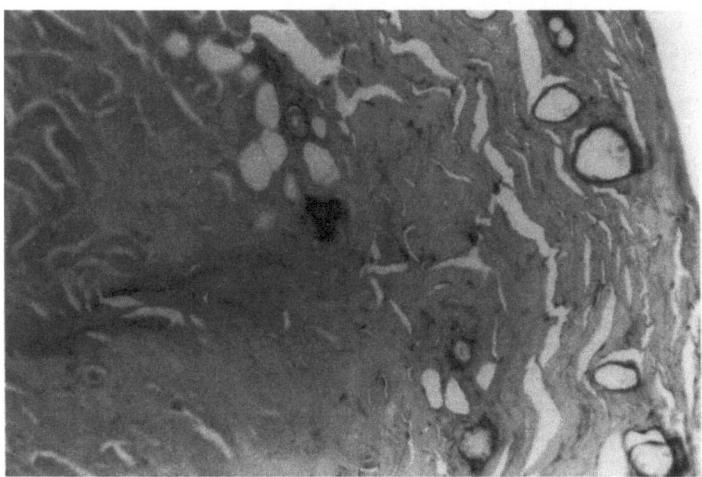

Fig. 5. Subcutaneous application: The surface is
intact; the subcutaneous coagulation area
is visible

The histological analysis also shows the layers of the skin of the rats down to which the laser energy penetrated. The histomorphometric and the histopathological evaluation was statistically made by an independent biometric institute (Datenservice Hönig, Rohrbach). The details obtained were translated into arithmetic average values and a cone-shaped laser spot was calculated in geometrical values based on the depth and the width. We obtained the significant results, above all that the coagulation produced in the subcutaneous way is remarkably higher when compared with the percutaneous application, provided the administered laser dose was the same.

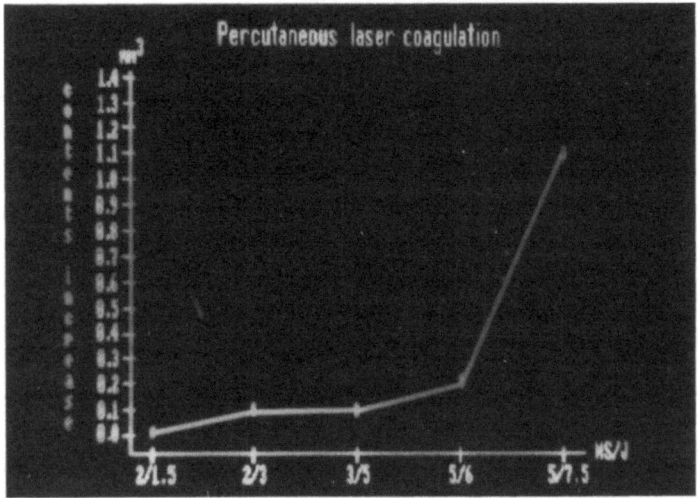

Fig. 6. Percutaneous application: Slight coagulation extent, not more than 1,1 mm^3

That allows the assumption that in the subcutaneous way essential lower doses can be applied to get the same effect.
A survey as to which layers we reach with the percutaneous and a subcutaneous laser application showed that the two applications are quite different. In the case of the percutaneous application mainly the surface layers are reached, in the case of the subcutaneous application the deeper layers are reached. Whereas the percutaneous application only reaches the penetration range, the range of the subcutaneous application depends on the position of the applied cannula. Thus directions in all dimensions and depths are possible.

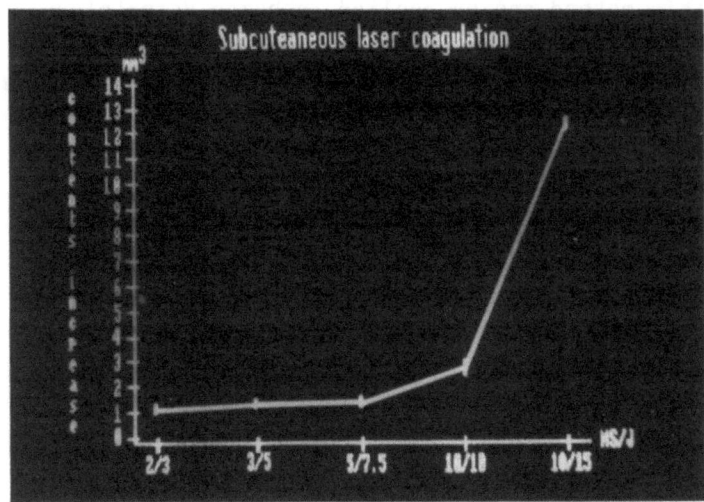

Fig. 7. Subcutaneous coagulation: High effect between 2 to 12 mm^3

The analysis of the animal experiments showed that
1. Subcutaneous laser application is technically feasible.
2. After the subcutaneous laser application the coagulation is definitely stronger than in the percutaneous mode.
3. The laser beam can reach any skin layer through the subcutaneous application.
4. The surface of the skin will not be injured.

Our animal experiment allows us to have our thoughts move as to the possibility of the subcutaneous laser application on the human skin. In the first place it must be mentioned that the subcutaneous laser application will most probably be applied by a small surgical intervention - under the necessary surgical precautions and conditions - as a cut and the undermining of the skin is necessary. It is assumed that the cut is made in a place where it is not noticed. Due to the fact that the subcutaneous application does not injure the surface, a certain new significance can be attributed to this way of application. Also the possibility of starting the laser coagulation in deeper skin layers may mean new indications for the laser therapy, for instance laser-epilation, therapy in the layer of the sweat glands, in the region of the arteriovenous plexus of the subcutis, subtle cosmetic therapy and last not least skin welding. We will examine with our further tests to what extent this method can be applied in human dermatology. It is just possible that in some cases that are treated in the percutaneous way today, a subcutaneous application would show better results.

We have also started tests in the human dermatology, and we intend to try to find the answers to the following questions:
1. Which lesions that have been treated up to now through the percutaneous method might be treated better in the subcutaneous way?
2. Which new indications are suitable for the subcutaneous Nd-Yag laser application?

The way to seizable results is longer than expected. So, we cannot make any statements about our experience which is today in an early stage.

New Diode Laser for Immediate Pain Attenuation Following Snowy Dry Ice Treatment for Naevus of Ohta

Toshio Ohshiro, M.D.*, J. Kubota, M.D.**,
K. Iwahira, M.D.***, I. Tanaka, M.D.****

* Japan Medical Laser Laboratory
  TBR Bldg. #607, 5-7 Kojimachi, Choyoda-ku, Tokyo 102, Japan.
** Kyorin University, Japan
*** Toho University, Japan
****Keio University, Japan

ABSTRACT

Snowy dry ice application followed by epithelial peeling is an effective treatment for Ohta's naevus. However, it is quite painful. The GaAlAs diode laser has been found to be effective in pain attenuation. A retrospective study of 452 patients is presented, using the diode laser for immediate pain attenuation following snowy dry ice application and epithelial peeling. One group of 100 patients participated in an additional separate study to determine the time course for pain recovery after dry ice application alone _without_ laser or peeling. A second group of 100 patients participated in a second study to evaluate recovery and determine the time course following peeling without laser irradiation. In all cases the laser proved effective in attenuating the perceived pain by 60%, and shortening the overall recovery time by 37%, with minimal (0.7%) and controllable side effects.

INTRODUCTION

Naevus of Ohta, or Ohta's (Ota's) naevus, is a particularly oriental disease, consisting of a bluish-brownish-gray pigmented lesion in the periorbital region, possibly extending into surrounding areas and even the eyeball itself. It consists of two separate entities: Hypermetabolic melanocytes exist in the epidermal basal layer, with the simultaneous existance of abnormal undifferentiated melanocytes in the underlying dermis. The different depths of the melanin granules account for the varying colour layers. It is therefore a difficult disease to treat successfully. Many therapeutic methods such as skin graft or radiation therapy have been tried, but with little success.

We evolved snowy dry ice and epithelial peeling treatment (DIET) over 10 years ago. DIET has now been successfully indicated in over 3,000 patients. The treatment, while effective, requires several repeat visits, and is quite painful. Children, and others with a low pain threshold, find it too painful, and may stop the treatment before it is complete. The GaAlAs diode laser has been used in our clinic for pain attenuation with success for the last 6 years. We decided to try the diode laser in low level laser therapy (LLLT) following both the application and peeling phases of DIET.

In order to evaluate the data objectively, two further trials were run simultaneously. One group of 100 patients received dry ice application only, without laser treatment or epithelial peeling. This gave the value for longest overall recovery time. A second group of 100 patients had laser treatment for the dry ice application, but received no laser treatment following the epithelial peeling phase of DIET. With these aditional data we were able to compare the effectiveness of the LLLT in overall pain attenuation and also its effect on the patients' overall recovery times after DIET.

MATERIALS & METHODS

The laser used for all patients was the PANALAS-4000, developed in conjunction by the Japan Medical Laser Laboratory and Matsushita Electronics Co., Ltd., Japan. The system delivers 60 mW at a nominal 830nm with an irradiated area of aprroximately $0.3cm^2$.

Snowy dry ice is manufactured daily as required by venting carbon dioxide gas under pressure into a chamois bag. A solid CO frost forms on the inside of the bag, which is collected and compacted in equipment developed in the Japan Medical Laser Laboratory. The equipment is capable of producing snowy dry ice applicator sticks of different diameters.

The applicator stick is pressed against the epidermis in a previously outlined treatment area, and removed after blanching is seen. The blanching is due to cryogenic vasoconstriction in the treated area, and is accompanied by a sharp burning sensation which resolves into a dull ache. Serum exudation as part of the body's repair process then collects in the treated area, rupturing the epidermal tonofibrils and aiding separation at the dermo-epidermal junction, forming a large, serum-filled vessicle. At the 1 hour mark, the epidermis is then easily peeled from the dermis, complete with hair sheath and sweat gland linings as part of the complete external integument.

The diode laser is applied in contact technique during and after dry ice application to the periphery of the treatment area, with multiple irradiations in 3-4sec exposures, until the pain has been removed, usually 5-10min. A second laser irradiation is given as before just before peeling, to remove the pain which has gradually built up during the serum exudation, and a third irradiation session immediately following peeling, to remove the sharp pain caused by detaching the epithelium complete with its hair sheath and sweat gland lining.

Treatment invariably requires 3 or more visits. Accordingly all informed and consenting patients in the main study had DIET both with and without LLLT in a double-blind trial. For the first of the secondary trials, as for the second, patients were selected on the basis of their requiring more than 4 treatment sessions. The trial involved receiving the dry ice application only, without laser therapy, and without peeling. The patients were asked at 10 minute intervals how their pain was, and the results plotted to find the standard time it took for total recovery. Selection for this trial disqualified them for selection for the second trial. This involved dry ice application, laser therapy, pre-peeling laser therapy, and epithelial peeling only. This was to arrive at the time to recovery from the peeling pain. The results were charted and the mean average time plotted.

RESULTS

Figure 1 is the graph plotted from the data gathered in the main and subsidiary trials. The three periods at which the laser was irradiated were the application of the dry ice, with the post irradiation point A; B, the laser treatment given before peeling; and C, the treatment given after peeling. Table I shows the data in tabular form. In order to reach a value for the pain attenuation, patients were asked to grade the difference between no irradiation at point A and the pain intensity with irradiation, on a scale from 1 to 10, with 1 being the highest pain level. Almost all patients reported a 6 for the application with irradiation, and all but 3 from the total group reported total pain removal at point A. Those 3 had received laser irradiation directly over the subocular nerve, and reported an intensifying of the pain, which gradually died down. All of the subjects reported total pain removal with irradiation at points B and C. Total recovery time without diode laser therapy and peeling was approximately 3 hours. Recovery time with laser therapy after application but not after peeling was

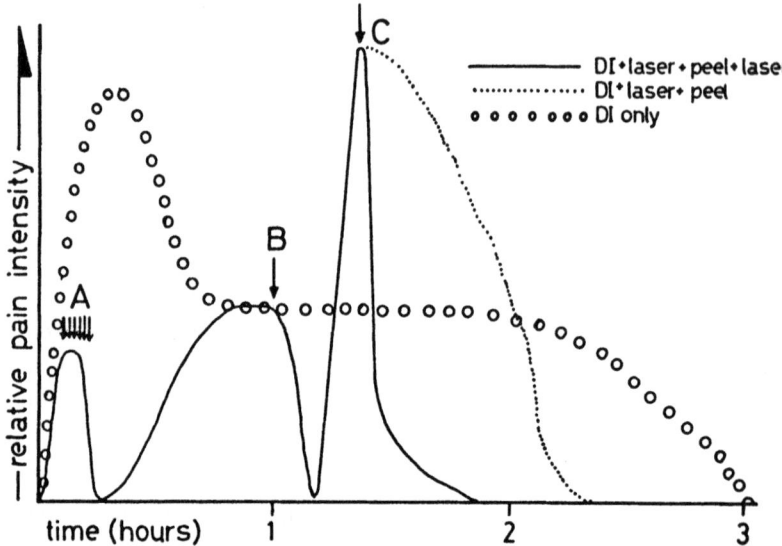

Fig 1. Graph from data on trials. Note shorter recovery times following laser application, and lower pain at point A.

Table I. Data from Fig 1 in tabular form. Patients who took part in test A did not participate in Test B. A, B, and C correspond to the same points in Fig 1

	NUMBER	AVERAGE PAIN ATTENUATION	TIME 1	TIME 2	PAIN REMOVAL (N /%)		
					A	B	C
TOTAL POPULATION	452	60% less	1.9hrs	0.7hrs	449 99.3%	452 100%	452 100%
TEST A	100	N/A	3hrs	N/A	N/A	N/A	N/A
TEST B	100	60% less	2.3hrs	1.2hrs	100%	100%	100%

※ N/A = NOT APPLICABLE

2hrs 20min. Total recovery time after both laser treatment at application and peeling was 1hr 54min. Recovery time at point C without laser was 1hr 12min, and with laser was 42min.

DISCUSSION

The success rate for the application of snowy dry ice followed by epithelial peeling is very high, but the process is very painful, as it involves application of the snowy dry ice, which causes a burning pain, the pain caused by the pressure build-up of the serum, and the extremely sharp pain on peeling the epidermis from the dermis. As the hair sheath and sweat gland linings are also removed with the epithelial sheet, this stimulates an inflammatory response in the dermis, thus elevating the macrophage level. The undifferentiated melanocytes are then recognised as foreign to the dermal matrix, and are macrophaged.

The effectiveness of the diode laser in pain attenuation has been reported by the author and others over the last six years. It seemed a logical step to apply the diode laser to the pain caused in the various stages of DIET, as the treatment results are so good compared with other methods, the pain being the only adverse side effect. It has been shown that the diode laser works at two levels, a local cellular level and a systemic level, through the blood, lymphatic and neural systems. The action here would appear to be a purely local anaesthetic one, with some possible after-benefits from heightened circulatory response, and cessation of the exudate response after peeling, thus assisting better wound healing with less exudate to cause adhesion of the dressing to the wound.

The reduction in recovery time, both overall and at the point of peeling speak for themselves. The patients unanimously agreed that there was a real lessening of the pain, and they are able to leave the clinic sooner, thus representing a double benefit to them and to any institution.

In conclusion, the authors recommend the use of the diode laser as an adjunct to DIET for Ohta's naevus, as a safe, effective and noninvasive pain attenuating instrument.

Abnormal Skin Microcirculatory Reflex in Diabetic Patients with Autonomic Neuropathy Detected by the Use of Laser Doppler Flowmeter

L.T. Ho, Kam-Tsun Tang, Jeng-Tao Wang, Hing-Chung Lam, Shing-Hung Li, Li-Chuan Hsiao, Jing-Cherng Perng, Yueh-Fen Liu
Department of Medicine, Veteran General Hospital
Shih-Pai RD., Taipei, Taiwan, R.O.C.

INTRODUCTION: Autonomic neuropathy (DAN) is a well-recognized complication of diabetes. Because it is often asymptomatic[1] in the early stage and has a higher mortality risk,[2,3] it is very important clinically. Since the first introduction of cardiovascular reflex (CVR) tests on 1973,[4,5] they have been widely used for detecting DAN. With increasing understanding of the pathophysiology of DAN, more aspects of autonomic dysfunction have been explored.[6] In the present study, we wanted to characterize the skin microvascular reflex (MVR) changes in diabetes using newly available technology - The laser Doppler flowmeter,[7,8] and compare the MVR between patients with and without cardiac autonomic dysfunction, as determined by CVR tests.

MATERIALS & METHODS: Seventy NIDDM patients, aged 42 to 72 years (mean 59.7 yr), with duration of diabetes ranging from 3 mo to 30 yr were evaluated. The control group consisted of 20 healthy age-matched (40-73 yr, mean 56.1 yr) volunteers. None of the participants had heart, renal, liver, thyroid, or neurological diseases, or were treated with drugs known to interfere with autonomic nervous function. After overnight fasting participants were tested in an air-conditioned room (22-25°C) with a 30 min rest prior to testing. No smoking or medication was allowed before the examination. The CVR tests were performed with a Grass polygraph (7P8 EKG/Sphygmomanometer preamplifier-Tachograph and 7DA driver amplifier, with appropriate accessories). The limb lead II of EKG and blood pressure by Korokoff's sounds (detected by sphygmomanometer and piezoelectric microphone) are fed into the polygraph, in which the impulses are automatically converted to instantaneous heart rate and blood pressure curves throughout the following procedures:[9] 1) Single deep breath (SDB), 10 sec for the whole cycle. 2) 12 consecutive deep breaths (12DB), 10 sec for each cycle. 3) Valsalva's maneouvre (VM), keeping positive thoracic pressure at 40mmHg by blowing a barometer via a mouth piece. 4) Position change lying-standing (ST) and sitting-standing. We measured the heart rate variability (HRV) of SDB (normal [N] $\geq$ 15 b/m), 12DB (N, mean $\geq$ 11 b/m), VM (N $\geq$ 20 b/m), ST (N $\geq$ 17 b/m) and the blood pressure changes from sitting to standing (N, systolic fall $\leq$ 25mmHg & diastolic fall $\leq$ 10mmHg) in each subject.[10] If 2 or more of the above tests were abnormal, we regarded them as having cardiac autonomic dysfunction.[1] After the CVR tests, the patients were tested by a periflux laser Doppler flowmeter (PLDF, Perimed, Stockholm). The method involves conducting a 2mW He-Ne laser via an optic fiber to the pal-

mar surface of the 1st metacarpal area. The scattered laser light reflected from the underlying red blood cells is transmitted back and transformed into analogue voltage by electronic processing. The output is proportional to the number of RBCs in the measuring volume (radius 1-1.5mm semisphere) multiplied by their average velocity. However, due to the different skin characteristics in the measuring volume of different individuals, there is a large variation between different subjects, and in the same subject at different areas, and over time.[12] Quantitative comparison of absolute values of blood blow between patients are unreliable, but semiquantitative estimates can be made by determining the relative changes in blood flow under the following stimulations:[13]
1) Autonomic vasoconstrictive stimulations: a) SDB. b) VM. c) Contralateral hand cold stimulation (ICE), placing the contralateral hand in ice for 15 sec.
2) Local vasodilatory stimulations: a) Local heat stimulation (HEAT), warming the test area to 40°C for 1 min by the heat producing thermostat. b) Reactive hyperemia (RH), applying pressure (200mmHg) to the testing arm for 1 min by a pressure cuff and releasing abruptly.

The relative changes in skin blood flow (changes in energy gain at the recorder output) after stimulation is expressed as percent remaining value (%RV): Flow value after stimulation X 100% / Basal flow value. The %RV of SDB, VM and ICE, in addition the reciprocal (1/X) of the %RV of HEAT and RH tests were analyzed by Student's t test and linear regression after arcsine transformation.

RESULTS & DISCUSSION: Fifty of the 70 diabetics were diagnosed as having cardiac autonomic dysfunction (DAN +) and the rest were DAN - as determined by CVR tests. The heart rate changes in each of the individual CVR test correlated with each of the other CVR tests (P < 0.01). This implies that these reflexes may share similar pathways, particularly the parasympathetic system as suggested by other workers.[9] The low incidence of postural hypotension (8%) in our study population is compatible with other studies,[11,14] in which it was considered to be abnormal only with more extensive and widespread sympathetic damage. The mean %RV of microvascular reflex tests in different population subgroups are shown in figure 1. No difference was found among any of the population subgroups in local vasodilatory stimulation tests (RH & HEAT), although denervative hypersensitivity was expected initially. However, in autonomic vasoconstrictive stimulation tests, the %RV in all diabetics was significantly higher than in normals (SDB, VM & ICE, P < 0.01). After further analysis, the subgroup of DAN + patients had significantly higher %RV than either normal controls or DAN - patients (P < 0.01), except in VM test. In this test, DAN - patients had significantly higher %RV than normals (P < 0.05), and no difference compared to the DAN + patients. This condition was not seen in SDB or ICE tests, in which DAN + patients had higher %RV than DAN - patients (P < 0.01 in SDB & P < 0.05 in ICE). A higher %RV indicates a lesser vasoconstrictive responses. We do not know whether this implies that the abnormal MVR may precede the cardiac autonomic dysfunction, or simply reflects the fact that the CVR tests are more sensitive for parasympathetic evaluation.[11] The %RV of each microvascular autonomic stimulation test correlat-

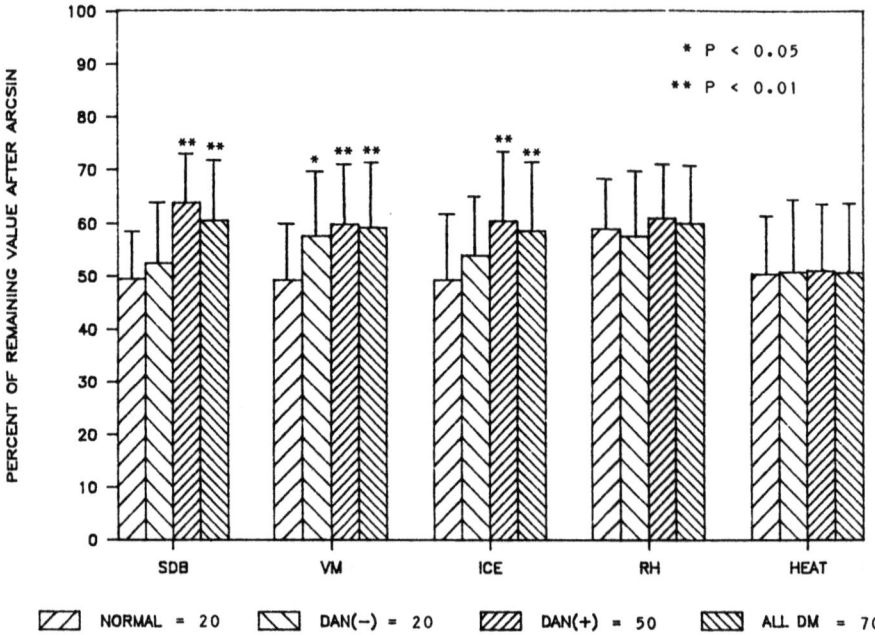

Fig. 1. The mean %RV of microvascular reflex tests in different population subgroups

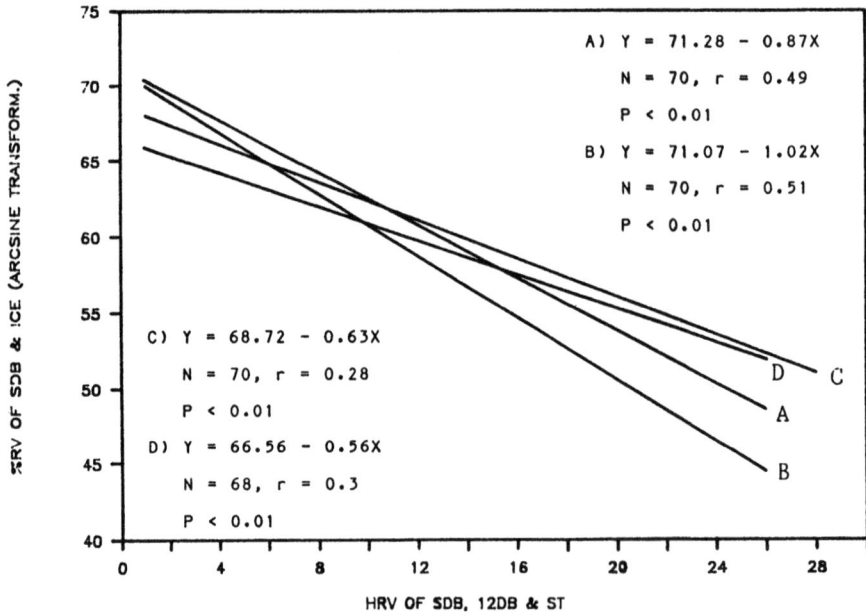

Fig. 2. Relationships between microvascular reflex tests and cardiovascular reflexes tests. A) %RV of SDB vs HRV of SDB. B) %RV of SDB vs HRV of 12DB. C) %RV of SDB vs HRV of ST. D) %RV of ICE vs HRV of SDB

ed with each of the other microvascular autonomic stimulation tests (P < 0.01). Figure 2 illustrates the relationships between CVR tests and MVR tests. The %RV of SDB test correlated with the HRV of SDB, 12DB and ST tests (P < 0.01). The %RV of ICE test corrlated with only the HRV of SDB test (P < 0.01). In summary, both CVR and MVR may be abnormal in diabetics. There are some correlations between these two types of reflex tests. Some evidence suggests that abnormal MVR may precede the CVR. We cannot document any denervative hypersensitivity in our results that we had expected initially. The laser Doppler flowmeter is a simple, noninvasive tool in the detection of abnormal MVR, especially for the study of peripheral autonomic neuropathy and follow up care.

REFERENCES

1. Pfeifer MA, Weinberg CR, Cook DL, et al. Autonomic neural dysfunction in recently diagnosed diabetic subjects. Diabetes Care 1984; 7:447-453.
2. Ewing DJ, Campell IW, Clarke BF. Mortality in diabetic autonomic neuropathy. Lancet 1976; III:601-603.
3. Page MMcB, Watkins PJ. Cardiorespiratory arrest and diabetic autonomic neuropathy Lancet 1978; I:14-16.
4. Wheeler T, Watkins PJ. Cardiac denervation in diabetes. Br Med J 1973; IV:584-586
5. Ewing DJ, Campell IW, Burt AA, Clarke BF. Vascular reflexes in diabetic autonomic neuropathy. Lancet 1973; 12:1354-1356.
6. Ewing DJ, Clarke BF. Diabetic autonomic neuropathy: present insights and future prospects. Diabetes Care 1986; 9:648-665.
7. Nilsson GE, Tenland T, Oberg PA. A new instrument of continuous measurement of tissue blood flow by light beating spectroscopy. IEEE Trans Bio-Med Eng 1980; 27: 12-19.
8. Nilsson GE, Tenland T, Oberg PA. Evaluation a laser Doppler flowmeter for measurement of tissue blood flow. IEEE Trans Bio-Med Eng 1980; 27:596-604.
9. Ewing DJ, Clarke BF. Diagnosis and management of diabetic autonomic neuropathy. Br Med J 1982; 285:916-918.
10. Ho LT, Chou TY, Chan RL, et al. The diagnostic criteria of diabetic autonomic neuropathy. Proc Natl Sci Counc ROC 1982; 6:286-291.
11. Ewing DJ, Martyn CN, Young RJ, Clarke BF. The value of cardiovascular autonomic function tests: 10 years experience in diabetes. Diabetes Care 1985; 8:491-498.
12. Johnson JM, Taylor WF, Shepherd AP, Park MK. Laser-Doppler measurement of skin blood flow: comparision with plethysmography. J Appl Physiol 1984; 56:798-803.
13. Wallin G. Intraneural recording and autonomic function in man. In: Bannister R, ed. Autonomic failure. A textbook of clinical disorders of autonomic nervous system. Oxford UK: Oxford Univ Press, 1983:37-51.
14. Tarazi RC, Fouad FM. Circulatory dynamics in progressive autonomic failure. In: Bannister R, ed. Autonomic failure. A textbook of clinical disorders of the autonomic nervous system. Oxford UK: Oxford Univ Press 1983:97-114.

PDT

PDT – State of the Art

P.Spinelli, M,Dal Fante
Divisione Endoscopia, Istituto Nazionale
Tumori, Milan, Italy

Photodynamic therapy is an experimental treatment for solid tumors. Photodynamic therapy (PDT) consists of the activation of a photosensitizing agent by light. This photodynamic reaction produces damage to the tissue containing the photosensitizer and exposed to light and in presence of oxygen. The idea of treating tumors by photosensitizers is as old as the early '900; already in the 1903 topic application of eosin and esposition to sunlight was known to produce response by skin tumors (1). On the other hand Policard, 1924, observed reddish fluorescence in animal and human tumors observed under Wood lamp. The presence of fluorescence was attributed to endogenous porphyrins accumulated after infection of the observed tissue by hemolytic bacteria (2). In 1942 Auler and Banzer (3) reported animal tumor fluorescence after systemic administration of Hematoporphyrin (HP) and in 1960 Lipson and coworkers prepared the Hematoporphyrine derivative (HPD), a mixture of porphyrins obtained treating HP with acetic and sulphuric acids (4). They demonstrated that HPD was selectively accumulated by malignant as well as by actively proliferating tissues and realized the first demonstration of endoscopic diagnosis of malignant tissues by detection of fluorescence in the respiratory and in the upper digestive tract (5). After the development of laser, fluorescence diagnosis and particularly PDT have been furtherly studied and the advantage of laser on filtered lamp light has been demonstrated by the possibility of obtaining the necessary power of light with a very narrow band (630 nm wavelength).

Photosensitizer: after the initial observations HpD has been the most widely utilized photosensitizer among the various photosensitizers known (6). Biologically photoactive agents can be distinguished in (a) natural phluorochromes, like porphyrins, (b) exogenous phluorochromes, like acridine orange, phluorescin, rhodamine, (c) endogenous phluorochromes, like flavoproteins and keratine. Most studies deal with first group of natural phluorochromes and their derivatives, because of their activation with a wavelength (600-690 nm) more deeply penetrating in the biological tissues than shorter wavelengths necessary to activate other phluorochromes. Particularly important appear studies regarding phtalocyanine-induced phototoxicity (7,8). Also other drugs are actually under study (9) and will be reported later.

Instrumentation: there are different possibilities òf obtaining the sufficient amount of light of a tissue-penetrating wavelength to be used for PDT. Light of 600-700 nm wavelength is the most penetrating and penetration increases with wavelength. We can obtain these wavelengths by filtered lamps to be used for surface application (10) but, when an intracavitary tumor must be treated by endoscopic systems and light must be trasmitted on fiberoptics it needs special characteristics such as intensity, coherence and monochromaticity. Lasers are the best sources so that the photobiological responses produced by laser-tissue interaction can be quantitatively and qualitatively different from those caused by conventional light sources (11). The advantages of lasers can be summarized as follow: a) intensity: important to produce effects requiring large energy doses; varying peak and average power separately one can induce thermal or photodynamic effects. High peak powers can produce localized thermal damage and high average powers are more likely to produce thermal damage over larger tissue volumes than photodynamic effects. b) coherence: important for direction and focusing on small areas. c) monochromaticity: allows chromophores selection within tissues and selective photobiologic responses.

The most used lasers for PDT are: 1) Ar-laser: (488-514 nm), limited penetration 2) Dye lasers, namely Rhodamine-B laser (630 nm, tunable) the most extensively used for PDT. 3) Gold vapour laser (628 nm); a comparison of gold-vapour and dye-lasers for PDT has been done (12) and the gold-vapour laser appears to be simpler and easier to install and run although it requires a larger diameter fiber for light delivery. The wavelength of the dye laser is tunable, whereas that of the gold vapour is fixed; it can be turned in a copper vapour laser at 510 and 578 nm and used to pump a dye laser.

Methods for irradiation: Irradiation of tumors can be done keeping the fiber distant from the tissue or inserting the fiber into the tissue itself. The evaluation of the energy delivered by the fiber is different in the two situations: if the fiber is kept at distance the energy is expressed in Joules/cm^2; if a sharp cut fiber is inserted into a tissue the energy is expressed simply in Joules; if a circularly radiating fiber is inserted into a tissue the energy is expressed in Joules/cm of fiber inserted. Between the extremity of the fiber and the tissue different light diffusing devices can be used, like diffusing solution, sapphire tips or microlenses (13). Diffusing solutions can be contained into diffusing balloons attached to the end of a fiber or to the end of an endoscope.

Fields of application for PDT: 1) Skin: indication for PDT is extensive, multicentric or critically sited primary cancers, in whom traditional methods of treatment are considered inappropriate (14). Also cutaneous and subcutaneous metastases from breast carcinoma have been treated. 2) Gynecological tumors (15): a) Primary vaginal carcinoma, specially when located in the upper third, is difficult to treat with conventional modalities of treatment because the anatomical relationship with rectum and bladder can cause fistulas. b) Carcinomatous ulcers of the vulva superficially infiltrating also if very wide c) Intraepithelial cancer of the uterine cervix has been treated. The problem of the possible involvement of the deep parts of the cervical glands in the neoplastic process mantains under evaluation this area of PDT. The effectiveness of PDT in completely destroying the cervical glands must yet be demonstrated. 3) Head and neck: cutaneous and mucosal cancers in this area, specially when sited in critical positions. Cases of face, tongue, nasopharynx, larynx and vocal cords carcinomas have been reported as responders to PDT (16). 4) Eye: different interesting application for PDT have been proposed for ophtalmologic treatments a) malignant melanoma of the choroid and retinoblastoma responded to therapy. In the case of highly pigmented melanomas a thermal effect is suspected to be a very important therapeutic factor owing to the high quantity of energy used to treat these lesions. Particular indications such as control of lens epithelial proliferation secondary to cataract surgery have been recently proposed (17). 5) Brain (18): clinical studies involving patients with malignant brain tumors irradiated by the surface or by optic fiber implantation both stereotactically or surgically have been reported but it is too early to assess the results. Photosensitizer can be administered topically or intravenously. 6) Vascular system: Atheromatous plaques show porphyrin uptake (20). It can be demonstrated by fluorescence methods by violet light illumination. This is probably due to the rich vascularization of human plaques that allows porphyrin to reach the plaques, but also other different mechanisms are supposed to be involved in the uptaking of the photosensitizer by atheromatous plaques. Clinically, these bases appear to be useful for PDT of arteries occluded by atheromas, by removing or reducing plaques, with methods of treatment superimposable to those used for PDT in other districts of the body. Also if PDT appears efficacious for atheromas many problems arise in the clinical applications. 7) Endoscopic treatments: PDT has demonstrated particular usefulness in endoscopic treatments particurarly in cases of small tumors with macroscopically undefined borders or in cases of multicentric tumors. These conditions are mostly present in the upper and lower digestive tract, in the bronchi and in the bladder. Hayata, in Tokyo Medical College, started with clinical endoscopic applications of PDT in 1980 and has up to now accumulated the largest experience in the world in the various fields (19). In two international enquiries proposed in the 1984 and in the 1986 we collected data from respectively 467 and 912 patients. Tables are reported; the enquires suggest that the number of centers working in the area of PDT is increasing. Geographically the centers expanded all over the world during the last years. Up to 1984, 467 patients have been treated in 8 centers, between 1984 and 1986 the total number raised up to 912 and the number of centers to 20. The laser sources used show that 4 groups are using the new gold vapor lasers and that activation by Nd:YAG laser photoradiation has been abandoned. Pratically unchanged are a) the photosensitizers used, b) the time interval between drug injection and irradiation, c) the modality of irradiation. Regarding the anatomical areas irradiated the number of bladder treatments is increasing. Regarding the stage, the early tumors are more than the advanced ones; the power and the energy of treatments tend to decrease, probably because of a relative optimization of treatment parameters. If we consider the overall results they can appear worse in the last than in the previous enquiry but we must take into account that 135 patients from the previous enquiry have been referred as complete response (CR) only after a macroscopic evaluation (for example: the reopening of a bronchus). The results of the 1986 enquiry show a CR in 61% of early stage and in 7% of advanced tumors treated, partial response (PR) in 33% early and 80% advanced and no response (NR) in 6% early and 13% advanced.

Perspectives: looking forth to the perspectives of PDT one must separate the different problems being on the table: a) photosensitizers, b) laser light. c) therapeutic combination protocols. a) Photosensitizers: the most used photosensitizer is hematoporphyrin as hematoporphyrin derivative (HPD) and dihaematoporphyrin ether or ester (DHE), its active form. These drugs have two kinds of limitations: skin photosensitization and low tissue penetration of the light at wavelength used for the activation of the sensitizer. The approach to the first problem, due to the uncleared drug present in the body up to 3-4 weeks after injection, can be that of finding a more selective drug and consequently using smaller amounts reducing cutaneous sensitization. Furthermore new drugs, now under experiment, having a high absorption coefficient in the near infrared would improve light penetration into the tumor (8). Between the new drugs, some are compounds resulting from modification of porphyrins: modifying the structure of DHE by converting one or more of the porphyrin rings to chlorin (DHEC), and linking HP to chlorin. Of great interest is also the use of phthalocyanines, which are porphyrin like compounds with a main absorption band in the red; and have experimentally demonstrated to be very efficient as photosensitizers. The action spectrum for chloroaluminium phtrhalocaynine (ClAlPC) is a narrow band centered around 680 nm. ClAlPC appears to be about 50 times more efficient than HPD and the red-shifting of its action spectrum allows a better light penetration into the irradiated tumors.

b) New lasers and irradiation modalities: new laser devices are actually under study; special interest have tunable dye lasers, allowing to produce different wavelengths and new modalities of irradiation by short pulses.

c) Selection of patients and combined protocols: indications for PDT are changing from the first attempts. PDT seems to be more reliable in treating small cancer lesions, superfially extended on large areas, multicentric. PDT can be used as curative and as palliative treatment. It can treat cancer at various stages, from precancer lesions, to cancer in situ and invasive cancer both at "early" (21) and at advanced stages (22). The future tendency is developing treatments in the field of early cancer and precancer lesions. Treatment protocols, involving combination of traditional therapies are actually submitted to international evaluation.

Table 1. Laser sources

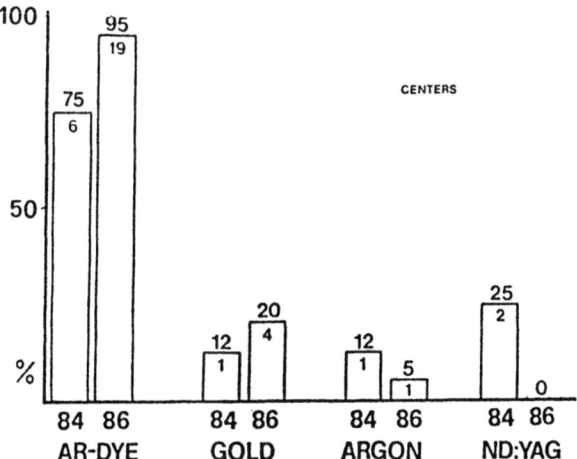

Table 2. Anatomical site of treated lesions

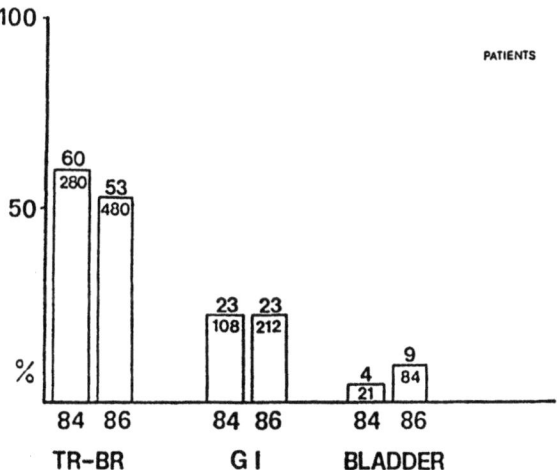

Table 3. Stage of tumors

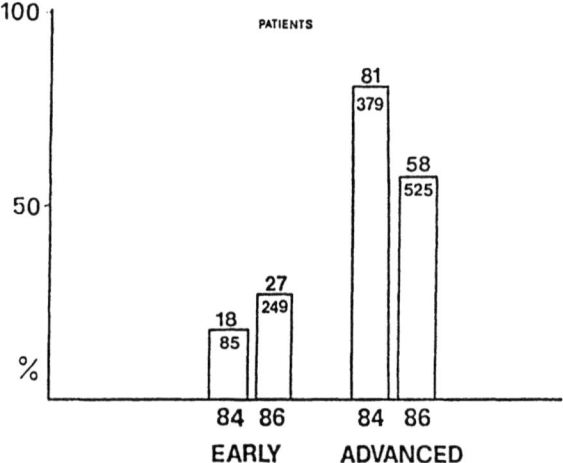

Table 4. Results

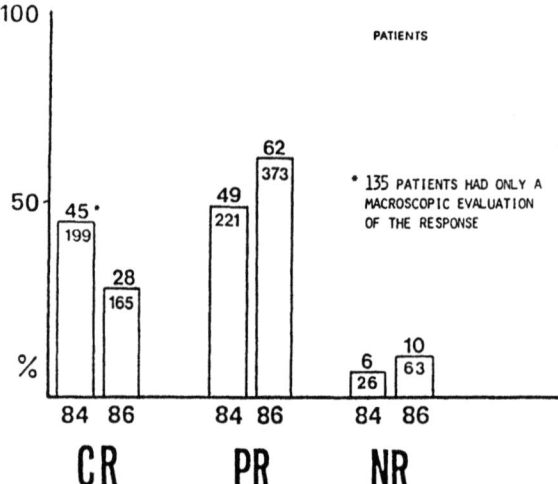

REFERENCES

1. Tappenier H., Jesionek A.: Therapeutische versuche mit fluoreszierenden stoffe. Muench.Med.Wochenschr. 1: 2042, 1903.
2. Policard A.: Etudes sur les aspects offerts par des tumeurs experimentales éxaminées à la lumieère de Woods. Cr.Soc.Biol. 91: 1423, 1924.
3. Auler H., Banzer G.: Untersuchungen uber die rolle der prohpine bei geschwulstkranken menschen und tieren. Z.Krebsforsch. 53: 65, 1942.
4. Lipson R.L., Baldes E.J.: The photodynamic properties of a particular hematoporphyrin derivative. Arch.Dermatol. 82: 508, 1960.

5. Lipson R.L., Baldes E.J., Olsen A.M.: Hematoporphyrin derivative: a new aid for endoscopic detection of malignant disease. J.Thorac.Cardiovasc.Surg. 42: 623, 1961.
6. Spinelli P.: Endoscopic laser-fluorescence and photochemotherapy of cancer. Acta Endoscopica 13: 201, 1983.
7) Ben-Hur E., Rosenthal I.: Action spectrum (600-700 nm) for chloroaluminium phtalocyanine-induced phototoxicity in chinese hamster cells. LLSCES 1: 79, 1986.
8) Kol R., Ben-Hur E., Riklis E., Marko R., Rosenthal I.: Photosensitized inhibition of mitogenic stimulation of human lymphocytes by aluminium phthalocyanine tetrasulpohnate. Las.Med.Scie. 1: 187, 1986.
9. Cubeddu R., Ramponi R., Sacchi C.A., Bottiroli G., Croce A.C., Spinelli P., Dal Fante M., Truscott T.G., Keir W.F.: Photophysical properties of hematoporphyrin compounds for tumor diagnosis and therapy. Photochem.Photobiol., in press.
10. Dougherty T.J., Kaufman J.E., Goldfarb A., Weishaupt K.R., Boyle D.G., Mittleman A.: Photoradiation therapy for the treatment of malignant tumors. Cancer Res. 38: 2628, 1978.
11. Parrish J.A.: Photomedicine potential for lasers. An overview from lasers in photomedicine and photobiology. R.Pratesi and C.A. Sacchi eds., Springer, Berlin, 1980 pag.2.
12. Mc Kenzie A.L., Carruth J.A.S.: A comparison of gold-vapour and dye lasers for PDT. Lasers Med.Sci. 1: 117, 1986.
13. Russo V.: Optical fiber delivery systems for laser medical applications. In: Photodynamic Therapy of Tumors and other Diseases. G.Jori, C.Perria eds., Progetto Publ., Padova, 371, 1985.
14. Gregory R.O., Goldman L.: Application of PDT in plastic surgery. Lasers Surg.Med. 6: 62, 1986.
15. Soma H., Nutahara S.: Cancer of the female genitalia in lasers and hematoporphyrin derivative. In: Lasers and Hematoporphyrin derivative in Cancer. pag. 97, Hayata Y. Dougherty T.J. eds. Igaku-Shoin, Tokyo, 1983.
16. Carruth J.A.S., McKenzie A.L.: Pilot study of photodynamic therapy for the treatment of superficial tumors of the skin and head and neck. In: Photodynamic Therapy of Tumors and other Diseases. G.Jori, C.Perria eds., Progetto Publ., Padova, 1985, pp. 289.
17. Parel J.M., Cubeddu R., Ramponi R., Lingua R., Sacchi C.A., Haefliger E.: Endocapsular rinsing with photofrin II as a photodynamic therapy for lens epithelial proliferation. Abstr. Third Congress of ELA, Lasers Med.Scie. 1: 289, 1986.
18. Laws E.R., Wharen R.E., Anderson R.E.: Photodynamic therapy of brain tumors. In: Photodynamic Therapy of Tumors and other Diseases. G.Jori, C.Perria eds., Progetto Publ., Padova, 1985, pp 311.
19. Hayata Y., Kato H., Konaka C., Ono J., Takizawa N.: Hematoporphyrin derivative and laser photoradiation in the treatment of lung cancer. Chest 81: 269, 1981.
20. Kessel D., Sykes E.: Porphyrin accumulation by atheromatous plaques of the aorta. Photochem.Photobiol. 40: 59, 1984.
21. Tajiri H., Daizukono N., Joffe S.N., Oguro Y.: Photoradiation therapy in early gastrointestinal cancer. Gastrointest.Endosc. 33: 88,1987.
22. Mc Caughan J.S., Williams T.E., Bethel B.H.: Palliation of esophageal malignancy with photodynamic therapy. Am.Thor.Surg. 40: 113, 1985.

Endoscopic Nd: YAG Laser Photocoagulation in Oncology: A 5 Year Experience

P.Spinelli, M.Dal Fante,
Divisione Endoscopia, Istituto Nazionale Tumori (INT), Milan, Italy

Introduction: Actually the best we can do for patients with non-curable cancers is to improve their life expectancy and to give them a better quality of life by treating the most distressing symptoms. Lasers allow palliation of bleeding and obstruction in the respiratory, digestive, and urinary tracts, applied as unic therapeutic resource or in combination with radio- and chemo-therapy or with other endoscopic procedures. Besides palliation Endoscopic Laser Therapy (ELT), has curative indications, firstly in high risk patients with cancers at early stages and then in accurately selected cases, as an alternative to traditional therapeutic methods. Also sessile adenomas of the digestive tube can be treated by laser.

Patients and Methods: Five hundred eleven patients have been submitted to 2025 treatments from 1981 to 1986. All lesions were proven by biopsy. Number, duration and energy of treatments are indicated in tables referred to the different tracts such as Upper Gastro-Intestinal (U.G.I.), Lower Gastro-Intestinal (L.G.I.), Respiratory (R) Tab.I. Laser equipments used were: Cooper Laser Sonics Mod. 8,000 (Santa Clara, CA, U.S.A.), Pilkington Fiberlaser 100 (Glasgow, England), Medilas 2, Medizintechnik GmbH (Munich, West Germany), with a maximum power output of 100 W, and, more recently, Surgical Laser Technologies CL 40 (Malven, Pennsylvania, U.S.A.), with a maximum power of 60 W, U.G.I.: 130 patients have been submitted to laser treatment. palliation of bleeding 5, and obstruction 125, lesions were divided in relation to the length of the stenotic tract evaluated on a barium meal in group 1 (less than 5 cm) 48; group 2 (5-10 cm) 59; group 3 (more than 10 cm) 18. In 5 cases bleeding was indication to treatment. Laser treatment has been associated to dilation in 41 and to intubation in 25 cases Tab.II. Treatment has been performed after insertion of a naso-trans-stenotic tube, its esternal end was plunged into water to avoid over-distension by coaxial flow of gas. Bulking lesions are partially removed by electro-snaring and then treated up to the base by laser. Infiltrating lesions are treated by laser after they have been dilated. The treatment starts from the most central parts and concentrically extends towards the periphery; it continues until a sufficient passage for food (1,5 cm or more) is obtained; nine patients have been treated by contact-laser probes. L.G.I.: in out of 97 carcinomas, 94 were located in the recto-sigmoid. In presence of bulky tumors, as much as possible of the mass was removed by electric snare and the remaining was coagulated by laser from the top to the base. Similar techniques have been used in 95 adenomas. The base of adenoma has been photocoagulated with the surrounding mucosa appearing as healthy. Adenomas has been divided in 3 groups: I, smaller than 1 cm (9), II, from 1 to 4 cm (53) and III, larger than 4 cm (33). Histology showed that 13 were tubular adenomas, 40 tubulo-villous adenomas, 37 villous adenomas and 5 villous adenomas with focal malignancy. The rectal stump after colectomy in 27 patients affected with familiar colorectal polyposis has been treated. R. tract: 128 patients with histologically proven malignant tumors, 38 in trachea and carina, 60 in main and 23 in lobar bronchi have been treated.

Results: U.G.I.: data concerning the number of sessions and energy delivered as well as overall results, and complication rate are shown in table III, IV, V. L.G.I.: results of treatments for malignancies are shown separately: the first group deals with obstruction and the second with bleeding. They are presented in tab. VI, VII, VIII. Those concerning adenomas are reported in tab. IX, X. R. tract: treatments data, results and complication are shown in Tab. XI, XII, XIII.

Discussion: Endoscopic laser therapy is a good method of palliation for advanced cancers and of treatment for early malignant and premalignant tumors as adenomas and adenomas containing foci of carcinoma. UGI tumors are generally diagnosed when symptomatic; in most cases that corresponds to very advanced stages of the disease and to the presence of not curable tumors (1). The palliation regards treatment of dysphagia, chest pain and malnutrition. Endoscopic palliation of dysphagia can be obtained by dilation, prosthesis, electrocoagulation, photocoagulation, photo-radiation therapy and gastrostomy. Laser photocoagulation is efficacious in establishing quick and durable oesophageal and cardial patency with a low rate of complications. Polypoid tumors are directly irradiated by laser but, in infiltrating and stenotic lesions, dilation allows passing of the scope through the stenosis and treating relevant parts of tumor so achieving a more durable patency of the lumen (2-3). Contact-laser probes can avoid the need for dilation introducing the contact-probe through the stenosis (4). Introduction of a prostesis after laser photocoagulation can make the treatment definitive, but increases the risk of complications: these include migration, bleeding and perforation (5). Best results have been achieved in stenosis shorter than 10 cm; in the group 1 complications are absent. Sometimes after achieving the patency of the lumen patients can't swallow mainly because of severe oesophagitis: that is the reason why we separated successful treatment from those followed by good clinical results. In the LGI tract tumors, laser treatment is effective in palliation of bowel obstruction. It can avoid a colostomy in non-operable patients, and allows operable patients to be submitted to elective surgery, avoiding emergency treatment. In our series of 79 patients treated in order to relieve an obstruction, sufficient luminal patency has been obtained in 70. In our series of 18 patients, rectal bleeding, has been stopped in all. The treatment can be repeated in case of need in out-patient clinic. Lasers seem to be more efficacious than X-therapy and endoscopic electrocoagulation for bleeding tumors (6). In the R tract Nd:YAG laser allows palliation of obstruction and care of small malignancies with little tendency to submucosal and lymphatic invasions (7,8). There are two indications for laser palliative treatment: the first is to obtain patency of the airway, the second aims to avoid the tumor to invade a larger and proximal segment of the airway i.e. a tumor arising from the upper lobe bronchus to invade the main bronchus or a tumor of a main bronchus to cross the carina and invade the controlater bronchial tree. Of the 44 successful cases in the main bronchi in 43 we obtained patency of the bronchial lumen. In tracheal tumors success has been achieved in 92% of the treated cases, since the success rate falls to 70% in lobar bronchi.

Tab. I. 5-year experience in endoscopic laser therapy (e.l.t.) 2025 nd:yag and argon laser treatments
(argon treatments are marked with *)

	u.g.i.	l.g.i.	respiratory
malignant tumors			
n. of patients	130	97	128
n. of treatments	384	368	363
benign tumors			
n. of patients	3	125	–
n. of treatments	10	785 + 9*	–
vascular lesions			
n. of patients	10	13	2
n. of treatments	12 + 41*	6 + 15*	2 + 2*
others			
n. of patients	2	–	11
n. of treatments	2	–	26

Tab: II. e.l.t. in u.g.i. cancer associated therapy

	group 1	group 2	group 3
bougienage	13/48 (27%)	20/59 (34%)	8/18 (44%)
prosthesis	4/48 (8%)	18/59 (31%)	3/18 (17%)

Tab. III. e.l.t. in u.g.i. cancer data of treatments

	group 1	group 2	group 3
n.sessions	1.4	1.5	2.2
days	2.7	5.2	8.9
energy (J)	7,362	11,993	14,153

Tab. IV. e.l.t. in u.g.i. cancer - results

	group 1	group 2	group 3
successful treatments	43/48	57/59	15/18
(%)	(90)	(97)	(83)
with clin. improvement	33/43	46/57	12/15
(%)	(77)	(81)	(80)
complications	-	2/59	2/15
(%)	-	(3)	(13)

Tab. V. u.g.i. - complications

1 hemorrhage
  conservative management
1 perforation
  endosc. prosthesis: dead 7 days
2 fistulas after treatment
  1 surg.therapy: alive 1 month
  1 endosc. prosthesis: alive 3 m

Tab. VI. e.l.t. in l.g.i. cancer data of treatments

	obstruction	bleeding
n.sessions	1.7	1.1
days	8.7	2.4
energy (J)	11,404	4,929

Tab. VII. e.l.t. in l.g.i. cancer results

	obstruction	bleeding
successful treatments	71/79	18/18
(%)	(90)	(100)
further treatments	47/71	9/18
(%)	(66)	(50)

Tab. VIII. e.l.t. in l.g.i. cancer complications

2 early hemorrhages:
  medical treatment
2 late hemorrhages:
  medical treatment
3 perforations:
  1 surgery
  2 medical management

Tab. IX. e.l.t. in colorectal adenomas data of treaments and results

	group 1	group 2	group 3
disappeared	9/9	40/53	14/33
n. of sessions	1	2	6.5
weeks	1 day	9	52
recurrence	1	18	6
time interval (wks)	26	44	40
non-recurrence	8	22	8
time interval (wks)	38	45	30

Tab. X. e.l.t. in colorectal adenomas - complications

3 hemorrhages during treatment:
  interm.
    endoscopic therapy
3 late hemorrhages:
  medical management
9 invasive ca. during therapy

Tab. XI. e.l.t. in tracheo-br. tree data of treatments

	trachea & carina	main bronchi	lobar & bronchi
n.sessions	1.4	1.8	1.5
days	3.7	7.4	5.7
energy (J)	7,019	8,364	4,605

Tab. XII. e.l.t. in tracheo-br. tree results

	trachea & carina	main bronchi	lobar bronchi
successfull treatm.	35/38	44/60	16/23
(%)	(92)	(73)	(70)
complications	1/38	7/60	1/23
(%)	(3)	(12)	(4)

Tab. XIII. e.l.t. in tracheo-br. tree complications

trachea & carina:
  1 oedema: tracheostomy
main bronchi:
  1 pnx: spontaneous recovery
  2 perfor: 1 septic shock, 1 med.tr.
  2 late hemorr: endosc. treatment
  2 hypertensive crisis: 1 TIA,1 coma
lobar & intermediate bronchi:
  1 early hemorr.: endosc. treatment

REFERENCES

1. Boyce M.Y.: Palliation of advanced esophageal cancer. Semin.Oncol. 11:186, 1984.
2. Riemann J.F., Ell Ch., Lux G., Demling L.: Combined therapy of malignant stenoses of the upper gastrointestinal tract by means of laser beam and bougienage. Endoscopy 17:43, 1985.
3. Mellow M.H., Pinkas H.: Endoscopic therapy for esophageal carcinoma with Nd:YAG laser: prospective evaluation of efficacy, complications, and survival. Gastrointest. Endosc. 30: 334, 1984.
4. Spinelli P., Dal Fante M.: Contact laser surgery with sapphire micro-probes. Proceedings of the European Conference on Optics, Optical Systems and Applications, ECOOSA, 1986, in press.
5. Ogilvie A.L., Dronfield M.W., Ferguson R., Atkinson M.: Palliative intubation of oesophagogastric neoplasms at fibreoptic endoscopy. GUT 23: 1060, 1982.
6. Mathus-Vliegen E.M.H., Tytgat G.N.G.: Nd:YAG laser photocoagulation in gastroenterology: its role in palliation of colorectal cancer. Lasers Med. Scie. 1:75, 1986.
7. Kao S.J., Shen C.Y., Hsu K.: Nd:YAG laser application in pulmonary and endobronchial lesions. Lasers Surg.Med. 6:296, 1986.
8. Toty L., Personne C., Colchen A., Vourc'h G.: Bronchoscopic management of tracheal lesions using the neodymium yttrium aluminium garnet laser. Thorax 36: 175, 1981.

The Effects of Photoradiation Therapy and Hyperthermia on Mice Bearing Subcutaneous Tumor

D.M. Hau[1], H. Chang[2], M.C. Kao[3] and H.Y. Hsu[4]

[1] Institute of Radiation Biology, National Tsing Hua University Hsinchu, Taiwan R.O.C., [2] Department of Chemistry, National Tsing-Hua University, [3] Department of Surgery, National Taiwan University, College of Medicine, [4] Department of Radiology, KMC

INTRODUCTION. Hematoporphyrin derivative (HPD) is a photosensitizer and has strong affinity to quickly growing tissues and tumors (1). After HPD is excited by light, the energy can transfer to oxygen which may cause the tumor cells lysed (2). Photoradiation therapy, the application of HPD and light irradiation, is a good modality for cancer therapy. The therapeutic effect of photoradiation therapy in subcutaneous tumor for BALB/C strain mice had been studied in this laboratory (3).

Hyperthermia is also a good modality for cancer therapy. Leith had investigated the clinical application of local hyperthermia by 43 to $45^{\circ}C$ (4). The block of capillaries and other factors were the causes for the lysis of tumor cells (5,6). The treatment of subcutaneous tumor for ICR strain mice by hyperthermia had also been studied in this laboratory (7).

Waldow and Dougherty combined the hyperthermia and photoradiation therapy to treat tumor and led a better result (8). This paper showed that the combination of photoradiation therapy and hyperthermia have better therapeutic effect in tumor therapy for mice bearing subcutaneous tumor.

MATERIALS AND METHOD. Seven to eight week old BALB/C and C3H strain mice were used in this study. Ehrlich ascites tumor cells (1×10^7) were inoculated into the subcutaneous tissue in the femoral part of mice. When the subcutaneous tumors grew to 10 ± 2 mm in diameter, the animals were divided into normal control group, experimental control group and experimental groups. Different treatment of photoradiation therapy or/and hyperthermia were applied.

The treatment condition of photoradiation therapy and hyperthermia are listed in Fig. 1. The method of preparing HPD and the radiation source had been described elsewhere (3). All the equipments had been reported too (7). For the combination treatments, hyperthermia was applied immediately after the photoradiation therapy.

All the treatments were applied to each mouse once a day for three successive days. Mice were examined every tenth day for a period of 120 days after the treatments. The experimental responses were recorded by measuring the tumor volume ($\pi/6 \times D_1 \times D_2 \times D_3$), body weight, mortality rate, tumor control rate and mean survival time.

RESULTS. The factors which varied were the total irradiation energy, the amount of HPD injected, the hyperthermia temperature and the duration of the hyperthermia treatment. Figure 1 shows the mean survival time of all experimental groups for both BALB/C and C3H strain mice observed in this study. From the results of the experimental group treated by varying one of these factors, the best conditions were followings: (1) 300 and 400 J for total irradiation energy for BALB/C strain mice and 200 and 300 J for C3H strain mice, (2) 7.5 and 10 mg HPD/kg body weight for BALB/C strain mice and 7.5 mg HPD/kg body weight for C3H strain mice for the HPD injected, (3) 44 and 45°C for hyperthermia temperature in the tumor and (4) 30 min for the duration of hyperthermia treatment. The experimental condition for the combination of photoradiation therapy and hyperthermia were limited to the above conditions.

Body weights and tumor volumes are two criteria for evaluating the therapeutic effect. The results were summarized as following. The body weight in the normal control group increased steadily. For the experimental control group, it increased rapidly in the first 60 days due to the growth of the tumor. In the experimental groups, it increased slowly and finally was close to that of the normal control group.

The tumor volume in the experimental control group increased very rapidly in the first 60 days. It increased much less in the experimental groups. The tumor became non-detectable earlier in the groups treated with combination of photoradiation therapy and hyperthermia.

For BALB/C strain mice, the mean survival time was improved by photoradiation therapy. Hyperthermia gave better results. However, the combination treatment of photoradiation therapy and hyperthermia showed even a higher mean survival time. The group had the best therapeutic effect was treated by 400 J of total irradiation energy, 7.5 mg HPD/kg body weight and 45°C for 30 min. In that group, the tumor control rate, the mortality rate and the mean survival time were 90.0%, 10.0% and 114 days, respectively. Other groups treated with both photoradiation therapy and hyperthermia also had longer mean survival time than had the group treated by photoradiation therapy or hyperthermia.

For C3H strain mice, the best conditions were: 300 J for total irradiation energy, 7.5 mg HPD/kg body weight, 45°C and 30 min for hyperthermia. The tumor control rate, the mortality rate and the mean survival time were 93.3%, 7.1% and 114 days, respectively. Although the group with best result in the combination of photoradiation therapy and hyperthermia had the similar mean survival time with the group treated by hyperthermia (45°C for 30 min). However, the results for the combination treatment were in gerenal good for other experimental groups.

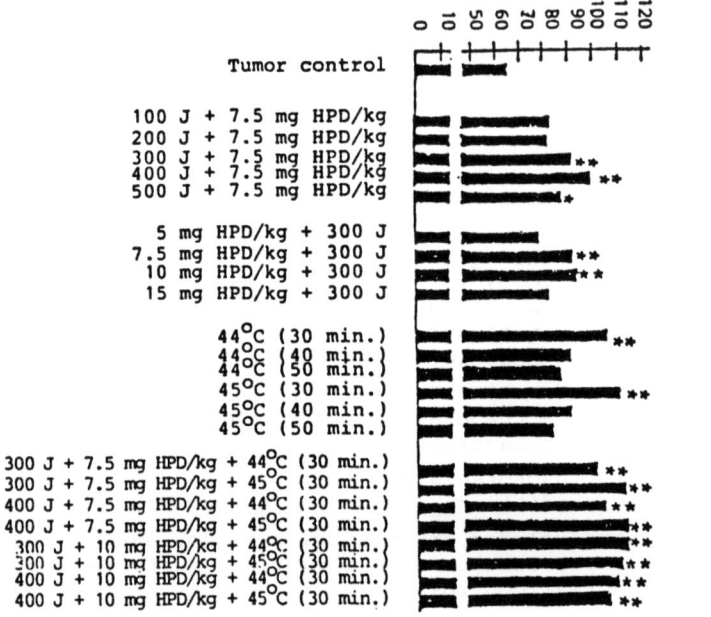
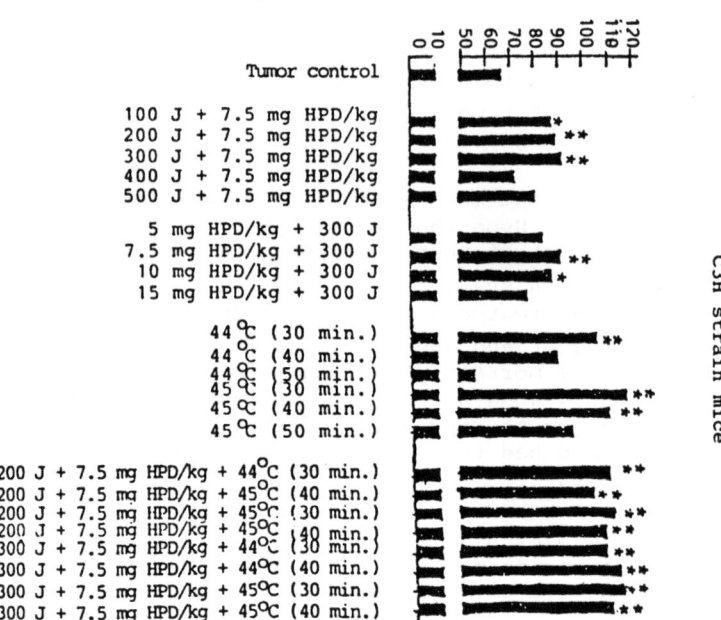

FIG. 1. THE MEAN SURVIVAL TIME OF VARIOUS TREATMENTS OF BALB/C AND C3H STRAIN MICE. * : P < 0.05, ** : P < 0.01 (Student's t-test; compared with tumor control group).

DISCUSSION. Goldman et al noted that the temperature raised in solid tumor during the laser irradiation due to the absorption of photon energy (9). The rise of the temperature also depended on the power of the laser beam (10). Martin et al found that the temperature inside the tumor depended on the irradiation time because of the accumulation of photon energy (11). Another important factor was the concentration of HPD in the tissue because HPD has high absorpting (12). They were also observed in this study. However, the temperature rise due to the HPD and laser irradiation was not fast nor high enough for hyperthermia in this study.

In the previous reports, for photoradiation therapy the best therapeutic effect (70.6% tumor control rate) was observed in the group of BALB/C strain mice treated with 7.5 mg HPD/kg body weight and total irradiation energy of 400 J of 514.5 nm argon ion laser light (3). Some good therapeutic effect of hyperthermia was also observed in treating subcutaneous tumor of ICR strain mice with 44.4°C for 30 min or 44.4 and 45.4°C for 45 min (7). The results in this study showed that the best conditions for combination treatment of photoradiation therapy and hyperthermia on both strain mice were similar to those in photoradiation therapy or hyperthermia. The results for combination treatment were much better than photoradiation therapy, but similar to hyperthermia. However, the therapeutic effect did not decrease much if the treatment conditions changed. This may be important because the therapeutic conditions were not critical if photoradiation therapy and hyperthermia were combined to treat tumors.

References

1. Figge, F. A.T. et al., Proc. Soc. Exptl. Biol. Med. 68:640-641, 1948
2. Dougherty, T. J. J. Natl. Cancer Res. 52:1333-1336, 1974.
3. Hau, D. M. et al., J. Formosan Med. Assoc. in press.
4. Leith, J. T. et al., Cancer Res. 39:766-779, 1977.
5. Hume, S. P. et al., Br. J. Radiol. 55:438-443, 1982.
6. Warters, R. L. et al., Radiat. Res. 93:71-84, 1983.
7. Hau, D.M. et al., Bull. Chin. Oncol. Quart. 5:9-17, 1984.
8. Waldow, S. M. et al., Radiat. Res. 97:380-385, 1984.
9. Goldman, L. et al., J. Am. Med. Assoc. 198:173-176, 1966.
10. Kinsey, J. J. H. et al., Cancer Res. 41:5020-5026, 1974.
11. Martin, S. et al., J. Am. Med. Assoc. 187:154-159, 1964.
12. Peter, J. B. et al., Cancer Res. 41:4606-4612, 1981.

Laser Inactivation of Blast Lymphocytes by Photodynamic Effect with Hematoporphyrin Species

S. Satomi*, T. Taguchi*, H. Inaba**,***,

S. Mashiko***, S. Sato**

* IInd Department of Surgery, Tohoku University
School of Medicine

** Research Institute of Electrical Communication,
Tohoku University

*** Bio-Photon Project, Research Development
Corporation of Japan

* 1-1 Seiryo-cho, Sendai, 980 Japan

Photodynamic effect caused by combination of hematoporphyrin (Hp) and photoradiation on malignant cells, which is cytocidal, has been used as a new therapeutic modality of malignant disease. We found that cytotoxic T-cells (CTL), which play a prominent role in rejection episode in clinical organ transplantation, also possess an affinity for Hp like malignant cells. Therefore, photoradiation after administration of Hp can destroy CTL, and if we can destroy the activated CTL selectively, it has a possibility to become a new rejection therapy. We report here for the first time the photodynamic effect of Hp on human Concanavarin A (Con A) activated blast lymphocytes and mouse CTL.

Materials and Methods

Normal lymphocytes derived from healthy people are stimulated in a medium containing Con A (10 μg/ml) at 37°C for 3 days to obtain blast lymphocytes. Then both the normal and blast lymphocytes are incubated with the varying concentration of Hp for 60 min. For the excitation, all emission line of Ar laser is employed. Thus the survival rates of both the sample cells are measured after the irradiation. Also the fluorescence intensity of Hp uptaken to the cells is measured by flow-cytometry.

Mouse CTLs are gained by using mixed lymphocyte culture and are kept as CTL line (CTLL) with exogenous IL-2. The experimental method is almost similar to the previous Con A blast lymphocyte study.

Results

A three dimentional graphic display of fluorescense intensity distribution across the cell is demonstrated (Fig.1). Upper one is obtained from blast lymphocyte containing hematoporphyrin dihydrochroride and lower one is from normal lymphocyte. And it is found that the fluorescence intensity is greater in cytoplasma than the

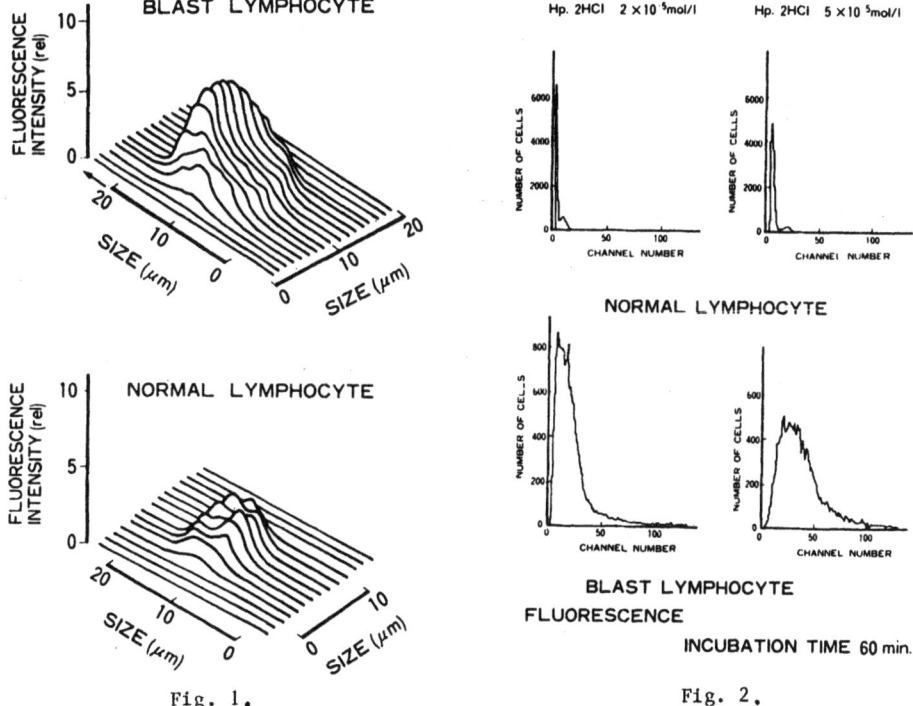

Fig. 1.

Fig. 2.

nuclear portion. Furthermore, the difference of dye concentration can be seen distinguishly. Fluorescence intensity of blast cell is almost four times greater than that of normal one. Fig. 2 shows fluorescence intensity measured by flowcytometry. Both normal and blast lymphocytes are incubated with the varying concentrations of Hp for 60 min. Vertical axis is cell number and horizontal axis is fluorescence intensity. It has been found that the concentration of Hp depends on the uptake of Hp. Also when the both lymphocytes are incubated with same concentration of Hp (5×10^{-5} Mol/l) for varying period of time, the fluorescence intensity depends on the incubation period (Fig. not shown). Fig. 3 & 4 show survival rate of both lymphocytes uptaken with varying Hp concentrations. The irradiation times of laser ranges one to five minutes. The survival rate shows a linear decrease with the irradiation time in general and the photodynamic effect is more appreciable for higher dye concentration. In addition, even for the same dye concentration and irradiation time, the survival rate of normal lymphocyts is higher than that of blast ones. Fig. 5 shows inactivation coefficients of both lymphocytes. In this expeiment, we defined the gradient of survival rate as the inactivation coeffecient. The inactivation coeffecient for the blast lymphocyte is larger and steeper than that of normal one. From these findings, laser induced photodynamic effect on Con A blast lymphocytes is likely to be associated with the fact that the blast lymphocytes uptake more Hp than normal lymphocytes uptake.

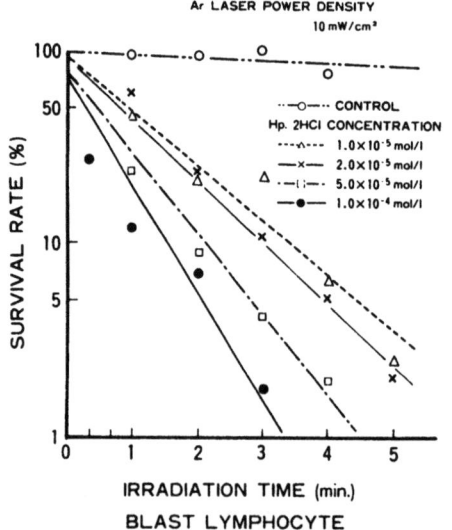

Fig. 3.

Fig. 4.

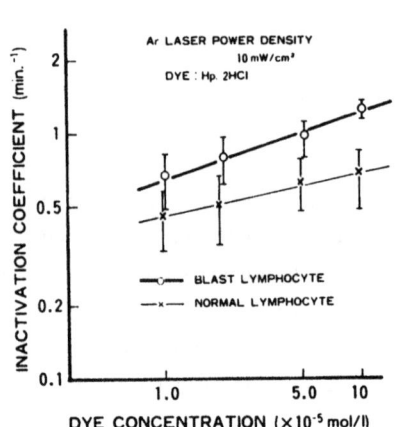

Fig. 5.

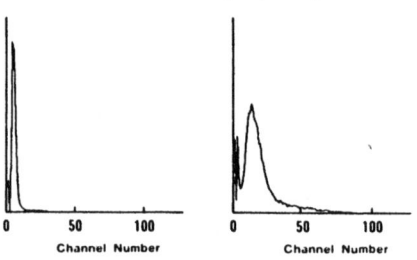

Fig. 6.

In the transplantation immunology the most important cell is cytotoxic T-cell. Because, these cells have an important function in graft rejection. Therefore, as the next step, photodynamic effect of the CTL are investigated. Since to make a cytotoxic T-cell line in human is difficult, a mouse CTLL is used in this experiment.

Fig. 6 shows fluorescence intensity measured by flowcytometry. Both cells are incubated with the varying concentrations of Hp for 60 minutes as shown in the Con A

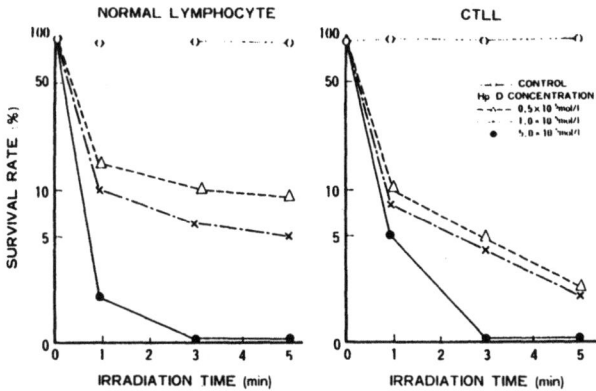

Fig. 7.

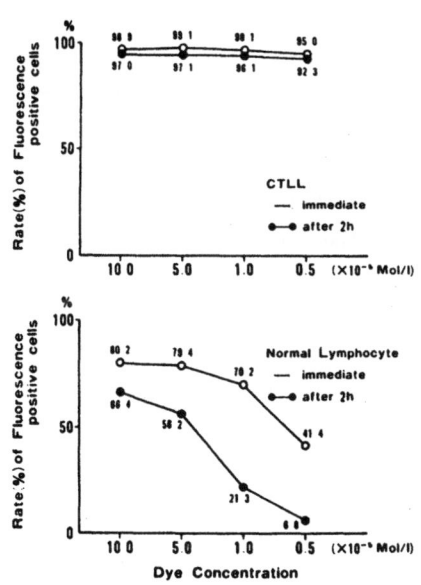

Fig. 8.

blast lymphocyte study. The higher concentration of Hp is the greater uptake is obtained. Fig. 7 shows the survival rate of the both cells after 10 mW/cm^2 laser power density irradiation. For the both cells, almost 90% cells are killed by 1 minute irradiation.

In order to investigate excretion of dye from cells, both lymphocytes containing Hp are washed out completely and then incubated for additional 2 hours at 37°C. Fig. 8 shows the rate of fluorescence positive cells. Though both the normal lymphocytes and CTL decrease fluorescence intensity after additional 2 hour incubation (Fig. not shown), as far the rate of fluoresence positive cells, cytotoxic T-cells keep 90% positive rate after 2 hour incubation.

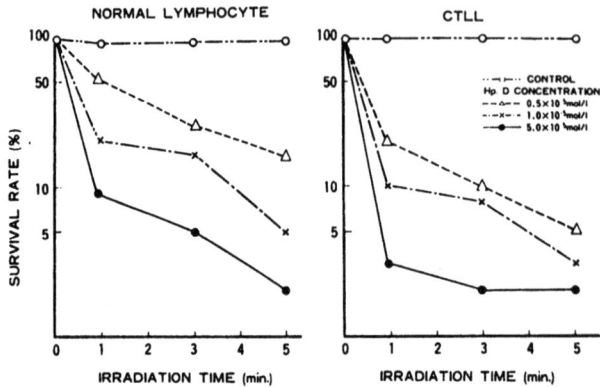

Fig. 9.

Meanwhile, positive rate of normal ones decrease within a short period of incubation. It is supposed that normal lymphocytes excrete Hp easier than CTL excrete. Fig. 9 shows the survival rate of both cells incubated for additional 2 hours and then irradiated for varying period of time. Since mouse lymphocyte is sensitive to photodynamic effect, 90% of both cells are killed by 5 minute irradiation. But survival rate of normal lymphocyte containing lower Hp concentration has increased up to 50% from 15% following one minute irradiation. On the other hand, changes in survival rate of CTL are minimal. These findings seems to be the influence of different dye excretion from the both cells.

Conclusion

It is well known that the lymphocyte depletion is effective immunosuppression which results prolonged graft survival. So, many materials and methods, such as ALS treatment, thracic duct drainage, irradiation, and lymphopheresis, are used for the therapy in clinical transplantation. But these methods are not selective lymphocyte depletion. Therefore, if we can destroy the activated blast lymphocyte selectively, there would be a possibility to become a more effective rejection therapy. The phenomena found in this experiment seem to be associated with the fact that there are different uptake and excretion of Hp between the normal lymphocyte and activated blast lymphocyte such as Con A blast lymphocyte and CTL. For the selective depletion of CTL, it is nescessary to investigate more clearly, optimum dye concentration, incubation time, irradiation power density and irradiation time. We think that it has a possisility to use the photodynamic therapy as a new rejection therapy in clinical organ trasnplantation in near future.

Two-Photon Excited Visible Fluorescence and Photodynamical Effect of Pheophorbide a on Cultured Tumor Cells Using a Nd: YAG Laser

S. Mashiko[*], H. Inaba[*,+], S. Sato[+], Y. Taguchi[#] and S. Kimura[**]

[*]Biophoton Project, Research Development Corporation of Japan (JRDC), Yagiyama-minami 2-1-1, Sendai 982, [+]Research Institute of Electrical Communication, Tohoku University, [#]The 2nd Department of Surgery, School of Medicine, Tohoku University, and [**]Department of Food Chemistry, Faculty of Agriculture, Tohoku University, Sendai 980, Japan

Photodynamic therapy (PDT) represents a new approach to treatment of a variety of malignant tumors in man and animals[1]. A nontoxic, photosensitizing drug with fluorescent properties, such as the hematoporphyrin derivative (HpD), is first injected systemically. After 2-3 days, this drug exhibits a higher retention in the cancerious region than in the surrounding normal tissue. Subsequent irradiation at a proper optical wavelength, mainly red light around 630 nm, results in rapid necrosis of the neoplastic tissue.

The attenuation depth of 630 nm light in living tissues is estimated to range generally from 2 to 4 mm, which lies between those for Ar and Nd:YAG laser wavelengths. Typically tumor necrosis occurs to 2 or 3 times the attenuation depth, that is, possibly, 5 to 15 mm at that wavelength. However, this depth is usually smaller than that of Nd:YAG laser light, which seems to be several times or more greater than that of the red light. Hence we have exploited for the first time the new possibility of achieving deeper activation depth using a Nd:YAG laser emitting at 1.064 μm for a photodynamic therapy incorporating hematoporphyrin species, based on a two-photon excitation process[2,3].

As a further extension of this research, we report the first time spectroscopic studies including absorption and fruorescence of pheophorbide a (PPa) solutions excited by Q-switched Nd:YAG laser output and in vitro experiments on survival rates of cultured cancer cells associated with the new kind of two-photon PDT[4].

The activation mechanism which is generally recognized for PDT involves the intermediacy of the cytotoxic agent, singlet oxygen $^1O_2$, generated by electronic energy transfer, or intersystem crossing, from the upper triplet state of a specific dye, such as hematoporphyrin derivative(HpD), through its excited singlet state by the direct transition from the singlet ground state. However, Nd:YAG laser radiation can cause the singlet-singlet transition only by simultaneous absorption of two photons[2,3]. This process is called simply two-photon absorption, as is well known in the field of nonlinear optics[5], because no energy level exists between them.

Pheophorbide a which is one of the decomposition products of chlorophyll a, has a structure as shown in Fig.1. We have already demonstrated that PPa ex-

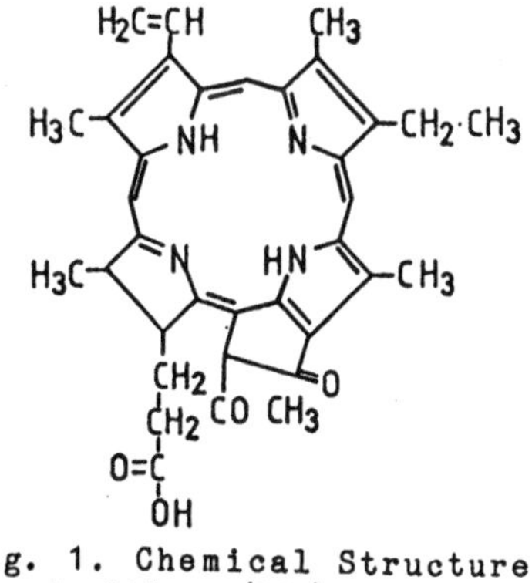

Fig. 1. Chemical Structure of Pheophorbide a (PPa)

hibits more effectively the photodynamic action in cultured cancer cells than the hematoporphyrin species in conditions of nearly the same concentrations and the same laser output irradiation time employing visible lasers[6].

In order to examine a two-photon transition, spectroscopic studies were first performed by exciting PPa dissolved in PBS and ethanol with a Q-switched Nd:YAG laser output and its second harmonic beam at 532 nm. The absorption spectrum of PPa shows a strong absorption band near 380 nm and also exhibits another absorption bands around 690 nm characteristic of a chlorin structure. Both the visible fluorescence spectra were found to have similar distributions with peaks near 690 nm, with a relatively minor differences around 750 nm.

Figures 2(a) and (b) show the measured fluorescence intensity of PPa in PBS and ethanol solution at a concentration of 10^{-4} mol/l as a function of the second harmonic pulse energy (a) and the fundamental pulse energy (b) from a Q-switched Nd:YAG laser. After a linear increase with pulse energy, the fluorescence intensity generated by the second harmonic pulse saturates for higher excitation energies. However, the fundamental pulse excited fluorescence was observed to increase with the square of the Nd:YAG laser energy, as is seen in Fig. 2(b). This quadratic dependence is definitely indicative of the occurrence of two-photon absorption[5] in the case of Nd:YAG laser pulse excitation. However, this intensity was found to be about four orders of magnitude smaller than that for the single photon absorption process due to the second harmonic pulse with the same excitation energy of 1 mJ/pulse.

Based on this spectroscopic evidence, in vitro experiments were performed with cultured esophagus cancer cells. Before irradiation the cells were incubated at 37 °C for up to 2 hours with different concentrations of PPa in the culture medium. Samples in a 3.5 cm diameter quartz cuvette were uniformly irradiated with either the fundamental Nd:YAG laser pulses at 1.064 μm or second harmonic pulses at 532 nm.

In Fig. 3(a), the measured dependence of the cancer cell survival rate on the irradiation time with the fundamental pulse at an energy density of 10 mJ/pulse.cm^2 and 10 pps pulse operation is shown for different incubation times of the 10^{-4} mol/l

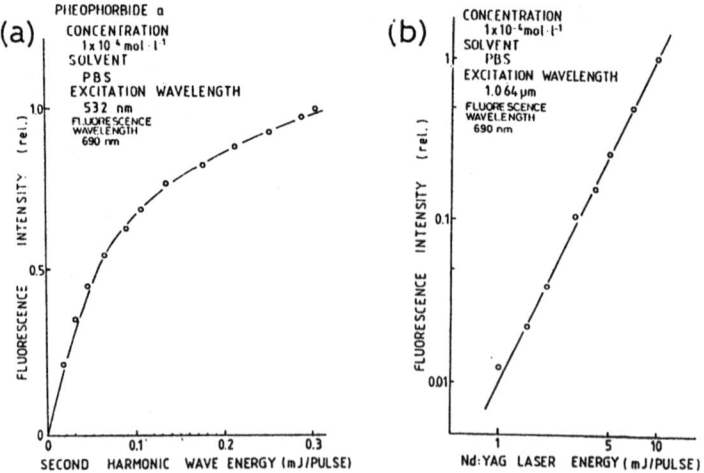

Fig. 2. Measured fluorescence intensity of pheophorbide a in PBS solution as a function of the fundamental pulse energy at 1.064 μm (right) and the second harmonic pulse energy at 0.532 μm (left) from a Q-switched Nd:YAG laser (PPa concentration : 10^{-4} mol/l)

PPa taken up cells. Fig. 3(b) presents the inactivation coefficient for these experimental conditions against the incubation time. We estimated the inactivation coefficient from the slope of the experimental linear curve in semi-log scale as drawn in Fig. 3(a).

Figure 4(a) also depicts the measured survival rate of the cancer cells as a function of the irradiation time with the fundamental Nd:YAG laser pulse at an energy density of 10 mJ/cm^2 and 10 pps pulse operation for different concentrations of PP a in PBS solution after 1 hour of incubation. Fig. 4(b) then gives the inactivation coefficient against PP a concentration under the same experimental conditions.

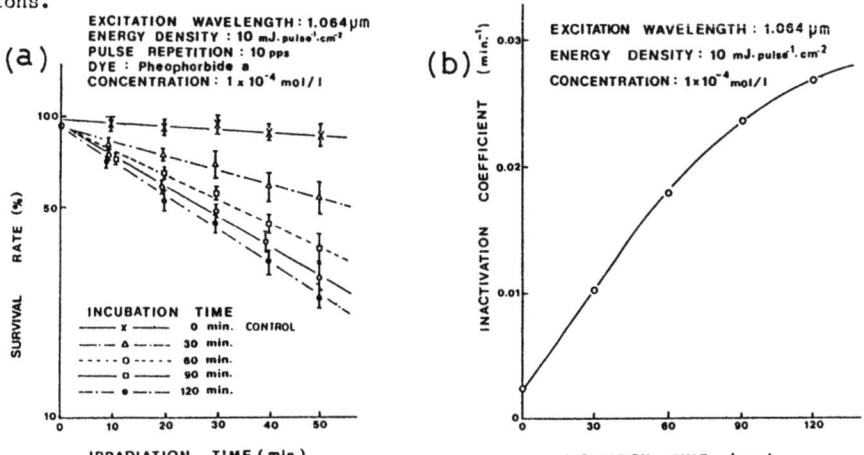

Fig. 3. Measured results of survival rate (a) and inactivation coefficient (b) of cultured esophagus cancer cells by changing the irradiation time of Nd:YAG laser pulses at 1.064 μm and incubation time in PBS solution containing pheophorbide a

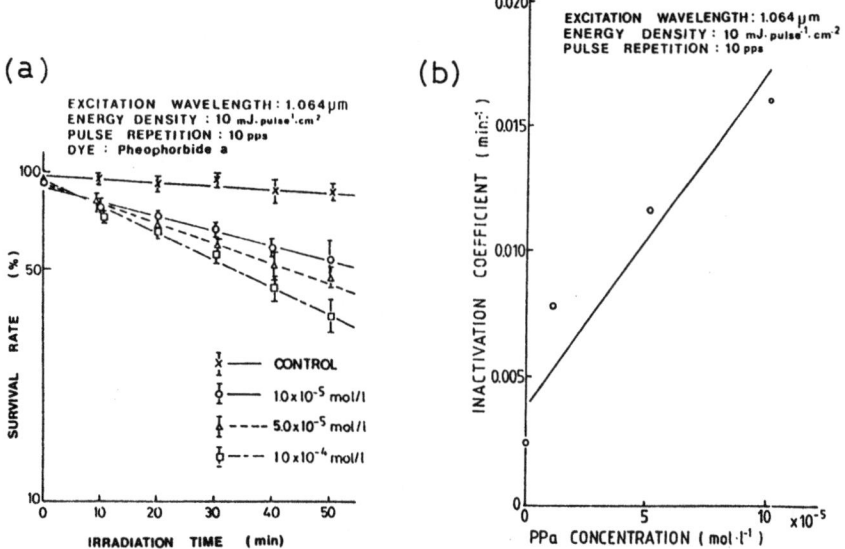

Fig. 4. Measured results of survival rate (a) and inactivation coefficient (b) of cultured esophagus cancer cells by changing the irradiation time of Nd:YAG laser pulses at 1.064 μm and pheophorbide a concentration in PBS solution for the case of 1 hour incubation time

Figure 5 shows a comparison of the measured survival rate of cultured, PPa and hematoporphyrin dihydrochloride (Hp.2HCl) taken up cultured esophagus cancer cells as a function of irradiation time with fundamental pulses and second harmonic pulses from a Q-switched Nd:YAG laser. The energy densities at a 10 pps repetition rate, and the PPa and Hp.2HCl concentrations are shown in the table of this figure. The inactivation coefficient for both the dyes in the case of a fundamental pulse energy density of 12 mJ/pulse.cm^2 was estimated from this measurement to be about 10^{-3} smaller than that for a second harmonic pulse energy density of 0.5 mJ/pulse.cm^2.

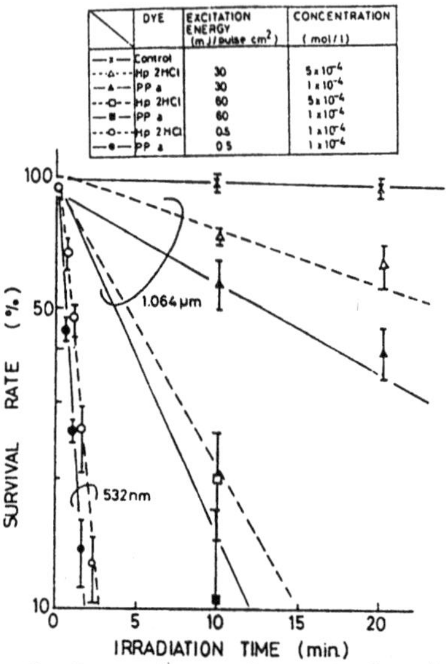

In summary, we have measured and examined for the first time the visible fluorescence properties of PPa in PBS and ethanol solutions excited by the fundamental pulse at 1.064 μm from a Q-switched Nd:YAG laser. This visible fluorescence intensity was found to be proportional to the square of the fundamental pulse energy at 1.064 μm and is attributed to a two-photon simultaneous absorption excitation process. Dependence of survival rate and inactivation coefficient of cultured esophagus cancer cells taken up PPa on irradiation time, incubation time, PPa concentration and laser energy density were measured employing Q-switched Nd:YAG laser output.

Fig. 5. Comparison of survival rate of cultured esophagus cancer cells taken up pheophorbide a and hematoporphyrin dihydrochloride as a function of irradiation time for fundamental pulses at 1.064 μm and second harmonic pulses at 0.532 μm from a Q-switched Nd:YAG laser

The inactivation coefficient provided by PPa was found to be approximately four times larger than that for Hp.2HCl under the same in vitro experimental conditions. Even though the photodynamic effect of these dyes associated with Nd:YAG laser pulse excitation is rather small compared to the case for the second harmonic pulse irradiation, these novel results suggest the possibility of inducing photosensitizing oxidation reactions employing near infrared lasers offering some potential basic and clinical implications for PDT.

References
1) Y.Hayata, T.J.Dougherty, Eds. : Laser and Hematoporphyrin Derivative in Cancer, Igaku-shoin, Tokyo (1983)
2) M.Shimamoto, S.Mashiko, S.Sato, H.Inaba, T.Kuwahara, Y.Taguchi, M.Kasai: J. Jpn. Soc. Laser Medicine, 5, 441(1985)(in Japanese)
3) H.Inaba, M.Shimamoto, S.Mashiko, S.Sato, T.Kuwahara, Y.Taguchi and M.Kasai: in Laser/Optoelectronics in Medicine W.Waidelich and P.Kiefbaher, Eds., 66, Springer Verlag, Berlin(1986)
4) S.Mashiko, S.Sato, H.Inaba, Y.Taguchi, M.Kasai and S.Kimura: J. Jpn. Soc. Laser Medicine, 6, 113(1986)(in Japanese)
5) E.g., Y.R.Shen: The Principles of Nonlinear Optics, John Willy and Sons, New York (1984)
6) S.Takahashi, S.Sato, H.Inaba, T.Akaishi, Y.Taguchi, M.Kasai: J. Jpn. Soc. Laser Medicine, 4, 57, 99(1984)

Intracellular and in vivo Composition of Hematoporphyrin Derivative by Various Fluorescent Components

H. Schneckenburger[1], M. Frenz[1], J. Feyh[2], and A. Götz[2]

[1] GSF Research Center, Institute of Applied Optics,
Ingolstädter Landstr. 1, D-8042 Neuherberg, F.R.G.

[2] Institute for Surgical Research, Klinikum Großhadern,
Marchioninistr. 15, D-8000 München 70, F.R.G.

Introduction

Due to a coincidence of tumor-localizing, fluorescent and photosensitizing properties, hematoporphyrin derivative (Hpd) and a purified version Photofrin II (containing mainly dihematoporphyrin ether or ester, DHE, with a large amount of aggregated compounds) are used for detection and photodynamic therapy of cancer /1/. Tumor localization and photosensitization, however, are attributed to different components of the porphyrin mixtures Hpd or Photofrin II. Dimeric and aggregated species were reported to be the main tumor localizers /1,2/, whereas the monomeric and dimeric components have the best photosensitizing properties /3/. Fluorescence is most pronounced for the monomeric species hematoporphyrin, hydroxyethyl-vinyldeutero-porphyrin and protoporphyrin /4/, less efficient by one order of magnitude for DHE, and very low for aggregated compounds.

A differentiation of porphyrin components in cells and tissues by conventional spectroscopic or other non-destructive means is almost impossible. However, by using the method of time-resolved laser microfluorometry, different components could be distinguished on the basis of their fluorescence lifetimes /5,6/.

In the present paper comparative time-resolved fluorescence measurements of Photofrin II in solution, cultured cells, and an in vivo hamster model are reported. It was to be proved whether certain components accumulate selectively in tumor cells or tissues, or whether a tumor specific conversion of the different components might take place.

Materials and Methods

Solutions of commercially available Photofrin II in phosphate buffered saline (PBS) were prepared at concentrations of 5 µg/ml, 50 µg/ml and 500 µg/ml. Cultures of malignant osteosarcoma and non-malignant muscle cells of mice were grown within Petri dishes and incubated for 48 h with solutions of Photofrin II in medium RPMI 1640 at concentrations of 5 µg/ml. After incubation the cells were kept in Photofrin II - free medium (Hank's solution) for variable times ranging from 1 h to 72 h, prior to microfluorometric detection. In addition, Photofrin II was measured from tumors (amelanotic hamster melanoma A- Mel-3) and the adjacent host tissues within the dorsal skin fold of Syrian golden hamsters, using transparent access chambers, as described elsewhere /7/. For this purpose the fluorescence of 10 animals was determined in vivo from well defined tissue areas (0.16 mm²) during a period of 6 - 8 days after i.a. application of Photofrin II.

All samples - droplets of Photofrin II solution, single cells or small groups of 5-10 cells, and hamster tissues - were excited in a fluorescence microscope by the picosecond pulses of a synchronously pumped dye laser system operated at 420 nm /8/. The irradiation density varied between 1 mW/cm² (tissues) and 40 mW/cm² (single cells) and was kept low enough to avoid photobleaching during the exposure times of 20 sec. The fluorescence was measured within the spectral range of 610 - 690 nm for Photofrin II detection, as well as 510 - 570 nm for correction of the superimposing autofluorescence. Besides single photon counting measurements at a time resolution of 0.3 ns /8/, picosecond fluorescence profiles were detected from cells and solutions after adapting a Hamamatsu synchroscan streak camera (time resolution 10 - 40 ps) to the microscopic system (Fig. 1, for details see /9/). A computer program for deconvolution and multi-exponential curve fitting was used to calculate the lifetimes and integral intensity contributions of the different components. No more than 3 components were so far distinguished.

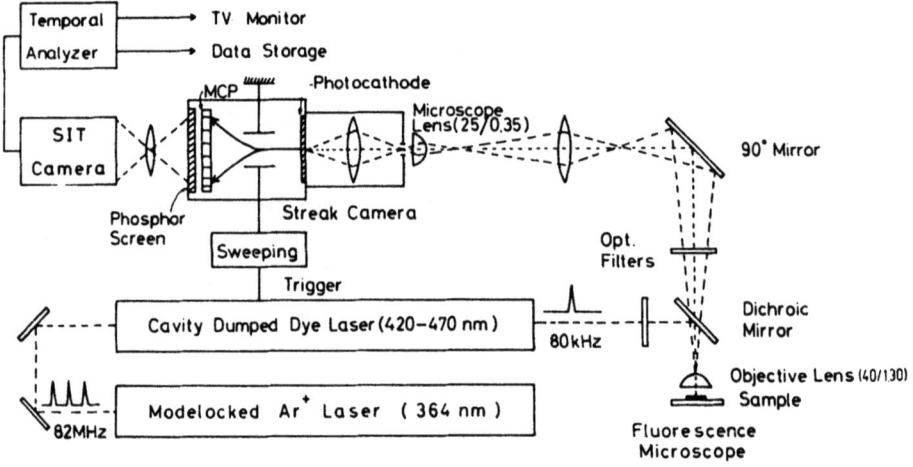

Fig. 1. Experimental setup for picosecond fluorescence microscopy

Results and Discussion
- Fluorescence lifetimes of $\tilde{\tau}_1$ = 1.7-2.3 ns ("short-lived component") and $\tilde{\tau}_2$ = 11-13 ns ("long-lived component") measured in solutions, cells and tissues (Fig.2), agreed with previous results of intracellular Photofrin II /6/. In addition, a more rapidly decaying component of $\tilde{\tau}_0$ = (90 ± 20) ps was detected only in PBS solution. The inten-

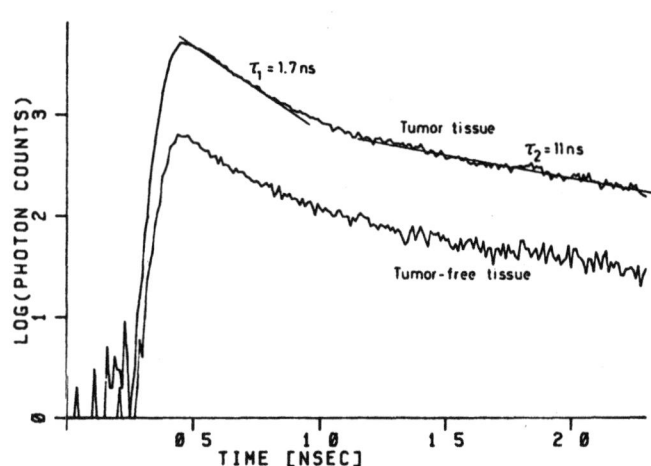

Fig. 2.
Fluorescence profiles of Photofrin II in tumor and tumor-free tissue, as obtained from time-resolved photon counting measurements (semilogarithmic scale) Picosecond laser pulse excitation at 420 nm, detection range 610 - 690 nm

sity contribution of this "very short-lived component" increased with Photofrin II concentration from about 2 % at 5 µg/ml to 5 % at 500 µg/ml. According to a previous discussion /10/ the lifetimes of the different components are concomitant with their fluorescence yields. Therefore, a correlation of τ_2, τ_1, and τ_0 with monomeric, dimeric and aggregated species, respectively, appears probable.

- The intensity contribution of the "short-lived component" in hamster tissues was 40 - 60 % of the total fluorescence intensity, as compared to 20 - 30 % for single cells, and an even lower value for cell nuclei and cells containing very high concentrations of mitochondria. This seems to prove a monomerization of porphyrins taken up by cells /3,11/ and indicates a further monomerization for those porphyrin molecules which enter the cell nucleus or mitochondria.

- Maximum intensity ratios of 1.5 -8.0 between tumor and tumor - free hamster tissues were obtained at 5 - 9 hours and 6 - 8 days after Photofrin II administration. No preferential accumulation of particular porphyrin components was found. The long-lasting fluorescence in alive tissues is in contrast to the rapid decrease of intracellular fluorescence (to about 10 % of its initial value within 2 days) and may be due to monomerization or dimerization of non-fluorescent aggregates.

- Using highly sensitive fluorescence imaging, preferential accumulation of porphyrins within and, in particular, at the edges of microvessels could be demonstrated within a time range of $\leq$ 6 hours after Photofrin II application (Fig. 3).

Acknowledgements
The authors thank H. Fißlinger and A. Kreisle for their skillfull technical assistance, as well as L. Schleinkofer and U. Denzer (Hamamatsu Photonics) for their stimulating co-operation.

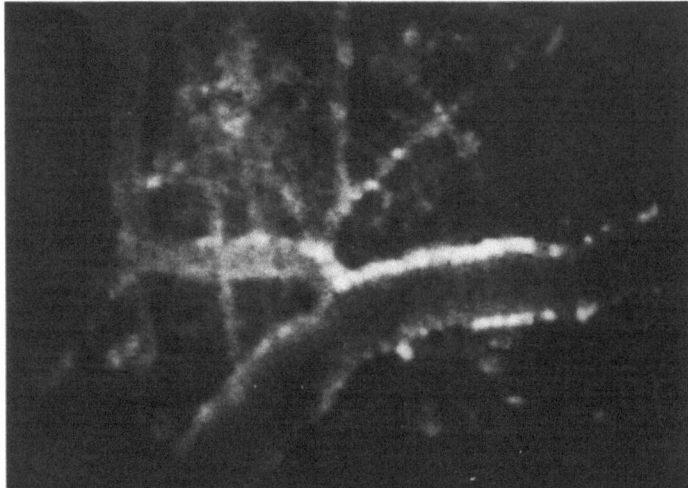

Fig. 3.
Fluorescence image of the tumor-free hamster tissue 2 hours after i.a. application of Photofrin II.
Detection range 580 - 800 nm; width of the screen 1 mm

References

/1/ T.J. Dougherty (1985) Photodynamic therapy. In Methods in Porphyrin Photosensitization (Edited by D. Kessel), pp. 313 - 328, Plenum Press, New York - London.
/2/ T.J. Dougherty, D.G. Boyle, K.R. Weishaupt, B.A. Henderson, W.R. Potter, D.A.Bellnier and K.E. Wytyk (1983) Photoradiation therapy - clinical and drug advances. In Porphyrin Photosensitization (Edited dy D, Kessel and T.J. Dougherty), pp. 3 - 13, Plenum Press, New York - London.
/3/ J Moan and S. Sommer (1984) Action spectra for hematoporphyrin derivative and Photofrin II with respect to sensitization of human cells in vitro to photoinactivation. Photochem. Photobiol. 40, 631 - 634.
/4/ J. Moan and S. Sommer (1981) Fluorescence and absorption properties of the components of hematoporphyrin derivative. Photobiochem. Photobiophys. 3, 93 - 103.
/5/ A. Andreoni, R. Cubeddu, S. de Silvestri, P. Laporta, G. Jori and E. Reddi (1982) Hematoporphyrin derivative: Experimental evidence for aggregated species. Chem. Phys. Lett. 88, 33 - 36.
/6/ H. Schneckenburger, F. Pauker, E. Unsöld and D. Jocham (1985) Intracellular distribution and retention of the fluorescent components of Photofrin II. Photobiochem. Photobiophys. 10, 61 - 67.
/7/ A. Götz, J. Feyh, H. Schneckenburger, P. Conzen, D. Jocham and E. Unsöld (1985) Quantitative in vivo measurement of Photofrin II in tumor and adjacent tumor-free tissues. In Photodynamic Therapy of Tumors and Other Diseases (Edited by G. Jori abd C. Perria>, pp. 405 - 408, Libreria Progetto, Padova.
/8/ H. Schneckenburger (1985) Time-resolved microfluorescence in biomedical diagnosis. Opt. Eng. 24, 1042 - 1044.
/9/ H. Schneckenburger, M. Frenz, Y. Tsuchiya, U. Denzer and L. Schleinkofer (1987) Picosecond fluorescence microscopy for measuring chlorophyll and porphyrin components in conifers and cultured cells. Lasers in the Life Sciences 1, 299 - 307.
/10/H. Schneckenburger, J. Feyh, A. Götz, M. Frenz and W. Brendel (1987) Quantitative in vivo measurement of the fluorescent components of Photofrin II. Photochem. Photobiol. (in press).
/11/D. Kessel (1986) In vivo fluorescence of tumors after treatment with derivatives of hematoporphyrin. Photochem. Photobiol. 44, 107 - 108.

Dynamical Processes Associated with Singlet Oxygen Generations in Porphyrin Solutions

Ichiro Tanabe, Hiroshi Fujimura, Yukinori Okazaki,
Tadayoshi Takemoto, Yoshihiko Kanemitsu*,
Yuichi Tanaka* and Hiroto Kuroda*
Yamaguchi University School 1st Dept. of Medicine
1144 Kogushi, Ube-shi, 755, Japan
*The ISSP, University of Tokyo
Roppongi 7-22-1, Minato-ku, 106, Japan

1. INTRODUCTION

Photoradiative therapy(PRT) has become one of attractive reliable method for cancer therapy nowadays. Since early work by Dougherty and his group[1] in the 1970's, a lot of medical and fundamental investigaters have been reported about it. Most of cases, the singlet oxygen has been postulated to play important role in PRT because of its powerful capacity to react on cell organerals chemically and this resulting in cell destruction. The energy transfer model from porphyrin to oxygen molecule is shown in Figure 1.

In this paper, we will present experimental proof of the singlet oxygen generation which are not so far clarified and will discuss on the dynamics of the singlet oxygen generation based on the rate equations.

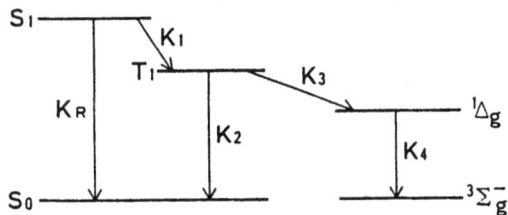

Fig.1. Schema of the energy transfer process

2. EXPERIMENTAL

The investigated substances were hematoporphyrin free base(Hp), protoporphyrin(Pp), uroporphyrin(Up), hematoporphyrin derivative(HpD), and dihematoporphyrin ester(DHE). Hp, Pp and Up were marketed by SIGMA Chemical Co. HpD and DHE were aquenous solutions which were obtained from Oncology Research and Development. Furhtermore, we used acridine orange, adriamycin and mitomycin C(MMC) which have been thought to form the singlet oxygen to make anti-cancerous effect.

For the solvent, we used water, ethanol, CCl_4, acetone and benzene. The concentration of each solution was 4×10^{-4} mol/l. We performed on experiments in the manner as shown here.

i) Experimental setup for confirming the singlet oxygen

For confirming the fluorescence of the singlet oxygen, we used the CW Ar laser for light source and detected the fluorescence by the fast responce Germanium detector and the lock-in amplifier system(Figure 2).

The laser beam released from oscillator is chopped and applied to quartz sample cell. The fluorescence is led to Ge detector passed through the monochromator. The output is fed to lock-in amplifier system triggered by synchronous photoelectric pulse from chopper.

ii) Experimental setup for measuring the fluorescence of the singlet oxygen

We measured the temporal change of the fluorescence from the singlet oxygen by using the picosecond pulse Nd:YAG laser system(Figure 3).

The second harmonic generation (λ =532nm) of the single pulse from the oscillator, pulse duration is 30ps, is applied to the quartz sample cell. The fluorescence from the singlet oxygen is led to the Ge detector passed through combinational band-pass filter consisted of 1.27 μm. The output is led to the fast response storage oscilloscope triggered with laser pulse.

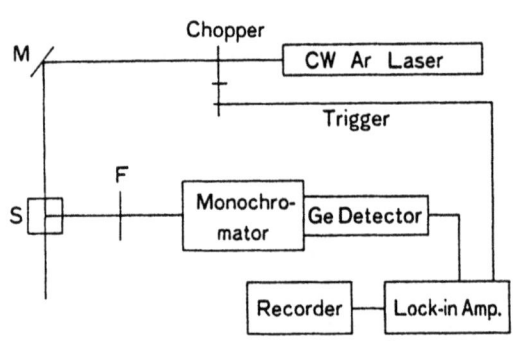

Fig.2. Setup of the experiment i)

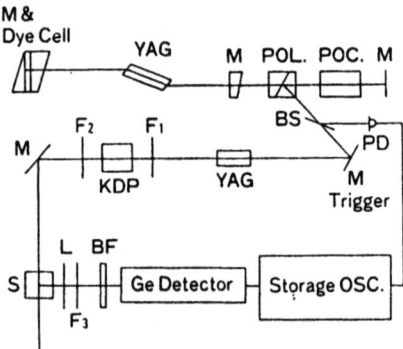

Fig.3. Setup of the experiment ii)

3.   RESULT

i) Experiment for confirming the singlet oxygen

In each solution except water and ethanol, we observed the sharp fluorescence of the singlet oxygen at 1.27 μm. We showed the pattern of fluorescence in Hp CCl_4 solution at Figure 4.   There was not any other fluorescence inspite of scanning from 1.0 μm to 1.5 μm.

The inset of Figure 4. is the time solved change of the fluorescence intensity during N_2 and O_2 bubbling to the sample solution. The fluorescence decreases gradually during N_2 bubbling and increases when O_2 bubbling starts again. It is one of the evidence that the origin of this fluorescence is due to the singlet oxygen.

We could not observe any fluorescence in acridine orange, adriamycin and MMC solutions. Of course, no fluorescence was observed in the case of solvent only.

ii) Experiment for measuring the fluorescence of the singlet oxygen

As to the direct observation of the fluorescence emitted from the singlet oxygen, we could observe rise and decay curve of fluorescence clearly in each solution other than water solution. The curve's pattern in Hp CCl_4 solution is shown in Figure 5. The results of other porphyrin solutions are summarized in Table 1. From this, it is confirmed that the rise time is regarding at about 40~80 μs and the decay time is about 100~200 μs.

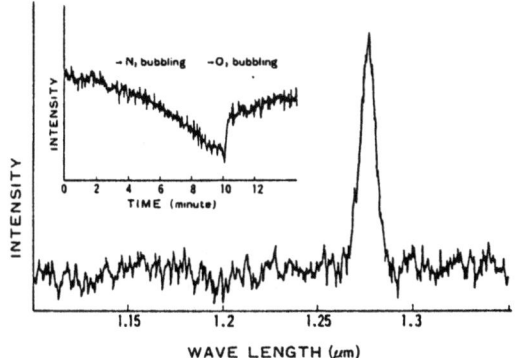

Fig.4. Fluorescence of singlet oxygen in Hp CCl_4 solution

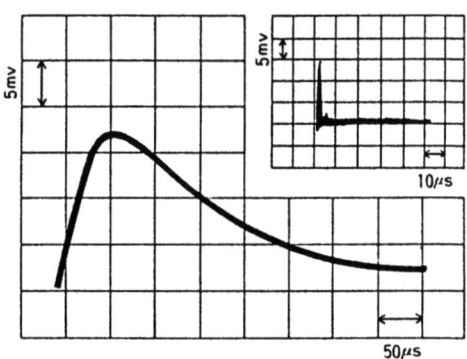

Fig.5. The decay curve of the singlet oxygen. The inset is the time response capasity of the Ge detector. It is within 1 μs

4. DISCUSSION

We previously reported[2] that the lifetime of the red fluorescence of porphyrin which wavelength was 630nm was about 10ns and could not observe any faster component than it. The reciprocal of its lifetime is the sum of k_R and k_1 which were presented in Figure 1. k_1 could be calculated theoretically from the absorption spectrum of porphyrin by using Einstein's A coefficient. From this, we could determine value of k_1 about $10^7 \sim 10^8$.

k_3 is the rate of energy transfer process from porphyrin to oxygen molecule and regarded it as the reciprocal of the risetime of the singlet oxygen's fluorescence. So its value was about 10^4.

Parker[3] determined the lifetime of T_1 state about several hundred nanosec. in porphyrin solution by the experiment of T-T absorption. We could think the reciprocal of this value as k_2 because there was another energy transfer process from T_1 state beside the process to oxygen.

k_4 is the reciprocal of the lifetime of the singlet oxygen's fluorescence and the value is about $10^3 \sim 10^4$.

As above mentioned, all rate constants of each process presented in Figure 1. were determined.

The rate equation of this each energy transfer process is as follows,

$$\begin{cases} \dot{S}_0 = k_R S_1 + k_2 T_1 \\ \dot{S}_1 = -(k_R + k_1)S_1 \\ \dot{T}_1 = k_1 S_1 - (k_2 + k_3)T_1 \\ {}^1\dot{O}_2 = k_3 T_1 - k_4 {}^1O_2 \\ {}^3\dot{O}_2 = k_4 {}^1O_2 \end{cases}$$

We assumed that the initial energy given to S_1 state was 1 and calculated the rate of the singlet oxygen generation by microcomputer quantitatively. From this analysis, we concluded that the energy reached to oxygen molecule was about $10^{-2} \sim 10^{-3}$ and the majority of the exited energy at T_1 state was escaped other than oxygen molecule.

solvent solute		Ethanol	CCl₄	Acetone	Benzene
Hp	RT	50	60	80	60
	DT	100	170	190	100
Pp	RT	50	60	60	60
	DT	70	120	120	130
Up	RT	40		60	
	DT	90		80	
HpD	RT		50	50	
	DT		90	100	
DHE	RT	50		60	
	DT	130		90	

RT = rise time (μs) DT = decay time (μs)

Table 1. Rise and decay time of the singlet oxygen in various solutions

Regarding this energy escape process, we point out two possible ways. The first is the non-radiative process from T_1 to S_0 state as the heat. Another possibility is the reabsorption by solvent[4] and this may be the reason of the undetection of the singlet oxygen's fluorescence in water solution. In vivo, the tissue component contains much water, so the energy reached to oxygen becomes much smaller.

These facts suggest the necessity to investigate the photoradiative effect from different points, for example, the thermal effect and radical reaction.

But it is important to elucidate the generation of the singlet oxygen in porphyrin solutions because we could not observe it in acridine orange and other antineoplasmic drug solutions. So, there is sufficient possibility to destruct tumor cell in small amount of the singlet oxygen.

5. CONCLUSION

In this report, we presented the clear evidence of the singlet oxygen's generation in vitro by direct observation and discuss the dynamical energy transfer process by analyzing the temporal change of its fluorescence.

REFERENCES

1) Dougherty TJ, et al : J Natl Cancer Inst 1975;55:115~121.
2) Tanabe I, et al : Nd : YAG Laser in Med. and Surg, 57~62, PPS, 1986, Japan.
3) Parker JG, et al : Johns Hopkins APL Tech. Dig. 1981 ; 2 : 196~199.
4) Merkel DB, et al : Chem. Phy. Lett. 1971 ; 12 : 120~122.

An in vitro Comparison of Laser Parameters for Photodynamic Therapy

B.W. Stewart, M. LaPlant[*], S.B. Kim, C. Distler

The Jewish Hospital, Cincinnati, OH
University of Cincinnati, Cincinnati, OH
Christ Hospital, Cincinnati, OH

Abstract

Although the use of Photodynamic Therapy (PDT) as a mode for the treatment of cancer is in an experimental stage, very little is known about the fundamental mechanism(s) behind the effect itself. The purpose of this study was to further characterize the light and/or heat induced destruction of cancerous cell in vitro. Comparisons were made of the effects of average irradiance, peak irradiance and energy fluence on cell kill.

Introduction

The etiology of tumor necroses in PDT is still unknown. It has been shown that HPD uptake is primarily within the vascular stroma verses intracellularly. (Ref. 1) It is felt that in the presence of radiation, energy is transferred to molecular oxygen causing it to go from a singlet state to an unstable triplet state which leads to irreversible oxidation of some tissue component causing cell death. (Refs. 2,3) From previous experiments it appears that one source of tumor necroses is damage to the tumor vasculature which leads to ischemia and eventual tumor necroses. (Ref. 4)

More information is needed to determine the actual effect of HPD and light on tumor tissues in order to fully exploit its anti-tumoral activity and minimize any harm it may have to surrounding tissues. It is not yet known how changes in different parameters in the administration of the laser light source itself may effect the degree of tumor necroses. A major goal of this research was to establish which of several laser parameters have an influence on the efficacy of PDT. The degree of influence and the optimum range of each are sought in order to eventually maximize the performance of this type of treatment.

Methods and Materials

Human epidermoid nasal pharyngeal carcinoma cells (H.Ep2, MA Bioproducts, Walkersville, MD) were grown in DMEM-10% FCS with penicillin and streptomycin and were harvested prior to confluency. Cells were washed in Dulbecco's Ca++ and My++ free PBS. Trypsin-versene (1:250) was added and the cultures incubated at $37^\circ C$ for 3 minutes. When the cells were loosened from the flask DMEM-10% was added. Cell viability was determined using the trypan blue exclusion. One half of the cell suspensions received dihematoporphyrin ether (Photomedica, Inc., Raritan, NJ) at a concentration of $1 \times 10^{-5} M$. The cell suspensions were then aliquoted to 5.0 ml/50 ml sterile polypropylene tubes for a final concentration of 1.25×10^6 viable cells per tube. Tubes containing DHE were allowed to incubate 3 hours before being irradiated.

Cell cultures were exposed in duplicate to average irradiances of 75, 200 & 350 mw/cm^2 at energy fluences of 100 and 150 J/cm^2 using the pulsed gold vapor laser (GVL) (Cooper Lasersonics, model 452) and the continuous wave argon-pumped dye laser (ADL) (Spectra Physics, models 375 & 170). Additional cultures were exposed to the mechanically chopped beam of the argon-pumped dye laser at 75 mw/cm^2, 100 and 150 J/cm^2. All cultures were agitated during laser exposures. Temperature readings were recorded every 15 seconds throughout the exposure period with a copper constantan thermocouple microprobe (Bailey Instruments, Saddlebrook, NJ). The trypan blue exclusion test was used to determine cell viability at 0, 1, 2, 4 and 8 hours post-irradiation.

Results

The results of the experiments are shown in the tables. With DHE present, there is clearly a greater cytocidal effect in the 350 mW/cm^2 GVL exposures than in the cw-ADL 350 mW/cm^2 exposures. Any differences between the ADL exposures (cw and chopped) don't appear significant at the irradiances used. Temperature increases during all exposures were less than $2^\circ C$, therefore hyperthermia wasn't a factor.

Additionally, we made a somewhat surprising observation. As the average power density increased, for fixed exposure energy density, the cell viability increased. This seems to imply a "time of ex-

TABLES

All laser exposures w/o DHE

	Reading time				
	Imm.	1 hr.	2 hr.	4 hr.	8 hr.
Mean viability(%)	93.3	92.7	92.1	93.4	92.5
Standard dev.	2.9	3.1	3.9	3.2	3.5

Controls: DHE w/o laser

	Reading time				
	Imm.	1 hr.	2 hr.	4 hr.	8 hr.
Mean viability(%)	97.5	96.3	96.6	95.3	67.3
Standard dev.	1.0	3.5	1.2	1.5	13.9

Controls: No DHE/ No laser

	Reading time				
	Imm.	1 hr.	2 hr.	4 hr.	8 hr.
Mean viability(%)	96.8	96.6	95.5	96.0	95.0
Standard dev.	1.6	1.5	1.3	1.0	2.8

Mean Viability Laser w/ DHE 100 J Exposures

Irr. / laser	Imm.	1 hr.	2 hr.	4 hr.	8 hr.
75 mW/CW ADL	67.5±1.5	46.5±6.5	41.5±1.5	37.5±3.5	23.0±2.0
75 mW/ CH ADL	72.5±.5	73.0±11.0	73.0±11.0	50.5±5.5	20.0±3.0
75 mW/ GVL	61.0±9.9	61.3±6.1	42.3±13.1	37.7±8.2	29.0±4.1
350 mW/CW ADL	88.0±2.0	66.5±5.5	60.5±10.5	44.0±5.0	35.0±2.0
350 mW/ GVL	78.0±3.0	62.0±14.0	57.0±19.0	47.5±11.5	23.0±0.0

150 J Exposures Mean viability

Irr. /laser	Imm.	1 hr.	2 hr.	4 hr.	8 hr.
75 mW/ CH ADL	72.5±10.5	71.0±1.0	57.0±8.0	57.5±11.5	50.0±0.0
350 mW/ CW ADL	81.7±4.1	60.7±9.8	55.3±8.8	24.3±3.7	27.0±6.4
350 mW/ GVL	66.0±4.0	46.5±10.5	38.0±12.0	28.0±3.0	24.5±2.5

posure" effect as the longer the exposure time, for a fixed energy density, the lower the cell viability as measured immediately after cessation of irradiation. All exposures without DHE present yielded identical results, within experimental error.

It appears, with this cell line and within the range of peak powers used in this experiment, that pulsed light alone is not directly cytotoxic. On the other hand when used in conjunction with DHE, the much higher peak power of the GVL pulses seem to activate an additional cytocidal mechanism. (This has been previously observed for laser exposures in the UV, Ref. 5.) Pulse repetition rate does not seem to be an important factor here. (This suggests that a laser capable of delivering energy of a joule per pulse over a few nanoseconds may be the best choice in even if only ten or so pulses per minute could be generated.)

The fact that time of exposure as well as exposure energy density seem important in both the GVL and ADL cases may indicate the presence of a cytotoxic transport mechanism. Although the cells were agitated during irradiation, if a slowly diffusing cytotoxic byproduct were produced during the irradiation one would expect a time effect similar to the one seen. It also seems that this effect is less important for the pulsed GVL exposures.

Preliminary studies using the Human Tumor Clonogenic Assay to determine cell viability after laser exposure produced results which were consistant with the trypan blue exclusion test approach used.

NOTE ADDED IN PROOF: It has since been brought to the authors' attention that a similar " time of exposure " effect was previously reported in Ref. 6.

This research was funded by the Charlotte Pennington Memorial Fund.

References

1. Bugelski PJ, Porter CW, Dougherty TJ: Autoradiographic distribution of neoplastic verses normal cells and tumor tissue of the mouse. Cancer Research, 41: 4606-4612, 1981.
2. Weishaupt KR, Gomer CJ, Doughtery TJ: Identification of singlet oxygen as the cytotoxic agent in photo-activation of a murine tumor. Cancer Research, 36: 2326-2329, 1976.

3. Grossweiner LI, Goyal GG, Richard P: Effects of aggregation and sensitizer binding on liposome membrane photosensitization by hematoporphrin and hematorphyrin derivitive. <u>Adstracts, Amer. Soc. Photobiol.</u>, p.91, 1982.
4. Henderson BW, Dougherty TJ, Malone PB: Studies in the mechanism of tumor destruction by photoradiation therapy. Alan R. Liss, Inc., p.607-612, 1984.
5. Andreoni A, Cubeddu R, De Silvestri S, Laporta P, and Svelto O: Two-Step Laser Activation of Hematoporphyrin Derivative. <u>Chem. Phys. Letters</u>, <u>88</u>: 37-39, 1982.
6. Camps JL, Jr., Powers SK, Beckman WC, Jr., Brown JT, and Weissman RM: Photodynamic Therapy of Prostate Cancer: An In Vitro Study. <u>J. Urology</u>, <u>134</u> P.1222, 1985.

Histological Analysis of Cottontail Rabbit Papilloma Virus-Induced Papillomas Treated with Hematoporphyrin Photodynamic Therapy

Mark J. Shikowitz, M.D., Bettie M. Steinberg, Ph.D., Rachel L. Galli, Allan L. Abramson, M.D.

From the Department of Otolaryngology and Communicative Disorders, Long Island Jewish Medical Center, New Hyde Park, NY 11042, U.S.A.

Our findings of papilloma regression following treatment with HPD-PDT have been reported recently (Shikowitz et.al., 1986). HPD has been shown to localize selectively in rapidly growing tissue such as malignancies and papillomas. Henderson et.al. (1980) demonstrated the ability of HPD to localize in both squamous cell carcinomas and chemically induced papillomas raised on the shaved backs of Swiss white mice by painting with 9,10-dimethyl-1,2-benzanthracene and croton oil. This prompted our initial investigation into the possible efficacy of HPD-PDT for the treatment of virally induced papilloma disease, utilizing CRPV as a model system. We successfully treated large cutaneous rabbit papillomas with intravenous administration of HPD followed by activation with light at 630 nm from an Argon pump dye laser. Two animals were maintained for 18 months following treatment. The animals were sacrificed and biopsies were taken from totally regressed papillomas, partially regressed papillomas, untreated papillomas and normal skin. The histological analysis with molecular analysis confirmation form the basis of this report.

Materials and Methods

Papillomas were induced in 4 distinct regions on the back of each of 5 Dutch belted rabbits by topical injection with 0.1 ml of a CRPV suspension. Photodynamic therapy was delivered at 630 nm. The materials and methods and clinical results at 6 months post treatment were reported previously (Shikowitz et.al., 1986). Two rabbits were maintained in separate stainless steel wire-meshed cages in a room controlled for temperature and humidity. Rabbit I was a control rabbit and received no HPD treatment, and Rabbit II underwent HPD phototherapy. At a pre-determined time of 18 months following treatment, both animals were sacrificed by a lethal intravenous injection of T-61. Excisional biopsies of involved and normal tissues were taken and divided into two portions. One portion was fixed in 10% Formalin, Paraffin-imbedded, and serially sectioned. Sections were stained with hematoxylin and eosin for histological examination. The second portion was immediately frozen in liquid nitrogen for later molecular analysis by Southern blots. Total genomic DNA was then extracted from powdered tissue according to the method of Krieg et.al. (1983). For each biopsy site 5 mg of DNA was digested with the restriction enzyme Sal 1 and 5 mg of DNA was digested with Hind III. The digests were electrophoresed, Southern blotted, and probed for the presence of CRPV DNA sequences as described by Brandsma et.al. (1986).

Results

Clinical Effects and Histological Analysis of HPD Phototherapy

Following administration of HPD (5 mg/Kg) and PDT the cutaneous papilloma and surrounding tissue showed a generalized hyperemia within 24-48 hours. At 96 hours, there was necrosis of the papilloma, leaving a flat eschar. During the following weeks, normal-appearing hair-bearing skin replaced the eschar from the periphery. The papilloma of the treated rabbit that had undergone initial total progression remained free from any recurrence. There was no evidence upon histological examination of any abnormality of the hair-bearing skin in this area. A papilloma adjacent to the treated area that had received a small amount of light had partially regressed initially. This papilloma persisted but did not increase in size during the 18 months observation period. Upon histological examination, the partially regressed papilloma showed normal papillary features with no signs of malignant transformation. An adjacent, shielded papilloma continued to grow, evidence that the rabbit had not mounted an immune response to the CRPV-induced lesions. Histological examination revealed normal papillary features.

Effects of HPD Phototherapy on CRPV DNA

Southern blot analysis of DNA from multiple biopsy sites was examined. Rabbit I, which received no treatment showed no viral DNA in samples from two biopsy sites of normal skin taken 5 cm away from any papilloma. DNA extracted from the normal papilloma revealed the expected findings and bands on Southern blot. Rabbit II was treated with HPD phototherapy. Most importantly, biopsies from the site of complete phototherapy-induced papilloma regression showed the complete absence of CRPV DNA by Southern blot analysis. DNA samples from an untreated papilloma and a partially regressed papilloma revealed approximately equal copy numbers of viral DNA.

Discussion

This study clearly demonstrated a strong correlation between the clinical findings of papilloma regression without recurrence following HPD phototherapy and replacement by histologicaly normal hair-bearing skin. These findings were confirmed by the complete absence of CRPV DNA on molecular analysis by Southern blot. The concept of phototherapy to kill tumor cells selectively after administration of a light sensitive dye is not new. Jesionek and Tappeiner (1903) were the first to utilize this technique by successfully treating human tumors with eosin. Despite their report no further studies on PDT immediately followed. It was not until the acid purified form of Hematoporphyrin or HPD was shown to be a better localizing agent in malignant tissues that a resurgence of interest in PDT occurred. The ability of HPD to act as a fluorescent marker to delineate papillomas and malignant tumors from the normal adjacent tissue has been well documented. When activated by appropriate wavelengths of light, this same HPD can destroy cells in which it is localized.

We have previously demonstrated the therapeutic potential of HPD as a selective photosensitizing agent to destroy papillomavirus-induced lesions. These same lesions were then followed for an 18 month period. The area of total aggression showed no signs of clinical recurrence. We have now confirmed these findings by histological and molecular analysis. Also of importance is the finding that a papilloma which received a sub-lethal dose of HPD-PDT, and underwent partial regression, only displayed benign papillary features upon histological examination without signs of malignant conversion. These findings were again confirmed by molecular analysis. HPD without light activation did not appear to have an adverse effect on the shielded papilloma, normal skin, or general health of the animals.

We began this study as a model for a possible future treatment of respiratory papillomatosis, caused by one or more of the human papillomaviruses (HPV). Additional studies are underway to confirm that phototherapy will be effective on latent infections and that there is no possibility of inducing carcinogenesis with this treatment. We believe that this therapy has great potential for the future cure of papillomavirus-induced diseases.

References

Brandsma, J.L., B.M. Steinberg, A.L. Abramson, and B. Winkler. 1986. Human papillomavirus sequences are found in verrucous carcinoma of the larynx. Cancer Res. 46:2185

Dougherty, T.J., G.B. Grindey, R. Fiel, K.R. Weishaupt, and D.G. Boyle. 1975. Photoradiation therapy. II. Cure of animal tumors with hematoporphyrin and light. J. Natl. Cancer Inst. 55:115.

Dougherty, T.J., J.E. Kaufman, B. Goldfarb, K.R. Weishaupt, D. Boyle, and A. Mittleman. 1978. Photoradiation therapy for the treatment of malignant tumor. Cancer Res. 38:2628.

Henderson, R.W., G.S. Christie, P.S. Clezy, and J. Lineman. Hematoporphyrin diacetate: A probe to distinguish malignant from normal tissue by selective fluorescence. Br. J. Exp. Pathol. 61:345.

Jesionek, A. and V.H. Tappeiner. 1903. Zur behandlung der hautcarcinomemet fluoresciecenden stoffen. Muench. Med. Wochenschr. 47:2042.

Krieg, P.E., Amtmann, and G. Sauer. 1983. The simultaneous extraction of high molecular-weight DNA and of RNA from solid tumors. Anal. Biochem. 134:288.

Schuller, D.E., J.S. McCayghan, and R.P. Rock. 1985. Photodynamic therapy in head and neck cancer. Arch. Otolaryngol. 111:351.

Shikowitz, M.J., B.M. Steinberg, and A.L. Abramson. 1986. Hematoporphyrin derivative therapy of papillomas: Experimental study. Arch. Otolaryngol. Head Neck Surg. 112:42.

Steinberg, B.M., W.C. Topp, P.S. Schneider, and A.L. Abramson. 1983. Laryngeal papillomavirus infection during clinical remission. N. Engl. J. Med. 308:1261.

Stevens, J.G. and F.O. Wettstein. 1979. Multiple copies of Shope virus DNA are present in cells of benign and malignant non-virus-producing neoplasms. J. Virol. 30:891.

Strong, M.S., C.W. Vaughn, G.B. Healy, and S.R. Cooperband. 1979. Recurrent respiratory papillomatosis: Management with the CO_2 laser. Ann. Otol. Rhinol. Laryngol. 88:192.

Biodistribution of Indium-III Dihematoporphyrin Ether in Papillomas and Body Tissues and its Relevance to Photodynamic Therapy

Mark J. Shikowitz, M.D., Rachel Galli, +Dibyendu Bandyopadhyay, Ph.D. and +Schlomo Hoory, Ph.D.

From the Department of Otolaryngology and Communicative Disorders and the +Division of Nuclear Medicine, Department of Radiology, Long Island Jewish Medical Center, New Hyde Park, NY 11042, U.S.A.

Hematoporphyrin derivative (HPD) and its newly purified form, dihematoporphyrin ether (DHE) have been shown to selectively localize in malignant tissues and virally induced papillomas (Shikowitz et.al.). Its use as a probe to distinguish tumors from normal tissues has been largely based on its fluorescence when activated by ultraviolet light. These findings are largely subjective, and a direct correlation to its use as a photosensitizing agent to selectively kill transformed cells when activated by an appropriate wavelength of light (630 nm) could not be made. We labeled DHE with Indium-111 and tracked its biodistribution through CRPV induced papillomas and normal body tissues.

Materials and Methods

DHE was labeled with Indium-111 as described by Wong (1984). Four Dutch belted rabbits, 3 with long standing, virally induced papillomas and one normal for control, were each administered Indium-111 DHE, 170 uCI/2 mg intravenously. Total body imaging was performed on a Siemans large field of view gamma camera (ZLC-370) equipped with a medium energy Collimater. Analog images were obtained in posterior and LAO positions for all four animals. Imaging was performed at 3, 16, 27 and 39 hours post injection. At 50 hours the animals were sacrificed with a lethal intravenous injection of T-61 and tissue biopsies were taken from selected sites for scintillation counting and biodistribution studies (see Table).

Results

During Indium-111-DHE imaging at 3 hours, no discernible difference is observed between papillomas and adjacent normal skin. At 16 hours, an increased retention is seen in the papillomas relative to the surrounding normal areas. The absorption and retention continues to increase in the papillomas from 27 to 50 hours (Figure 1). It is apparent that a large portion of Indium-111-DHE is absorbed and retained in the liver and excretory organs (see Table).

Discussion

The concept of utilizing a photosensitizing dye activated by light to selectively kill tumor cells is not new. This technique of PDT was first used by Jesionek and Tappeiner in 1903 with their treatment of human tumors with eosin. Despite success no further reports of PDT immediately followed.

Table. DISTRIBUTION OF INDIUM LABELED HEMATOPORPHYRIN
50 HOURS POST INJECTION

	Percent Injected Dose Per Gram of Tissue	Organ:Skin Ratio
Papilloma	0.026%	5.0
Skin	0.005%	1.0
Blood	0.009%	1.8
Bone	0.109%	22.9
Muscle	0.002%	0.4
Larynx	0.012%	2.4
Lung	0.034%	7.0
Heart	0.018%	4.1
Urinary Bladder	0.014%	2.7
Gall Bladder	2.690%	665
Kidney	5.340%	989
Liver	5.590%	1258

Early studies with hematoporphyrins showed promise but results with these crude mixtures were inconsistent. A resurgence of PDT was seen with the superior localization in tumors with increasingly purified forms of hematoporphyrin derivative (HPD) and now di-hematoporphyrin ether (DHE).

Our earlier studies (Shikowitz et.al., 1986) showed the ability of HPD to selectively localize in CRPV induced papillomas. These results were determined by relative fluorescence of tissue samples at various time periods. Based on these results, we have administered HPD-PDT to CRPV induced rabbit papillomas resulting in total regression of the papillomas. Despite good clinical correlation between the fluorescent localization of HPD or DHE and desired therapeutic result, it has been suggested that the "gross visualization of porphyrin fluorescence cannot be correlated with actual tissue concentrations of the dye" (Gomer and Dougherty, 1979). Our results clearly demonstrate an increased localization in the papilloma compared to the normal surrounding skin, confirming the therapeutic potential of DHE-PDT.

We have also shown that an even higher concentration of DHE is found in the liver and excretory organs. These findings confirm those previously reported by others. The higher concentration of the HPD or DHE in these organs must be taken into consideration if one plans to utilize PDT for intra-abdominal lesions. The possible destruction of normal vital organs by misdirected PDT may prove to be deleterious.

We believe that DHE-PDT shows great promise for obtaining a possible cure in virally induced papilloma lesions of the upper aerodigestive tract. Their superficial location makes them an excellent candidate for phototherapy.

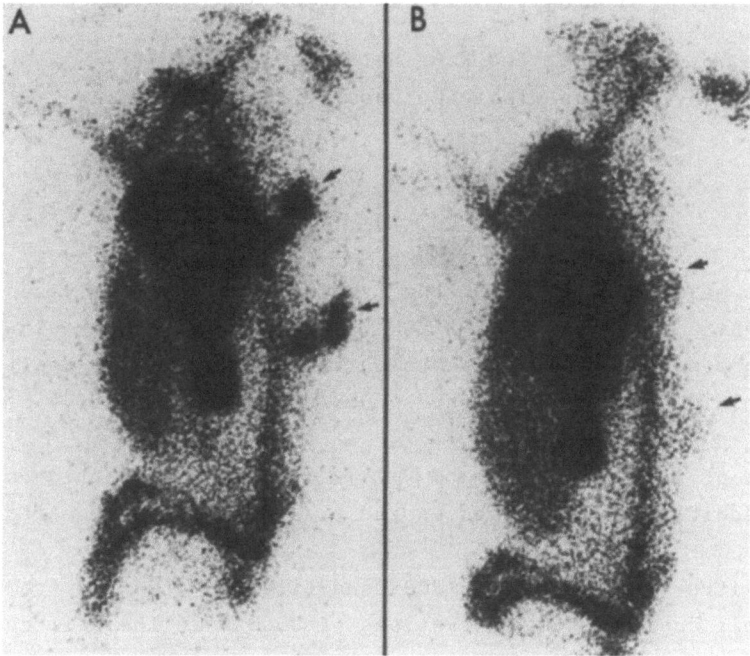

Figure 1: Indium-111-DHE imaging showing increased localization in the papillomas (Arrows). Figure A shows region of papillomas identified with Indium-111 marker. Figure B shows region of papillomas without marker.

References

Gomer, C.J. and T.J. Dougherty. 1979. Determination of ^1H and ^{14}C hematoporphyrin derivative distribution in malignant and normal tissue. Cancer Res. 39:146.

Henderson, R.W., G.S. Christie, P.S. Clezy, and J. Lineman. Hematoporphyrin diacetate: A probe to distinguish malignant from normal tissue by selective fluorescence. Br. J. Exp. Pathol. 61:345.

Jesionek, A. and V.H. Tappeiner. 1903. Zur behandlung der hautcarcinomemet fluoresciecenden stoffen. Muench. Med. Wochenschr. 47:2042.

Shikowitz, M.J., B.M. Steinberg, and A.L. Abramson. 1986. Hematoporphyrin derivative therapy of papillomas; Experimental study. Arch. Otolaryngol. Head Neck Surg. 112:42.

Wong, D.W. 1984. A simple and efficient method of labeling hematoporphyrin derivative with In-111. Int. J. Appl. Radiat. ISOF. 35:691.

Photodynamic Therapy (PDT) of Superficial Bladder Tumor

H.D. Nöske, J. Kraushaar and C.F. Rothauge
Dep. of Urology, Justus Liebig-University, D-6300 Diessen

The PDT is mainly suitable for the treatment of relatively superficial tumors.
This is an opportunity for the urologist to approach the healing or to diminish the tendency for recurrence of non-invasive bladder tumors.
The method of illumination of the whole bladder after injection of HPD may have additional advantages in the treatment of the multifocal disease.
First in vitro-tests made with HPD-sensitized tumor cells from the bladder well confirm the observations of JOCHAM in the cell culture (Fig. 1).

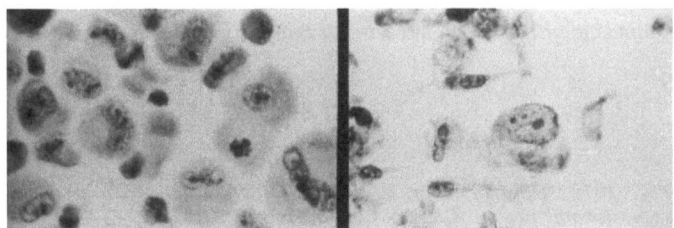

Fig. 1: Cell culture: On the left side untrated tumor cells, on the right cytology after PDT.

On the left-hand side of the microscopical picture you may see untreated tumor cells with disturbed nucleus-plasma relation and one mitosis.
On the right-hand side the cytological result after PDT: You can see only non-damaged stroma tissue cells and a pure tumor cell nucleus without any cytoplasma.
A pilot-study made on different urological tumors should confirm this experience especially for the bladder carcinoma.
According to the literature we injected HPD (PHOTOFRIN I) 48 hours before operation in a quantity of 2 mg/kg body weight.

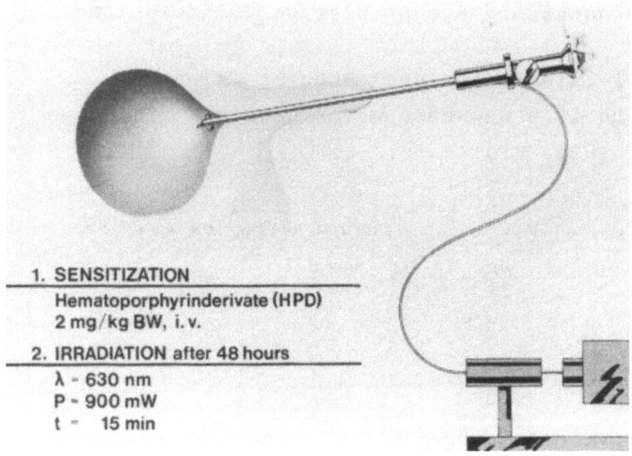

Fig. 2.
Operation-technic

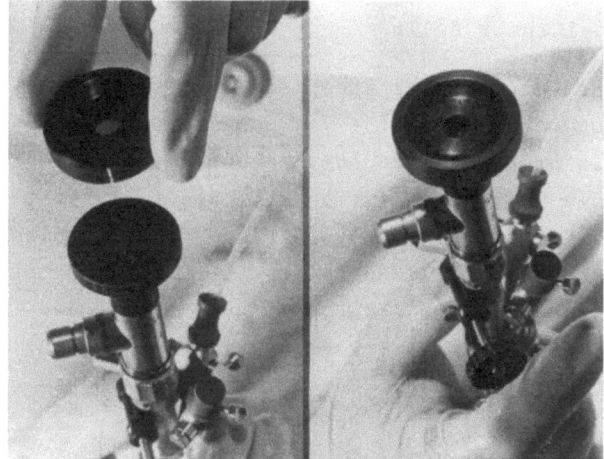

Fig. 3.
Eye protection

It is our understanding that the PDT should be a topical method for complete removal of any traces left following surgery.
Therefore, we undertook a macroscopical complete removal of the tumor by transurethral resection.
For the additional radiation of the tumorbed and its surrounding we use a COHERENT-Dye-Laser-system PRT 92. It delivers 630 nm and is therefore because of the greater penetration depth of red light a suitable light source for this application (Fig. 2).
On the next slide you can see, how the laser light is delivered into the bladder by the fiber through the working-channel of an operation-cystoscope. We use 800-1000 mWatts in an exposure time of 15 min. (Fig. 3).

The next slide shows the necessary eye protection filter on the optic of the cystoscope.

The human bladder is well illuminated even when it is not an 'Ulbricht-bowl'. But there is a decrease of brightness, if you go more to the bladder neck (Fig. 4).

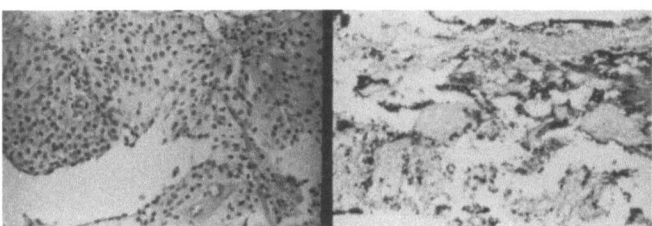

Fig. 4. Effect of treatment: On the left side untreated tumor tissue, on the right the same tumot tissue after PDT: No vital tumor cells

The next slide shows the efficacy of the treatment. It is a urothelium carcinoma T1G1: On the right-hand side you can see calcificaceous necroses as well as a group of granulocytes but no vital tumor structures. In this case, we left by intention a little tumor rest and removed it seven weeks after PDT. For evaluation of our clinical results we used a method published by SCHULMANN et al. 1982. By this method it is possible to calculate the recurrence rate before and after treatemnt of the same patient. This was done in dividing the total sum of all verified recurrences by the sum of the months in the follow-up and for better presentation multiplied by 100.
36 patients with bladder tumors -Tis, T1,T2- have been treated.
For these patients - treated with conventional methods before using PDT - the average recurrence rate was 4.5 relapses since the diagnosis of the primary tumor.
The period of observation lasted nearly three years. The checks moves at intervals of 3 to 6 months by using cytology, cystoscopy, intravesical sonography and biopsy (Fig. 5).
The slide shows the results from 33 patients. The recurrence rate R was before PDT 9.57 and afterwards 3.96. This is a significant difference.
For nearly all patients with a fast recidivation in spite of PDT we found an aneuploid distribution of DNA or an increased proliferation.
It may be possible that an integrated illumination of the bladder may lead in certain cases to improved results of the PDT.

RECURRENCE-RATE	R	NUMBER OF	
		RECURRENCES	MONTHS
BEFORE PDT	9,57	181	1892
AFTER PDT	3,96	13	328
	p < 0,04		

* Recurrence rate (Recurrences observed by cysto-scopy) x 100 / follow-up (Months)

Fig. 5: Recurrence rate before and after PDT

LITERATURE

KELLY, J.F. and SNELL, M.E., Hematoporphyrine Derivate: A possible aid in the diagnosis and therapy of carcinoma of the bladder. J.Urol.115,150-151 (1976)

TAPPEINER, H. von und JESIONEK, A., Therapeutische Versuche mit fluorezierenden Stoffen. MMW 1, 2042-2044 (1903)

JESIONEK, A. und TAPPEINER, H. von, Zur Behandlung der Hautcarcinome mit fluorezierenden Stoffen. Dtsch.Arch.Klin.Med.82, 223-227 (1905)

GOMER, C.J. and RAZUM, N.J., Acute skin response in albino mice following Porphyrin photosensitization under oxic and anoxic condition. Photochem.Photobiol. 40, 435-439 (1984)

MOAN, J.,SMEDSHAMMER, L. and CHRISTENSEN, T., Photodynamic effects on human cells exposed to light in the presence of hematoporphyrine. pH-Effects. Cancer Letters 9,327-332 (1980)

BOWN, S.G., BARR, H., TRALAU, C.J., COLERIDGE-SMITH, P.D. and SANDEMAN, D.R., How selective is PDT and which factors determine selectivity ? 7th Congr.Int.Soc.Laser Surgery and Medicine, Munich 1987

JOCHAM, D., STÄHLER, G. CHAUSSY, C. HAMMER, C. und LÖHRS, U., Laserbehandlung von Blasentumoren nach Photosensibilisierung mit Hämatoporphyrin-Derivat.Experimentelle Erfahrungen. Urologe A (Suppl.20) 340 (1981)

BORTZ, J., Eine faktorielle Varianzanalyse mit Meßwiederholung. Lehrbuch der Statistik für Sozialwissenschaften, Springer, Berlin/Heidelberg/New York, 1977

SCHULMANN, C.C., ROBINSON, M., DENIS, L., SMITH, P. VIGGIANO, G., de PAUW, M., DALESIO, O. and SYLVESTER, R., Prophylactic chemotherapy of superficial transitional cell bladder carcinoma: An EORTC randomized trial comparing Thiotepa, an Epipodophyllotoxin (VM 26) and TUR alone. Eur.Urol.8, 207-212 (1982)

HPD Mediated Photochemotherapy for Selective Treatment of Leukemic Cells VS Normal Cells

T. PATRICE, M.T. FOULTIER, V. PRALORAN, D. CLOAREC, L. LE BODIC,

DÉPARTEMENT LASER - HOPITAL G et R. LAENNEC

BP 1005 - 44035 - NANTES CEDEX - FRANCE

As photochemotherapy of solid tumors is rapidly develloping recent studies suggested that in-vitro photochemotherapy mediated by HPD could be more efficient on leukemic cells than normal cells (1), (2) and this represent a way of cell selection. In order to demonstrate this phenomenon we studied the phototoxicity on both leukemic cells (L1210) and normal syngeneic hemoprogenitors. We varied three culture parameters : time incubation of the cells with HPD, temperature of the medium during incubation and treatment of the cells, laser dose fractionation in 2 or 3. For each condition 3 separates experiments in triplicate have been performed, and each experiment involved simultaneously both cell types for 2 or 3 laser energy levels.

Results show a clear-cut selectivity, improved by an incubation temperature of 37°C and 4°C during laser exposure. Dose fractionation seems to protect normal cells. For both cell types and HPD, an incubation time, longer than 2 hours does not seem to increase the photosensitivity. Results concerning dose fractionation are in agreement with those found by MOAN et al on NHIK 3025 cell lines (3). Results concerning temperature during HPD incubation or laser treatment, indicates that HPD uptake is a function of cell activity as phototoxicity decreases with incubation temperature.

The increased PDT selectivity observed with an HPD incubation at 37°C and a laser treatment at 4°C, could be explained, by an increased level of repair of potentially lethal demages for normal cells Vs leukemic cells. As suggested by SIEBER et al (4) using merocyanine 540 as photosensitizer, photochemotherapy could represent a promissive way of selecting cells in bone marrow leukemic cells purging in the perspective of human autografts.

REFERENCES

Effects of laser irradiation on hematoporphyrin treated normal and transformed thyroid cells in culture.
A. ANDREONI, R. CUBEDDU, S. DESILVESTRI et Al
CANCER Res. : 43, 2076 - 2080. 1983

Uptake of hematoporphyrin derivative by normal and malignant cells :
Effects of serum, ph, temperature, and cell size
R. BOHMER, G. MORSTYN
CANCER Res. : 45, 5328 - 5334, 1985

Photodynamic inactivation of cancer cells in-vitro :
Effects of irradiation, temperature and dose fractionation
J. MOAN, T. CHRISTENSEN
CANCER Lett. : 6, 331 - 335, 1979

Dye-mediated photosensitization of murine neuroblastoma cells
F. SIEBER, M. SIEBER-BLUM
CANCER Res. : 46, 2072 - 2076, 1986

Indirect Appreciation of the PDT Effect on the Tumor Vasculature

T. PATRICE, M.T. FOULTIER, M.F. LE BODIC, L. LE BODIC
DEPARTEMENT LASER - HOPITAL G et R. LAENNEC
BP 1005 - 44035 NANTES CEDEX FRANCE

Some authors recently published papers evidencing the rôle of PDT on neovasculature of tumors. In order to appreciate the exact role of PDT on vasculature versus the tumor mass itself we realized 3 different vitro-vivo comparisons on our tumor model HT 29 grafted on nude swiss mice :

- HPD injection, tumor excision, in vitro laser irradiation, tumor "re-graft", VS tumor excision, in vitro delay (20' at 37°C), tumor "re-graft"

- HPD injection, tumor excision, in-vitro irradiation, tumor graft on a new nude mouse VS tumor excision, in-vitro delay, tumor graft on a new nude mouse

- HPD injection, tumor excision, laser irradiation of the tumor site of implantation, tumor "re-graft" VS tumor excision, delay, laser irradiation, tumor "re-graft".

The growth index study at 7 days (experiment) and 14 days (sacrifice) and the anatomo-pathologic study evidence a better effect of HPD-PDT treated groups VS mechanical anoxy. HPD-PDT efficacy is not only due to tumor vasculature damages.

"Rosette" Argon Laser Phototherapy with Rhodamine 123: A new Method for Eradication of Melanoma Tumors in Nude Mice

D.J. Castro, R.E. Saxton, H.R. Fetterman, P.H. Ward

Dept. of Head & Neck Surgery, U.C.L.A. Med. Center
10833 LeConte Ave., Los Angeles, Calif. 90024

Rhodamine 123 (Rh-123) is a mitochondrial specific dye that can be successfully used as a photochemosensitizing agent for the argon laser treatment of human melanoma in vitro. In this study a new technique of "Rosette" treatment with the argon laser was developed to completely eradicate human melanoma (M24) tumor transplants in nude mice after "sensitization" with a nontoxic dose of Rh-123. Each experimental group included 4 nu/nu mice injected subcutaneously with 10 millions cells/site for a total of 48 sites. Tumor take was >95% at one week with >10 mm^3 tumor volume at each site. Control groups of untreated M24 tumors and M24 tumors sensitized with 1ug/ml of Rh-123 demonstrated significant growth during the 10 weeks follow-up. Test groups were sensitized with Rh-123 (1ug/ml for one hour) by intratumor injection at one week then treated with the argon laser at 514.5 nm. To allow uniform delivery of energies to the tumors and its edges, a new "Rosette" technique was developed. The tumors were then exposed to non-thermal levels of 700J/cm^2 (36°C) or 950J/cm^2 (40°C) as determined by a reproducible method of dosimetry. All 16 tumors in this test group showed complete regression with excellent healing and no recurrences even after ten weeks follow-up. Control tumors treated with the argon laser alone, exhibited regrowth at 4 weeks after treatment. These results demonstrate that effective eradication of tumors can be achieved in vivo, only after chemosensitization with Rh-123 and specific argon laser treatment ("Rosette"), even at non-thermal levels of energies. The high effectiveness of this technique and low toxicity of Rh-123, may render its clinical use very attractive for the treatment of superficial malignancies.

Photodynamic Therapy of Oral Cancer in Hamsters

M. Herzog,[*] H.-H. Horch,[*] Th. Meier,[**]
S. Enders [***]
[*]Clinic of Oral and Maxillo-Facial
Surgery, Klinikum rechts der Isar,
Technical University of Munich,
Ismaningerstr. 22, D-8000 München 80
[**]Institute of Laser Technology, University of Ulm, Oberer Eselsberg 9,
D-7900 Ulm
[***]Institute of Pathology, Städtisches
Krankenhaus Bogenhausen, Engelschalkingerstr., D-8000 München 81

Oral cancer can arise from a primary multiple dysplastic epithelium. Therefore oral cancer can be surrounded by normal mucosa, but also by leucoplakial or sources of a carcinoma in situ. The multifocal origin is one of the reasons for the high recurrence rate and the bad prognosis of oral cancer. According to the statistics the 5-years-healing rate amounts to only 30%-40%. (FRIES 1978, NOLTENIUS 1987, PAPE 1985)

For therapy of oral cancer operative methods and radiotherapy are used as well as, in the stage of clinical studies, immunestimulating measures. The radical operation proved to be the most successful therapy. It is necessary to remove the tumor out of the normal tissue whereby the safety distance has to be at least 1 cm. This therapy means a mutilation of the patient which cannot be totally repaired, even not by the means of the plastic surgery of today. (REHRMANN 1973, SCHEUNEMANN and SCHMIDSEDER 1976)

The sole application of radiotherapy on oral cancer is only possible to a very limited extent. The side effects consist not only of the radiation reaction of skin and mucosa, but also dryness of the mouth caused by the obliteration of the salivary glands and the danger of osteoradionecrosis with imminent loss of the lower jaw. (HERZOG et al 1986, WANNENMACHER 1976)

The application of cytostatic drugs has been established first of all for the palliative therapy but a curative treatment of oral cancer is only possible in exceptional cases. This concerns also the combination of radiotherapy and chemotherapy, the socalled radio-chemo-therapy. (BITTER 1977, PHILLIPS 1982, SCHMITT et al 1983)

Considering this background and the growing incidence of oral cancer
the development of additional complementary therapy methods seems
to be urgent. Especially interesting should be treatment methods
which grant the destruction of visible and invisible tumor tissue,
preserves normal tissue and at the same time come into action at
another point than radiotherapy and chemotherapy.

Different photosensitising substances, i.e. hematoporphyrin-derivative (HpD) concentrate selectively in different tumors after systemic
administration and a fast clearance of normal tissue. Also the human
oral cancer including the carcinoma in situ accumulate HpD. The
mechanisms of this accumulation could not be explained totally
(DOUGHERTY, 1984, ARONOFF 1986).
HpD photosensitises tissue. During radiation with light specific
wave lenght which is absorbed by the porphyrin molecule, biological
aggressive singlet-oxygen, peroxide and hydroxyl radicals arise
which mainly damage the cell membrane, the tumor vessels, and the
tumor surrounding vessels.

A successful treatment is then possible when tumors proved to be
resistant against the two methods mentioned before (DAS et al 1985,
DUBBELMAN and v.STEVENINCK 1984, GROSSWEINER and GROSSWEINER 1982,
STAR et al 1984).

The tests were carried out with syrian hamsters, both male and female.
By the application of DMBA two times a week during 12 weeks, oral
cancer in the mucosa of the cheek pouch had been induced. Via dysplasias and carcinoma in situ, infiltrative and finally metastasi-
sing   tumors developed. Up to this
stage the animals general conditions was satisfactory. The animals
were killed at this stage at the latest.

HpD had been produced using the method which is recommended by
Kessel (KESSEL 1985, KESSEL and CHENG 1985).

24 hours before radiation of the animals it has been intraperitoneally
injected with a dose of 2.5, 5 and 10 mg HpD per gram of body weight.
The laser treatment was carried out with parallel laser light. The
red light emitted by the dye laser showed a maximum of 630 mm, laser
efficiency at the end of the light guide was 2 W. After a radiation
period of 4 and 8 minutes, the surface dose was 120J per cm^2 and
240J per cm^2, respectively. To avoid thermic damages the irradiated
areas had been intensively aircooled.

Immediately after radiation tumors didn't show any changes. After
4 hours a livid discoloration can be seen. Histological examination
now show a significant vascular filling and a beginning destruction
of tumor cells. This destruction is distinctly visible after 2 to
4 days. The limit of normal tissue constitutes a granulocytic border.
In the clinical examinations significant signs of necrosis can be
seen, the tumor begins to separate. After 10 days only inflammatory
tissue which is partly covered with fibrin is visible. No tumor can
be detected. After some time the mucosa forms a star shaped scar.
At the border of the radiation area new tumors grow. Signs of inflammation disappear and more connective tissue fibres can be seen.

Photodynamic therapy causes tin almost 90% of treated tumors severe
damages. Tumors with a diameter below 3 mm can be totally destroyed
nearly always by means of direct radiation. In tumors with a diameter of more than 3 mm partial radiation effect could be observed.
An influence on the success of the therapy by the applied different
HpD-doses could not be determined. Tumors which have not been photosensitised by HpD showed no reaction under the same conditions of
radiation.

The principle of photodynamic therapy is based on the increase of
photosensitivity of tissues by means of photosensitizing substances.
This reaction of the tissue is released by the radiation with an
appropriate light which is absorbed by the HpD-molecule and which is
deeply infiltrating tissues. As light absorption is mainly determined
by absorption of the haemoglobin, it ist necessary to work with the
absorption minimum of the blood to obtain a sufficient infiltration
of the tissue, in the red spectral range (DOUGHERTY 1984, TSE et al
1984).

The reason for the partial destruction of more extensive tumors lies
in the insufficient infiltration depth of the applied red light of
the dye laser. In most cases of squamos cell carcinoma the infiltration
depth has to be about 4 mm. Still different distribution and a smaller
concentration in the depth of tumors is possible (HERZOG et al 1987,
SVAASAND, 1984, BUGELSKI et al 1981, BOGGAN et al 1981).

Another explanation for the only partial destruction of large tumors may
be the insufficient oxygen supply, as photodynamic therapy similar
to radiotherapie and chemotherapie requires a sufficient oxygen
supply (GIBSON and HILF 1985).

An explanation of the ineffectiveness of therapy in some cases may be a primary resistance to photodynamic therapy or mistakes during the intraperitoneal administration of HpD.

As a conclusion it can be said that by means of the photodynamic therapy a regular destruction of small tumors (diameter below 3 mm) in the cheek pouch of hamsters is successful. Therefore this technique may be also very important for the therapy of human oral cancer.

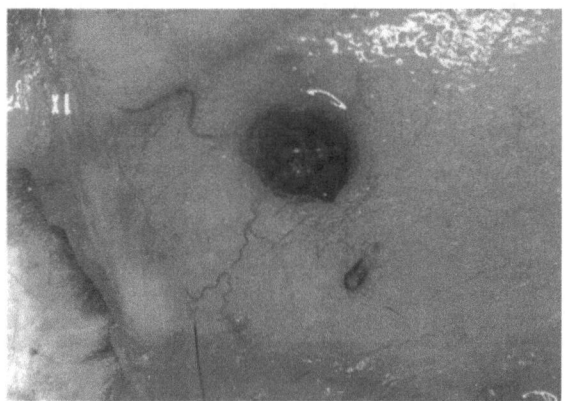

Fig. 1. Tumor 4 days after photodynamic therapy. The necrosis is shown by the dark colour. Surrounding the tumor unchanged mucosa

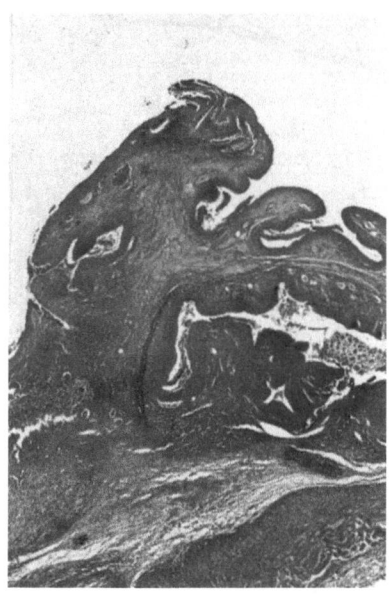

Fig. 2. Tumor necrosis. The necrotic tumor is separated by a granulocytic border of the normal tissues

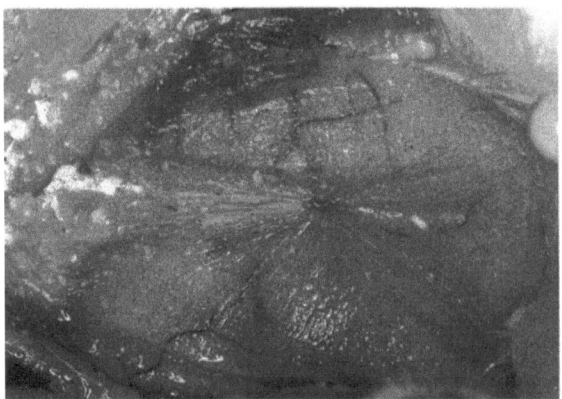

Fig. 3. Star shaped scar in dysplastic mucosa 4 weeks after photodynamic therapy

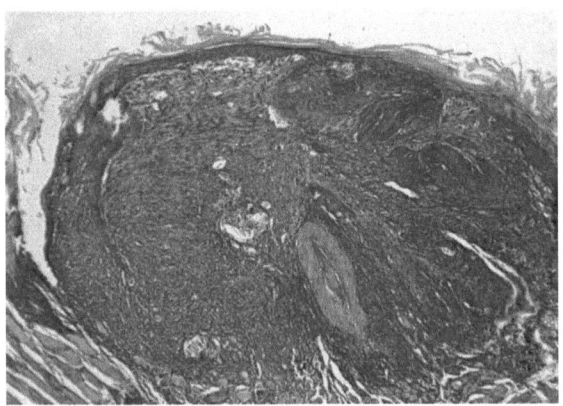

Fig. 4. The same scar as in fig. 3. Scar with connective tissue fibres. No tumor

REFERENCES

ARONOFF, B.L.: The state of art in general surgery and surgical oncology.
Lasers Surg. Med. 6, 376, 1986

BOGGAN, J.E., EDWARDS, M.S.B., BERNS, M.W., WALTER, R.J., BOLGER, C.A.: Hematoporphyrin derivative photoradiation therapy of the rat 9 L gliosarkoma brain tumor model
Lasers Surg. Med. 4, 99, 1984

BITTER, K.: Die Behandlung des Mundhöhlenkarzinoms mit der Kombination Bleomycin, Methotrexat, Telekobaldbestrahlung
Strahlenther. 7, 153, 1977

BUGELSKI, P.J., PORTER, C.W., DOUGHERTY, T.J.: Autoradiographic distribution of hematoporphyrin derivative in normal and tumor tissue of the mouse
Cancer Res. 41, 4606 , 1981

DAS, M., DIXIT, R., MUKHTAR, R., BICKERS, D.R.: Role of active oxygen species in the photodestruction of microsomal cytochrome P-450 and associated monooxygenases by hematoporphyrin derivative in rats
Cancer Res. 45, 608, 1985

DOUGHERTY, T.J.: Photodynamic therapy
Clin. Chest Med. 5, 219, 1985

DOUGHERTY, T.J.: An overview of the status of photoradiation Therapy. In: Doiron, D.R., Gomer, C.J.: Porphyrin localization and treatment of tumors
Alan. Liss. New York, 1984

DUBBELMAN, T.M.A.R., STEVENINCK, J.: Photodynamic effects of hematoporphyrin-derivative on transmembrane transport systems of murine L 929 Fibroplasts
Biochim. Biophys.Acta 771, 201, 1984

FRIES, R.: DÖSAK: Karzinome der Mundhöhle. Zur Frage der Abhängigkeit der Prognose von der Lokalisation der Primärtumors (Organe der Mundhöhle)
Dtsch Z Mund-Kiefer-Gesichtschir., 2, 63, 1978

GIBSON, S.L., HILF, R.: Interdependence of fluence, drug dose and oxygen on hematoporphyrin derivative induced photosensitization of tumor mitochondria
Photochem. Photobiol. 42, 367, 1985

GROSSWEINER, L.I., GROSSWEINER, J.B.: Hydrodynamic effects in the photosensited lysis of liposomes
Photochem. Photobiol. 35, 583, 1982

HERZOG, M., HORCH, H.-H., SENEKOWITSCH, R.,SCHRÖDER, E.: Experimentelle Untersuchungen zur Laser-Diagnostik und Therapie des Mundhöhlenkarzinoms nach tumorselektiver Photosensibilisierung mit Hämatoporphyrin-Derivat (HpD) - vorläufige Mitteilung
Dtsch. Z Mund-Kiefer-Gesichtschir. 11, 18, 1987

HERZOG, M., SAMEK, M., SIRANLI, F.: Zur Indikation der zahnärztlich-chirurgischen Sanierung bei Strahlentherapie
Dtsch. Zahnärztl. Z 41, 449, 1986

NOLTENIUS, H.: Tumor-Handbuch; Pathologie und Klinik der menschlichen Tumoren Bd. 2
Urban & Schwarzenberg, München-Wien-Baltimore, 1987

KESSEL, D.: Localization and photosensitization of murine tumors in vivo and in vitro by a chlorinporphyrin ester
Cancer Res. 46, 2248, 1986

KESSEL, D.:
pers. Mitt. 1986

KESSEL, D., CHENG, M.L.: On the preparation and properties of
dihematoporphyrinether, the tumor localizing component of HPD
Photochem. Photobiol. 41, 277, 1985

KESSEL, D., CHENG, M.L.: Biological and biophysical properties
of the tumor-localizing component of hematoporphyrin derivative
Cancer Res. 45, 3053, 1985

PAPE, H.-D.: Tumoren der Mundhöhle. In: Gross, R. Schmidt, C.G.
Klinische Onkologie
Thieme, Stuttgart-New York, 1985

PHILLIPS, T.L.: Radiation Sensitizers and Protectors
In: De Vita, V.T., Hellmann, S., Rosenberg, S.A..Cancer
Principles and Practice of Oncology
J.B. Lippincott, Philadelphia-Toronto, 1982

Rehrmann, A.: Operative Behandlung der Tumoren der Kiefer und
der umgebenden Weichteile einschließlich plastischer re-
konstruktiver Maßnahmen
Zahnärztl. Mitt. 27, 264, 1973

Svaasand, L.O.: Optical dosimetry for direct and interstitial
Photoradiation Therapy of malignant tumors. In: Doiron, D.R., Gomer,C.J.
Porphyrin Localization and Treatment of tumors
Alan Liss. New York, 1984

SCHEUNEMANN, H., SCHMIDSEDER, R.: Fortschritte und Schwerpunkte
der Geschwulstbehandlung im Mund-Kiefer-Gesichtsbereich
Fortschr. Kiefer-   Gesichtschir 21, 155, 1976

SCHMITT, T., SCHETTLER,D., SCHERER, E., HIGI, M., HAUENSTEIN, H.G.:
Present interdisciplinary treatment regimen for advanced
head and neck tumors at the West German Tumour Centre, Essen
J max-fac Surg 11, 51, 1983

Star, W.M. MARIJNISSEN, J.P.A., v.d.BERG-BLOK, A.E., REINHOLD, H.S.:
Destructive effect of photoradiation on the microcirculation of
a rat mammary tumor growing in "sandwich" obervation chamber
In: Doiron, D.R., Gomer, C.J. Porphyrin localization and
treatment of tumors
Alan Liss., New York, 1984

TSE, D.T., KERSTEN, R.C., ANDERSON, R.L.: Hematoporphyrin derivative
photoradiation therapy in managing nevoid-basal-cell carcinoma
syndrome
Arch   Ophthalmol   102, 990, 1984

WANNENMACHER, M.: Die Wirkung ionisierender Strahlen auf die
Gewebe im Mundhöhlenbereich
Hanser München-Wien, 1976

Low Power Laser/Biostimulation

Low Power Laser in Medicine and Surgery – State of the Art

Kazuhiko ATSUMI
Institute of Medical Electronics, Faculty of Medicine
University of Tokyo, 7-3-1 Hongo, Bunkyo-ku, Tokyo, 113, Japan

Introduction

Laser applications in medicine and surgery have been started by using high power to coagulate, to vaporize the biological tissues -- it means by use of thermal effect. Next application of laser is considered to be using pressure effect to destruct biological stone by application of short pulse laser. Recently, the use of low power is becoming one of the topics of laser applications in medicine. (Figure(1))

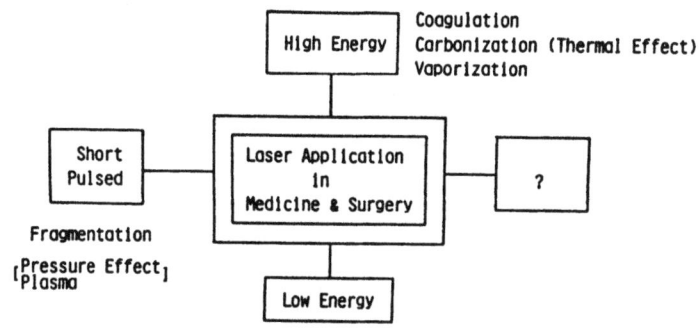

Figure(1). Bio-medical Application of Laser Energy

1) The Papers of "Low Power Laser in Medicine" in the Conferences

In 1985, the historical conference of laser in medicine and surgery was held in Bologna by presiding by Prof. Galletti. In this meeting, 35 papers of low power laser therapy were presented and 8 papers of pain laser were reported.

In the same year, the international congress of laser surgery and medicine was held in Jerusalem presiding by Prof. Kaplan. In this congress, the new session of low energy laser was organized and 24 papers were reported in the session.

The Figure(2) shows the papers reported in the Japanese Society of Laser Surgery & Medicine during last four years. The papers in the biostimulation sessions have been increasing year by year in the Figure(2).

The Figure(3) shows the papers reported in the American Society during last three years. Three years ago, no paper was reported in the session of biostimulation. However, the sessions of biostimulation were organized last year and in this year.

Until now, the definition of low power laser was not clarified. My definition is as follows; low power laser means non-thermal effect. Therefore, it must be said that low power are less 100 mW of output and 50 mW/cm^2 of power density of the power level. (Figure(4))

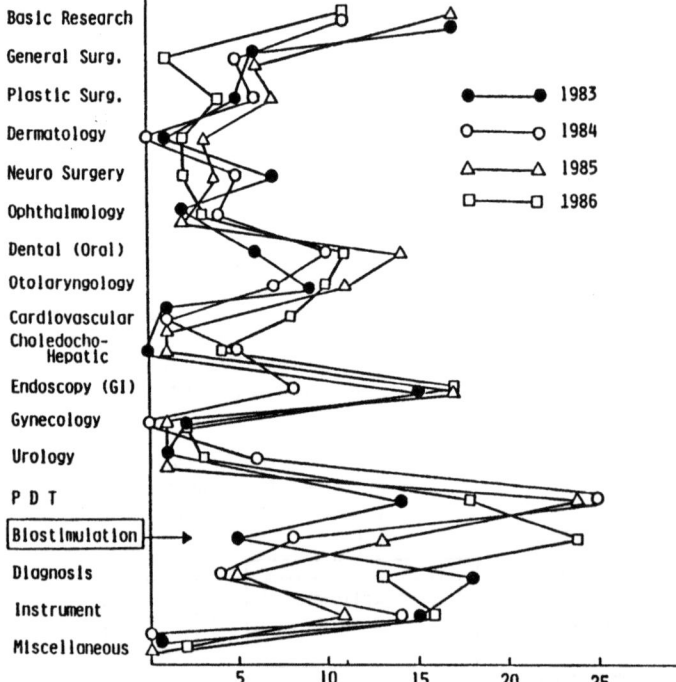

Figure(2). Classification of the Applied Medical Fields from the Reported Papers in the Annual Meeting of Japan Society for Laser Surgery & Medicine (1983 - 1986)

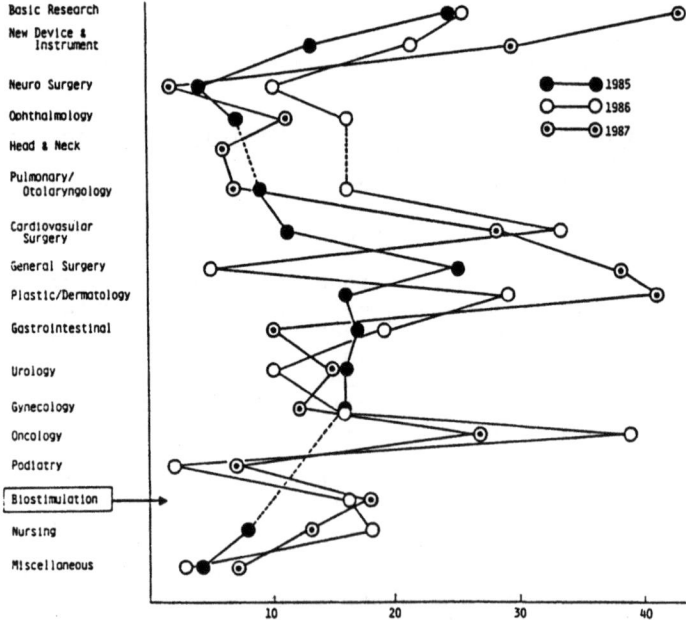

Figure(3). Classification of the Applied Medical Fields from the Reported paper in the Annual Meeting of American Society for Laser Medicine and Surgery (1985 - 1987)

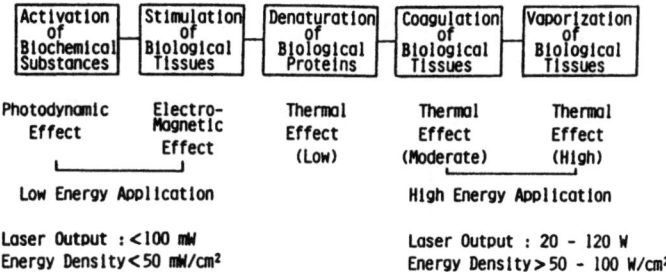

Figure(4). Biological Effects of Laser Energy Irradiation

The Table(1) shows the classification of low power laser applications in medicine reported in main medical laser conferences. In this Table(1), major topics are concerned on pain relief, basic research, wound healing and diagnosis.

Table(1). Classification of Low Power Laser Applications in Medicine Reported in Medical Laser Conferences

	International Congress on Laser in Medicine and Surgery (Bologna, 1985)	Annual Meetings of Japanese Society for Laser Surgery & Medicine (1985, 86, 87)	Annual Meetings of American Society for Laser Surgery & Medicine (1986, 87)	Total
General	0	0	2	2
Basic Research	9	10	1	20
Instrument	2	0	0	2
Cultured Cell Stimulation	1	0	3	4
Wound Healing	9	7	2	18
Hormonal Stimulation	3	0	0	3
Neural Stimulation	1	0	0	1
Acupuncture	2	0	2	4
Pain Relief	7	13	14	34
Bacteriocidal Effect	2	0	0	2
Vascular Anastomosis	0	2	1	3
Diagnosis	4	11	0	15
Miscellaneous	1	1	1	3
Total	41	44	26	111

In 1985, the first international symposium on low energy laser in medicine and surgery was held in Tokyo in 1985. The Figure(5) shows the topics of this symposium which are biostimulation, PDT, wound healing, tissue welding, acupuncture, pain relief, sports medicine, orthopedics, dentistry and medical diagnosis.

2) The Environment of Laser Biostimulation

The Figure(6) shows the environment of laser biostimulation. Laser radiates on the biological tissues and several interactions were occured between laser energy and biological tissues. In the factors of lasers, wave length, power, duration and mode are related in the interactions. As the biological factors, homeostasis should be essentially considered. It means that living body is keeping the living conditions under the principle of homeostasis. Placebo effect should be considered, in regards to normalization, by one of the action of homeostasis. Arndt-schulz's law is also should be considered as the principle of the physiology of living body.

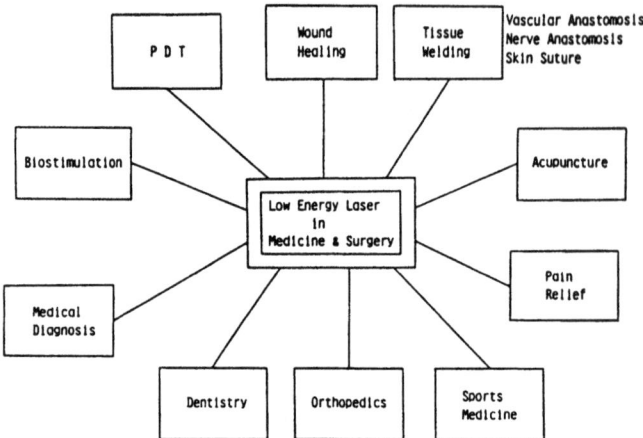

Figure(5). *International Symposium on Low Energy Laser in Medicine and Surgery, Tokyo '85*

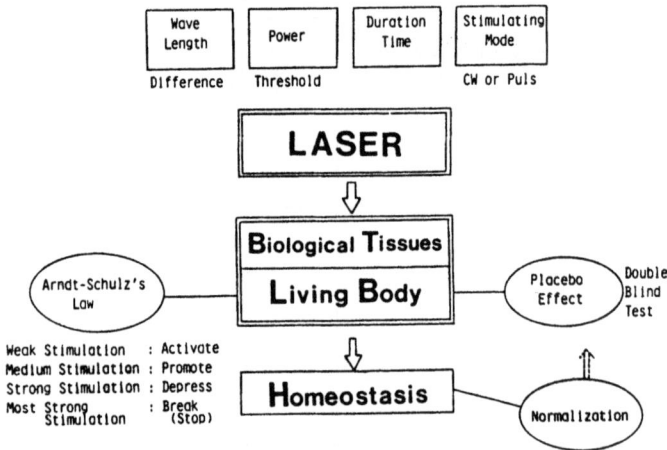

Figure(6). *Environment of Laser Biostimulation*

3) Pain Relief by Diode Laser

As the one of the typical example, I would like to introduce the pain relief effect of diode laser.

The diode laser -- 820 nm of wave length, continuous wave and 60 mW -- has been used in the animal experiments and in clinical trials which was developed by Matsushita Electric Industrial Co., Ltd.

The preliminary studies were done by using infrared thermography and some positive findings were revealed.

Therefore, the double blind test was performed by using the random number generator. In this test, the medical doctors, engineers and patients could not detect the stimulation by the actual laser radiator or by the placebo (Dami).

The double blind tests were carried out in the two facilities -- Tokyo University Hospital and Keio University Hospital --.

The result of 200 clinical cases is as follows; the effective ratio using active diode laser stimulation is 80.3 %, however, the effective ratio using dami is 41.5 %. (Photo(1))

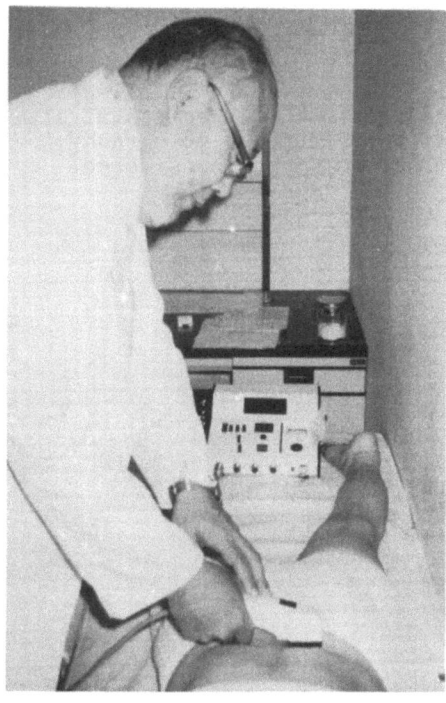

Photo(1).
Biostimulation by diode laser was carried out for the patient of lumbago

The result is positive according to the statistical analysis, however, the further studies should be continued for the placebo effect.

4) The Biomedical Applications of Low Power Laser

The Figure(7) shows the biomedical applications of low power laser -- therapeutics, diagnosis, rehabilitation & health care, and miscellaneous -- .

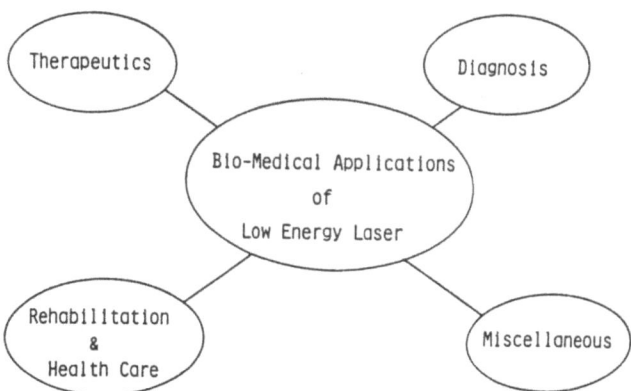

Fig.(7). Bio-Medical Applications of Low Energy Laser

The Figure(8) shows therapeutic applications -- photodynamic, electromagnetic and mild thermal effect --. Each effect has important applications. Mild thermal effect seems to be contrary to the definition, however, it has been included in low power laser application.

The Figure(9) shows diagnostics applications -- spectroanalysis, interference, doppler method, stimulation threshold, holography, speckle pattern, microscope and illumination -- are considered.

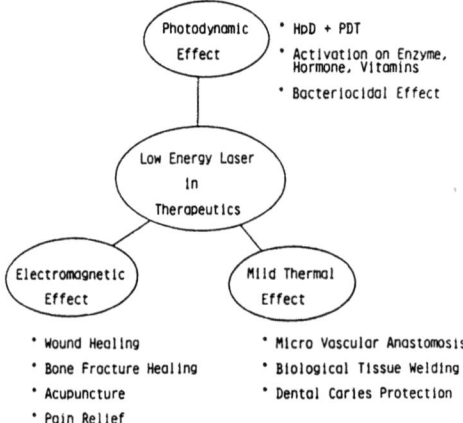

Fig.(8). Low Energy Laser Applications in Therapeutics

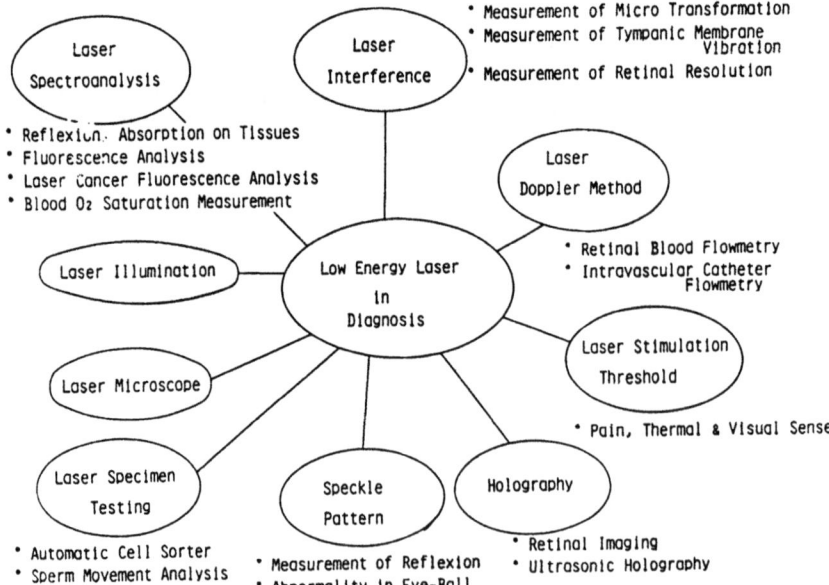

Fig.(9). Low Energy Laser Applications in Diagnostics

The Figure(10) shows rehabilitation and health care applications in which biostimulation, sensory, prosthesis, health care system are comprized.

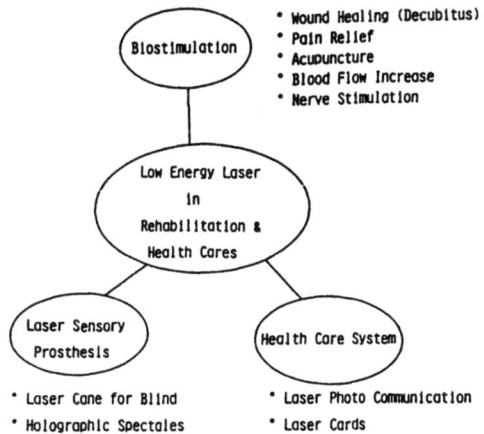

Fig.(10). Low Energy Laser in Rehabilitation & Health Care

5) The Future of Low Power Laser in Medicine

In future, essential mechanism of laser biostimulation should by clarrified. (Figure(11))

In order to complete this purpose, basic researches are to be investigated. For wound healing, enzyme biochemistry, for pain relief, neurophysiology and neuropharmacology, for antiphlogistic effect, enzyme chemistry, blood flow measurement, etc. are to be investigated. For laser acupuncture, comparison of laser stimulation with needle are to be investigated.

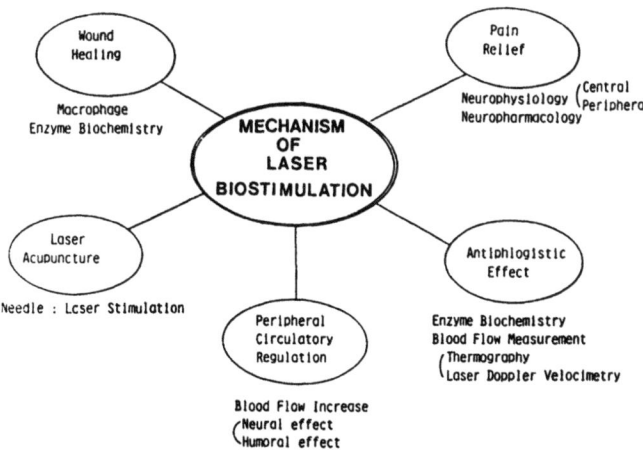

Fig.(11). Analysis of Essential Mechanism of Laser Biostimulation Effects

The future of laser surgery and medicine will challenge to change the impossible diagnosis and therapy in past to possible one as follows.
1. Noninvasive, bloodless surgery
2. Precise diagnostic and selective treatment of cancer
3. Ultramicrosurgery
4. Laser genetic engineering
5. Specific diagnosis by laser immunology
6. Subcellular biomedical research
7. Sensitive diagnosis by laser doppler flowmetry
8. Online, three-dimensional imaging of the whole body by x-ray holography
9. Medical data processing by optical fibers
10. Medical data bank and networking by laser communication

It is meaningful that almost of these future applications will be achieved by using low power lasers.

Effects of Low Dose Laser Radiation on Bacterial Growth

M.Džinić, N.Nanušević, O. Nanušević
Military Medical Academy
ul. Crnotravska 17, 11oo2 BELGRADE, Yugoslavia

Two years ago, we demonstrated inhibitory effects of sublethal doses of laser radiation on bacterial growth (1). In the range of laser radiant exposures below 4 J/cm^2 our results were inconclusive. As this range is of a great importance for laser application in biostimulative medicine, we repeated our investigation using a more sensitive experimental model.

Material and method

In these experiments we used Staphylococcus aureus, lab strain ATCC 25923 as a representative of Gram-positive bacteria, and Escherichia coli, lab strain ATCC 25922 as a representative of Gram-negative bacteria. The bacteria were cultivated for 24 hours as single colonies on two kinds of nutrient media: blood agar (which is red) and Mueller-Hinton agar (which is witish transparent). Each colony, except controls, was thereafter irradiated by Argon laser ("Cooper Medical" model 77o) with the beam expanded to cover 1 cm^2 i.e. the whole colony. Radiant exposures (or doses) were: 0.1 , 0.2 , 0.5 , 1 , 2 , 3 , 4 , 6 , 8 , 1o , 3o , 4o , 6o , 8o , and 1oo J/cm^2. These doses were reached using 1 W power, 0.1 etc. seconds exposure times, and 1 cm^2 spot size.

After irradiation the bacteria were transfered to the Abbott's culture medium diluted to be 4×10^6/ml. During incubation at $37^\circ C$ in the "Abbott MS-2 Research System", bacterial growth was registered as optical density difference between irradiated and non-irradiated cultures. The registration period lasted 1245 minutes.

Results

Optical density differences, calculated by the "Abbott's MS-2 Research System" computer, were analysed as longitudinal kynetics of bacterial growth in the period of 1245 minutes for each dose of radiation, and also, comparison of bacterial growth between various consecutive doses was done. The analysis also included investigation of the nutrient medium colour influence to the effect of irradiation, and the difference in response to laser radiation between the two sorts of bacteria: Gram-positive and Gram-negative.

Generally, at the low doses of laser irradiation, differences in the rates of bacterial growth between irradiated and non-irradiated cultures were quite slight but consistent.

Starting from the lowest dose applicated, Staphylococcus aureus presented inhibition of growth, developing during the phase of exponential bacterial growth in the first hours of cultivation, and thereafter some negative difference persisted till the end of the observation period (Fig. 1.). Colour of the medium did not influence the response of Staphylococcus aureus to the low doses of irradiation.

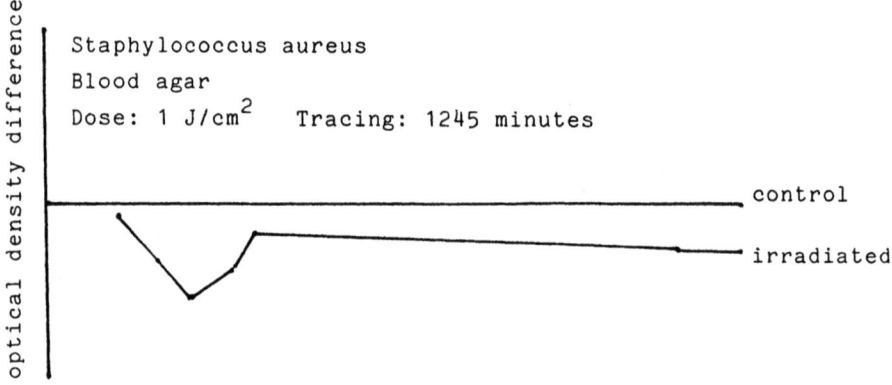

Fig. 1.

Escherichia coli at the same dose of irradiation responded differently: the low doses of laser radiation provoked stimulation of the bacterial growth (Fig.2.). This effect was less pronounced when the bacteria were on the red nutrient medium as compared to the witish one.

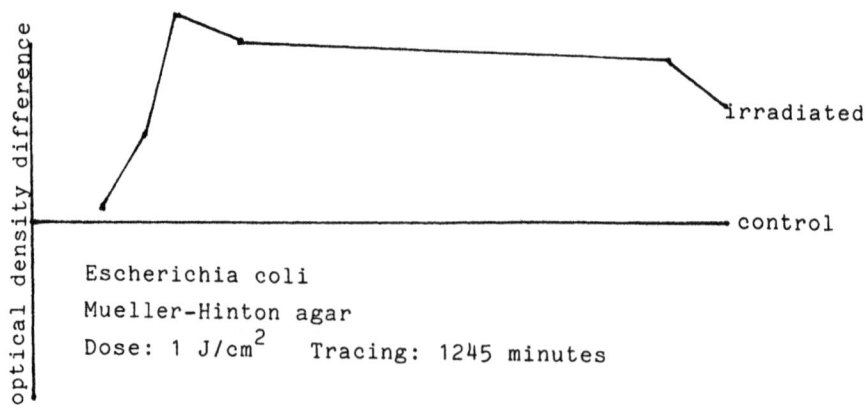

Fig. 2.

Comparison of the response to low dose laser radiation between various consecutive doses revealed approximately equal values, independently upon the doses (Fig. 3.). At the median doses (above 1o J/cm²) reversion of stimulative to inhibitory effect was observed in Escherichia coli on blood agar (Fig. 4.), and Staphylococcus aureus presented potentiation of inhibition.

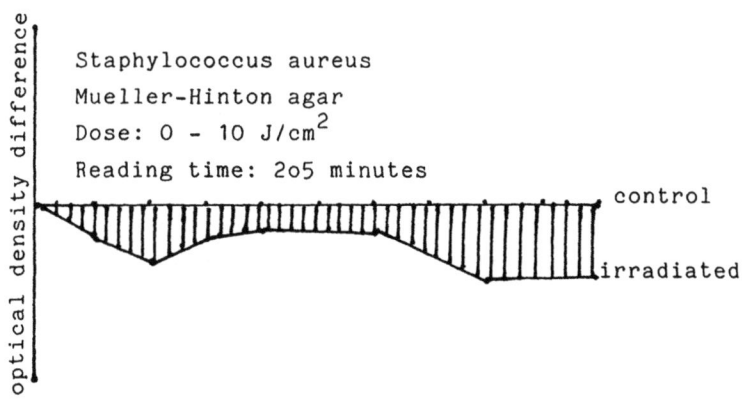

Fig. 3.

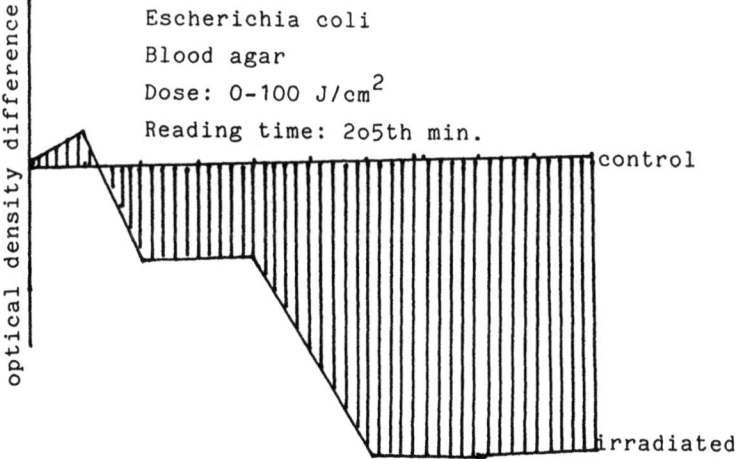

Fig. 4.

Comments and conclusion

Difference in the response to low dose laser radiation between Gram-positive and Gram-negative bacteria can be attributed to important difference in their cellular wall composition (2). The wall of a Gram-positive organism is thick and dense, containing glycopeptide as the main layer, while Gram-negative bacteria have 2-8 times thinner walls containing a good deal of lipopolysacharide and possibly lipoproteins. Our results suggest that the most important biological effects of laser radiation on bacteria exert on the cellular walls, what is in accordance with Mester`s hypothesis related to multicellular organism (3).

Another interesting observation is non-linear effect of low dose laser radiation on bacteria, which is related to electric and magnetic fields of laser rays (4). With so low doses, resonant interactions between electromagnetic energy and biological molecules are only explanation. Abrupt potentiation of the inhibitory effects observed at median doses is probably related to the influence of thermal effects. This occurrence comes sooner when a bacterial colony is irradiated on blood agar because red medium better absorbs energy of Argon lasser wavelength

At last, the observation that low dose laser radiation stimulates growth of Gram-negative bacteria raises a question why this phenomenon does not promote development of an infection during medical application of low dose laser radiation. A quite possible answer lies in the fact that this stimulative effect on bacterial growth is slight, and on the other hand, this effect is compensated by simultaneous stimulation of the patient`s immunological defence mechanisms which has also been proved (3,5).

Literature

1. Džinić M., Nanušević O.: Effects of laser radiation on bacteria. In: Laser/Optoelektronik in der Medizin, Springer-Verlag, Berlin, 1986. pp. 184-187.
2. Davis B. D. et al.: Microbiology. Hoeber Medical Division, Harper and Row Publishers, New York, 1967.
3. Mester E. et al.: The biostimulatory effect of laser beam. In: Optoelectronics in medicine, Springer-Verlag, Berlin, 1982. pp. 146-151.
4. ... Lasers and optical radiation. WHO, Geneva, 1982.
5. Nanušević N., Milićević S.: Changes of some of the immunological parameters in persons exposed to laser radiation. Period. biol., 81:2, 3o5-3o7, 1979.

Preliminary Observation and Approach of the Laser Biological Effect of the Immune Liver RNA in the Action of Malignant Tumor

FU-SHOU YANG, DA-WEN XU
Department of Laser Medicine, Shanghai Seamen's Hospital
505, Dong Changzhi Rd 200080, Shanghai, China.

I. Introduction

The methods now being used in the treatment of tumors may be basically classified into two broad categories: One is the direct killing of cancer cells and the other is the inhibiting of the cancer cells growth by strengthening the function of immunity surveillance to cancer cells. But in this paper, we try to probe into the technology of laser treatment of cancer by both the two main methods mentioned above and the way in which the "reversion" of the cancer cells takes place.

II. Biological effect of immune liver RNA by Laser

1. Observation on the inhibiting action of immune liver RNA irradiated by laser on animal liver cancer cells in vitro

    (1) Materials and Method

    a. The mouse ascitic type liver cancer cells, after being properly treated, were used as a antigen to immunize the mouse of C57DL series[2], and then the RNA was extracted by disecting its liver[1].

    b. The RNA-water solution (5mg/ml) was made in four test tubes which then were respectively irradiated by lasers of different wavelength and power density (3250Å = $8J/cm^2$, 3371Å = $6J/cm^2$, and 5145Å = $9J/cm^2$). For an even laser irradiation over the immune liver RNA, each test tube was put on the same high-frequency vibrating stand with a timing stirrer above it, and its rotation speed was 30 seconds per circle.

    c. The immune RNA in four tubes that had gone through the above steps (hereafter referred to as simply 3250RNA, 3371RNA, 4416RNA, 5145-RNA) were respectively cultured with the ascitic type liver cancer cells of mouse for 12-16 hours at the temperature of 0-4°C, then, these cultured cancer cells (5 x 10 cells/mouse) were inoculated into the abdominal cavity of C57DL series mouse, ten mice for each RNA group. Besides, normal saline was mixed with cancer cells under the same conditions which were used as a contrast group.

(2) Results and Discussion

These experimental results showed us that all the ten inoculated mice in contrast group suffered from ascitic cancer but no one in each laser group. Our experimental results also showed that the complete disappearing of growth ability of liver cancer cells cultured with RNA in vitro was related with the action of RNA being introduced into liver cancer cells. Besides, in the view of the fact that the liver cancer cells in each laser group had no dyeability to the intravital stain by Eosin method, we had good reason to believe that the RNA inhibiting action on cancer cells was not due to its direct killing action. Moreover, the 3250RNA, 3371RNA, 4416RNA and 5145RNA would not have the inhibiting action on the growth of asctic type liver cancer cells any longer when they had been treated with ribonuclease, which means the RNA inhibiting action on cancer cells truly resulted from the laser-irradiated RNA macromolecules themselves.

2. Observation on the inhibiting action of 3250RNA, 3371RNA, 4416RNA and 5145RNA on the growth of animal liver cancer cells in vivo

(1) Materials and Method

a. The mice of C57DL series, supplied by Shanghai Pharmaceutical Research Institute, Academia Sinica, were divided at random into eight test groups: contrast group (o.9% NaCl solution group), independent immune RNA + PVS group, 3250RNA group, 3371RNA group, 4416RNA group and 5145RNA group ten mice in each group.

b. The ascitic type liver cancer cells were injected into the abdominal cavity of mice in each group (6×10^6 cells/mouse) for inoculation for eight hours, then the different drugs, corresponding to each group, were respectively injected into the abdominal cavity of mice (the drug for contrast group was normal saline; the RNA capacity for each laser group was 0.5mg/mouse and the PVS capacity was 0.15mg/mouse. etc.). This same experiment was carried out once a day, for three successive days. After a week, the mice were killed to count the number of their cancer cells. The experimental results showed in table I.

(2) Table I.

The inhibiting action of immune RNA irradiated by laser on the growth of ascitic type liver cells of C57DL series mice

Group	Number of mice	Number of cells	Inhibition rate	Condition
contrast	10	4.98×10^8	-------	0.9% NaCl sol. / mouse
3250ARNA	10	1.70×10^8	66 %	0.5 mg

3371ARNA	10	1.76×10^8	65 %	0.5 mg
4416ARNA	10	2.98×10^8	41 %	0.5 mg
5145ARNA	10	3.60×10^8	28 %	0.5 mg
P V S	10	4.56×10^8	8 %	0.15mg
PVS + immune RNA	10	2.83×10^8	44 %	PVS 0.15 mg + immuneRNA 0.5 mg
immune RNA	10	4.20×10^8	16 %	0.5 mg

As the rebonuclease in the mouse would destroy the exogenous RNA, the inhibiting action on liver cancer cells could not be attained, when the liver RNA was directly injected into the abdominal cavity of mice suffering from ascitic type liver cancer. It has been reported that the ribonuclease activity was successfully inhibited by PVS and thus the inhibiting action of liver RNA on ascitic type liver cancer of mouse was strengthened[3].

The results listed in table I showed us, the inhibiting action of both 3250RNA and 3371RNA on liver cancer cells in vivo could run into 65% or so which means it was quite possible that the biological effect of ultraviolet wavelength laser provided the immune liver RNA with the function resisting the ribonuclease of mouse, and as a result, the percentage of RNA inhibiting the growth of liver cancer cells was increased. Encouraging as these findings may be, this experiment was only preliminary and needed further confirmation. In view of these points, the results showed in this experiment are only for reference.

(3) Observation for histology

Through the comparison between the sections of all the groups, the shape of lymphaden under the microscope for all the laser groups displayed the striking proliferation of small lymphocytes in lymphaden subcortex, and the germinal centre of lymphocyte was enlarged with its reactive proliferation. Besides, the endothelial cells in lymph sinus-space swelled, the post-capillary venules were highly dilated and congested, the MGP staining showed, the immune blast-cells increased in number. The small lymphocytes surrounding central lienalis proliferated and the number of multinuclear giant cells in laser groups was about 5-10 times more than that in contrast and PVS groups. Moreover, the sections of thymus gland showed that the thymic corpuscles hypertrophied and grew in with the lymphatic tissue proliferating among them.

All the histological changes mentioned above may bring us the conclusion that the immune RNA was able to stmulate the defensive action of mouse immune function.

3. The killing action of HPD(c) and laser on animal liver cancer cells cultured with 3250RNA and 3371RNA (experiment in test tube)

(1) Materials and Method

a. The HPD(c) was an improvement of Lipson's HPD[4].

b. 3250RNA, 3371RNA and the 0.9% NaCl solution (contrast) were respectively cultured with ascitic type liver cancer cells according to the method introduced in part 1, then 3 ml of liver cancer cells suspension (2.5×10^5 cells/ml) of each group were put in a small Beijing bottle together with HPD(c) of different concentrations (0.5; 1.0; 10; 50; 100μg/ml). These bottles were kept from light for an hour at the room-temperature and then were irradiated by He-Ne laser for 5 min. at the power density of 5 mw/cm^2. At this moment, with the surveying technique of ^{125}IudR isotope marking[5], 9 μl of 10^{-3}M FudR and 7.5 μci of ^{125}IudR were put into each bottle to be cultured for another 2 hours at the temperature of 37°C away from light. After a centrifugal process, the upper clear liquid was drawn off, the cells were washed twice with Hank's fluid, the quantity of cpm in the remaining cells was determined with the results expressed by inhibiting percentage of ^{125}IudR penetration. The formula of calculation is shown as follows:

$$\text{Inhibiting rate of } ^{125}\text{IudR penetration \%} = \frac{\text{contrast group cpm} - \text{laser group cpm}}{\text{contrast group cpm}} \times 100\%$$

(2) Results

When the HPD(c) concentration was at 1 μg/ml, the inhibiting rate of ^{125}IudR penetration could respectively run into about 92% and 87% for both the 3250RNA and the 3371RNA groups, but only when the HPD(c) concentration was up to 50 μg/ml could the inhibiting rate 96% be reached for 0.9% NaCl solution group as showed in the table II.

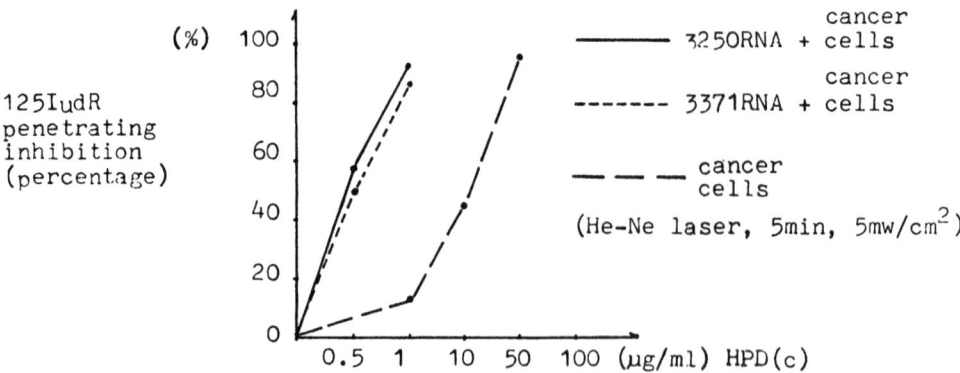

Table II. The HPD(c) photosensitive effect on the ascitic type liver cancer cells cultured with 3250RNA and 3371RNA.

III. Discussion

1. These experimental results showed us, that the biological effect of immune liver RNA by ultraviolet laser would likely have the resisting effect on the rebonuclease activity in mouse, and, it had been observed that the chemical changes on histology indicated the increase of immune function in mouse. Consequently, the inhibition rate on the growth of ascitic type liver cancer cells considerably increased.

2. The results, obtained in an experiment on the inhibition action of normal liver RNA on ascitic type liver cancer cells in vivo and in vitro made by Jian-Ren Gu et al. in 1966 and in 1977, proved that the introduction of normal liver RNA into cancer cells was capable of inhibiting the growth and proliferation of cancer cells instead of direct killing action[1,6]. These experiments meant that the changes of radical characterizations in cancer cells as well as the phenotypical reversion to normal cells could take place through the exogenous RNA by means of both the mRNA template action and the radical regulation of cancer cells. We observed, however, in an experiment on mouse in vitro, the biological effect of immune RNA irradiated by ultraviolet laser beam, with the above similar action,[8] further increased the inhibition rate on the growth of cancer cells.

3. The HPD(c) photosensitive effect on the ascitic type liver cancer cells cultured with 3250RNA and 3371RNA in vitro gave the strength of synthetical killing effect 50 times more than the independent HPD(c) group's under the same laser irradiation.

4. Our experiment being only a preliminary work on the treatment of cancer, some important details need further verification to attain final confirmation. We believe our findings will go their way in theoretical research and clinical practice.

References

1. K.S.Kirdy: Biochem. J.64, 1964
2. Cancer. 26(4): 737 - 754, 1970
3. Jian-Ren Gu et al: Chinese Medical Journal 52:209, 1966
4. Lipson R, et al: Cancer. 20:255, 1967

5. Qiu-Da Wang: Shanghai Immunology Correspondance 4:63 - 68, 1980
6. Shanghai Tumor Research Institute: Experiment on Normal Animal Liver Cytoplasm RNA and Clinical Research (to be published)
7. Shanghai Medical Journal. 1:6 - 12, 1978
8. Fu-Shou Yang et al: Medical Laser Research & Clinic 1:28 - 31, 1987

Low Power CO$_2$-Laser Treatment of the Facial Neoplasm – 3,000 Cases

Fu-Shou Yang
Department of Laser Medicine, Shanghai Seamen's Hospital
505, Dong Changzhi Rd 200080, Shanghai, China.

Since 1985 we have been using a small size portable (gross weight 5Kgs) low power CO$_2$ laser treatment apparatus, its wave length 10.6 μm, output power 0 — 3 W, controllable. The surgical operation apparatus is in revolver form, the trigger controls the laser beam output, its operation is easy and safe. We have treated 3,000 cases of facial neoplasm with this apparatus, the curative effect has been satisfactory.

Of 3,000 cases of facial neoplasm, 841 were of nevus, 998 of wart, 369 of pigmented spots, 240 of sebaceous adenocele (2 — 20 mm diameter), 155 of eyelid neoplasm, 81 of freckles, 316 of others. These patients were 100% healed in one period, the facial skin basically had no remnant mark. For the sebaceous adenocele, we first opened a small hole of 1 — 2 mm at the adenocele on the facial surface with laser beam, then gently squeezed the content and took out the whole hydatid wall with surgical tweezers; as for the hydatid wall and what was adherent to the surrounding tissue, we used the laser beam to destroy the hydatid wall, during the operation basically there was no bleeding or a little bleeding. Because the wound was small, there was no infection, the healing was rapid.

This simple quick laser treatment is welcome by the patients for the facial plastic operation, it is more so for the medical home visit to families or for the patients in medium and small size towns and villages.

I. Introduction

The facial neoplasms, mainly the nevus, wart, pigmented spot etc. will not only annoy people with displeasing appearance, to same extent, bringing moral pressure on patients themselves, but also have the possibility of pathological change. An average of 15 — 20 nevoid neoplasms, according to statistics, could be found on the every one's skin and most of them appear benign while the percentage of malignant change into melanoma is only 0.027%.

For a long time, the cure of such nevoid neoplasms by means of various special medical measures has been stressing on both cure and prevention. The laser treatment, however from the view of cosmetology, has been developed in recent years and has been welcome by patients for its numerous advantages not available for the conventional therapies.

II. Apparatus and Methods

1. Low power CO_2 laser : output power 0 — 3 W, wavelength 10.6 μm, diameter of the focus area less than 0.2 mm, adjustable.
2. Local infiltration anaesthesia on the base of the affection with 2% of lidocaine. An intermittent projection of laser beam can be performed on minor nevi (less than 1 mm) directly without any anaesthesia.
3. Indication : The laser treatment is suitable for all kinds of nevus patients except those who have the record of serious diabetes, of abnormal skin scar formation, hyperchromatosis and other special skin diseases.

III. Results

A total of 3,000 cases of facial neoplasm (1600 men and 1400 women) had received our laser treatment from March 1985 to October 1986 with the age varying from 8 months to 76 years, but most of them were 20 — 45.

Indicated by the following table : of 7,021 out of 3,000 cases of facial neoplasm, 6,953 had been cured (99.03% of the total) by low power CO_2 laser treatment. Recurrences take place when a small scar on the edge of wounded surface of original affection is observed with a magnifying glass within 3 — 6 following months, if any, then carefully burn it off with low power CO_2 laser beam and satisfactory result could be reached as soon as the wounded surface is healed. The affection would have no possiblity of recurrence, if no remnant is found within six following months.

The laser treatment on sebaceous adenocele was characterized by its small wounded surface (bearing a diameter of 1 — 2 mm). If no adhesion existed between hydatid wall and surrounding tissues, the only thing you had to do was to gently squeez the content that looked like bean drags, and then take out the whole hydatid wall with surgical tweezers. The facial skin basically had no remnant mark after the cure . It is evident that the effect of laser treatment was better than the conventional one's.

Table. Analysis on therapeutic effects of facial neoplasm by low power CO_2 laser

No.	Kind of diseases	Number of cases	Number of affections	Area (Or diameter) of the affection	Cure cases	Number of cures by laser after recurrence
1.	melanotic nevus	841	2,413	1 — 10 mm	2,394	19
2.	nevus compound	94	162	2 — 6 mm	162	0
3.	nevus vascularis	22	22	2 — 5 mm	18	4
4.	birth mark	84	105	5 — 20 mm	82	23
5.	eyelid neoplasm	155	155	1 — 4 mm	155	0
6.	pigmented spot	369	380	20 — 30 mm	380	0
7.	sebaceous cyst	240	240	2 — 20 mm	240	0
8.	common wart	458	816	3 — 10 mm	800	16
9.	flat wart	440	2,518	1 — 3 mm	2,518	0
10.	traumatic scar	45	45	5 — 20 mm	45	0
11.	capillary tumor	10	10	3 — 10 mm	6	4
12.	nevus pilosus	20	20	20 — 30 mm	18	2
13.	tattoo	3	3	10 — 20 mm	3	0
14.	pseudotragus	10	10	10 — 15 mm	10	0
15.	cutaneous neoplasm	122	122	3 — 30 mm	122	0
16.	freckle	87	not counted number	about 10~several hundreds (~1mm)	not counted number	
		3,000	7,021		6,953	68

IV. Discussion and Comprehension

1. The treatment of facial neoplasm by low power CO_2 laser was noted for the lack of bleeding and pain, and the swiftness of operation, its beams could be selected to take off the affection without damage to surrounding tissues, which was not available for the conventional treatment. A fine therapeutic effect could be reached by constantly clearing out the carbonized substance with cotton through magnifying glass examination.

2. The infiltration anaesthesia on the base of the affection before operation, besides its action of local anaesthesia, could protect surrounding tissues against heat damage by laser beam, the easy absorption of the CO_2 laser beam (10.6 um) by water, makes the repair of wounded surface easier after operation.

3. The facial neoplasm will not only annoy people with displeasing feelings bringing certain moral pressure on patients themselves, but also have the possibility of pathological change. A healthy and good looking face can reappear, when the neoplasms were burnt off by laser. The laser treatment apparatus, which had been welcome by patients, was noted for its light weight, handiness, practicalness and safety.

Studies of Laser-Induced Cell Growth with Yeast in Continuous Culture

A.Gfrörer, J.Spahn, W.-D.Wagner and W.Waidelich
Institut für medizinische Optik d.Universität München/D

Most of the studies concerned with biostimulation are subject to large statistical uncertainties. Thus it was our aim to develop a very precise and reproducible method to measure the multiplication rates of two simultaneous growing cultures, one of them being irradiated with laser, the other one kept in the dark.
The disadvantages of conventional batch cultures are the quite limited time available for observation and the fact that the different stages of cell growth are not very well separated from each other. In a continuous culture, as we used it, however, the cell cultures are kept at constant concentrations throughout the experiment. Therefore it is in principle possible to observe an unlimited number of cell-generations at constant cultivation parameters. Consequently both precision and reproducibility are better than in a batch culture. Control tests with both cell cultures kept in the dark indeed proved the very high reliability of our experimental setup. In none of twelve experiments did the relative differences of the two multiplication rates exceed 1.6%. The standard deviation of 0.6% was another convincing proof of the high quality of the method applied.

Method and Material

The experimental setup is illustrated in figure 1. For continuous measurement of the cell concentration via the registration of extinction we established an enclosed flow-through system with peristaltic pumps and flow-through cuvettes. In this way continuous observation of concentration changes could be combined with continuous irradiation.
Whenever concentration reached a specified threshold an automatic dilution system began to work. A small quantity (1-2 ml) of fresh medium was transported via a peristaltic pump into both cultures. Simultaneously, the same amount of old medium was removed from the cultures. To achieve a direct comparison of the multiplication rates of irradiated and non-irradiated cultures in our system only the

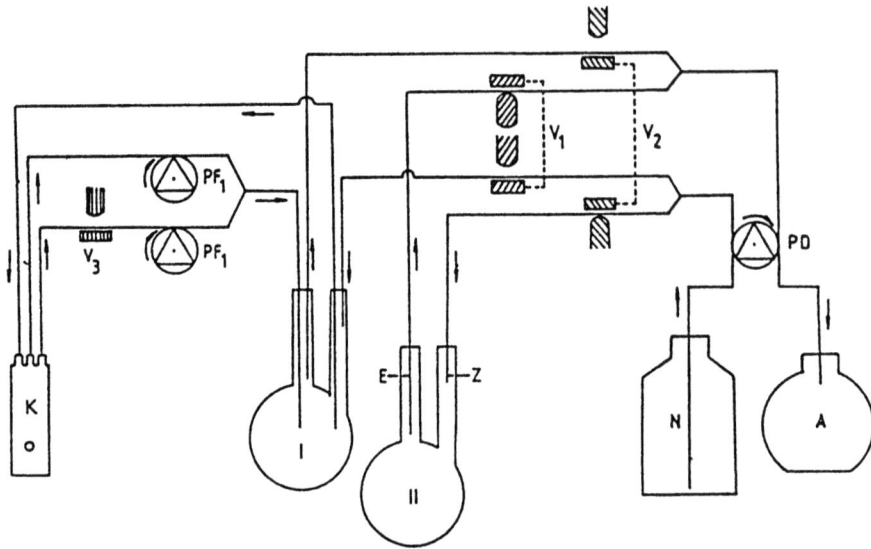

fig.1. left:flow-through system for continuous measurement of cell con
centration (PF:peristaltic pump;C:flow-through cuvette; V3:valve to
eliminate gas bubbles from the light path inside the cuvettte)
centre:culture flasks for probe and reference (I,II) right:system for
continuous dilution (N:fresh medium, A:old medium, PD:peristaltic
pump, V1/V2:valves to ensure equal dilution rates for both cultures)

nonirradiated culture was kept strictly at a constant concentration level. The second culture, however, was diluted with exactly the same dilution rate. When it exhibited the same rate of multiplication as the first culture, its concentration also remained constant. On the other hand, at slower (faster) multiplication rates the dilution did not correspond to the cell growth and the concentration decreased

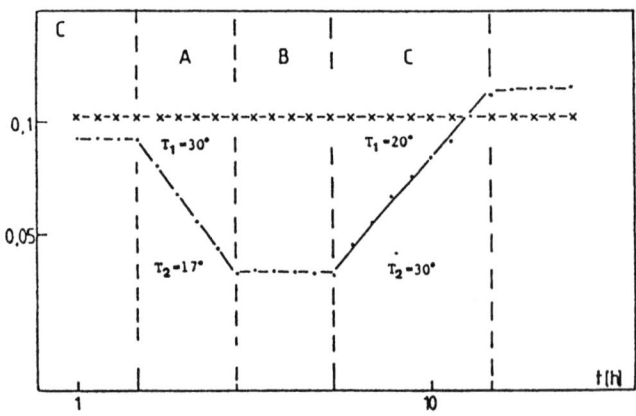

fig.2. experiment to
demonstrate the prin-
ciple of measurement
culture 1 (x-x-x):
strictly controlled
concentration (dilution
rate: $D=dV/dt*(1/V)=\mu 1$)
cuture 2 (-·--·-): same
dilution rate D, but
with lower (A) or
higher (C) rate of mul-
tiplication ($\mu 2$) than
culture 1, induced by
temperature difference

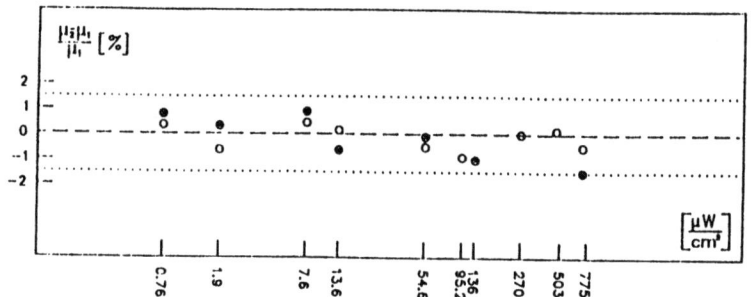

fig 3. irradition with He-Ne-laser (632.8nm) abscissa:relative differences of multiplication rates (○:medium with glucose; ●:medium with ethanol); ····: max. range of control tests

(increased). In this way, differences of multiplication rates can be seen directly from the concentration curve of culture 2 (fig.2). This culture grows with an effective multiplication rate that is equal to the difference of the two multiplication rates.

$$C2(t)=C02(t)*\exp(\mu1-\mu2)t$$

The cell type we used in all of our experiments was Saccharomyces cerevisiae 211 (wildtype). The medium contained glucose (21g/l) or ethanol (0.1% Vol.), yeast-extract (5,2g/l) and buffers (KH_2PO_4, Na_2HPO_4).

Results

Figure 3 shows the results of irradiation experiments with the He Ne-laser. The intensity was varied from 0.76µW/cm² to 775µW/cm², but in none of the experiments could any stimulating or inhibiting effect of irradiation be discerned. All of the results were entirely within the range the control tests.

Using the Kr^+-and Ar^+-laser, experiments with 676,647,514,488,and 458 nm were performed. The results, depicted in figs.4 and 5, demonstrate the absence of an irradiation effect at these wavelengths.

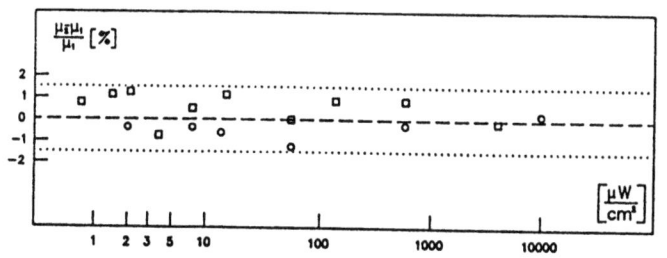

fig.4. irradiation with Kr^+-laser; ○:647.1nm; □:676.4nm; ····: max. range of control tests

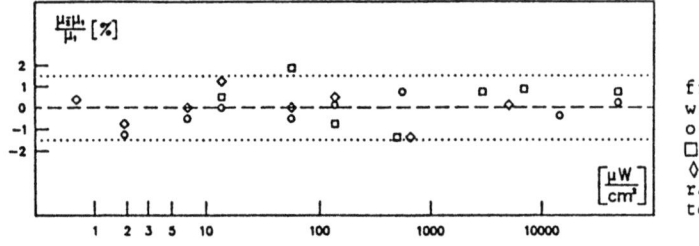

fig.5. irradiation with Ar⁺-laser
o: 514.5nm
□: 488.0nm
◊: 457,9nm; ....: max. range of control tests

In all of the experiments reported so far the culture was irradiated continuously throughout the experiment. To examine the influence of irradiation time and overall energy dose we also tried short-time irradiation. The results are summarized in fig.6. Four different intensities at two wavelengths were used. The irradiation times varied between 5s and 900s, but again no irradiation effect could be seen.

In a further series of experiments, ethanol was used instead of glucose as energy source. In the experiments presented above, the cell respiration decreased to less than 10% due to the high glucose concentration. On being exposed to ethanol instead of glucose, the cells were forced to activate their respiratory chain, where cytochromes, absorbing in the visible, are involved. However, as is evident from fig.3, also in this case no influence of laser irradiation could be discerned.

Thus we can rule out any stimulating influence of laser radiation in the blue and red region on the exponential growth of our cells. If influences exist at all, they would more likely be due to adaptation processes than to normal and fully adapted exponential cell growth.

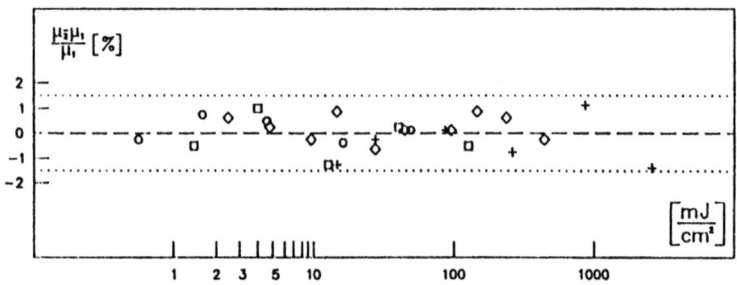

fig.6. short time irradiation   o:632.8nm, 0.05mW/cm²; □:632.8nm, 0.15mW/cm²; ◊:632.8nm, 0.5mW/cm²; +:676.4nm, 2.9mW/cm²; energy dose regulated by irradiation time

The Concept of "Biologon" and the Influence of Laser Light on Vital Activities

P. Greguss
Applied Biophysics Laboratory, Institute of Precision Mechanics and Optics,
Technical University Budapest, P.O.Box 91
Budapest, Hungary H-1502

Introduction

The purpose of this study is to present a theory with some new features for the analysis of the behavior of the living matter in the case when one ore more parameters of its environment change. The first part deals with the fundamental problem of what the precondition is that turns any change into a signal, into a stimulus which, when processed, becomes "vital" information provoking responses which manifest themselves either in an attempt to preserve the structure status quo existing before the change in the environment, or in creating a new type of dynamic structure status quo. It will be followed by application to clear up confusion in the interpretation and comparison of the responses of living matter to laser light.

The living material - as any material - has to be considered as a 3-D structure of atoms, molecules and molecular aggregates in space, however, it differs from the nonliving material in so far as it is ruled not only by the laws of physics and/or chemistry but also by homeostasis, the degree of which depends upon the evolutionary stage the living material has reached. Thus, the living material reacts to the changes in the parameters of its environment in a different way from nonliving material since in the first case the signal pattern representing these changes propagates in a permanently changing substrate structure, i.e., living material has a "functional mobility", while signal patterns in the nonliving material propagate in a constant substrate structure, i.e., nonliving material shows "functional stability". One should never forget that this is a basic difference between signal processing by a von Neumann-type machine and that by a living matter, independently from where it stands in the line of evolution or function.

Homeostasis means that the living material is structured in interacting sub-regulatory schemes which all are of oscillatory nature, i.e., from the point of view of the living matter, parameter changes of the environment - i.e., signals - have a definite "time pattern" as well as "frequency pattern". Therefore, if we wish to discuss and/or interpret correctly, e.g., the interaction of radiations with living material at its level of evolution, we have to solve the problem of the mutual exclusive formulation of "time analysis and frequency analysis".

The "biologon"

Let us consider the effects which can be produced by a signal s having the form of a time function s(t), assuming that power and energy associated with the signal are proportional to its square (i.e., in first approximation, the nature of the signal carriers is linear). Since the living matter is built up by interacting homeostatic subscheme patterns, it has to analyze the time-frequency diagram into rectangles which have shapes dependent upon the nature of the living matter, and areas of the order unity, but not less than one-half, if we follow the reasoning of the "Theory of Communication" of Gabor. (1) He introduced the concept of elementary signal, and named it "logon". This is a signal which occupies the minimum area $\Delta t \Delta f = 1/2$, which is the modulation product of a harmonic oscillation of any frequency with a pulse of the form of a probability function, and where $\Delta f = [2\pi(f - \bar{f})^2]^{1/2}$ is the "effective" signal bandwidth, and $\Delta t = [2\pi(t - \bar{t})^2]^{1/2}$ is the "effective" signal duration.

Following the steps of Gabor we introduced the concept of "biologon" (2), i.e., the elementary quantum of the change in any parameters of the environment of the living matter which produces a signal, i.e., a stimulus. In our model the living matter is analyzing not a function of one variable, i.e., time or frequency, but a function of two variables, time and frequency at a time. Thus, it cannot process the signal with any degree of accuracy only beyond a certain limit, which is in good agreement with the functional mobility of the living matter. Therefore, it is sometimes rather difficult to decide whether a response of the living matter can be provoked only but only by the stimulus in question or not.

By introducing the concept of biologon we assume that the living matter uses a signal processing scheme, i.e., a treatment of frequency and time which mirrors that of coordinates and momenta in quantum mechanics leading to the Heisenberg uncertainty relation between momentum p and position x: $\Delta p \Delta x \geq \hbar/2$, where $\hbar = h/2$, and h represent Planck's constant. However, by mentioning this resemblance we do not intend to explain "life" by means of quantum theory, we only wish to present a model which may help us to decide whether an observed result in the interaction of radiation with a given living matter may be specific or not.

Returning to the concept of biologon we have to remind again that t and f can be processed simultaneously only if the "coherence length" of the signal carriers is taken into account, which recognition leads us to a number of uncanny predictions of biological behavior. Without pretending to be exhaustive, but in order to characterize our model, we have to outline a few features of this biological signal processing concept, according to which the strategy of the living matter is based on the formation of an information diagram of minimum area defined by the r.m.s. duration of the signal and its r.m.s. frequency-width. Assuming that the living material uses a numerical factor $\sqrt{(2\pi)} = 2,506$, the resulting information diagram will be equal to the number of independent data which the homeostatic scheme involved in the processing can handle. It consists of "cells" of size one half which transmit exactly one datum of information, a "logon", either a "sine type" or a "cosine type" one. Consequently, the unit cell in the time-frequency space of the living matter is represented in two orthogonal logons with carrier $90°$ in phase. Further, it follows that the signal will be processed only if the living matter "knows" not only the past but also the future, i.e., a situation emerges which in modern physics has often been called "the breakdown of causality". Life solves the problem of "converting the future into past" by delaying the transmission of $s(t)$, however, the accuracy of the processing depends upon the delay time. Indeed, there are some experimental hints that "life" really works this way. (3, 4)

Laser Light and Vital Activities

From the existence of homeostatic substrate structure, further, from the nature of signal processing via biologons, it follows that temporal and spatial coherence may play a definite role in the functioning of the living matter. In relation to laser light, which differs from thermal light only in being highly coherent and polarized, two rather distinct questions have to be answered. First, how many biologons must be transmitted per second to achieve coherent excitation in a biological system. The second is the corresponding question whether coherent excitation is the only way to achieve the biological response in question.

Before attempting to answer these questions, we have to investigate: when can the living matter perceive a change in the parameters of its environment as a signal? Since the processing of biologons supposes coherence, we can use the formalisms of holography. If I_S is the intensity of the stimulus proportional to the intensity of the signal carrier and I_R that of the stimulus involved in signal processing, we can write for the energy terms: $E = E_S + E_R + (E_S E_R)^{1/2} \cos\psi$. The right side of this equation carries the signal pattern but, if $E_S < E_o$, this term becomes smaller than the square of the random deviation of the reference background, $\overline{E_S E_R} < \overline{(\Delta E_R)^2}$. In this case $\Delta(\overline{E_R^2}/E_o) = \overline{E_R}/E_o$, thus, since both sides are dimensionless, we can write: $\overline{\Delta N^2} = N$, which is the Poisson formula for the alternation of "seldom events", indicating that the monochromatic signal carrier become stimulus only if its energy exceeds a given value, otherwise the living material behaves itself as a nonliving system only. Therefore, when analyzing the effect of monochromatic signal carriers, not the intensity of the signal carrier but rather its spectral irradiance $(mW.cm^{-2}.nm^{-1})$ should be considered.

The first question is difficult to answer since one has to know not only which homeostatic scheme is involved in signal processing but also those conditions which preserve a given type of dynamic status quo, nevertheless, some considerations should be mentioned. Let us assume that the signal processing homeostatic substrate structure is a biomolecule, and the spectral irradiance of the signal source is that of a cw HeNe low- or mid-power laser. Calculations show that the phase relaxation time of the homeostatic substrate structure is 10^{12}-10^{13} times higher than the rate of coherent state generation under these spectral irradiance conditions. (5) This means that the coherent property of the laser light is negligible, i.e., the same response can be expected from thermal light of equal spectral irradiance. This conclusion is in good agreement with the findings of Maroti et al. (6) who observed that there was no difference between the observed bioeffects of visible monochromatic light originating from a laser and an incoherent light source, provided that the interaction time was longer than 50 microseconds. Naturally, homeostatic schemes other than biomolecules have different rates of coherent state generation, but to our present knowledge they are several orders of magnitude lower or higher than those offered by the frequencies of the visible spectrum, e.g., 10^{11} Hz (millimeter wave region) in the case of membrane-like structures. (7, 8) Therefore, in the frequency range of 10^{14} Hz one cannot expect any primary coherent excitation effect in the case of cw laser irradiation but - at least theoretically - it may be possible to find a pulse width and repetition rate which matches the needs of one or another homeostatic subsystem. So, e.g., Dyson (9) has recently demonstrated that biological effects may be different if the repetition rate of a 9.10^{14} Hz radiation is 200 Hz or 1.2 kHz. But this difference shows up only and only on some days, which observation is in good agreement with what we have said about "functional mobility" of the living matter.

Conclusions

The presented biologon model of biological signal processing clearly suggests the necessity that, before proposing laser light to solve biological problems, one must be sure that the proposed application requires one or more of the unique properties of a laser. If this is not the case, a conventional light source of the same spectral irradiance may do the same job. (10)

Literature

1. Gabor, D.: Theory of communication. J. IEE 93:429, 1946.
2. Greguss, P.: Manifestation of Gabor's holographic principle in various evolutionary stages of the living material. Proc. of the International Conference on Holography Applications, Beijing, P.R.C. 1986.
3. Greguss, P.: Bioholography - a new model of information processing. Nature 219: 482, 1968.
4. Pollen, D.A., Ronner, S.F.: Science 212:1411, 1981.
5. Lobko, V.V., Karu, T.I., Letokhov, V.S.: Is low intensity laser light coherence essential when biological objects are affected? Biofizika 30:366, 1985 (In Russian).
6. Maroti, P. et al.: The effect of time dependent coherence of excitation on the primary processes of photosynthesis. Acta Univ. Szegediensis 22:155, 1977.
7. Fröhlich, H. and Kremer, F. (Eds.): Coherent Excitations in Biological Systems. Springer Verlag, Berlin, Heidelberg, New York, Tokyo 1983.
8. Polk, Ch., and Postow, E. (Eds.): CRC Handbook of Biological Effects of Electromagnetic Fields. CRC Press, Inc., Boca Raton, FL 1986.
9. Dyson, M.: Effects of the Space Mix Mid Laser on the healing of full thickness excised lesions in CD1 mice. Medical Laser Report 4:2, 1986.
10. Smith, K.C.: Common misconceptions about light, In: Lasers in Photomedicine and Photobiology. Ed. Pratesi, R., Sacchi, C.A. Springer Verlag, Berlin 1980.

Low Energy Laser Irradiation Prevents the Early Morphological and Electrophysiological Effects of Optic Nerve Injury

M. Rosner, M. Belkin, M. Erlich, J. Friedman and M. Schwartz
Goldschleger Eye Research Institute, Tel-Avive University,
Sackler Faculty of Medicine, Sheba Medical Center, Tel-Hashomer 25621,
and Neurobiology Department, Weizmann Institute of Science, Rehovot, Israel.

The present study provides evidence that low-energy laser irradiation causes, at least temporary prevention of degeneration of mammalian central nervous system (CNS) axons after moderate compression injury.

Injuries to the CNS cause severe, permanent loss of function because injured axons of the mammalian CNS undergo posttraumatic degeneration and are incapable of functional regeneration (1-4). Low-energy laser irradiation was reported to alter growth and regenerative parameters of various cells and tissues (5-8) including the peripheral nervous system (9).

In the present study we evaluated morphologically and electrophysiologically the effect of low-energy He-Ne laser irradiation on posttraumatic processes in injured optic nerves of adult mammals which represent the nonregenerative mammalian CNS (10).

The morphological evaluation of the laser effect on injured optic nerves was carried out in adult rabbits. The optic nerves were exposed and crushed for 30 seconds by a hemostat, 8 mm distal to the eyeball. He-Ne laser (632.8 nm, 15 mW) irradiation was given for 5 to 14 minutes daily, beginning immediately after the crush injury and repeated for 8 to 14 days. The irradiation was either through the cornea or through the skin above the upper lid in animals in which the orbital bony roof was removed. Morphological evaluation was performed using Horse Radish Peroxidase (HRP) which stains viable nerves.

In the control group of nonirradiated injured nerves, no HRP labeled fibers were found from 8 days after injury onwards. In the irradiated groups. The injured optic nerves maintained their morphological integrity, when studied 14 days after injury. It should be noted that at longer period of time after injury, signs of degeneration were noticed, thus suggesting that the primary effect is in delaying the degeneration ruther than it's prevention.

The electeophysiological evaluation of the laser effect on crushed optic nerves was performed in adult rats. The severity of the crush injury was calibrated by recording the in-vitro effect of the crush on excised normal optic nerves. The crush was adjusted to a level which was followed by immediate disappearance of the action potential and it's recovry, 30 minutes later, to only about 20-50 µV (a thousandth part of the normal amplitude). In such level of injury the laser irradiation was found to have maximal effect.

The low energy (4.5 or 15 mW) He-Ne irradiation was given transcorneally, beginning half an hour after the crush injury and repeated for 10 or 14 consecutive days. Electrophysiological evaluation was carried out by measuring the compound action potential of the excised optic nerves between the injury site and the chiasm, using suction electrodes.

In normal, noninjured optic nerves of rats, the average action potential amplitude was found to be 5382.6 $\pm$ 1621.2 µV. The action potential which was recorded 14 days following injury in nonirradiated nerves, was very low and avereged 600$\pm$341 µV. The action potentials of irradiated injured nerves recorded 10 and 14 days following injury showed signifficantly higher action potentials than nonirradiated injured nerves. These action potential amplitudes reached 2000-5000 µV, close to those of noninjured nerves. Preliminary studies showed that the effect is not unique to the He-Ne laser and to coherent radiation.

Irradiation did not have an effect if started 3 days after injury or on transsected nerves. These observations further support our hypothesis that the laser effect is in arresting the process of neural degeneration.

When CNS injury involve nerve compression which leads initially to functional block but leaving the nerve otherwise structurally intact, such injured nerves might be rescued if treated promptly and properly. Such treatments would probably have to be given in the critical period between the initiation of the conduction block and the commencement of disintegration, which otherwise could result in irreversible retrograde degeneration and secondary cell death. We suggest that treatments with low-energy laser might have a role in promoting the survival of injured CNS at the early posttraumatic critical period.

Low-energy laser irradiation probably affects primarily the glial cells. It was found that the irradiation caused a decrease in the Ca^{++} efflux from these cells, which might suggest an elevation in bounded Ca^{++} in the cells. Further studies are currently carried out to find out the significance of these changes to the cellular behavior.

REFERENCES

1. Attardi, D.G. and Sperry, R.W.: Preferential selection of central pathways by regenerating optic nerve. Exp. Neurol. 1963, 7: 46-64.

2. Clemente, C.D.: Regeneration in the vertebrate central nervous system. Int. Rev. Neurobiol. 1964, 6: 257-301.

3. Guth, L. and Windle, W.: The enigma of central nervous system regeneration. Exp. Neurol. Suppl. 1970, 5: 1-43.

4. Kiernan, J.A.: Hypotheses concerned with axonal regeneration in the mammalian nervous system. Biol. Rev. 1979, 54: 155-157.

5. Vacek, A., Bartonickova, A., Vesela, Z. and Perto, F.: Increase in colony forming capacity of the haemopoetic stem cells in the bone marrow exposed to the He-Ne laser irradiation in vitro. Folia Biol. 1982, 28: 426-430.

6. Mester, E., Mester, A.F. and Mester A.: The biomedical effects of laser application. Laser Surg. Med., 1985, 5: 31-39.

7. Poon, A.M.L. and Yew, D.T.: Low dose laser and the lens protein analysis and mitotic rate. Acta Anat. 1980, 107: 114-120.

8. Abergel, R.P., Meeker, C.A., Lam, T.S., Dwyer, R.M., Lesavoy, M.A. and Vitto, J.: Control of connective tissue metabolism by lasers: recent development and future prospects. J. Am. Acad. Dermatol. 1984, 11: 1142-1150.

9. Rochkind, S., Bartal, A., Razon, N., Nissan, N. and Schwartz, M.: The long-term effect of He-Ne laser irradiation on repairative processes in peripheral nerve and denervated tissue in normal and crushed sciatic nerve in the rat. Proc. 6th Cong. Int. Soc. Laser Surg. Med. 1985. p. 78.

10. Schwartz, M., Doron, A., Erlich, M., Lavie, V., Ben-Bassat, S., Belkin, M. and Rochkind, S.: Effects of low-energy He-Ne laser irradiation on post-traumatic degeneration of adult rabbit optic nerve. Laser Sur. Med., 1987 (In Press).

Application of the CO₂ Laser in the Rheumatoid Hand

H.R. Herrera, J.R. Hinshaw, R.J. Lanzafame
Department of Surgery and Division of Plastic
Surgery at Rochester General Hospital and the
University of Rochester School of Medicine
and Dentistry, Rochester, N.Y.

One of the major goals in tendon reconstruction is the restoration of the gliding motion of the tendon. This is particularly difficult in the complexity of the healing process in the rheumatoid hand.

During our research in the lab with welding of chicken tendons using the CO_2 laser, we observed a smooth process of healing around the tendons with less adhesions. We have used the CO_2 laser in the rheumatoid hand when synovectomy and tendon release were indicated. The CO_2 laser was used with a 125mm lens with 8-10 Watts in a continuous mode. Although we have not accumulated large numbers of patients, we have obtained excellent results in the process of healing in our patients. We have observed less bleeding, pain, and edema. This has allowed us to initiate early physiotherapy and improvement in the clinical outcome of these patients.

REFERENCES

Herrera, H.R.: Use of CO_2 Laser in Tendon Welding. Six Congress of the International Scoiety for Laser Surgery and Medicine, Israel.

Lindsay, W.K.: The fibroblasts in flexor tendon healing. Plast. Reconstr. Surg., 34:223, 1964.

Peacock, E.E., Jr.: Biological principles in the healing of long tendons. Surg. Clin. North Am., 45:461, 1965.

Potenza, A.D.: Critical evaluation of flexor tendon healing and adhesion formation within artificial digital sheaths. An experimental study. J. Bone Joint Surg., 45A:1217, 1963.

Na$^+$-K$^+$ Transport, Cotransport and Cell Volume of Rats Erythrocytes Submitted to Helium-Neon Laser Radiation

Hugo Juri M.D.* Jose Palma M.D.* Frank Frank Phd.** Ron Lapin M.D.***
Jose Lillo M.D.*** Sham Yung M.D.***

* National University Of Cordoba-LaserCenter H.Espanol-Argentina
** M.B.B. Munich- W. Germany
*** Coast Plaza Medical Center Norwalk, California USA

ABSTRACT: It has been studied the Na$^+$-K$^+$ transport, cotransport, and cell volume in erythrocytes of rats irradiated with Helium-Neon laser. It has been observed an increase in the passive diffusion of Na$^+$ and K$^+$ compensated by higher Na$^+$-K$^+$ pump activity. There was not observed alterations in Na$^+$ and K$^+$ cotransport, cell volume, as well as in the Na$^+$ and K$^+$ intracellular content.

Every day is more frecuent the use of different types of lasers in medicine and biology, and this fact makes increasingly neccesary the knowledge of its effects on the cell.

Alterations has been observed at cellular and subcellular levels by effect of laser radiation (1-5). It has been also reported depolarization at the cellular surface (6); alterations of the contractility of cardiac cells (3); increase of osmotic fragility of erythrocytes (7-8); alterations of fibroblast membranes and stimulation of fibroblast proliferation (9), etc.

The reason of this investigation is to study transport and cotransport of Na$^+$ and K$^+$ in red cells "in vitro" submitted to He-Ne laser radiation.

The Helium-Neon laser is widely used in medicine in ophthalmologic diagnostic; retinal Doppler velocimetry; physioterapy, etc. It is also used in other industrial and entertaintment area with direct human exposure to its radiation. According to the results of this study, the He-NE laser radiation increase the passive permeability of erythrocyte membrane to Na$^+$ and K$^+$ which is compensated by an increase on the activity of Na$^+$-K$^+$ pump.

---

*Address for Correspondence: Dr. J.A.Palma, Cátedra de Física Biomédica. Santa Rosa 1085. 5000 Córdoba. Argentina.

MATERIALS AND METHODS: It has been used heparinized blood extracted from the aorta of twelve female rats of Wistar strain, previously anesthetized with ether. Immediately after extraction, each sample was divided in two different aliquots. One of these aliquot was irradiated with a He-Ne laser (Biolas D, Messerschmitt, during five minutes (0.50 W/cm^2). Specimens were lasered in 5 ml polypropylene test tubes which were mechanically raised and lowered during the procedure to allow gentle mixing and uniform distribution of laser energy. The non irradiated aliquot of blood sample was used as control.

The method used to study transport and cotransport of Na$^+$-K$^+$ through the red cell membrane has been previously described by Duhm and Göbel (10-12). In brief, the erytrocyte were washed in a incubation medium (140 mM of ClNa-5 mM glucose), and then resuspended in the following conditions: a) without inhibitors b) with ouabain 5 mM c) with Furosemide 0.5 mM + ouabain 5 mM. After 15 minutes of pre-incubation period, it was added to the medium 2 mM of Rb Cl (the rubidium replace to the potassium at the cell membrane transport system). The mean hemoglobin concentration was determined in red cells hemolyzed with 5% butanol. The concentration and transport rates of Na$^+$ and K$^+$ in red cells were measured by spectrophotomer of atomic absorption. The red cell cation content and transport rates are refered to 5.6 µmol hemoglobin .ml^{-1} which is the mean hemoglobin content in 1 ml of erythrocytes of non irradiated rats (12).

Ouabain-sensitive sodium extrusion is a manifestation of sodium-potassium pump. Ouabain-sensitive-Rubidium uptake indicates the inward active K$^+$ transport by the Na$^+$-K$^+$ pump. With ouabain + Furosemide it was studied the cotransport of Na$^+$ and K$^+$ (ouabain resistant-furosemide sensitive flux). Rubidium leak is a manifestation of the passive diffusion of sodium (ouabain resistant-furosemide resistant flux). The statistical analysis was done using the Studen's "t" test (paired groups). P was considered significant when it was lower than 0.05.

RESULTS AND DISCUSSION: The results obtained to study Na$^+$ and K$^+$ Transport, Cotransport and cell volume are presented in Table 1.

Is well known that the electrochemical gradient across the cell membrane is maintened by the sodium-potassium pump. In the red cell the exchange between intracellular Na$^+$ and extracellular K$^+$ is done in approximately a 1.5 ratio. The blood irradiated with Helium-Neon laser shows a significant increase in both K$^+$ leak and K$^+$ active transport compared with K$^+$ diffusion rate and active K$^+$ transport in non irradiated cells. This fact leads us to think that the Na$^+$-K$^+$ pump compensate the increase of K$^+$ leak by passive diffusion, increasing the rate of inward active potassium transport. Accordings to the results obtained, practically all the K$^+$ leaked by the radiated red cells (due to an increment of the diffusion rate) is compensated by the Na$^+$-K$^+$ pump.

Intracellular K$^+$ concentration does not shows significant changes comparing radiated and non-radiated red cells (Table 3). Neither were observed

TABLE 1.

CHARACTERISTIC OF NET K⁺ TRANSPORT IN LASER IRRADIATED AND NON IRRADIATED ERYTHROCYTES

	POTASSIUM			
	RUBIDIUM UPTAKE			PASSIVE DIFFUSION
Transport System	Total	Ouabain Sensitive (K^+ pump)	Ouabain Resistant-Furosemide Sensitive -(K^+ Cotransport)	Ouabain and Furosemide Resistant
Control	4.67±0.32	4.02±0.18	0.40±0.09	0.28±0.06
Laser	5.59±0.36	4.43±0.20	0.46±0.17	0.71±0.08
	$p < 0.001$	$p < 0.001$	NS	$p < 0.05$

Mean ± S.D. - Net flux is given in µmol per 1 ml per h. Red cell transport are normalized to 5.32 µmol hemoglobin (ml.cell)⁻¹

TABLE 2.

CHARACTERISTIC OF NET Na⁺ TRANSPORT IN LASER IRRADIATED AND NON IRRADIATED ERYTHROCYTES

	SODIUM		
	EXTRUSION		PASSIVE DIFFUSION
Transport System	Ouabain Sensitive Na^+ pump)	Ouabain Resistant-Furosemide Sensitive (Na^+ Cotransport)	Ouabain and Furosemide Resistant
Control	5.96±0.24	0.70±0.12	5.30±0.24
Laser	6.60±0.30	0.70±0.10	5.91±0.18
	$p < 0.001$	NS	$p < 0.001$

Mean ± S.D. Net flux is given in µmol per 1 ml per h. Red cell transport are normalized to 5.32 µmol hemoglobin (ml cell)⁻¹

significant variations in Na⁺K⁺ cotransport, comparing ouabain resistant-furosemide sensitive fluxes in radiated and non radiated red cells.

The passive inward sodium diffusion (Na⁺ leak) is increased in the irradiated red cell (Table 2). On the other hand, it has been observed an

TABLE 3.

SODIUM, POTASSIUM AND MEAN HEMOGLOBIN CONTENTS OF RATS ERYTHROCYTES μmol (ml cell)$^{-1}$

	SODIUM	POTASSIUM	MEAN HEMOGLOBIN
Control	4.24±0.31	96.0±0.80	5.32±0.10
Laser	4.32±0.36	99.2±0.74	5.36±0.26

Values are Mean ± S.D. Red cell contents are refered to mean cellular hemoglobin contents (5.32 μmol ml . cell^{-1})

increase in the active extrusion of Na^+ (ouabain-sensitive flux) in the laser radiated blood compared with non irradiated blood.

The increment of active extrusion of Na^+ due to increase of Na^+-K^+ pump activity allows to the red cell to compensate the Na^+ passive diffusion. The intracellular concentration of Na^+ showed no significant change comparing radiated and non radiated blood (Table 2). According these results is discarded the participation of an increment of intracellular Na^+ content in the increase of activity of Na^+-K^+ pump.

It has not been observed statistically significant differences in Na^+ cotransport in radiated and non radiated erythrocytes. The stoichiometry (relation between outward Na^+ flux and inward K^+ flux by pump action) is approximately 1.5 in irradiated red cell, which coincide with the accepted values in normal red cells and indicates that the increase of active Na^+ extrusion by pump is proportional to the inward flux by passive transport. The increment is active transport of Na^+ and K^+ could mean higher activity of the Na^+-K^+ ATPasa. This increase of activity could be the result of a more rapid rate of cation translocation or a higher density of pump units.

It has not been observed variations in volume in erythrocytes mediated by He-Ne laser radiation. This fact coincide with the lack of alterations observed in the Na^+K^+ cotransport (variations in cellular volume interfere in normal erythrocyte cotransport in rat)(12). On the other hand, the lack of cellular volume changes in the Helium-Neon laser radiated erythrocytes indicates: 1) there is not net flux of water through red cell membrane 2) there is not change in the number of osmotically active particles inside the red cell. The lack of alterations in mean hemoglobin content and cation concentration in lasered and non lasered rats indicates no changes in red cell volume (12).

The results of this investigations may represent functional or structural alterations of the red cell membrane. It will be necessary to investigate different energies and types of laser radiations, applied in differents amounts of time, and correlate eventual morphological or functional changes in red cell membrane with changes in transport across it.

Utilizing other different types of laser radiation (Argon) and with more potency (2.5 W; 4-20 J) (13-14) it has been found red cell fragments (spherocytes) and red cell "ghost", hemolysis, etc. Also Neodymiun Yag (Nd:Yag) produce cell damage in spite of the poor absortion of it by the red cell (at difference to the argon laser effect). Some of this effects are attributed only to heat produced by laser radiation. We do not feel that this is the case in our study because He-NE laser (632 nm-red color) is poorly absorbed by the red cell and the low power used in this investigation make very difficult a significant increase in temperature of the red cells.

In spite of not doing electron microscopy studies in our investigation it will be probable to find structural changes with He-Ne laser as seen with the biologically more potent argon and Nd: Yag laser.

In conclussion, the Na^+-K^+ membrane transport in the rat's red cell is altered by He-Ne laser radiation. The observed alterations were: a) increase in passive diffusion of Na^+ and K^+, which was completely compensated by the activity of Na^+-K^+ pump. 2) There was not alterations in Na^+-K^+ cotransport, cell volume or in Na^+-K^+ intracellular content.

ACKNOWLEDGEMENT: to Laura Teisseire and Beatriz Ramos for excellent technical assistance.

REFERENCES

1. Moskalit, K. G., and Petrov, O. L. (1974) Citologija 10, 1284-1288.
2. Rattner, J. B., and Berns, M. W. (1974) J. Cell. Biol. 62, 526-533.
3. Burt, J. M., Strahs, K. R., and Berns, M. W. (1979) Exp. Cell. Res. 118, 341-351.
4. Berns, M. W., Aist, J., Edwards, J., Strahs, K., Girton, J., Mc Neill, P., Ratner, J. B., Kitzes, M., et al. (1981) Science 213, 505-513.
5. Kozlov, A. P., Moskalic, K. G., and Pospelova, I.I. (1981) Radiobiol. Radiother. (Berl) 22, 91-104.
6. Kitzes, M., Twiggs, G. and Bern M. W. (1977) J. Cell. Physiol. 93, 99-104.
7. Vzdensky, A. B. (1977) J. Cell. Physiol. 93, 99-104.
8. Ham, T. H., Shen, S. C., Fleming, E. M. and Castle, W. B. (1948) Blood 3, 373-403.
9. Kubasova, T., Kovács, L., Somosy, Z., Unk, P., and Kókai, A. (1984) Lasers Surg. Med. 4, 381-388.
10. Duhm, J., Göbel, B. O. (1982) Hypertension 4, 468-476.
11. Duhm, J., Göbel, B. O. (1982) Hypertension 4, 477-482.
12. Duhm, J., Göbel, B. O. (1984) Am. J. Physiol. 246, L20-L29.
13. Theis, J. H., Lee, G., Ikeda, R. M., Stobbe, D. Ogata, C., Lui, Mason D.T. (1983) Clin. Cardiol. 6, 396-398.
14. Gamaleya, N. F. (1972) Laser Biomedical Research in the URSS - In Wolbarsht (ed). Laser applications in Medicine and Biology, Vol. III Plemum Press - New York and London, pp 173.
15. Doerger, P. T., Glueck, H. I., Vander Bel-Kahn, J., Taylor, A., Golman, L. (1985) Lasers Surg. Med. 5, 457-468.

Biological Effects of Low Laser Irradiation on Cultivated Rat Brain Cells

Ming-Chien Kao, Jui-Chang Tsai, Teh-Cheng Jou*
Department of Surgery, College of Medicine
National Taiwan University Hospital
No. 1 Chang-Te Street, Taipei, Taiwan, R.O.C.
Institute of Neuroscience, National Yang-Ming
Medical College*, Taipei, Taiwan, R.O.C.

A well-established neuroglial cell line obtained from the dissociated culture of normal neonatal rat (JAR-2 F-51) brain tissue was used as a model to investigate its biological effects resulted from the irradiation of low power lasers. These lasers are conventionally used for "bioregulation" or "acupuncture". This culture shows a relatively constant morphological characteristics of the cell and presents a steady growth and proliferation in the monolayer system. The monolayer culture was exposed to the irradiation of various lasers in low power density of various situations. The effects on cellular morphology, proliferation and other functional activities after various conditions of irradiation will be studied.

In recent years, there is a rapid increase of reports concerning the clinical effects of the use of low power lasers in enhancement of wound healing and alleviation of functional disorders especially relief of pain.[1,2,5-11] However, the reliability or reproducibility of their advocated results requires further critical evaluation and the exact underlying mechanism of the "laser bioregulation" remains undiscovered and needs furthermore scientific and basic investigation.[1,2,5-11] The study of laser-tissue interaction particularly its biological effect on the cultivated tissue may be substantially contributory to the understanding of this attractive field. In this study, the biological effects of the monolayer neuroglial cells cultivated from neonatal rat brain tissue [3] after exposure to various lasers in low power density were observed. The effect on cellular growth, morphology and proliferation and other functional activities after various conditions of irradiation will be presented.

Materials and Methods

The cell line used in this study was a well-established neuroglial cell in monolayer system. It was the passage culture derived from the dissociated culture of normal neonatal rat (JAR-2,F-51, 2-10 days old) brain tissue. This culture shows a relatively constant cellular morphology and presents a steady growth and proliferation in the monolayer system. It is suitable as a model to investigate its biological effects resulted from the irradiation of low power lasers. [4]

The lasers used in this study were those conventional ones for "laser biostimulation" or "laser acupuncture".

Initially, He-Ne laser, Argon laser and CO_2 laser were used as the source of irradiation, since these are the only available laser systems with low power facility in our service. The incident energy density used in this study was first according to the dose of exposure currently used in "laser acupuncture". The exposure energy was then adjusted, usually increased, gradually in order to obtain a demonstrable biological effect on the culture cells. However, when the incident energy was high enough to cause a rise of temperature in culture media above 42°C, it was discarded to exclude the obvious thermal effect. The power density of He-Ne laser was around 10 mW/cm^2 and the subsequent incident energy density was 3-18 J/cm^2. The power of argon laser was 0.4-1.6 W and the energy density was 0.4-16 J/cm^2.

The power of CO_2 laser used was 400-800 mW and the energy density was around 0.4-16 J/cm^2.

The cell density was around $2-8 \times 10^4$/ml and the culture plates used were 24-well and 96-well type.

When the cell density is 2×10^4/ml at inoculation, it will increase to 50×10^4/ml at the 5th day and 101×10^4/ml at the 8th day, and when 5×10^4/ml at inoculation, it will become 91×10^4/ml at 5th day and 125×10^4/ml at 8th day.

The laser irradiation was applied to the culture well 24 hours after the inoculation and obervation of the laser biological effect was done, each at 4th and 7th day after irradiation.

The He-Ne laser and argon laser were directly applied to the culture plate with the cover in place, but for the CO_2 laser, irradiation was performed in the laminar flow chamber because the cover of the plate should be opened so that the culture system could be exposed to CO_2 laser directly.

The study of DNA Synthesis with thymidine technique was also measured at the 2nd and 8th day after laser irradiation.

Result

No significant change of the morphology, growth and proliferation rate of the culture cells was observed after exposure to the laser irradiation in low power range without causing a rise of temperature above 42°C in the culture. The irradiation dose of He-Ne laser was 3 to 18 J/cm^2. Argon and CO_2 laser was 0.4-16 J/cm^2 with single irradiation. The observation was done at the 4th and 7th day after laser irradiation. The synthesis of DNA was also not obviously affected by the same sequential study. However, the above results were in fact the observation data which were obtained only after 2 or 3 times study in each group.

The results will be evaluated after more times of study in due time and the biological effects resulted from the repeated cumulative irradiation will also be studied in due course.

Discussion

Although there are many enthusiasts who advocated the exciting clinical results with the use of low power laser in enhancing wound healing or relieving pain syndrome, the exact underlying mechanism was still not elucidated.

In this study, we try to study the biological effects of the cultivated rat brain cells by exposing them to the conventional medical lasers in low power range. This range of irradiation or this laser energy was conventionally used for "bioregulation" or "acupuncture". Unfortunately we are still not able to demonstrate any significant biological change of the culture cell after exposing to this low power range of He-Ne laser, Argon laser and CO_2 laser in one single irradiation.

The biological effects, either chronic or acute, resulted from a single laser exposure or repeated cumulative irradiation may be substantially different and need further investigation. Meanwhile, the incident laser energy actually received by culture cells is practically difficult to be measured and it is substantially reduced by passing through the culture medium. The water content of culture medium may absorb a great portion of CO_2 laser, therefore the culture fluid is removed as much as possible before it is exposed to irradiation.

Acknowledgement:
This study was supported by a research grant NSC-76-0412-B-002-84 from the National Science Council, R.O.C.

Literature References

1. Abergel RP et al: Nonthermal effects of Nd:YAG laser on biological functions of human skin fibroblasts in culture. Lasers Surg Med 3:279-284, 1984
2. Hunter J et al: Effects of low energy laser on wound healing in a porcine model. Lasers Surg Med 3:285-290, 1984
3. Jou T C: Rat brain tissue cells intissue culture. I. Light microscopic studies. Proceedings of National science council 7:181-193, 1983
4. Jou T C et al: Immunofluorescence characterization of astrocytes in monolayer culture using antiserum to glial fibrillar acdic protein J. Formosan Med Assoc 82:1115-1125, 1983
5. Kamikawa K: Development of laser acupuncture systems and their clinical application in New Frontiers in Laser Medicine and Surgery by K. Atsumi, Ex. Medica pp 498-505, 1983

6. Kamikawa K et al: Low power laser therapy for pain relief. J. Japan Society for Laser Medicine 5:215-220, 1985
7. Kubasova T. et al: Biological effects of He-Ne laser, Lasers Surg Med 4:381-388, 1984
8. Mc Caughan J S st al: effect of low dose argon irradiation on rate of wound healing. Lasers Surg Med 5:607-617, 1985
9. Mester E et al: Effects of laser rays on wound healing. Am J. Surg. 122:532-539, 1971
10. Mester E et al: The biomedical effects of laser application. Lasers Surg Med 5:31-39, 1985
11. Nakajiima M et al: Effect of argon laser on mammalian cell. In Laser Tokyo '81, pp 7:32-33, 1981

Immunological Aspects of Laser Therapy

H.Klima *,   L.Schindl **,   D.Adamiker ***

*   Atomic Institute of the Austrian Universities
    A-1020 Vienna, Schüttelstraße 115
**   Hanusch Hospital, A-1140 Vienna, Heinrich-Collin-Straße 30
*** Versuchstierzucht und -haltung der Universität Wien
    A-2325 Himberg, Brauhausgasse 34

Abstract

Human polymorphonuclear leukocytes and macrophages emit light of low intensity during phagocytosis with maxima near 630 nm and near 760 nm. Singlet oxygen is one of the toxic agents, which are released from phagocytes in order to destroy strange particles or cells. In addition to that, singlet oxygen produces or mediates the photon emission of phagocytes during immune defense. Typical emission bands of singlet-oxygen are at 1060 nm and 1270 nm, but also at 480, 570, 634 and 760 nm steming from dimolar oxygen transitions. The wavelengths of 633 nm and 760 nm seem to be mainly involved in immune reaction of phagocytes.

On the other hand, laser light of specific wavelengths (e.g.633 nm He-Ne-lasers light), of relatively low emission intensity (mWatt range) and of low dose (Joule/cm2 range) has been successfully applied in various medical laser therapies during the last 15 years. Experimental investigations on the effects of low dose laser light and monochromatic light support these photomedical observations. Recent studies on cell division of low level light result in favorite wavelength near 630 nm and 760 nm.

Comparing these two immunological aspects of light in biological systems, the following hypothesis is formulated and discussed: Photon emission of phagocytes might play an important role in immune system regulation and, on the other hand, appropriate laser light supports the natural immune reaction by simulating phagocytosis, thus leading to healing or improvement of deseases.

This hypothesis is in agreement with our recent knowledge in nonequilibrium thermodynamics of open systems: even weak stimuli (e.g. some photons) can create new order in cases of weak instabilities of the system. This can be examined by various methods. By using thermocouples, the kinetics of the heat production of rabbits after the injection of pyrogenic substances changed by the additional influence of weak 633 nm laser light. By using radiochemical methods and by counting white blood cells,immune suppressive effects of 633 nm laser light on lymphocytes and an immune stimulating effect on neutrophils have been found.

Introduction

The interaction of light and living systems has two aspects: the aspect of energy dissipation through an open system and the aspect of a trigger function for structural changes. Photosynthesis of plants and stimulation of their flowering by only few 660 nm photons are examples for these aspects (1).

The phenomenological experiences of morphological changes have found their theoretical explanation in nonequlilibrium thermodynamics and weak instabilities of open biosystems (2).

A further example of the trigger function of light was given by Karu et al., who observed that weak light (100 J/m2) has increased cell dividing effects near 630 nm and 760 nm (3).

Stimulation of the immune system by laser light

A great variety of experimental studies in the field of laser therapy were done in the last decade. An overview was given by us in (4). A remarkable number of these works refered to immunological response induced by 633 nm He-Ne-laser light: Serum complement activity of patients underwent a change. Albumin synthesis was stimulated and phagocytosis of polymorphonuclear leukocytes was increased (5-9). From this aspect one can understand and accept the reports on wound healing in laser therapy (10-11).

But if 633 nm light has such immune stimulating and healing effects, why should'nt it be produced spontaneousely during immune reactions ? Is there any source of native bioluminescence within our body connected with immune reactions?

Light production of phagocytes

In 1972, Allan et al. discovered the photon emission of polymorphonuclear leukocytes (PMNL) during phagocytosis (12) and in 1976, Nelson et al. completed to this invention the photon emission from macrophages (13). Allan was also the first, who proposed that singlet oxygen was present during phagocytosis, but only Rosen and Klebanoff provided experimental evidence (14). In 1977, Anderson et al. compared the photon emission spectrum of singlet oxygen with the photon emission spectrum of PMNL and found nearly identical spectra (15).

In 1984, Littarru et al. were able to quench the photon emission of singlet oxygen and also the photon emission of PMNL by using alpha-tocopherol (16). Therfore, one can assume that singlet oxygen contributes to the photon emission of phagocytes. The production of singlet oxygen during phagocytosis can be found in (17).

The red photon emission of oxygen was first produced by Blanchetiere in 1913. This reaction was later on rediscovered by Seliger (18) who found the maximum of the spectrum near 635 nm. The final prove for singlet oxygen as a source of this red light was given by Kasha and Khan in 1963 (19). Besides, Khan and Kasha interpreted the visible light as a cooperative transition of two oxygen molecules in the ground state (20).

Roschger et al. were the first who measured the native spectral photon emission of phagocytes without using luminol as an artificial light producing mediator of PMNL acitivity. By using interference filters with a broad full width we were able to differentiate the spectrum of luminol from the native photon emission spectrum of PMNL. Two maximas near 630 nm and 760 nm have been found (21).

The hypothesis: Singlet Oxygen triggers immune regulation

The experimental results and observations described above indicates that immunologically effective and healing light of 633 nm is produced within our body during a process which itself is strongly connected with immune reactions of our phyagocytes. This light is assumed to be emitted from pairs of singlet oxygen molecules. Therfore, we can state the following hypothesis:

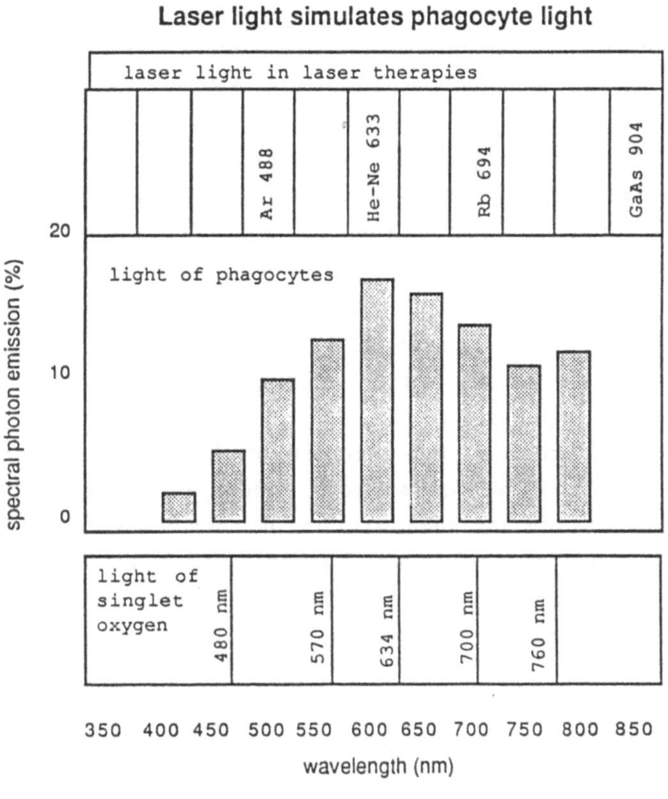

Fig. 1. The hypothesis: Singlet oxygen light of phagocytes can be replaced by appropriate light sources , e.g. by 633 nm laser light in laser therapy

Singlet oxygen light can be replaced by appropriate light sources as 633 nm-He-Ne-laser light, etc. Such a light may trigger the reduction of the activity of lymphocytes and stimulate the new differentiation of PMNL from stem cells. It is well known that PMNL have only a half life time of 4 - 8 hours in blood and must be produced from stem cells intensively after phyagocytosis.

These arguments are in good agreement with the findings of Mester et al. who observed a suppression of the activity of lymphocytes and a stimulation of PMNL activity after the application of 633nm-He-Ne-laser light. By using radiochemical methods, our own results on reduced 3-H-thymidin incorporation of lymphocytes after radiation with 633 nm laser light confirm these findings (22). But this argumentation does also agree with the activation of bone marrow described by Rachischev (23).

Besides, it should be possible to investigate this trigger function of singlet oxygen light, e.g. 634 nm, by using well known in-vivo-methods of laser puncture related to the stimulation of the immune system. Such an acupuncture method is reported by B.Hatai et al. They stimulated the immune system of rabbits by means of electro acupuncture (Pang-Gu). Amongst other results, they found a decrease of lymphocytes and an increase of neutrophils (24).

In addition, it should be possible to investigate some consequences of nonequilibrium thermodynamics of open systems. Special forms of open systems are biological systems. From this thermodynamical point of view, open biological systems are constantly dissipating heat according to their coherent state. A nonequilibrium measure of coherent states is the socalled " colour temperature" of the system. Usually, the measurement devices, which are measuring temperatures, need thermal equilibrium. Prigogine's concept is connect nonequlilibrium states with equilibrium ones. So it should be possible to measure the renewing of biological order by the alteration of the dissipated energy., i.e. the heat production. Besides, we know from nonequilibrium thermodynamics that very small stimuli can change the structure of coherent states in cases of weak instability, i.e. in cases of bifurcations. Therefore, the application of 633 nm laser light on biological systems might influence the morphological changes that are neasurable by the temperure of a biological system during its healing phase.

Some experimental results

In order to study the immune regulative effect of 633 nm light on lymphocytes and neutrophils in vivo, New Zealand white rabbits (average age 9 weeks, average weight 2,5 kg, male and female, sample number 6) were treated in a threefold manner:

a) The control group of the rabbits were held untreated for 90 minutes in their boxes at room temperature of 20 °C. After this period of time, 1 ml physiological NaCl solution/kg weight was injected in the ear vein of a rabbit. Then (1 hour after the injection) the laser tube touched the left and right acupuncture point Pang-Gu (new point NP 76) for 60 sec each, but it was not switched on (placebo puncture).

b) Another group of the rabbits were held untreated for 90 minutes in their boxes at the same room temperature. Afterwards 10 ng of an international pyrogen standard (25) E.coli endotoxin per kg weight were injected in the ear vein. One hour after the injection, the laser tube as a placebo puncture described above was applied to the left and right point Pang-Gu for 60 sec each.

c) The study group of rabbits were held untreated for 90 minutes in the same manner like the other groups. Afterwards 10 ng E.coli endotoxin per kg weight were injected in the ear vein. Then (1 hour after the injection) laser light (He-Ne-laser of 633 nm wavelength, laser power 5 mW) was applied to the left and right point Pang-Gu for 60 sec each.

Blood slides of each rabbit were taken at the beginning of this study. after 6 hours and after 24 hours from the beginning. The results significantly show an increase of the neutrophils and a decrease of lymphocytes (Fig. 2).

The 5 cm-rectal-temperature of each rabbit as a measure of fever production was investigated over a period of 270 minutes from the beginning by means of a Cu-Konstantan-thermoelement (producer P.Schenk, A-1212 Vienna, sensitivity +/- 0,1 oC) . Fig. 3 indicates the effects of the pyrogen standard E.coli Endotoxin and the influence of laser puncture on the rectal temperature of the rabbits.

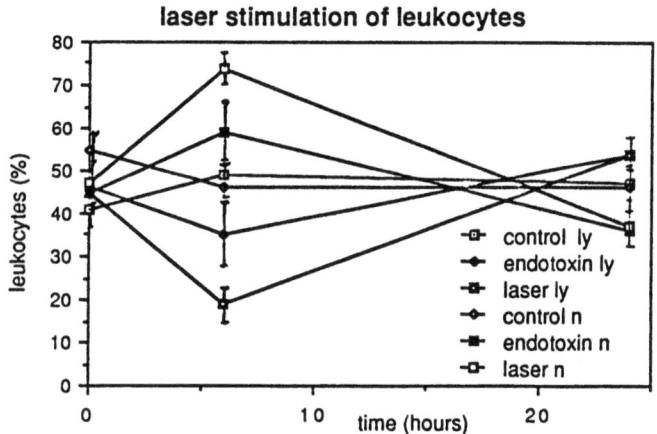

Fig. 2. The dependence of the ratio of lymphocytes (ly) and neutrophils (n) over leucocytes in the blood of New Zealand white rabbits (average age 9 weeks, average weight 2,5 kg, male and female, sample numer 6) after the injection of a) control ly, control n: physiol. NaCl-solution (1 ml/kg weight) and placebo puncture, b) endotoxin ly, endotoxin n: E.coli endotoxin (10 ng/kg weight) and placebo puncture, c) laser ly, laser n: E.coli endotoxin (10 ng/kg weight) and laserpuncture (NP 76 left and right, laser power 5 mW, irradiation time 60 sec each)

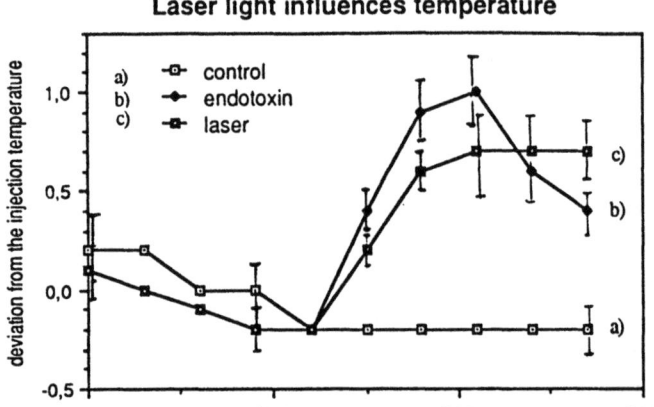

Fig. 3. Deviation of the rectal temperature from the injection temperature of New Zealand white rabbits (conditions and specifications of a, b and c   see Fig. 2)

Final remarks:

Further investigations on this topic are necessary. First of all, the influence of the wavelength due to singlet oxygen should be studied in laser therapy.

Secondly, the regulative effect of the singlet oxygen light on the immune system. especially on the differentiation of stem cells should be studied.

From a theoretical, but also clinical point of view it seems very interesting to investigate how the effects are dependent on the applied dose of the light. At this point, we appreciate the recent paper of Seichert et al. who found approximately the same biological effect by using low dose 633 nm He-Ne-laser light and middle dose 904 nm GaAs laser light (26). But we cannot follow their conclusions that the influence of 633 nm He-Ne-laser light compared to the sun light can be neglected, because we know from nonequilibrium thermodynamics that only small dosis are stimulating, but high doses are destroying. In addition, we know from photobiology and quantum optical interference that complementary wavelength like 660 nm and 730 nm can   compensate each other, finally showing no effect.

References

(1)   E.Strasburger, F.Noll, H.Schenk, A.F.W.Schimper; Lehrbuch der
       Botanik, Gustav Fischer V., Stuttgart 1978
(2)   G.Nicolis, I.Prigogine; Self-Organisation in Nonequilibrium
       Systems,John Wiley, New York 1977

(3) T.I.Karu, A.A.Tipklova, G.E.Fedoseyeva, G.S.Kalendo, V.S.Letokhov, V.V.Lobko, T.S.Lyapunova, N.N.Pomoshnikova; Laser Chem. 5(1984) 27

(4) H.Klima; Biophysikalische Aspekte von Lasertherapien, in "Laser- und Infrarotstrahlen in der Akupunktur"(Ed.J.Bahn, J.Bischko) Haug-Verlag, Heidelberg 1987

(5) E.Mester, S.Nagylucskay, S.Tisza, A.Mester, J.Toth; Z.Esp.Chir.10 (1977) 301

(6) E.Mester, S.Nagylucskay, W.Waidelich, S.Tisza, P.Greguss, D.Haina, A.Mester; Arch.Dermatol.Res.263 (1978) 241

(7) E.Mester, E.Jaszagi-Nagy, M.Hamar; Radiobiol.Radiotherap.6 (1974) 767

(8) E.Mester, S.Tisza, L.Csillag, A.Mester; Acta Chir.Acad.Sci.Hung.18 (1977) 141

(9) E.Mester, S.Nagylucskay, A.Döhlen, S.Tisza; Acta Chir.Acad.Sci.Hung.17 (1976) 49

(10) E.Mester; Über die stimulierende Wirkung der Laserstrahlung auf die Wundheilung; in "Der Laser"(Ed.K.Dinstl,P.I.Fischer) Springer Verlag, Berlin 1981

(11) I.S.Kana, G.Hutschenreiter, D.Haina, W.Waidelich; Arch.Surg. 116 (1981) 293

(12) R.C.Allan,R.L.Stjernholm,R.H.Steele; Biochem.Biophys.Res.Commun. 47 (1972) 679

(13) R.D.Nelson, E.L.Mills, R.L.Simmons et al.; Infect.Immun.14 (1976) 129

(14) H.S.Rosen, S.J.Klebanoff; Fed.Proc.35 (1976) 1391

(15) B.R.Andersen, A.M.Brendzdel, T.F.Lint; Infect. Immun.17 (1977) 62

(16) G.P.Littarru, S.Lippa, P.De Sole, A.Oradei, F.D.Torre, M.Macri; Biochem.Biophys.Res.Comm.119 (1984) 1056

(17) I.M.Roitt; Leitfaden der Immunologie, Steinkopf Verlag, Darmstadt 1984

(18) H.H.Seliger; Anal.Biochem. 1 (1960) 60

(19) A.U.Khan, M.Kasha; J.Chem.Phys.39 (1963) 2105

(20) A.A.Frimer; Singlet Oxygen, Volume I, Physical-Chemical Aspects, CRC Press 1985

(21) P.Roschger, W.Graninger, H.Klima; Biochem.Biophys.Res.Commun.123 (1984) 1047

(22) H.Klima, O.Haas, P.Roschger; in "Photon Emission from Biological Systems" (Ed.J.Slawinski, B.Kochel),World Publishing House, Singapur 1987

(23) A.Rachischev; Biologische Wirkungen von Laserstrahlen, Alma Ater 1976

(24) B.Hatai, T.Hashimoto, H.Ishizuka, M.Tany; Am.J.Acupuncture 5 (1977) 229

(25) S.Simon, M.Toth, Gy.Wallerstein, Zs.Remeny; J.Pharm.Pharmac.28 (1975) 111

(26) N.Seichert, P.Schöps, W.Siebert, W.Schnitzer, R.Liebermeister; Therapiewoche 37 (1987) 1375(1)

Low Power Laser Radiation Acts on Mast Cells Degranulation

Mayayo E.*, Trelles M.A.**, Miro L.***, Rigau J.**, Baudin G.***

* Serv. Anatomia Patológica del Hosp. Juan XXIII, Tarragona y Dpto. de Histología de la Fctad. de Medicina de Reus/Univ. Barcelona -E
** Instituto Médico Vilafortuny, Cambrils/Tarragona -E
*** Lab. de Biophysique Medicale. Institut Bouisson Bertrand, Centro Hosp. Univ., Nimes -F

INTRODUCTION

In a previous work (1) we reported that low power laser irradiation produce vasodilation and that this phenomenon could be associated to its direct or indirect action on mast cells (MC).

In this paper we communicate the results of our recent studies on the action of low power laser light on the physiopathology of MC.

MATERIAL AND METHOD

For irradiation we used two different output He/Ne lasers, emitting on the same wavelength (632,8 nm), but one of 4 mW and the other of 15 mW. The experiment was carried out on the swiss-laboratorium mice, all males, weighing 25 grs, normally bred at the stabularium.

Three groups of 8 animals each, were selected.
- Group 1 was kept as control. In these animals the whole procedure was performed but the beam was not lit (simulated treatment).
- Group 2 was irradiated with a 15 mW He/Ne laser during 2

minutes and 40 seconds. The energy reached per session was of 2.4 Joules (J).
- Group 3 was irradiated with a 4 mW He/Ne laser for 10 minutes. The energy reached by session was of same value as group 2.

Irradiation was carried out within the mouth cavity directly upon the tongue, the surface of exposure being approximatelly one quarter square cm. Immediately after the first irradiation two animals of each group were killed and their tongues were excised and processed by electronmicroscopy routine technique (inclusion into glutaraldehyde at 2,5 %, dissecation-inclusion into araldite). Cuts of 0,5 u were done and contrasted by lead citrat or stained by metachromatig technique with toluidine blue in order to examen the MC.

The rest of animals continued receiving one irradiation every second day during the experiment, the animals were normally kept and no local or general drug was given. On the 10th day, after five irradiations, all animals were killed. Immediately after death, the tongues were excised, weighed and polvorized in a mortar with 0,1 ml physiological serum and then frozen at $-30°$ Centigrade.

In order to analyse the functional reaction of MC under low power laser irradiation, histamin was analized by Radio Inmunological Assay (RIA) using the Inmunotech Kit.

RESULTS

- Concerning histological studies
  By using the Toluidine Blue Technique and examining the samples that have received only one irradiation, we observed a decrease

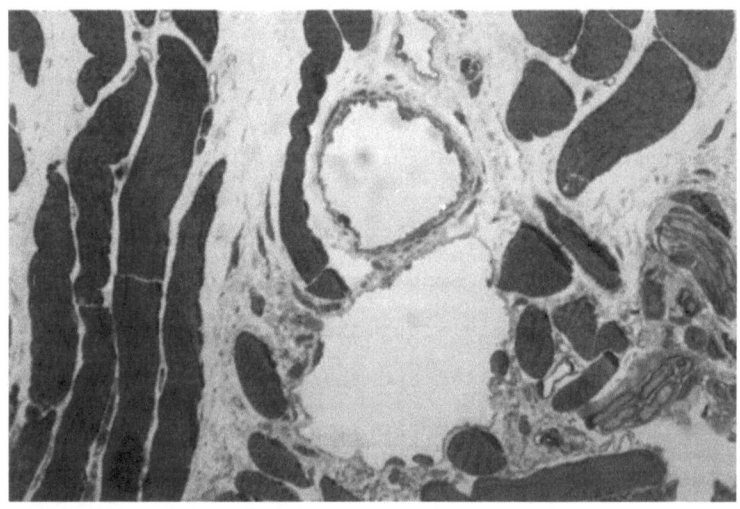

Fig. 1. Tongue tissue (Giemsa x 64). Note the muscular fibers and the fine vessels between them

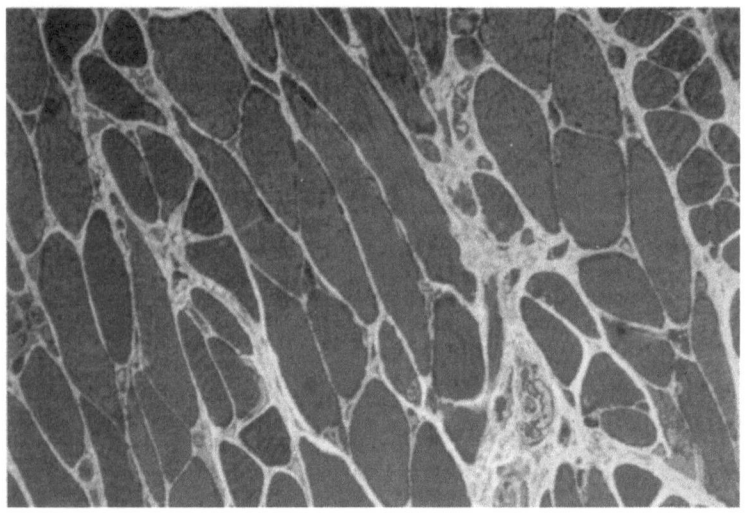

Fig. 2. Irradiated tongue tissue (Giemsa X 64). Observe the dilated vessels between the muscular fibers

in MCs number. MCs were not perceivible in equal number as in the control samples (Fig 1-2) at the same time. There was an important vasodilation in the irradiated tissue (Fig 3).

The ultrastructural studies of these cells showed a normal

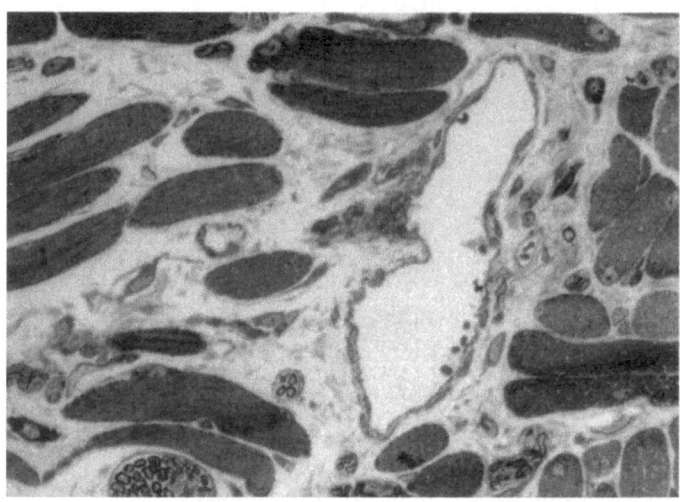

Fig. 3. Semifine cut. Great vasodilation with interstitial oedema in the laser irradiated tongue

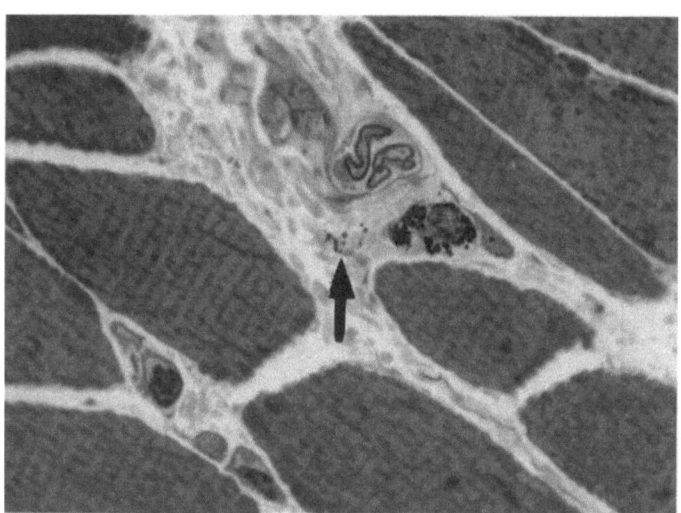

Fig. 4. Semifine cut. Irradiated tongue. A MC is degranulating. Observe that the granules appear in the interstitium (arrow). Degranulation is significantly more active comparatively to the non-irradiated control group

cytoplasm full of granules containing the various substances produced by MCs (Histamine, Heparine, Serotonine, etc.) which cause the Physio-pathological action of these cells.

In the tongues of animals irradiated by low power laser light, the MCs cytoplasm appear clear, totally or partially, of their granules; and some of these granules could be observed loose at the interstitial medium (Fig 4).

At greater microscopy magnification, this phenomenon was confirmed and we were able to observe some granules already drained out and other granules releasing MCs.

- Concerning histamine dosage.

The statistical study of the results using the Means Comparison Technique between small populations shows:

A decrease of histamine level on animals submitted to irradiation with a security coefficient of 95 % (Graph I).

No significant differences were concluded between the histamine level of groups 2 and 3, irradiated with different output lasers (but at same energy density of 2,4 J) contradictory to our previous results (2).

DISCUSSION

As far as two facts are concerned this study confirms and completes the results obtained in previous experiments:

- One irradiation of 2,4 J with He/Ne laser upon the tongue of the Swiss-mouse is capable of creating a vasodilation (Fig 3) and produces an active degranulation of the MC contents. At the same time MC become fewer in number and their granules are found at the intracellular medium and some of them could be observed draining-out of the cytoplasm.

- Six irradiations of 2,4 J each produce a decrease of histamine

Graph I

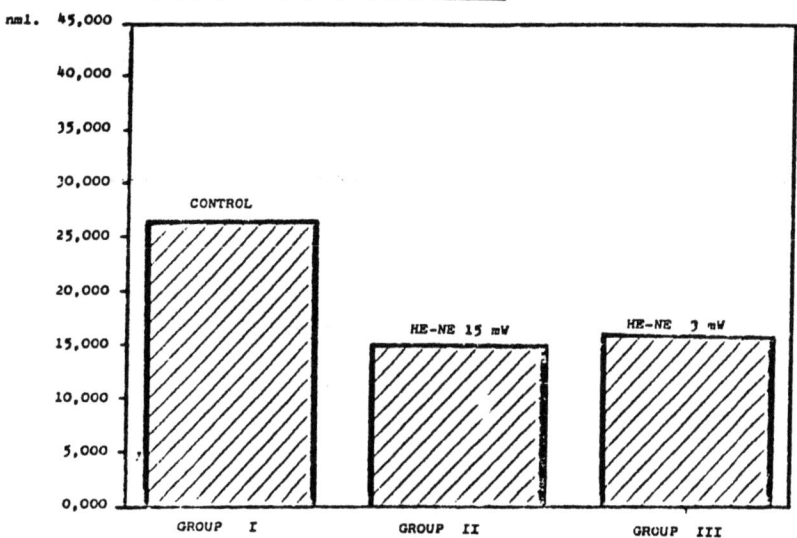

level in the tongue, in comparison to control samples. The differences in laser output seems to have no importance.

Although this experiment was carried out on few animals, the same results are shown in nearly all of them. This observation agrees with what we have observed in our previous experiments. Therefore we beleive that is reasonable to assure that these observations are valid.

Knowing the action of histamine in the vasomotricity physiology (3) it is also reasonable to assure that the observed vasodilation which occurs on tissues exposed to low-power-laser--light could be explained in part by the action of MC components. Histamine is not the only substance contained in MC granules; these cells also contain Serotonin, Prostaglandin, Heparine and other important amines (4). If MCs release histamine under low power laser irradiation it is obvious that the other substances contained in these cells might be released as well. We have analysed histamine only because it is easier to measure; Techniques for measurement of other amines are more complex and critical.

Nevertheless we consider that it is necessary to study the fluctuation level of all MC components under laser irradiation because of its physiopathological importance in human diseases. The analysis of their variations, eventually produced by low power laser irradiation, could help to understand better the action mechanisms of low power lasers on tissues and could also explain, to a certain extent, the clinical results obtained.

BIBLIOGRAPHY

1.- M.A. Trelles, E. Mayayo (1986) Mast Cells are Implicated in Low Power Laser's Effect on Tissue. A Preliminary Study. American Society for Laser Medicine and Surgery Abstracts, vol.6 n.2 pp277

2.- M.A. Trelles, E. Mayayo (1986) Mast Cells and Low-Power Laser: Analysis of its Components before and after Irradiation. Lasers in Medical Science Abstracts, vol.1 n.4 pp299

3.- F. Sagher, Z. Even-Paz (1967) Mastocytosis and Mast-cells. Bonlea S. Korger AG

4.- C. Cordon-Cardo (1985) La célula cebada o mastocito: biología celular y molecular. Medicina Clínica (Barcelona), 84 pp327:331

Data for Laser Biostimulation in Wound-Healing

Adam Mester, M.D.[+] and Andrew F. Mester, M.D.[++]

[+] Laser Research Laboratory, Postgraduate Medical University Budapest
Szabolcs 35, Pf: 112, Hungary 1389

[++] Department of Otorhinolaryngology and Human Communication
University of Pennsylvania, School of Medicine
3400 Spruce Street, Philadelphia, PA 19104, U.S.A.

Introduction and Basic Science

Since the first ruby laser was made in 1960, multiple applications of lasers have been identified. The special burning, coagulating, and vaporizing effects of high output lasers, together with their easy manipulation using optical systems, have resulted in extensive medical use. Additionally, there is much interest in the nonthermic effects of lasers in photodynamic tumor therapy and in biostimulation.

Early research demonstrated that several biological systems and physiologic processes are influenced by a variety of low-output lasers, and the biophysical law of Arndt-Schultz was found applicable to the laser: stimulation by low incident energy density (IED) and inhibition by high IED of radiation (Mester et al., 1967; 1968; 1969; 1970; 1971; 1972). Basic experiments were carried out with the ruby and later using continuous operating He-Ne, argon-ion and GaAlAs diode lasers.

Carcinogenicity was not observed by repeated ruby laser irradiaton of the skin, but hair growth increased in depilated mice by an IED of 1 Joule/cm^2 applied twice weekly for 3 to 5 weeks. Following the 10th irradiation hair loss occurred. The hystology showed inflammation and atrophic changes in hair follicles, which was the apparent cause of hair loss (Mester et al., 1967; 1968).

Phagocytosis of bacteria (Staphylococcus Pyog. aureus) by human and rat leukocytes was increased with the IED of 0.05 Joule/cm^2 while it decreased with 2 to 4 Joule/cm^2 (Mester et al., 1967; 1968). These effects were increased with methylene blue and Janus B green staining and decreased with acridine orange staining (Mester et al., 1970; 1972). When the supernatant of the laser-irradiated leukocyte suspension was added to fresh normal leukocytes, a significant increase in phagocytosis was observed within 1 hour, followed by a rapid decrease after 2 hours, with inhibition occurring between 3 and 4 hours. This suggests the involvement of an active extracellular and transferable substance (Mester et al., 1975).

Small bowel activity is sensitive to laser irradiation (Mester et al., 1969). The spontaneous movement of jejunal villi in dogs increased with IEDs of 1 to 3 Joule/cm^2 and decreased with IEDs of 4 to 7 Joule/cm^2 (Mester et al., 1970). Amino-ethylthiouronium (AET), an X-radiation protective substance, administered prior to laser irradiation prevented both stimulation and inhibition of bacterio-phagocytosis by leukocytes as well as intestinal mucosal micromotility (Mester et al., 1971; 1972). Another experiment on guinea-pig ileum demonstrated increased acetylcholine release following ruby laser exposure, suggesting possible effects on neurotransmitter release (Vizi et al., 1977).

The effect of ruby laser (0.05 to 26 J/cm^2 IED) in hemoglobin synthesis was studied in short-term rat bone marrow cultures, measuring 59 Fe and 14 C glycine incorporation. Low IED increased and higher IED inhibited hem synthesis, while the increase of globin synthesis was found by relatively higher IED. The IED differences between the two hemoglobin components were assumed to be related to the absorption parameters of these proteins (Mester et al., 1971).

DNA and RNA content (as measured by labeled thymidine and uridine incoroporation) and cell counts increased in 1 $Joule/cm^2$ ruby laser irradiated Escherichia coli CR54 cultures in the presence of the exogenic light stabilizer, methylene blue, when compared to the control. Higher IEDs decreased cell counts (Mester et al., 1971; similar results have been obtained by Dzinic et al., 1985).

Retinal pigment epithelium cultured on chorioallantoic membrane and irradiated with the He-Ne laser was observed to increase mitosis (Yew et al., 1982) and thymidine uptake and incorporation (Tsang et al., 1986).

Body weight of mice inoculated with laser-irradiated Ehrlich's ascites tumor cells increased 10 to 16%, and the number of tumor cells increased 19 to 30% compared to controls. Survival time following inoculation with laser-irradiated cells was shorter than in the control group (Mester et al., 1968). Electron microscopic subcellular changes observed in the laser-irradiated Ehrlich's tumor cells were not observed after acridine orange staining (Mester et al., 1971). The biostimulating effect of argon-ion laser irradiation on human squamous carcinoma cells was reported recently (Castro, et al., 1987).

The remote effect of laser irradiation on vessel formation in the rabbit cornea was observed. The angiogenesis promoting effect of adrenal gland total extract was decreased with 1 to 3 $Joule/cm^2$ IED (He-Ne laser) and increased with 5 $Joule/cm^2$ IED. The latter effect was also observed in the contralateral cornea, which received adrenal gland total extract only (Mester et al. 1970; Kiss et al., 1972).

Low-output laser irradiation has been reported to stimulate wound healing (Mester et al., 1968; 1969; 1971; 1973; 1975; 1983; 1984; 1985; 1986; 1987; Haina et al., 1981; Kovacs et al., 1981; Trelles et al., 1982; 1984; 1987; Iupatov et al., 1982; Kahn, 1984). Microscopic investigation revealed numerous dividing cell forms in the area of the irradiated wound, which healed faster than the control wounds.

Electronmicroscopy of granulation tissue was studied. After the first He-Ne laser irradiation the number of collagen fibres increased, and the cellular substance diminished. In addition, vesicles having electron-dense nuclei were found in both cytoplasmic and intracellular materials. Following the second laser irradiation the number of lysosoma-type bodyes increased in the intracellular area and mitochondria became swollen. In the intercellular space further multiplication of collagen and of vesicles were observed. After the third irradiation further multiplication of collagen, and of vesicles were found. Similar but less changes were detected at various dates in the samples excised from nonirradiated areas of the wound surface (Mester et al., 1973; 1974).

Collagen production in rat granulation tissue was studied. The incorporation of ^{2}C-glycine did not change, but that of ^{3}H-proline exceeded the control by 50% (Mester et al., 1972; 1973). Incorporation of ^{3}H-thymidine in human fibroblast culture irradiated with ruby laser increased reproduction by 53%, compared to the control (Toth et al., 1975). This information about the number of cells in phase S of the cellular cycle demonstrates an increased reproduction in the laser treated cultures. A stimulating effect on procollagen production was observed recently following low output Nd-YAG laser (Abergel et al., 1984; 1987) and by He-Ne and GaAs lasers (Lam et al., 1986; Boulton et al., 1986; Saperia et al., 1986; Lyons et al., 1987).

Enzymatic events in the early stages of wound healing have been studied. Activity of succinic acid dehydrogenase was significantly greater 8 to 48 hours after wounding in the basal epithelial cells within the sound tissue zone next to the wound lips compared to control wounds. Additionally, activity of the lactic acid dehydrogenase and nonspecific esterase was higher in laser-irradiated fibroblast tissue than in the control tissue (Bacsy et al., 1974).

Regeneration of microcirculation in rabbit ear (Sanders' ear chamber method) is significantly affected by laser irradiation, inasmuch as a significant increase in revascularization has been observed in He-Ne laser-irradiated wounds compared to controls (Kovacs et al., 1974). Laser stimulation on lymphatic vessel regeneration and circulation has been also described (Lievens 1985). Regeneration of muscle fiber (posterior great adductor of rat), injured through open skin, healed faster when irradiated by 1 Joule/cm^2 IED ruby laser every third day through the sutured skin compared to control animals (Mester et al., 1975).

Tensile strength (TS) of He-Ne laser-irradiated wounds in rat's skin was studied. TS of clipped wounds were not different on the 3rd postoperative day. On the 8th postoperative day the laser-irradiated wounds were 47% stronger, and on the 12th postoperative day 21% stronger compared to the control animals (Kovacs et al., 1974; similar results have been obtained by Abergel et al., 1986).

An immunosuppressive effect of laser-irradiation has been reported. The mean survival time (MST) of skin allotransplant in mouse treated with antithymocyte serum (ATS) rose by 56.2% compared with that of the control animals. Treatment with ATS and He-Ne laser irradiation resulted in a 84.7% MST increase (Namenyi et al., 1975), while laser irradiation alone had no significant effect.

In phytohemagglutine (PHA)-stimulated lymphocyte cultures 60 to 80% of the cells went through blast formation, while in cultures stimulated with PHA and irradiated with 1 Joule/cm^2 ruby laser, blast formation increased 20% when compared to unlased but PHA-stimulated cells (Mester et al., 1976).

The model experiment of the immunosuppressive effects of low-output laser irradiation on T and B lymphocytes (Mester et al., 1976, 1977, 1978) was applied to study the effect of noncoherent light sources. The monochromatic light had no effect, but with planopolarization 80% of the effect produced by coherent beam was found (Mester et al., 1977; 1978).

Prostaglandin (PG) content in wounded dorsal skin of the rat was studied. Both of the two tested PGs showed an increase in 4 day old wounds. After 8 days the value of PGE_2 dropped below the level observed with the control group, while that of PGF_{2a} continued to rise (Cseh et al., 1978).

Clinical Results

Because of evidence of laser biostimulation in experimental circumstances, in 1971 Mester and his group started treating patients with nonhealing ulcers. Some patients early in the study were treated with ruby laser (694.3 nm), later He-Ne (632.8 nm, 5-50 mW), argon-ion (457-514 nm, 100-150 mW), and GaAlAs diode lasers (820 nm, 15 mW) were used.

From 1971 to December 1985 1361 patients were treated with laser in our center. Patients' data were inputted in the computer and analyzed. We also analysed the clinical data of 806 conservative treated cases with leg ulcers during the last two years (1984-1985).

The patient population with 63 principal diseases made up of four groups: leg ulcers, other wounds and ulcers, non ulcer laser biostimulation, laser coagulation.

Treatment Protocol:

Healing wounds were not treated by laser. Patient population treated in our center went through all kinds of conservative and surgical treatments without success. Laser therapy was applied only in cases without any improvement and healing. However in some cases laser biostimulation started forthwith, because of life danger (i.e. coumarin caused skin necrosis), or because of the well known characteristic course of the disease (i.e. X-ray ulcer, amputation stump ulcer, diabetic ulcer on the sole, stomatitis causing incapacity of drinking in children). Laser treatments were carried on twice a week, later once a week, while in acute septic cases daily. The IED of laser irradaitons were 4 $Joule/cm^2$.

Results

Conservative treatment was running on till the patient healed. If there was no improvement for a period of three months laser therapy started. The healing rate with the conservative therapy in leg ulcers was 73.9%, and 22.4% of the patients were subjects for laser therapy, while 3.7% didn't show up again.

Total healing in the laser treated leg ulcer group was 81.4% (of thoose 22.4% who didn't heal with the conservative therapy). Healing in the ulcer not on the leg group was 76.0%, and in the non ulcer biostimulation group 42.9%. The average length of healing was 5.5 months excluded 3 months fruitless conservative therapy.

Discussion

In summary, biostimulatory effects of low-output laser irradiation have been demonstrated at a variety of molecular and cellular levels, as well as at whole organ and tissue levels. Under certain circumstances, synergistic effects with laser irradiation have been found as demonstrated in the immune system. There is evidence that effects remote to the irradiated site occur, suggesting the presence of a circulatory active substance. Furthermore, the biostimulatory effects of low-output laser irradiation is dose dependent and, with sufficient intensity, the stimulatory effect disappears and inhibition occurs.

According to our previous research studies laser biostimulation, inhibition, and coagulation depend on the IED, therefore the time-honoured protocol didn't change since 1971. The output of the laser determines the biological effects, while the wavelength influences the absorption. Our indication of the laser type in use depends mostly on the extension of the treated area. Smaller ulcers were treated with He-Ne, larger with argon-ion, and small deep with infrared lasers.

Non of the laser treated patients had side effects or complications as a result of laser therapy. Lesions suspect for malignancy were investigated histologically and patient became subject for laser biostimulation only after negativ results.

The experiments to elucidate the bioregulative process of wound healing and the clinical results has convinced us to recommend the use of lasers to stimulate wound healing.

Reference

Mester E, Szende B, Gartner P. Die Wirkung der Laserstrahlen auf den Haarwuchs der Maus. Radioboil Radiother 1968;9:621-626.

Mester E, Ludany G, Vajda G, Razgha A, Karika G, Tota JG. Uber die Wirkung von Laserstrahlen auf die Bakterienphagocytose der Leukocyten. Acta Biol Med Germ 1968;21:317.

Mester E, Ludany G, Sellyei M, Szende B. Untersuchungen uber die Biologische Wirkung der Laser-Strahlen. Bull Soc Int Chir 1968;26(1):1-6.

Mester E, Sellyei M, Tota GJ. Laserstrahlenwirkung auf das Wachstum des Ehrlichschen Ascitestumors. Arch Geschwulstforsch 1968;32:201.

Mester E. Clinical results of wound-healing stimulation with laser and experimental studies of the action mechanism. Laser '75 Optoelectronics Conference Proceedings Munich 1975 pp 119-125.

Mester E, Jaszsagi-Nagy E. The effect of laser radiation on wound-healing and collagene synthesis. Studia Biophysica 1973;35(3):227-230.

Mester E, Ludany G, Vajda G, Tota JG, Karika G, Hejjas M. Untersuchungen uber die Wirkung von Laserstrahlen auf die Bakterienphagocytose von Leukocyten. Acta Biol Med Germ 1970;25:927

Mester E, Ihasz M, Karika G, Tota JG. Effect of laser beam on the micromotility of the intestinal mucosa. Acta Biol Acad Sci Hung 1970;21(2):171-174.

Mester E, Nagylucskay S, Tisza S, Mester A. Neuere Untersuchungen uber die Wirkung der Laserstrahlen auf die Wundheilung - Immunologische Aspekte. Laser '77 Opto-electronics Conference Proceedings Munich 1977 pp 490-500.

Mester E, Neumark T, Tisza S, Mester A, Toth J, Mate L. Neuere elektronenmikroscopische Untersuchungen uber die Wirkung der Laserstrahlen auf die Wundheilung. In Waidelich W (ed): Laser '79 Opto-Electronics. IPC Science and Technology Press 1979;pp 330-337.

Mester E, Hazay L, Fenyo M, Kertesz I, Toth N, Jaranyi Zs, Toth J. The biostimulating effect of laser beam. Proceedings Laser Optoelectronics '81 Munich pp:146-152.

Mester E, Torok A, Nikolits I, Mester A, Simoncsics P, Borzsonyi M, Toth J. New experimental and clinical results of laser biostimulation. In: Waidelich W. Ed. Opto-electronics in Medicine 1984. Springer Verlag, Berlin-Heidelberg-New York. pp: 201-207.

Mester E, Mester AF, Mester A. The biomedical effects of laser application. Lasers Surg Med 1985;5:31-39.

Mester AF, Mester A. Mester's method of laser biostimulation. In: Waidelich W, Kiefhaber P. Ed. Laser Opto-electronics in Medicine 1986. Springer Verlag, Berlin-Heidelberg-New York-Tokyo. pp:103-109.

Waidelich W. In memoriam Professor Dr. med. Endre Mester. in: Waidelich W. Laser Opto-electronics in Medicine 1986. Springer Verlag Berlin-Heidelberg-New York-Tokyo, p: 3.

Clincial Experience on Mix HeNe and IR Low Energy Laser – A Review of 404 Cases

Peter Hasan, Agus Rijadi, Santoso Purnomo, Hendrik Kainama
Husada Hospital, Faculty of Medicine, Univ. Kristen Djaya
Jalan Raya Mangga Besar No. 137, Jakarta 10730. INDONESIA

Since 1971 Mester(31) had reported that he observed biostimulative effect of low energy laser beam. Thereafter, plenty of studies had been performed which included experimental studies on animals(7,14,16-,20,21,22,23,25,26,28,35,39,40,42,43), experimental invitro and invivo studies on human cells culture(1,24,25) and clinical studies(2,5,6,8,-9,11,13,15,17,19,27,29,31,32,33,34,35,36,37,38,41,44,45,47,48,49). All these studies comfirmed that the low energy laser had a nonthermal effect so called BIOSTIMULATION. Though studies on intracellular changes with electron microscope as well as studies on biochemical reaction and cellular enzymatic activity showed significant changes after low energy laser beam irradiation, the mechanism of this biostimulative effects remain unclear.

Recently low energy laser has been widely applied clinically for various indications such as:
- Pain attenuation(3,11,15,19,27,32,36,37,38,41,45,47)
- Wound healing promotion(5,13,31,34,44,48)
- Bloodflow and lymhflow enchancement(28,35)
- To reduce edema and inflammation(32,35)
- To soften scar(35)
- Nerve stimulation(35)
- Accupuncture(8,9,10,17,18,49).
- etc.

Those disorder treated with low energy laser were reported to have high success rate and free from side effect.

MATERIAL AND METHOD

474 cases in 413 patients, 181 male and 232 female were treated with mix HeNe laser (632 nm.) and Diode Infrared laser (904 nm.) at Husada Hospital from January 1986 to January 1987. The laser beam was irradiated mainly at the site of the disorder but for nerve and vascular involvement, short lasting irradiations were added along the path, and

for headache was added with distant accupoints irradiation. All cases were irradiated every two days but severe case initiated with daily irradiation for 5 consecutive days.

Cases who discontinued laser irradiation after the first or second session were excluded. No other medication was administered to each patient except antibiotic for infection cases and patient who had been taking analgesic previously should continue taking it, then after several session reduced and finally discontinued.

CRITERIA FOR EVALUATION

- A = Very Good to Excellent (81 - 100 % improvement)
- B = Good (41 - 80 % improvement)
- C = Slight (10 - 40 % improvement)
- D = No Improvement
- E = Worse

RESULT

70 cases of the 474 cases were excluded. The 404 cases reviewed consist of 11 groups of cases as seen in table 1.

Table 1. Case treated with low energy laser

Case Grouping	Cases Treated	Cases Evaluated
Gr. 1 = Infection/Inflammation	35	30
Gr. 2 = Postoperative Wound	57	52
Gr. 3 = Other Wound	44	43
Gr. 4 = Pain Attenuation	185	147
Gr. 5 = Nerve Stimulation	26	24
Gr. 6 = Vascular Insufficiency	31	28
Gr. 7 = Infertility	15	13
Gr. 8 = Flap Survival	6	6
Gr. 9 = Hair Growth Stimulation	6	6
Gr.10 = Softening Scar	12	8
Gr.11 = Miscellaneous	57	47
Total	474	404

The overall result of this series were:

- Very Good to Excellent : 22.8 %
- Good : 38.8 %
- Slight : 28.0 %
- No Improvement : 10.1 %
- Worse : 0.3 %

Treatments with mix HeNe and I.R. low energy laser were effective in 61.6 % of the total cases (good to excellent) and not effective in 38.4 % (slight improvement to worse). Best results were observed in Gr.7 (flap survival) = 100 %, Gr.2 (postoperative wound) = 86.5 %, and Gr.3 (other wound) = 74.4 %.

Table 2 . Result

Group	A	B	C	D	E	TOTAL	A + B	C + D + E
1	3	11	13	3	0	30	14(46.7%)	16(53.3%)
2	28	17	7	0	0	52	45(86.5%)	7(13.5%)
3	9	23	9	2	0	43	32(74.4%)	11(25.6%)
4	32	59	42	13	1	147	91(61.9%)	56(38.1%)
5	4	7	9	2	0	24	11(50.0%)	11(50.0%)
6	3	8	14	3	0	28	11(39.3%)	17(60.7%)
7	0	4	6	3	0	13	4(30.8%)	9(69.2%)
8	3	3	0	0	0	6	6(100 %)	0(0 %)
9	0	1	2	3	0	6	1(16.7%)	5(83.3%)
10	1	3	3	1	0	8	4(50.0%)	4(50.0%)
11	9	21	8	9	0	47	30(63.8%)	17(36.2%)
TOTAL	92	157	113	41	1	404	249	155
%	22.8	38.8	28.0	10.1	0.3	100.0	61.6 %	38.4%

SIDE EFFECTS

Out of the 404 cases in 351 patients, side effects were observed in 11 patients (3.1 %). One patient experienced skin rash (photosensitivity ?) after 5 session of laser irradiation; symtoms disappeared two days after cessation of the laser treatment. Six months later he was again treated with the same mix laser beam but without any side effects. The other side effects as seen in table 3 were minor and only temporary.

Table 3 . Side Effects

Type of side effects	No. of cases
Photosensitivity (?)	1
Dryness of the skin	4
Traffic photophobia (night time)	1
Temporary Post irrad. tenderness	5
T O T A L	11/351 (3.1 %)

DISCUSSION

Unlike other reports which had high success rate of 80 - 95 %, our series revealed only 61.6 %. Anyhow this supports the confirmation of laser biostimulation.

Most of the reports on clinical application of low energy laser are free from side effects but in our series we observed a 3.1 % which although mostly are minor and temporary, attention should be paid for the possibility of other more serious side effects.

It is concluded that mix HeNe and Diode Infrared low energy laser beam have a distinct biostimulative effects and also a powerful analgesic and anti-inflammatory effects. This will serve to the medical profession an alternative modality of treatment or at least a supplement to the conventional treatment.

It was very interesting that we also observed an increase in sexual potency and libido which possibly due to an increase in androgen production after low energy irradiation at the testicle of the infertile male. An increase in thyroid function had also been observed by colleague in Italy (personal communication). This finding suggest that a further investigation on the possibility to treat hormonal insufficiency with laser is expected in the future.

REFERENCES

1. Basleer, C. : Human articular chondrocytes cultivated in three demensions: Effects of I.R. Laser Irradiation. Preceedings of The International Congress on laser in Medicine and Surgery, Bologna 1985, p. 381-385.
2. Bieglio, C. : A report on experience in treatment of pain of spinal origin by low power laser. Preceedings of the International Congress on Laser in Medicine and Surgery, Bologna 1985, p 343-347.
3. Bieglio, C. : Physical Treatment for Radicular pain with low Power Laser Stimulation. Laser in Surg. and Med. vol 6 (2) : 173. (1986).
4. Bolognani, L., et. al. : Effects of GaAs pulsed laser on ATP consentration and ATP ase activity in vitro and in vivo. Preceedings of The International Congress on Laser Medicine and surgery, Bologna 1985, p 47-51.
5. Cabero, M.V., et. al. : Laser Therapy as a generator and healing wound tissue. Preceedings of The International Congress on Laser in Medicine and Surgery, 1985. p 187-193.
6. Coufalik, E.D., et. al. : Effects of Low Energy Diode Lasers in chronic vaginal discharge. 6th Congress of The International Society for Laser Surgery and Medicine, Jerusalem 1985.
7. Dyson, M., et. al. : Effects of laser therapy on wound contraction and cellularity in Mice. Laser in Medical Science vol 1 : 31-39 (1985).
8. De-Min, L., et. al. : Studies on mechanism of Laser accupuncture : Regulation of function. Preceedings of The International Congress on Laser in Medicine and Surgery, Bologna 1985, p. 255-258.
9. De-Min, L., et. al. : Studies on the mechanism of laser puncture promotion of defense immunofunction. Preceedings of The International Congress on Laser in Medicine and surgery, Bologna 1985, p. 259-262.

10. De-Min, L. and Yuan-Yu, Q. : Investigation into mechanism and clinic of laser accupuncture. Laser in Surg. Med. vol 3 (2) : 190 (1983).
11. England, S.M., et. al. : An observer blind trial of I.R. ceb Mid-Laser Therapy in bicipitaltendonitis and supraspinatus tendonitis. Preceedings of The International Congress on Laser Medicine and Surgery, Bologna 1985, p. 413-414.
12. Emmanoilidis, O., et. al. : C.W. I.R. Low Power Laser Application Significantly Accelerates Chronic Pain Relief Rehabilitation of Professional Athletes. A double Blind Study. Laser in Surg. and Med. vol. 6 (2) : 173 (1986).
13. Goujor, C., et. al. : Preliminary results of Mid-Laser Treatment of chronic ulceration of the legs. 6th Congress of The International Society for Laser Surgery and Medicine, Jerusalem 1985.
14. Haina, D., et. al. : Animal experiments on light-induced wound healing. Preceeding of The 4th Congress of The International Society for Laser Surgery, Tokyo,81. p. 22-1-22-3.
15 Hasan, P.H.W., et. al. : Low Energy Laser in Pain Treatment. International Symposium on Laser Medicine and Surgery, Jakarta 1986.
16. Kami, T., et. al. : Effect of Low Energy Diode Laser on Flap Survival. Annals of Plastic Surgery, 14 : 278-283 (1985).
17. Kamikawa, K. : Application of Low-Energy Laser to accupuncture. International Symposium on Low Energy Laser in Medicine and Surgery, Tokyo'85.
18. Kamikawa, K. : Development of Laser Accupuncture Systems and Their Clinical Applications. New Frontiers in Laser Medicine and Surgery. Ed. Kazuhiko Atsumi, Excerpta Medica, 1985, p. 498-505.
19. Kamikawa, K. and Kyoto, J. : Double Blind experiences with Mid-Laser in Japan (1985). Proceedings of The International Congress on Laser in Medicine and Surgery, Bologna 1985, p. 165-170.
20. Kartadinata, H. et. al. : Laser Biostimulation on Wound Healing. International Symposium on Laser Medicine and Surgery, Jakarta 1986.
21. Kokino, M., et. al. : An investigation of the stimulating effects of laser on callus in the treatment of fracture. Preceedings of The International Congress on Laser in Medicine and Surgery, Bologna 1985, p. 387-393.
22. Kokino, M., et. al. : Effect of Laser irradiation of tendon healing. Preceedings of The International Congress on Laser in Medicine and Surgery, Bologna 1985, p. 405-411.
23. Kovacs, L., et. al. : Experimental investigation of Photostimulation effect of low energy HeNe Laser Radiation. Preceedings of the 4th Congress of The International Society for Laser Surgery, Tokyo '81. p. 22-14-11-16.
24. Kubasowa, T., et. al. : Biological Effect of HeNe Laser : Investigation on Functional on Morphological alteration of cell membranes in vitro. Lasers in Surg. and Med. 4 : 381-388 (1984).
25. Lam, T. S. : Stimulation of collagen production by low Energy Laser in Human Skin Fibroblast. Lasers in Surg. and Med. 3 (2) : 189 (1983).
26. Lievens, P. : The influence of Laser irradiation on the motricity of lymphatical systems and on the wound healing process. Preceedings of The International Congress on Laser in Medicine and surgery, Bologna 1985, p. 171-174.
27. Lonauer, G. : Controlled Double Blind study on the Efficacy of HeNe Laser beams versus HeNe plus infrared Laser beams in the therapy of activited osteoarthritis of finger joints.
Lasers in Surg. and Med. vol 6 (2) : 172 (1986).
28. Maruyama, Y. : Effect of low Energy Diode Laser on Flap Survival. International Symposium on Low Energy Laser in Medicine and Surgery, Tokyo '85.
29. Mayordomo, M. M., et. al. : Laser in painful processes of locomotor system : Our Experience. Preceedings of The International Congress on Laser in Medicine and Surgery, Bologna 1985, p. 349-355.
30. Mc. kibbin, L. S., et. al. : A preliminary report on the use of a HeNe Laser to cause collateral axon sprouting into denerved tissue. Lasers in Surg. and Med. vol 5 (2) : 185 (1985).
31. Mester, E., et. al. : Biomedical Effects of Laser Application. Laser in Surg. and Med. 5 : 31-39 (1985).

32. Morselli, M.,et. al. : Very low energy density treatment by co2 Laser in Sport Medicine. Lasers Surg. and Med. vol 5 (2) : 150 (1985).
33. Motegi, M. : Application of Low Energy Laser in orthopedics. International Symposium on Low Energy Laser in Medicine and Surgery, Tokyo '85.
34. Ohara, I. : Application of Low Energy of Laser and light Emmeting Diode on Wound healing. International Symposium on Low Energy Laser in Medicine and Surgery, Tokyo '85.
35. Ohshiro, T. : Application of Low Energy laser to Living Tissue. International Symposium on Low Energy Laser in Medicine and Surgery, Tokyo '85.
36. Ohshiro, T. : Lumbago and Thermography. 6th Congress of The International Society for Laser Surgery and Medicine, Jerusalem 1985.
37. Ohshiro, T. : The diode Laser for Sports related and other types of pain : a review of 836 cases. 6th Congress of the International Society for Laser Surgery and Medicine. Jerusalem 1985.
38. Oyamada, Y. and Izu, S. : Application of Low Energy Laser in chronic rheumatoid arthritis and related rheumatoid disease. 6th Congress of The International Society for Laser Surgery and Medicine. Jerusalem 1985.
39. Palmieri, B., et. al. : Experimental Study on Wound Healing in the Rat. Medical Laser Report 2 : 6-8 (1985).
40. Pasariello, N., et. al. : Laser treatment and microcirculation. Medical Laser Report 3 : 11-12 (1985).
41. Shiroto, C., et. al. : Laser Stimulation Therapy using a diode laser : 1600 patients. Laser in Surg. and Med. vol 6 (2) 172-173 (1986).
42. Tang, X. M., and Chai, B. P. : Effect of CO2 Laser irradiation on experimental fracture healing. Lasers in Surg. and Med. vol 6 (3) : 346-352 (1986).
43. Trelles. M.A. and Mayayo, E. : Low Intensity Laser irradiation promotes more rapid repair of bone fracture : Experimental demonstration. Preceedings of The International Congress on Laser in Medicine and Surgery, Bologna 1985, p. 395-399.
44. Vuksic, M., et. al. : The use of the HeNe Laser for treating Bedsores in Elderly patients with Psychiatric disorder. Medical Laser Report 3 : 11-12 (1985).
45. Walker, J. : Laser Therapy for pain of Rheumatoid arthritis Laser in Surg. and Med. vol 6 (2) : 171 (1986).
46. Warnke, U. : An Elementar working mechanism of a semiconductor Laser effect on catalytic and redoxprocesses. Preceedings of the International Congress on Laser in Medicine and Surgery, Bologna 1985, p. 59-61.
47. Willner, R. et. al. : Low - Power infrared Laser biostimulation of chronic osteoarthritis in hand. Lasers in Surg. and Med. vol 5 (2) : 149-150 (1985).
48. Zalesskiy, V.N., et. al. : Treatment of the chronic venous ulcer of legs with low energy Laser Stimulation. Laser in Surgery and Medicine. Vol 5 (2) 143-144 (1985).
49. Zhou, Y. C. : Tooth extraction under laser accupuncture anesthesia. International Symposium on Low Energy Laser Medicine and Surgery, Tokyo '85.

---oOHKOo---

Laser Treatment of Backpain and Enthesiopathy in Ankylosing Spondylarthritis

Christian GÄRTNER, M.D. and M. BECKER, M.D.
Rheumatological Department, Krankenhaus Porz, Köln

Ankylosing spondylarthritis is one of the diseases which cause chronic pain, not only during the day, but often more severe during the night and in some cases nearly intolerable in the very early morning. Depending on stage and extension pain is localized at back, at the tendons (as enthesiopathy) and in about 30 % at joints because of peripheral arthritis. Common treatment uses NSAIDs and daily physiotherapy. The outcome with this concept of management for most patients is fair. Still not solved problems include: 1. loss of range of motion 2. management of iridocyclitis 3. side-effects of NSAIDs and 4. in some cases ineffectiveness of pain releaving drugs. Two years ago we reported our study with therpy-resistant tendonitis which we treated with low-power-laser. The immediate effect (87 %) and the long-term-outcome (80 %) of these patients has been as convincingly that we performed another preliminary study on 16 patients (10 male/ 6 female) with enthesiopathies (8 x achillestendon, 5 x periarthropathia coxae, 3 x plantar fasciitis) as manifestations of ankylosing spondylarthritis (12 x) or psoriasisarthritis (4 x). Treatment was performed with infrared-laser 904 nm (IR CEB Space) or IR mixed with He-Ne 632.8 nm (M 3 UP Space), the energy-density varied between 600 and 960 Joule/m^2, irradiations were daily up to 20 times as monotherapy. We registered pain at rest, on motion and during local pressure on a 10 cm scale, walk-distance and long-term-outcome after 5 to 15 months. 14 of 16 patients improved in all registered cathegories definitely. We closed this study in June 1986 but saw all successive patients once more:

none had relapsed ore needed any further treatment due to this condition

Therefore we now use this low-power-laser-method as treatment of choice in enthesiopathes. Up to may 1987 we have treated (all included) 43 enthesiopathies of different localisations with similar good results whereby only 9 of 43 did not response to this method.

Back pain resistant to common NSAIDs or intolerance of drugs is another problem managing ankylosing spondylarthritis. As enthesiopathies can be treated with low-power-lasers we have to discuss how much of the back pain is due to the arthritis of the small joints of the vertebrae themselves, which we shurely cannot reach directly with our laser equipment. A certain part of this pain may originate in the paravertebral soft tissue structures. And there we have a chance to reach them with infrared-lasers. Nevertheless is there place for a lot of scepticisme wether we are able to apply enough laser-energy locally that it can be effective in deeper regions. However we started a further preliminary open study on patients with back pain due to ankylosing spondylitis. The 24 patients (22 x ankylosing spondylitis, 2 x psoriasisspondylitis; 2 in stage I, 5 in stage II, 9 in stage III, 8 in stage IV; all fulfilled New-York-Criterions) who entered this study all had back pain despite the standard management described above. The used equipment was the M 3 UP, which is able to scan his beam over a widespread area. All patients were treated 30 minutes i.e. IR energy density was between 300 an 120 $Joule/m^2$; irradiations were 20 to 30 times daily within 4 to 6 weeks sparing the weekends. All of them continued their physical exercises and at first they took the same dose of their previous NSAID. We allowed to change the doses but not the drug itself and requested them to keep a diary with regard to 1. pain expressed in per cent compared to that during a preperiod of 14 days 2. the dose of NSAID per day 3. hours of morning stiffness and 4. frequency of waking ups at night due to back pain. Physical examination by a rheumatologist took place before the first and after the last treatment and after a further 2 and 6 weeks.

Results : P a i n could be reduced to zero or nearly zero in 21 /24 patients in this study. Three did not respond, neither directly nor the weeks after. This result could be held over months, the longest time after treatment without a relapse is now 18 months.
D r u g   c o n s u m p t i o n has been the same in our 3 nonresponders and 5 more patients, who needed the same dose, but then were free

from pain. Another 7 did reduce their NSAID to about the half of the original dose and remained during the controls after the treatment-periode at the same level. 9 of 24 have been able to stay without any NSAID or analgetic drug and are still free from pain.

Both effects (the pain reducing and the drug reducing) occured during the second and third week of treatment and became complete in the 5. and 6. week.

M o r n i n g   s t i f f n e s s   and times of w a k i n g   u p in the night went striktly parallel with pain releave.

R e d u c t i o n   o f   m o b i l i t y was measured in the three regions of the spine (lumbar, thoracic and cervical part) as flexion, retroflexion, sideflexion and rotation and as tip-to-floor-distance, SCHOBERs and OTTs signe and so on as common. Only two patients improved in these parameters of motion significantly, the others remained unaltered even instead beeing free from pain.

Finally we couldt not register any sideeffects in this studies neither in clinical nor in the biochemical parameters which we examined.

The previous reported short neuralgias occured with higher doses (more than 2000 Joule/m^2) in energy density, which we did not reach during this investigation.

C O N C L U S I O N

1. In this preliminary study of low-power-laser treatment of enthesio-pathies this method seems to be as effective as in tendonitis of other origin

2. Even severe back pain due to ankylosing spondylarthritis, which was therapy-resistant to the common regimen with NSAIDs and physical exercise can be releaved through a serie of low-power-laser-irradiations

3. It can economize consumption of antirheumatic drugs (NSAIDs)

4. The known side-effects are rare

After these preliminary studies we see necessity of further studies in that manner

SUMMERY

Our experience with Infrared-Laser-Treatment (IRL) of previously unsuccessfully managed chronic tendonitis encouraged us to introduce this method in the management of enthesiopathies and back pain due to ankylosing spondylitis. 16 patients suffering from enthesiopathies (8 x achillestendonitis, 5 x periarthropathia coxae, 3 x plantar fasciitis) were treated with IRL (device: I.R. CEB or M-3-UP from SPACE/ Turin/Italy). Local irradiations of 1o to 20 min for 5 to 20 times were performed. Usually pain relief occured locally after 4 - 6 min, which was sustained after the first time for over 6 hours and than longer from session to session. Examination of all patients 5 - 15 months later showed 14 / 16 having complete pain relief and improvement of function.

Another 24 patients with ankylosing spondylitis suffering from severe back pain were treated with IRL (only sacroileitis: 2x, stage II: 5x, stage III: 9x and stage IV 8 x). Irradiations were given over the whole painful area during 3o min daily 2o to 3o times. Exerciseprograms and NSAIDs have been the same, the dose of NSAID, pain score, morning stiffness, frequency of waking up night and measurements of spine-motion were registered. As in enthesiopathies pain relief occured during treatment in 21/24 patients and allowed 9/24 to omit drug treatment completely. 7/24 to reduce it to 5o%. 3/21 did not achieve any improvement. Spine mobility was not altered and basic lab was not changed. The result of this preliminary first study is important enough to be further studied in a double-blind trial.

Key words: Infraredlaser, Mid-Laser, enthesiopathy, ankylosing, spondylitis, pain therapy.

LITERATUR

1. ABERGEL, P., MEEKER, Ch., LAM, T.,DWYER, R., LESAVOY, M. and UiTTO, J. "Control of connective tissne metabolism by Lasers: recent development and future prospects" I. Am. Acad. Dermatol, Vol. 11 1984 pp. 1142-1150

2. BASLEER, C.: Effets du Laser Infra-Rouge sur des cultures de chondrocytes articulaires humains en trois dimensions. Int. Kongres Lasertherapie II VUB 1985 Middelkerke

3. DYSON, M.: Effects of the Space Mix 5 Laser on the healing of fullthickness excised lesions in CDI mice. Medical Laser Report 4 (1986) 2-7

4. ENGLAND, S., G. STRUTHERS, P. BACON: An observer blind trial of the IR-CEB-Laser in the treatment of bicipital tendonitis. Int. Cong. on Laser, Bologna (1985) 195

5. GÄRTNER, Ch. "Behandlung therapieresistenter Insertionstendinopathien mit Infrarot-Laser" Arthritis und Rheuma 8 (1986) p. 27-33

6. HOPKINS, G. O.: Double blind cross over trial of infrared-Laser in the treatment of tennis elbow. Int. Congres on Laser Bologna (1985) 210

7. LIEVENS, P.: De invloed van Laser Therapie op het wondgenezingsproces (regeneratie van lymfevaten). Int. Kongres Lasertherapie II VUB 1985 Middelkerke

8. MESTER, E. et al.: Effect of Laser-rays on wound-healing. Am. J. Surg. Vol. 122 (1971) p. 352

9. MEEUSEN, R.: Lasertherapie en pijn. Int. Kongres Lasertherapie II VUB 1985 Middelkerke

10. PALMIERI, B.: A double-blind stratified crossover study of amateur tennis players suffering from tenniselbow using infrared Lasertherapy. Med. Laser Rep. 1 (1984) 2-14

11. PALMIERI, B.: Mid Laser action mechanisms: facts and hypotheses. Med. Laser Report 2 (1985) 3-5

12. PALMIERI, B.: Effects du Laser sur la douleur. Int. Kongres Lasertherapie II VUB 1985 Middelkerke

13. PREHN, H.: Objective and quantitative proof of sensomotiric action of Mid-Laser therapy in man, by reflexsometry and somatosensory evoced potentials (SEP). Medical Laser Report 2 (1985) 9-17

14. SEICHERT, N. SIEBERT, B., SCHÖPS, P. " Die Soft-und Mid-Lasertherapie in der Physikalischen Medizin" Z. Phys. Med. Baln. Med. Klim. 15 (1986) 400-404

15. VOLPI,N.,E. DAVOLIO, P. LENZI, L. BOLOGNANI, G. MAINI: Effetti del Laser I.R. ad impulsi sull attivita enzimatica in vitro ed in vivo. Med. Laser Rep. 4 (1986) 9-15

16. WARNKE, U.: Ein elementarer Halbleiter-Laser- Wirkmechanismus bei katalytischen Prozessen und Redoxvorgängen. Int. Congress on Laser Bologna 1985 Monduzzi Edit. p. 225

17. WANDERKA, H.: Persönliche Mitteilung 1986

A Double Blind Study of Low Power He-Ne Laser Therapy in Rheumatoid Arthritis

Y. Oyamada, Div. of Orthopaedic Surgery, National Hanamaki Hospital, Hanamaki 025-03/Japan
R. Satodate, J. Nishida, Dept. of Pathology and Orthopaedic Surgery, Iwate Medical Univ. School of Medicine, Uchimaru 19-1, Morioka 020/Japan
S. Izu, Y. Aoki, Senko Medical Instrument Mfg. Co.,23-12, Hongo 3-Chome, Bunkyo-ku, Tokyo, Japan

SUMMARY

We have studied the effectiveness of He-Ne laser (8.5mW) in treatment of RA, OA, and cervical spondylosis of totally 92 patients. Placebo irradiation was applied to 37 patients,and He-Ne laser to 55 patients. The irradiation was performed 20 times in 10 weeks on each subject. The length of irradiation was 15 minutes per each treatment. During the experiment period, the assessment to tenderness, pain on motion, circumference, range of motion, grip strength, duration of morning-stiffness, hydrops, and ESR was performed. Urine 5-HIAA, thermograph, and other laboratory tests were also assessed. The general assessment by the doctors showed significant clinical difference ($P<0.01$) in the intergroup comparison. In the assessment of the patients' personal impression, significant improvement was recorded too ($P<0.01$).

INTRODUCTION

We started applying He-Ne laser to clinical evaluations since 1983. Since we obtained its significant anti-inflammatory and analgesic effects during the evaluations, we often reported that He-Ne laser therapy would be effective as a preservative treatment of RA. Recently, we have made a statistical analysis through a double blind study using He-Ne and dummy laser units.

PATIENTS

The patients attended the study are indicated on Table I. The criteria for selection and exclusion of the patients basically comply with those defined by the Japan Rheumatism Foundation Drug Evaluation Committee. During the experiment, analgesics, immunosuppressants and immunomodulators were not allowed. Neither physiotherapy was newly applied. Gold, D-penicillamine and corticosteroid which have not reached the stage of maintenance dose were allowed under the same conditions. Even analgesics without effects so far were allowed to use under the same conditions.

TABLE I.   THE PATIENTS IN THE STUDY

parameter	placebo Gr.	He-Ne Gr.
classical RA	24	32
definite RA	8	13
OA	2	6
cervical spondylosis	3	4
female	29	41
male	8	14
total	37	55
mean age	59.1	55.4

METHOD

The He-Ne laser unit used in the experiment: medium: helium-neon gas, output power: 8.5mW, wavelength: 632.8nm, spot size: 0.2mm, Model PDT manufactured by Senko Medical Instrument Mfg. Co., Tokyo, Japan. The outer shape of the placebo unit was completely same as the He-Ne unit. A neon lamp with non-thermal effect which was covered wtih a red filter was incorporated at the end of the dummy laser tube. Black caps were attached to the distal end of both the tubes so that the patients could not see the output power emission ports. In principle, points tender to pressure on the swollen joints or the roots of nerves were irradiated 20 times, 15 minutes per one treatment. The treatment period of both groups was 10 weeks. The placebo and He-Ne laser irradiations were performed by two experimenters who did not know to which group each patient had been assigned by the controller.

The items evaluated by the doctors were tenderness, pain on motion, circumference, range of motion, grip strength, duration of morning-stiffness, ESR, CRP, and RA test. The test items described in Lansbury Index were not evaluated because we are applying He-Ne laser as a way of local therapies. The standards of judgement on each evaluated item are as follows: TENDERNESS--0: not tender, +1: tender, +2: tender winced, +3: tender winced and withdrew, PAIN ON MOTION--0: no pain, +1: slight pain (ADL possible), +2: ADL difficult, +3: spontaneously painful at rest, CIRCUMFERENCE--judged by change of over 0.5 cm, RANGE OF MOTION--judged by change of over 10 degrees, GRIP STRENGTH--measured only in the cases of wrist joints, DURATION OF MORNING-

STIFFNESS--judged by improvement rate of more than 50%, HYDROPS--
judged by existence of hydrops, ESR--measured for one hour and judged
by change of over 20mm, CRP--judged by change of over 1mg/dl, RA TEST
--assessed into four steps, (-), (±), (+), (++), URINE 5-HIAA--mea-
sured throughout the experiment and judged by the frequency of the
peak values exceeding the baseline of 5mg/day. The standards of rating of final overall improvement are as follows: +3: SIGNIFICANTLY
IMPROVED--improvement observed in more than 5 evaluated items, +2:
IMPROVED--improvement in 3 to 4 items, +1: SLIGHTLY IMPROVED--impro-
vement in 1 to 2 items, 0: NO CHANGE--no change observed in the evaluated items, -1: SLIGHTLY EXACERBATED--exacerbation in 1 to 2 items,
-2: EXACERBATED: exacerbation in 3 to 4 items, -3: SIGNIFICANTLY EXA-
CERBATED--exacerbation in more than 5 items. The standards of rating
of the patients' personal impression are as follows: 1: MUCH BETTER
THAN BEFORE, 2: BETTER THAN BEFORE, 3: NO CHANGE, 4: WORSE THAN BEFORE
5: MUCH WORSE THAN BEFORE.

RESULT

Each parameter, the ratings obtained in the doctors' assessment and
the patients' personal impression were compared with each other between the two groups under the methods of statistical analysis (Wilco-
xon's test, chi square test, and t-test). The general assessment by
the doctors showed significant improvement in the He-Ne group (P<0.01)
(Table II). In the assessment of the patients' personal impression,
significant improvement was observed in the He-Ne group too (P<0.01)
(Table II).

TABLE II. THE GENERAL ASSESSMENT BY THE DOCTORS AND PATIENTS' PERSONAL IMPRESSION

items / methods	placebo Gr.	He-Ne Gr.	P (Wilcoxon)
nos. of cases	35	55	
Doctors' assessment: +3: significantly improved	2 (5.7%)	15 (27.3%)	P<0.01
+2: improved	2 (5.7%)	21 (38.2%)	
+1: slightly improved	4 (11.5%)	8 (14.5%)	
0: no change	6 (17.1%)	9 (16.4%)	
-1: slightly exacerbated	4 (11.5%)	2 (3.6%)	
-2: exacerbated	11 (31.4%)	0	
-3: significantly exacerbated	6 (17.1%)	0	
Patients' impression: 1: much better than before	1 (2.9%)	14 (25.5%)	P<0.01
2: better than before	10 (28.6%)	29 (52.7%)	
3: no change	13 (37.1%)	12 (21.8%)	
4: worse than before	8 (22.8%)	0	
5: much worse than before	3 (8.6%)	0	

In the intergroup comparison of each parameter, significant improvement was observed in tenderness, pain on motion, circumference, and range of motion (P<0.01), and also in CRP (P<0.05).

CONSIDERATION

In this double blind study, we observed improvement in CRP, although we observed no significant change in ESR. This fact seems to show that the He-Ne laser therapy could produce a good effect not only on the factors in the local therapy such as tenderness, pain on motion, circumference, range of motion, but also on some factors in the systemic therapy. In some cases, we noticed improvement in immuno-serum globulin, and immuno-complex in synovial fluid, and we are now under further investigation.

CONCLUSION

The result of this double blind study concretely showed that significant analgesic (improvement in tenderness, and pain on motion), and anti-inflammatory (improvement in circumference) effects could be obtained by He-Ne laser therapy, and eventually improvement in ADL could be obtained. This test result almost complys with our findings in the previous report.

REFERENCES

1) Mester E et al: Laser stimulation of wound healing. Acad Sci Hung, 17: 49-55,1976
2) Goldman TA: In the biomedical laser. Springer Verlag, 293-311,1981
3) Walker J: Relief from chronic pain by low power laser irradiation. Neuroscience Letters, 43:339-344,1983
4) Oyamada, Y.,et al: Application of low energy laser in chronic rheumatoid arthritis and related rheumatoid diseases J. Japanese Soc. Laser Med. 6: 375-378,1986 (in Japanese)

Postoperative Helium-Neon-Laser Irradiation in the Face and Neck Region

PORTEDER H.[1], RAUSCH E.[1], JASKULKA U.[1], VINZENZ K.[1],
SCHENK P.[2]

[1] Department for Maxillo-Facial Surgery,
University Vienna (Head:Prof.S.Wunderer,M.D.,D.M.D.)
1090 Vienna, Alserstraße 4
[2] Department for Oto-Rhino-Laryngology,
University Vienna (Head:Prof.K.Burian,M.D.)
1090 Vienna, Garnisongasse 13

Introduction

Soft lasers (i.e. He-Ne lasers of 2 mW and 5mW output respectively, lent by the firm of Silberbauer) have been in use at this clinic for the last six years. Beside our own animal experiments (Strassl et al. 1983) and electron microscopy studies (Schenk et al. 1986, Porteder et al. 1986) and on the basis both of relevant literature (Kovacs et al. 1974, Mester et al. 1974, Haina et al. 1981, Silberbauer 1984, Mester A.F. and Mester A. 1986, Hubacek et al. 1986, Kövy et al. 1986, Benedicenti 1986) and of initial clinical results (Porteder et al. 1983), which would seem to indicate that healing is promoted, we have been using the low-power laser to an increasing extent in clinical practice.

Material and method

A He-Ne laser with an output of 2 mW was used for four years until we were given the use of a He-Ne laser with an output of 5 mW. Apart from lesions of the oral mucosa, such as postoperative wounds, scares, prosthesis pressure sores (mucosal ulcera), aphthae or herpes simplex, the skin in the neck and face region is also irradiated. The new laser has been used to date on 82 patients (45 w, 37 m), with ages ranging from 17 to 69. This low-power laser has a wavelength of 632,8 nm and a beam diameter of 0,7 mm. It emits tracked beam, red monochromatic light with parallel phase waves.

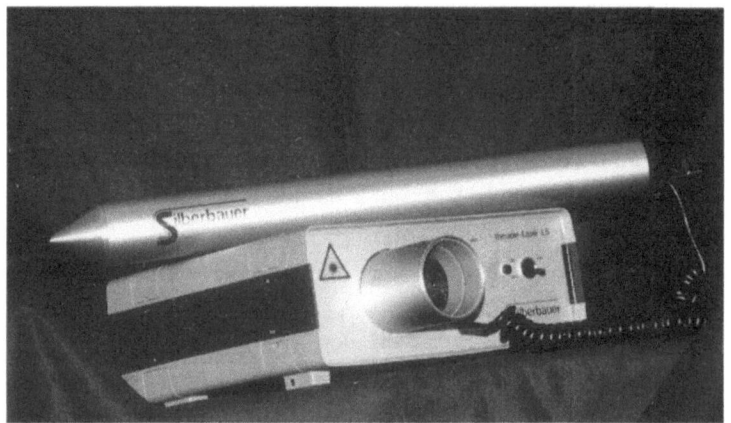

Irradiation was applied 2 to 3 times daily in the first 3 days, then 1 to 2 times daily. Exposure time per session and irradiation field was on average between 60 and 150 seconds. Irradiation was carried out over a period of at least four days to a maximum of eight days. It was carried out without any other local treatment.

TABLE I.   Distribution of lesions

Postoperative wounds of the oral mucosa	16
Prosthesis pressure sores (decubital ulcers)	19
Aphthae *	8
Herpes simplex	15
Neck and facial scares	24

* Not all aphthae were irradiated in each patient. Thus irradiated and non-irradiated aphthae could be compared in the same patient. Similar procedure was observed after surgical removal of gum tissue on opposite sides of the jaw. (l.h.upper jaw:r.h.upper jaw,l.h.lower jaw:r.h.lower jaw).

Results

All the patients tolerated the laser irradiation very well. No undesirable side-effects or subjectively unpleasent sensations were reported. The irradiated lesions of the oral mucosa displayed a clearly accelerated tendency to heal only two to three days after irradiation as compared to the non-irradiated regions (e.g.irradiation was only performed on one side after surgical removal of gingival pockets in the upper and lower jaw respectively). This effect was especially noticeable with the prosthesis pressure sores and decubital ulcers on the alveolar ridge mucosa.

Apart from four cases where the prosthesis had to be ground down, and one patient who had to have an alveolar ridge redressement, in all other patients granulation and epithelisation of the mucosal lesions were accelerated by this treatment.

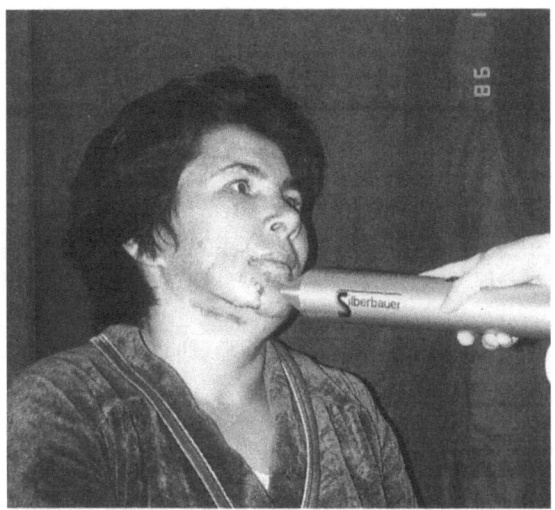

With the irradiated aphthae (n=8) rapid fading of the halo with significant alleviation of pain was observed, as compared to the non-irradiated aphthae.

Laser therapy has proved effective in the treatment of herpes simplex. From the second or third day of treatment onwards, the erythema and blisters were already observed to be remitting. Subjective discomfort began to subside fast. In the case of 4 patients we were able to commence treatment in the initial phase of the affection, here the development of blisters was inhibited.

Postoperative lesions of the face and neck healed more quickly after laser therapy. The scares were on average less conspicuous compared to those of a group of patients who had not undergone laser therapy.

Discussion

Our results and observations coincide with those of other authors (Chlebarov 1986, Benedicenti 1986, Mester E. 1981, etc.). The results of animal experiments (Kana 1981, Haina 1981) and electron microscopy experiments (Porteder 1986,Schenk1986) indicate the effectiveness of He-Ne lasers on various tissue and cell structures.

Assuming a critical stance towards these results, we agree with Pratzel (1986) in his demands for precise, reproduceable studies to qualify and quantify the effect of laser irradiation on biological tissue. We see these demands as a matter of concern regarding basic research in general. We have already taken a step in this direction with our electron microscopy and biochemical studies (Strassl et al. 1983).

In conclusion it can be said that the clinical results obtained give support for the therapeutic use of soft lasers, even if the effective principle has not yet been fully clarified.

Literatur

BENEDICENTI A.:Laser treatment of Periodontopathies,Laser-Optoelectronics in Medicine Eds:Waidlich W.,Kiefhaber P.,Springer Verl.,1986,136-139
CHLEBAROV S.:Dermatologische Indikationen für die Laser-Reiztherapie,Laser-Optoelectronics in Medicine,Eds.:Waidlich W.,Kiefhaber P.,Springer Verl.,1986,110-115
HAINA D:,R.Brunner,M.Landthaler,W.Waidlich,O.Braunfalco:Stimmulierung der Wundheilung mit Laserlicht-Klinische und tierexperimentelle Untersuchungen.Hautarzt (Suppl. V),32,(1981),429.
HUBACEK J.,J.Pospisilova,Z.Hlozek:Effect of He-Ne-Laser on healing of Wounds,Laser-Optoelectronics in Medicine,Eds.:Waidlich W.,Kiefhaber P.,Springer Verl.,1986, 199-203
KARNER J.S.,G.Hutschenreiter,D.Haina,W.Waidlich:Effect of low-power density laser radiation on healing of open skin wounds in rats.Arch.Surg.116,(1981),293.
KOVACS I.B.,E.Mester,P.Görög:Stimulation of wound healing with laser beam in the rat. Experientia 30,(1974),1275.
KÖVY M.B.,S.Tisza,A.Eöry:Veränderung der Parameter auf der Hautoberfläche infolge der Einwirkung von Softlasern,Laser-Optoelectronics in Medicine,Eds:Waidlich W., Kiefhaber P.,Springer Verl.,1986,144-148.
MESTER A.F.,A.Mester:Mester's Method of Laser Biostimulation,Laser-Optoelectronics in Medicine,Eds:Waidlich W.,Kiefhaber P.,Springer Verl.,1986,103-109.
MESTER E.:Über die stimulierende Wirkung der Laserbestrahlung auf die Wundheilung. In:Der Laser.Dinstl K.,P.L.Fischer (Hrsg.),Springer Verl.,(1981),109.
PORTEDER H.,H.Strassl,G.Stanek,K.Vinzenz:Einsatz des Helium-Neon-Lasers zur Förderung der Wundheilung,Österr.Zschr.Stomatol.,9,(1983)333-339.
PORTEDER H.,P.Schenk,K.Zetner:Tierexperimentelle elektronmikroskopische Studie über die Wirkung des Helium-Neon-Lasers,Laser-Optoelectronics in Medicine,Eds: Waidlich W.,Kiefhaber P.,Springer Verl.,1986,161-164.
PRATZEL H.:Biochemische Lichteffekte durch Laser,Laser-Optoelectronics in Medicine, Eds.:Waidlich W.,Kiefhaber P.,Springer Verl.,1986,140-143.
SCHENK P.,H.Porteder,K.Zetner:Helium-Neon-Laser-Effekt auf Haut und orales Schleimhautgewebe.Laryngol.-Rhinol.-Otol.,3,(1986),146-150.
SILBERBAUER G.,1984,Personal communication.
STRASSL H.,Porteder H.,Zetner K.:Tierexperimentelle Studie über den Einsatz von Laserstrahlen zur Beeinflussung der Wundheilung,Acta Chir. Austriac.15,(1983)33-42.

Acknowledgements

We would like to express our thanks to the firm Dipl.Ing.Silberbauer - Medizinische und physikalische Elektronik- for its generosity in lending us a Helium-Neon Laser.

Authors address

Univ.Doz.Dr.Hubert Porteder, Dept.f.Maxillo-Facial Surgery, University Vienna, 1090 Vienna, Alserstraße 4.

Laser Stimulation Therapy Using a Diod Laser

*CHIYUKI SHIROTO, KEIICHI ONO
**TOSHIO OHSHIRO
*IInd Dept. of Surg. School of Med.
Hirosaki University
**Japan Medical Laser Laboratory

For more than 3 years, we have been continuing pain-alleviating therapy using a low-power diode laser and made a clinical estimation of the efficacy of this method. We have presented the results at several conferences and meetings, either domestic or international.

on this occasion, I would like to present the summary of this therapy applied to 2,544 patients.

The instrument used was 'Panalas 4000', a portable low-power diode laser pain attenuator designed and manufactured by Japan Medical Laser Laboratory and Matsushita Electric Company. It operates at a wavelength of 830 nanometers and has a power output of 60 mW. In order to protect the eyes of a patient, the instrument is designed to operates only when the touch-sensor, built in the probe, comes in contact with the skin. A sound and light signals indicate the emission of laser beam. The instrument also contains a power meter that allows a easy of the power level. The laser light converges into a focussed beam two millimeters ahead the tip of the probe. Usually, the probe is directly applied to tender points, 'tsubo' or acupuncture points.

The patients included in this study were treated in a period of from April 1984 to December 1986. The total number of the patients were 2,544, 1058 male and 1486 female. The average age of the patients was 53.4 years. As most of the patients complained of more than one painful lesion, we took each one lesion as one case. Therefore, 3,876 cases (from 2,544 patients) are presented here.

The cummurative number of the performances summed to 29,002. The number of shots given to each case ranged from one to 289. The average length of each irradiation was 316 seconds.

A variety of painful symptoms or diseases which we treated are listed in the Table. Muscular were further categorized into five. These were stiff shoulder, lower extremity pain, upper extremity pain, back and chest pain and generalized whole body pain.

We ranked the efficacy of this laser treatment as excellent, good, slight, no change and aggravation, depending on the responses of the patients to this method. The result was, excellent in 34.6% of all cases, good in 49.4%, slight in 12.7% equivocal in 3.4% and aggravation in 0.1%. The Japanese sometimes feel it quilty to declare no efficacy of a therapy especially when a doctor in charge is very enthusiastic with his method he applies to them. We should, therefore, ignore the ranking of 'slight effect'. Nevertheless, positive responses, either excellent or good, were obtained in 84.0% of all cases treated. And so far as muscular pain was concerned, the efficacy amounted to 85%. Although the estimation of the efficacy of this laser therapy solely depends on a subjective judgement of the patients, the fact remains that most of the patients expressed a satisfaction with this therapy.

The painful regions with a relatively short history were much easier to treat compared to those with a old history. Characteristically, few patients mentioned an immediate effect of the therapy. They often reported their relief from the pain several hours later the treatment or even on the following day. The relief lasted for only 5 or 6 hours to as long as one month.

Two symptoms, periarthritis scapulohumeralis and lumbago, allowed a rather objective analysis of the effectivity of this laser therapy. Before administrating this treatment, the patients with either of these symptoms were often unable to raise their arm or unable to sit up. But after this, they could do so. Therefore, we felt these cases might be a good indicator to measure the efficacy of our diode laser therapy.

In conclusion, although there was no case where a single shot of irradiation sufficed to relieve the pain completely, this laser therapy, when repeated over a certain period of time, did provided a relief from pain that had not been given by other methods of treatments.

Duration of Experiment

April,1984-December,1986(32 months)

No.of Patients	2,544 (M.1,058 ; F.1,486)
No.of Symptoms	3,876 (M.1,465 ; F.2,411)
Aver.of Age	53.4 (M.50.9 ; F.54.5)
Actual No.of Treatments	29,002
Treatments per Patient	11.4
Minimum No.of Treatments	1
Maximum No.of Treatments	289
Aver. Time per Session(sec.)	316 (5' 16")

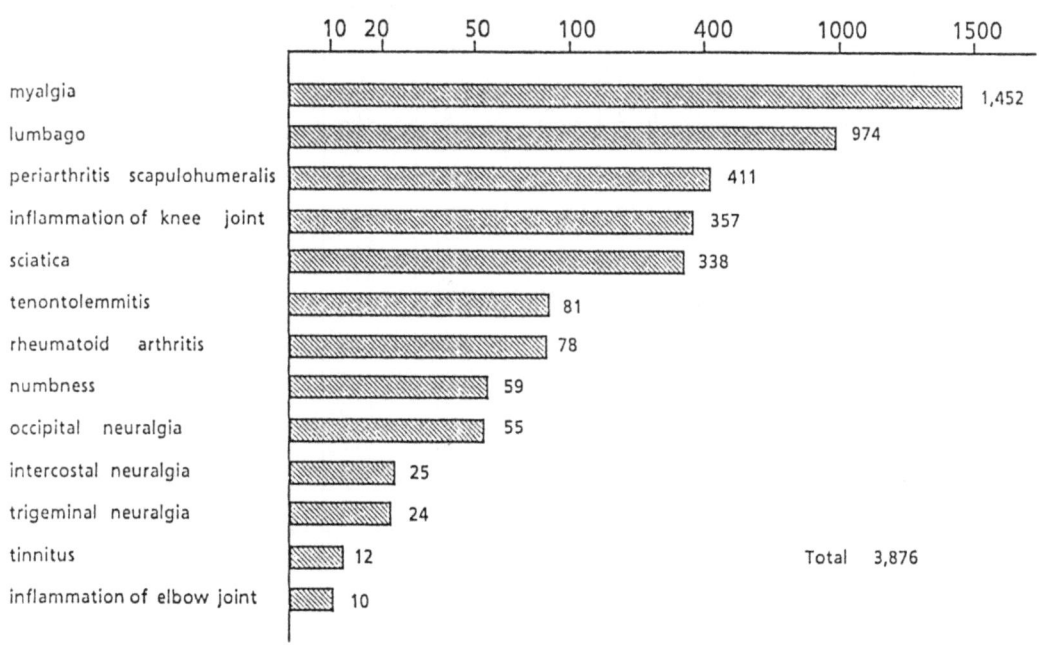

No. of Cases Treated

myalgia	1,452
lumbago	974
periarthritis scapulohumeralis	411
inflammation of knee joint	357
sciatica	338
tenontolemmitis	81
rheumatoid arthritis	78
numbness	59
occipital neuralgia	55
intercostal neuralgia	25
trigeminal neuralgia	24
tinnitus	12
inflammation of elbow joint	10

Total 3,876

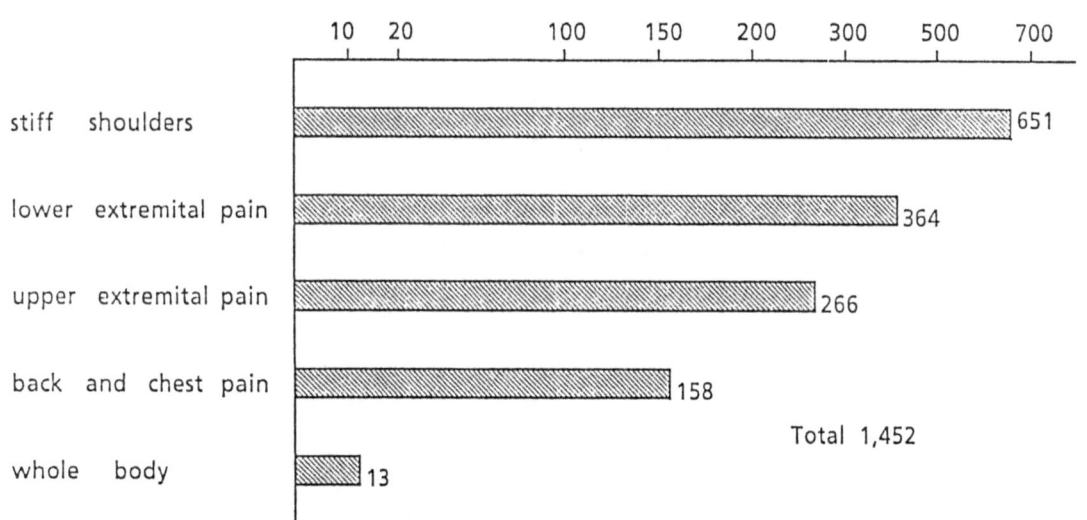

Muscular Pain : No. of Cases Treated

stiff shoulders	651
lower extremital pain	364
upper extremital pain	266
back and chest pain	158
whole body	13

Total 1,452

No. of Cases Treated

Symptoms	No.of Cases	Male	Female	Aver. of Age	Aver.Time per Session (sec.)	Aver. Treatments Per Patient	Aver. Effect
myalgia	1,452	509	943	51.9	282	10.7	4.2
lumbago	974	424	550	53.5	336	10.9	4.2
periarthritis scapulohumeralis	411	204	207	55.5	338	9.5	4.2
inflammation of knee joint	357	76	281	58.7	287	12.6	4.2
sciatica	338	133	205	55.1	334	11.2	4.1
tenontolemmitis	81	22	59	49.6	244	11.9	4.0
rheumatoid arthritis	78	15	63	52.2	524	22.7	3.8
numbness	59	26	33	53.6	399	17.2	4.0
occipital neuralgia	55	22	33	49.8	336	5.6	4.1
intercostal neuralgia	25	10	15	53.6	297	10.8	4.3
trigeminal neuralgia	24	12	12	64.3	277	13.6	3.9
tinnitus	12	7	5	56.0	303	10.4	3.9
inflammation of elbow joint	10	5	5	53.1	306	5.7	4.1
total	3,876	1,465	2,411	53.4	316	11.4	4.15

No. of Cases Treated

Symptoms	No.of Cases	Therapeutic Effects(%)					(卌) + (卄) %
		Excellent (卌)	Good (卄)	Slight (+)	No change (±)	Aggravation (−)	
myalgia	1,452	35.5	49.5	12.1	2.9	0	85.0
lumbago	974	36.5	48.5	12.3	2.7	0	85.0
periarthritis scapulohumeralis	411	36.0	49.6	12.0	2.2	0	85.6
inflammation of knee joint	357	35.8	50.7	10.6	3.1	0	86.5
sciatica	338	31.7	48.5	13.0	6.5	0.3	80.2
tenontolemmitis	81	26.0	50.6	18.5	4.9	0	76.6
rheumatoid arthritis	78	16.7	48.7	25.6	9.0	0	65.4
numbness	59	30.5	47.5	18.6	3.4	0	78.0
occipital neuralgia	55	32.7	49.1	14.5	3.6	0	81.8
intercostal neuralgia	25	40.0	44.0	8.0	8.0	0	84.0
trigeminal neuralgia	24	18.2	45.5	36.4	0	0	63.7
tinnitus	12	8.3	75.0	8.3	8.3	0	83.3
inflammation of elbow joint	10	30.0	50.0	10.0	10.0	0	80.0
total	3,876	34.6	49.4	12.7	3.4	0.1	84.0

Muscalar Pain (No.0f Cases Treated)

Symptoms	No.of Cases	Therapeutic Effects(%)					(卌) + (卄) %
		Excellent (卌)	Good (卄)	Slight (+)	No change (±)	Aggravation (−)	
stiff shoulders	651	36.0	52.4	9.3	2.3	0	88.4
lower extremital pain	364	36.4	46.2	13.9	3.4	0	82.6
upper extremital pain	266	30.5	50.7	15.1	3.7	0	81.2
back and chest pain	158	36.9	50.6	10.0	2.5	0	87.5
whole body	13	46.0	46.0	8.0	0	0	92.0
total	1,452	35.5	49.5	12.1	2.9	0	85.0

Treatment of Peripheral and Central Nervous Systems After Injury Using Low Energy Laser Irradiation: Experimental Results

S.Rochkind, M.Nissan, L.Barr-Nea, R.Lubart,
N.Brusovalnic, N.Razon, Y.D.Heilbronn, A.Bartal
Neurosurgery Dept. Tel-Aviv Medical Center, Ichilov Hospital
Center for Technological Education, Holon
Tel-Aviv University and Bar-Ilan Univ. ISRAEL

Our group has been working on various aspects of Low Energy Laser Irradiation - LELI - and its effects on the Peripheral Nervous System - PNS - during the last 8 years. In this work we used HeNe lasers to irradiate, directly or transcutaneously, the sciatic nerve of rats in vivo.

Action Potential - AP - was measured for immediate assessment of LELI effects, and histology was used to assess degenerative and regenerative processes. Our scope covered normal, healthy nerves, crushed and cut nerves. We published already a number of clinical, electrophysiological and histological results related to this work (1,2,3,4,5).

We found LELI to prevent the degeneration of the injured nerve that usually follows a crush to the PNS and to enhance regeneration. These findings encouraged us to apply LELI directly to the nerve cell in the spinal cord instead of the injured site. We caused a crush injury to the sciatic nerve in a group of rats and closed the wound. Next we irradiated transcutaneously the corresponding segments in the spinal cord using a CW HeNe laser (16mW). The injured site was not irradiated at all.

The short term effects were assessed electrophysiologically. A Grass stimulator delivered the needed stimulus to the nerve vicinity proximally to the crush and a Beckman Dynograph recorded the resulting AP distally to the crush site. We started irradiation the day after the crush and continued for 20 consecutive days, Figure 1.

Figure 1.

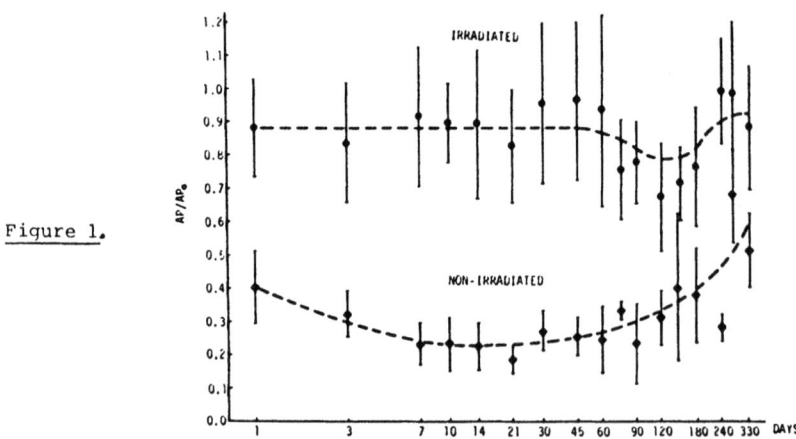

The encouraged findings in the PNS led us to look for possible effects of LELI on the CNS proper. During the last two years we developed a model and an operation procedure for assessing such effects in-vivo. Our injury model is a complete transaction of the spinal cord in the dog at the D_{10}-D_{11} level. This kind of injury causes an irreversible, complete paralysis of the lower body including both legs.

Some recent publications (6) claimed that an autologous graft of a peripheral nerve into the transected area encourage regeneration. We decided to combine grafting and LELI in our method. We used two groups of dogs: 7 dogs had only grafting and serve as controls while 10 other dogs had LELI using 16mW CW HeNe laser over the transection and grafting site. Otherwise both groups were treated identically.

Of the 7 non-irradiated dogs 4 died within a month and all the others were paralysed with minimal improvement within the test period.

In the irradiated group we found totally different results:

Only 1 dog died in the first 3 months and all the others started to use their hindfeet. After 1 month the dogs were trying to stand, Figure 2, for short periods and 2 months later the dogs were walking again, Figure 3.

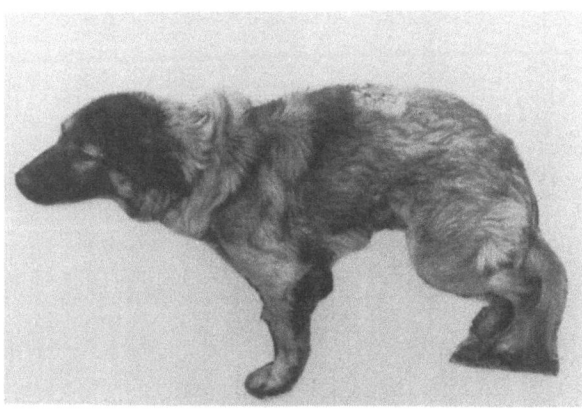

Figure 2.

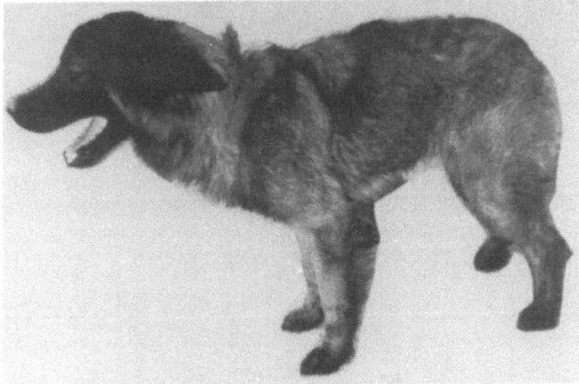

Figure 3.

I would like to emphasize that these last findings were similar in all the irradiated dogs (9 out of 10) and the pictures are not from the best performing animal. Histologically we looked on the grafted area in the irradiated dogs 21 days after the transection and grafting.

We found almost no scar tissue, no gliosis and no cysts. Instead we found new axons to cross the injured area.

At the end I would like to express our hope that our work will be used on human patients shortly and will contribute towards the cure of a major medical problem in a world with so many wars and accidents.

This work was supported by a joint grant from the Ministry of Industry and Commerce and Ramot, Tel-Aviv University.

References

(1) S. Rochkind: Stimulation effect of laser energy on the regeneration of traumatically injured Peripheral nerves. The Kim National Medical Inst., Morphogenesis & Regeneration, (1978), 73:48-50.

(2) S. Rochkind, M. Nissan, N. Razon, M. Schwartz, A. Bartal: Electrophysiological effect of HeNe on Normal and Injured Sciatic Nerves in the Rat. Acta Neurochir (Wien) (1986) 83:125-130.

(3) S. Rochkind, N. Razon, A. Bartal, M. Nissan: HeNe Low Energy laser - is it completely harmless? J. Biomed. Engineering (1986), 8(1):77

(4) M. Nissan, S. Rochkind, N. Razon, A. Bartal: HeNe laser irradiation delivered transcutaneously: its effect on the Sciatic nerve of Rats. Lasers in Surgery and Medicine (1986) 6:435-438.

(5) S. Rochkind, M. Nissan, L. Barr-Nea, N. Razon, M. Schwartz, A. Bartal: Response of peripheral nerve to HeNe laser: experimental studies. Submitted: Lasers in Surgery and Medicine.

(6) P.M. Richardson, U.M. McGuinness, A.J. Aguayo: Axons from CNS neurons regenerate into PNS grafts, Nature, 284, 264-265, 1980.

Investigations on Different Laser Wavelengths and Power in Peripheral and Central Nervous System

R. Lubart, S. Rochkind, M. Nissan, L. Barr-Nea

Bar-Ilan University. Neurosurgery Dept. Tel-Aviv Medical Center
Ichilov Hospital. Center for Technological Education, Holon
Sackler Faculty of Medicine, Tel-Aviv University. Israel

Introduction

In recent publications (1,2,3,4) we have reported the effect of Low Energy Laser Irradiation -LELI- on the regeneration of peripheral nerves in rats following a crush injury and using a He-Ne laser (632,8nm). We were looking into various parameters affecting the efficacy of so-called soft lasers on the biological material in vivo. In the work presented here we report our results comparing 3 wavelengths: 465nm, 520nm and 588nm. According to Olson (5) and others, the wavelength is probably one of the most critical factors.

Experiments and Results

in order to investigate the influence of various wavelengths on the electrical activity of nerves, the sciatic nerves of 16 rats were crushed and subsequently irradiated transcuteanously for 7 minutes daily and for 20 consecutive days. The rats were divided into four groups of 4 and each group was irradiated by one of the following laser sources:

1. C.W He-Ne laser - 632nm, 16mw
2. C.W Ar laser - 465nm, 40mw
3. C.W Ar laser - 520nm, 40mw
4. Pulsed dye-laser - 588nm, 20mw, $10H_3$

Thirty days post operation the rats vertebral columns were removed and the spinal cord prepared for light microscopy. The degree of chromatolysis was determined in each spinal cord. The results showed that all types of laser irradiation had a positive effect on the spinal cord, manifesting itself in the prevention of chromatolysis and in the increase of Nissl bodies in the nerve cells. The magnitude of the effect decreased with wavelength from 632nm down to 465nm. This is probably due to the poor penetration of the shorter wavelenghts through the biological tissues. the effect of penetration was measured by us in another experiment.

To avoid this handicap, and to measure the net effect of the influence of various wavelengths on the nervous system we intend to use a direct method, as described in the following paragraph.

The nerve of the rat is exposed under a surgical microscope and hook-shaped electrodes are attached to it. A Grass stimulator is used to stimulate the nerve and the resulting compound A.P. (Action Potential) is recorded on a Beckman Dynograph.

We used this method for measuring the effect of He-Ne and obtained the following results:

Test no 1.   After establishing the normal A.P. for 10 minutes, the exposed nerve was irradiated for 7 minutes with a 0.3m.w C.W He-Ne laser. The A.P. was then measured for 10 minutes. The nerve was crushed by closing a standard haemostat on it for 30 seconds and the A.P was measured again (Fig 1).

Fig 1.

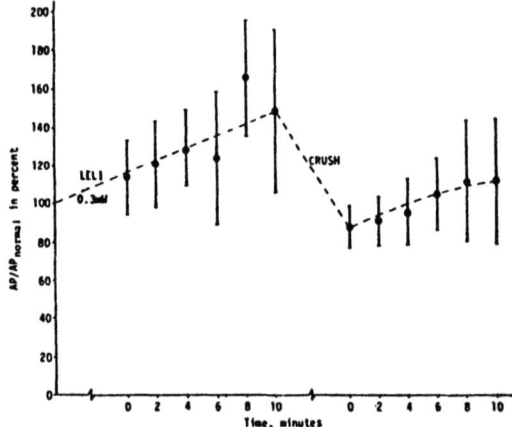

One can see that the application of the laser to the normal naked nerve causes an increase in A.P. by up to 150%. This indicates clearly that LELI affects the nerve itself. The crush induced a sharp decrease in the nerve electrical activities, which remains however around the normal value.

Test no 2.   After establishing the normal A.P. the nerve was crushed. A reduced A.P. was then measured for 10 minutes. The crushed nerve was irradiated for 7 minutes and an increase in A.P. was recorded (Fig 2).

Fig 2.

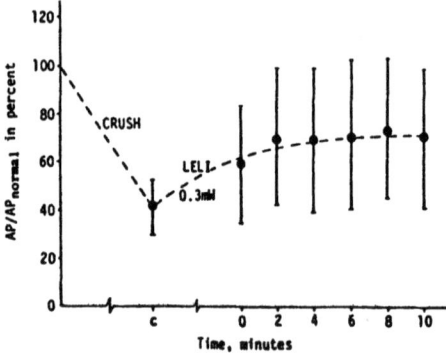

Here we see that a crush injury causes the A.P to fall to about 40% of the normal value. The application of LELI to the nerve in vivo, causes the A.P. to increase to nearly 70% of its normal value.

We repeated Test no.2 with 17 m.w He-Ne laser with effect on A.P . see Fig. 3.

Fig.3.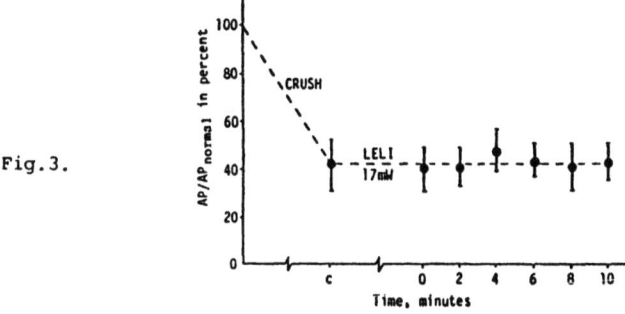

As can be seen, this system is a very convenient one for measuring the influence of different parameters on nerve regeneration.

References

1. Nissan M., Rochkind S., Razon N., Bartal A. HeNe laser irradiation delivered trancutaneously: its effect on the sciatic nerve of rats. Lasers Surg.Med. 1986.
2. Rochkind S., Barr-Nea L., Razon N., Bartal A., Schwartz M. Stimulatory effect of He-ne loe dose laser on injured sciatic nerves of rats. Neurosurger 20:843-847, 1987.
3. Rochkind S., Nissan M., Razon N., Schwartz M., Bartal A. Electrophysiological effects of He-Ne laser on normal and injured sciatic nerve in rats. Acta Neurochir. 83:125-130, 1986.
4. Rochkind S., Nissan M., Barr-Nea L., Razon N., Schwartz M., Bartal A. Response of peripheral nerve to HeNe laser: experimental study. Lasers Surg. Med. (In press).
5. Olson J.E., Schimmerling W., Tobias C.A. Laser action spectrum of reduced excitability in nerve cells. Brain Research 204:436-440, 1981.

Effect of Low Power Laser Radiation on Experimental Burns and Their Application in Clinics

M.A. Trelles, M.D.*, E. Mayayo, M.D.**, F. Dalmases, M.D.***, C. Romero, M.D.***

* Instituto Médico Vilafortuny, Cambrils/Tarragona -E
** Serv. Anatomía Patológica del Hosp. Juan XXIII, Tarragona y Dpto. de Histología de la Fctad. de Medicina de Reus/Univ. de Barcelona -E
*** Cátedra de Física Médica, Fctad. de Medicina de la Univ. de Valencia -E

INTRODUCTION

A number of different procedures are currently used with the aim of accelerating the healing of burns, as one of the direct consequences of the frequent complications accompanying burns is the need for xenografting, artificial skin grafting and other costly modes of therapy. A safe and secure therapeutic procedure which would avoid the need for such treatments would constitute a marked advance in the management of lesions resulting from burns (1).

The present study was undertaken in an attempt to determine the effect of low intensity laser beams on burns, induced with a standarized burning device, investigating the repairing process of the lesion comparatively to a control group.

MATERIAL AND METHOD

1) _Description of a prototype unit to produce standarized burns_: A burning device was used for this experiment. It consists of an aluminum head fixed to a mobile arm which was attached to a non-mobile column. The column stood on a platform on which the experimentation animal was placed (Fig 1).

The mobile arm of the burning device falls down vertically at a constant speed to the area previously designated for

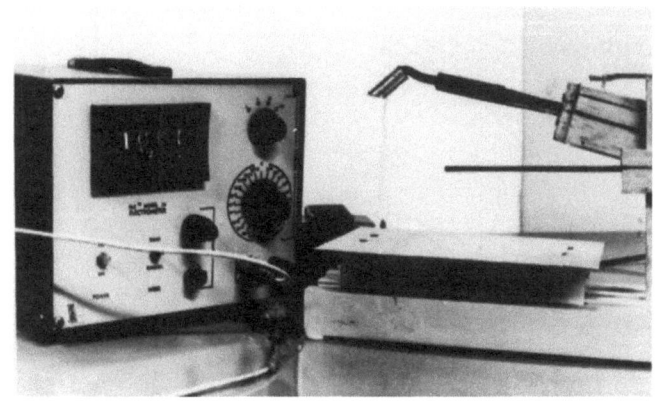

Fig. 1. Display of the thermoelectric-par, connected to the digital voltimeter for heat temperature measurement of the head of the burning device

burning. Burning was produced for a fixed time (in this experiment it was of 5 seconds). The platform on which the animal was placed was able to be moved horizontally and vertically so that the animal could be placed at the desired limit for burning procedure. The burning area was circular and of 1 cm. diametre.

The burning device stabilizes its temperature at $160°$ Celsius after 30 minutes of being connected to an electric current of 220 volts (Graph I).

2) Animal_selection: Two groups of mice were used. Group (A) was treated with laser and group (B) was kept as control. The mice were of the hair-less type MRL25, of 15 to 20 grms in weight. They were kept under the same living conditions.

Before burning, the animals were anaesthetisized by injecting 1 mg Kethamine (Ketalar -R- Parke Davis). Thirty minutes after burning, the animals of group (A) were irradiated with He/Ne 632 nm laser light, beamed directly on center of the lesion from approximately 10 cm. (Fig 2-3).

Graph I.

Curve of stabilization of burning divice measure in centigrade at room temperature related to time (minutes).

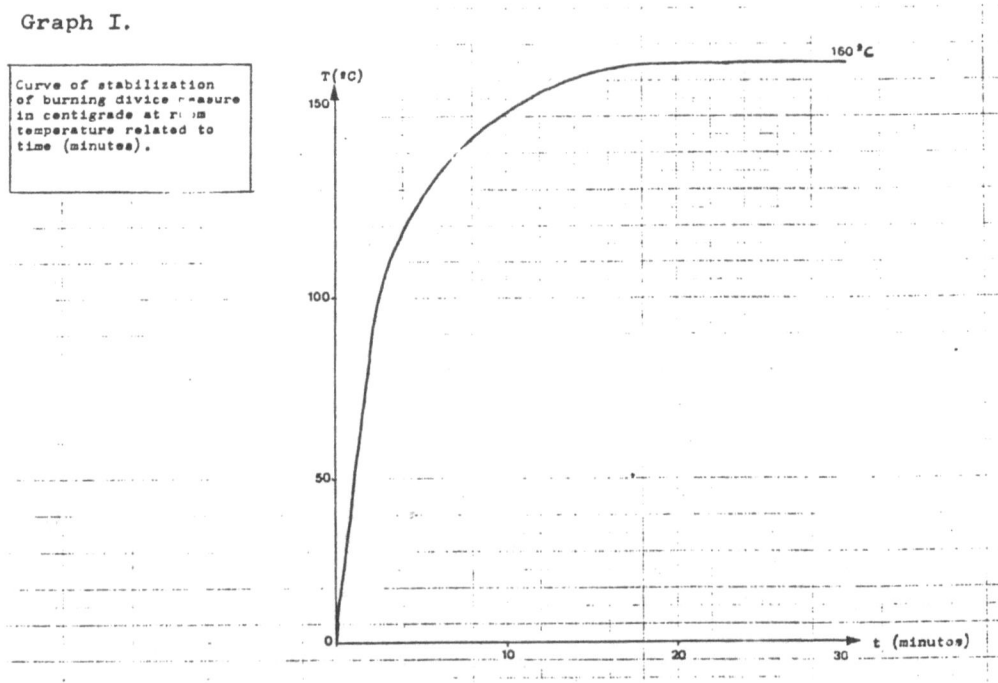

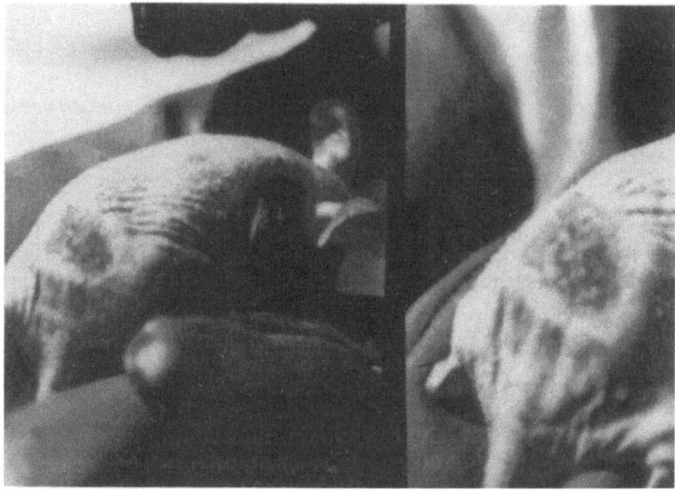

Fig. 2. Detail of the animal immediately after a standardized burn

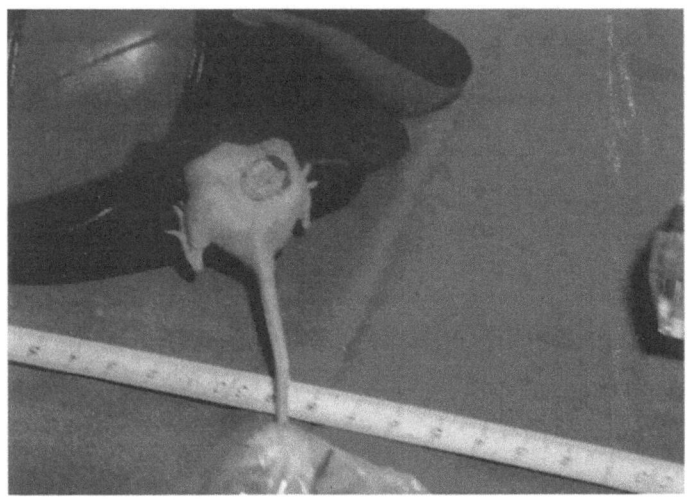

Fig. 3. Laser irradiation of the experimental burn

Output of laser was 4 mW, applied for 10 minutes (beam of 1 mm diametre). Irradiations were done every day-up to a total of 27. In control group (B) the whole treatment was simulated. Neither group (A) nor (B) received any local or general medication.

3) Examination of tissue samples: A photographic control of the evolution of the burnt lesion was carried out, as well as a bacteriological screening every 8 days. Samples of burnt tissue were taken on the 10th day after burning as well as on the 27th day-the end of the experiment. The histological examination was undertaken by optic microscopy after processing by routine technique and stained by Hematoxiline and Eosine.

RESULTS

1) Macroscopic examination.

Immediately after burning, the area of lesion showed an

Graph II.
BURNS UNDER LOW POWER LASER IRRADIATION

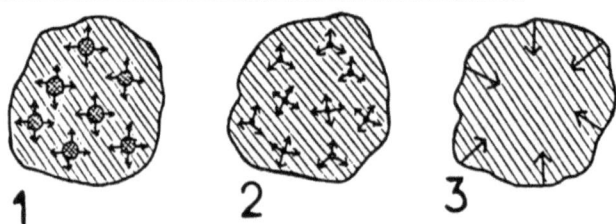

1-. Burn of superficial dermis, active centrifugal cicatrization
2-. Burn of deep dermis
3-. III degree burn, centripetal cicatrization

aspect of tanned leather (Fig 2), softly depressed in comparison to the healthly skin around the edges, which appear with oedema. At the 10th day, the burnt lesion of group (A), treated with laser, became darkened, developing a crust that progressively advanced from the periphery to the center during the following days (Graph II). The crust completely fell away between 18 to 20 days after burning. In control group (B) evolution was slower, and on day 20 the crusts still remained on the lesions.

At day 8, in group (A), the lesion showed a rich granulation tissue of a vivid red colour and, at the same time, in control group (B) the lesion was pale and of irregular aspect (Fig 4-5).

At day 27 when the experiment had finished, group (A) presented a fine cicatrization tissue, well constituted and of a good cosmetic appearance on the same day, while group (B) appeared with irregular zones of cicatrization, and the lesion had, macroscopically, a certain fibrotic component (Fig 6-7).

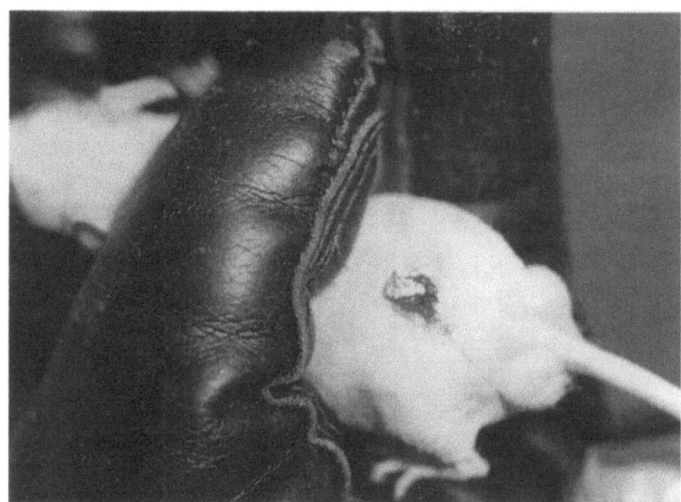

Fig. 4. Burn of the control group at 14 days

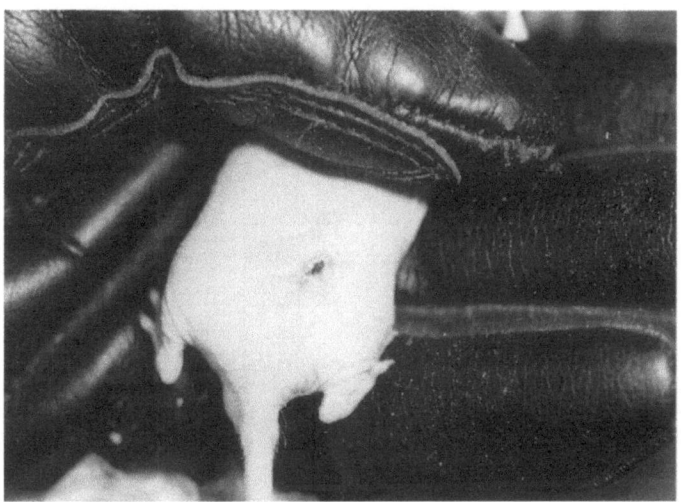

Fig. 5. Burn at 14 days irradiated with He/Ne laser. Observe, comparing with fig. 4, the greater speed of reparation

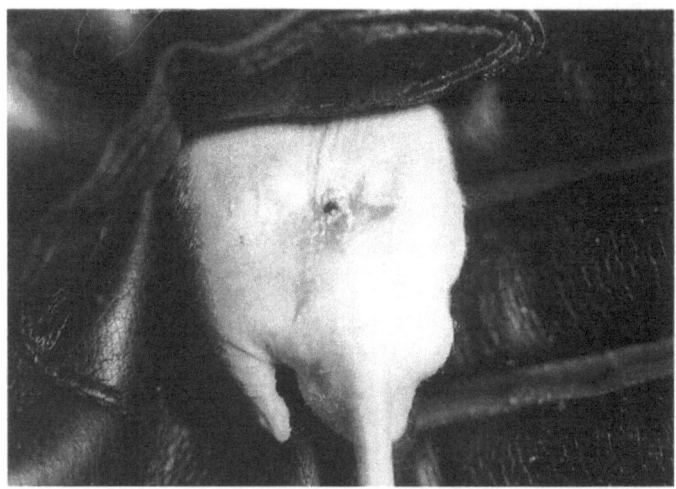

Fig. 6. Burns of the non-irradiated control group at 27 days (end of experiment)

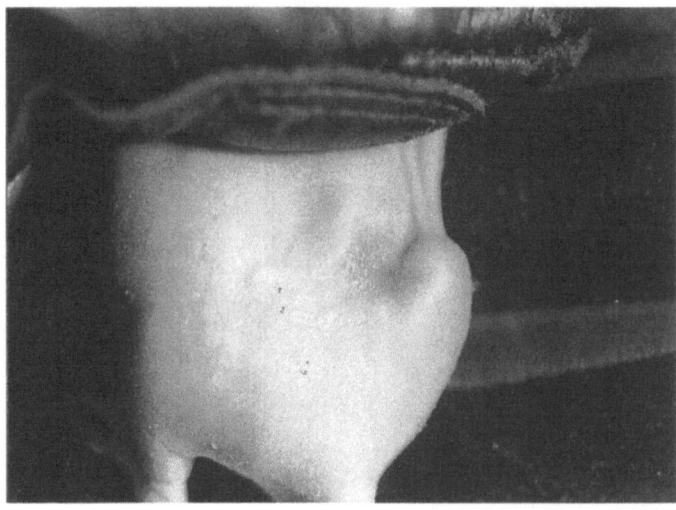

Fig. 7. Irradiated burn (He/Ne laser) at 27 days (end of experiment). Note better aesthetic quality of the tissue, compared to fig. 6 (non irradiated animal)

2) Microscopic examination

Ten days after burning it could be observed in both groups (A and B) that the epidermis and dermis had similar characteristics. The epidermis showed a regenerative aspect with increase of cellular layers and a prominent basal sheet. On the dermis an increase of collagen was noted together with regenerative fibrosis of low inflammatory component. In the irradiated group (A) was observed at this stage of treatment a slight vascular neoformation that did not exist in the control group (B) which appeared without hipodermis, cutaneous anexes and capillars.

In histological samples corresponding to the 27th day (Fig 8-10), at the end of the experiment in both groups (A and B) it was observed that the epidermis had fewer layers compared to tissue samples of the 10th day.

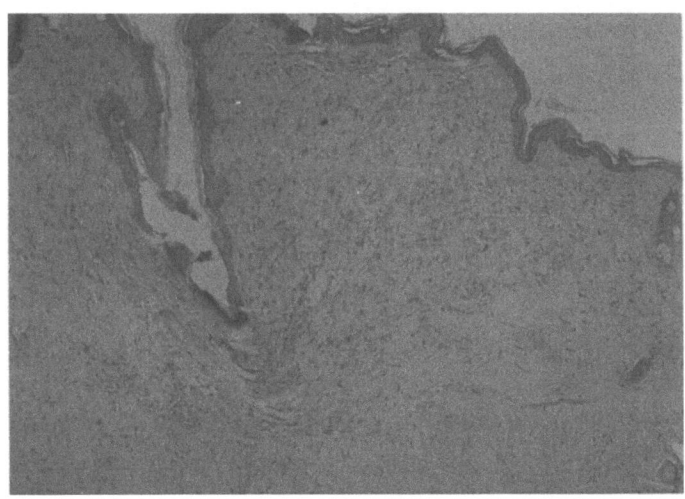

Fig. 8. Histological sample (X 32 Hematoxiline/Eosine-H.E.) The epithelium is well constituted and cells are well matured. The dermis is not organized and there exist few vessels

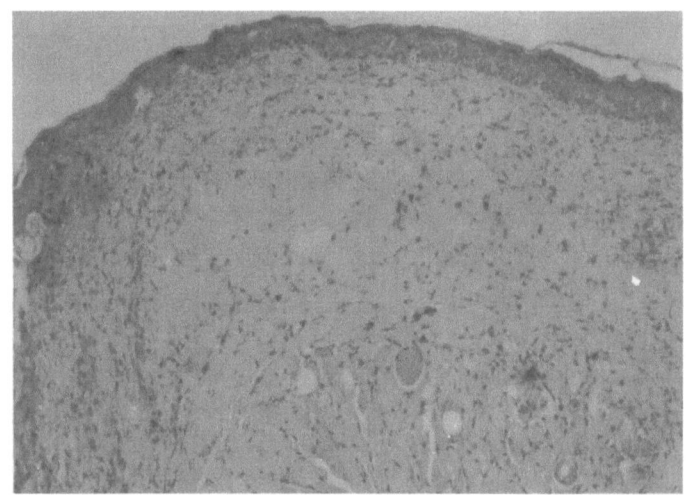

Fig. 9. X 32 H.E. Burn treated with He/Ne laser. The epithelium is prominent and it is of reactive type. The collagen in the dermis is more organized and with abundant and fine vessels

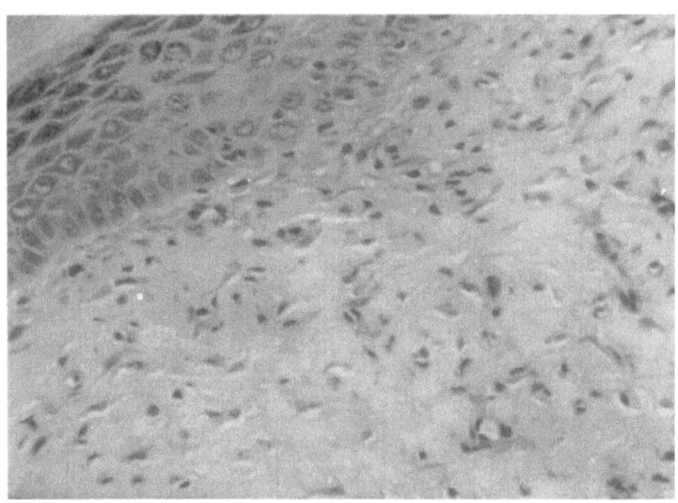

Fig. 10. Same histological sample as fig. 9, but at greater magnification (X 320 H.E.)

In group (A) the irradiated dermis presented a well defined structure of collagen fibres, significantly superior to group (B). In group (B) capillars were fewer and fine, and in group (A). They were abundant and neoformed on the superficial and deep dermis.

From a histological point of view, on day 27 after burning the lesion had not totaly recovered but, nevertheless, group (A) presented a more advanced stage of regeneration and the tissue had better quality than the control group (B), non-irradiated with laser.

COMMENTS AND CONCLUSIONS

Burn depth is related to the temperature of the agent which produces it, and varies according to the time of tissue exposure to heat. This circumstance defines the characteristics of cicatrization regarding major and minor complications. The practice of standarized experimental burns on animals using a burning prototype device facilitates the study of how these lesions react to diverse therapies.

Several papers report the interesting results that can be obtained when burns are irradiated with He/Ne laser, particularly those burns of I and II degree, in which an excellent reepithelization and protection against internal and external infection can be obtained. These effects have been related to a probable immunitary mechanism activated by laser irradiation.

In 1984 Interlandi (2) et al published their experience when burns of II and III degree were treated with laser. They obtained more rapid healing of the lesions without complications in comparison to conventional therapeutic methods used before. By using laser treatment it was possible to avoid the risk of queloids, fibrosis, and retractil scarring as well as to minimize the risk of infections. Later, these facts were confirmed by Teich-Alasia (3) et al on a large casuistic. We ourselves, communicated in 1985 (4) our observations on experimental burns of II and III degree on the MRL25 mouse, noting the benefits that could be obtained by using He/Ne laser irradiation.

Obviously our experiment does not consider the extensive burn cases in which some other important precautions, such as the rehydratation procedure should be taken into account as well as the antibiotic prophilaxis, and convenient lesion covering.

According to what we have observed laser irradiation should be done as soon as possible after burning in order to obtain best results against oedema and exudation. At the same time laser irradiation promotes rapid cicatrization and revascularization of lesion. The early granulation and reepithelization observed on the irradiated animals could avoid the formation of scarring and contractures.

The analisis of experimental burn reparation lead us to speculate that the more rapid cicatrization on irradiated animals does not only occur because of the increased blood circulation produced by low power laser. It might be assumed that another factor exists, which could be the heparine. This substance is released by mast cells degranulated more actively under laser irradiation (5). This hipothesis would favour those observations published by Moore and Saliba (6) on the beneficial effects of heparine for treatment of burns. According to these authors heparine avoids formation of microthrombs which intensifies cellular destruction. Heparine possesses strong qualities against inflammation, antialergic effects, effects against and proteolitics enzimes. All these effects collaborate in the rapid restoration of inflammated tissues. Heparine minimizes liquid accumulation and oedema formation, decreasing pain. From their clinical observations, Saliba et al, have noted that coagulation time is not altered even by using important quantities of heparine on burn patients. This fact agrees with Mayayo's (7) observations that on laser-irradiated tissues, vessels are dilated but without thrombotic or hemorragie phenomena.

On the other hand it has been noted on patients with important burns that blood has hipercoagulating characteristics, which indicates lack of heparine. Oraveskii and Pleshanov (8) have observed that laser irradiation of plasma and their components, which participate directly on the coagulation processes, increases their time of normal recalcification, showing 15 to 20% of free heparine.

From our casuistic we conclude that I degree burns which (epidermic burns) are, along with superficial dermic burns, that produce important pain, the principal indications of low power laser radiation. For deep dermic burns, laser radiation should be applied to regenerate the dermis and to afterwards produce an active epithelization and cicatrization by second intention. In case of subdermic burns we estimate that, before laser treatment, a surgical cleansing should be performed as early as possible. In these cases general care of the patient also should being taken.

REFERENCES

1.- Nubiola Calonge, P. (1983) Los Quemados. Mèdica Rural, 347 pp16:20

2.- Interlandi F., Roccia L. (1984) Nota clinica sui primi risultati nel trattamento delle ustioni con il laser He/Ne. Rev. Minerva Riflessoter. e Laserter., vol.I n.1 pp39:42

3.- Teich S., Alasia G., Magliacani G. (1984) La terapia laser nel trattamento delle ustioni. Rev. Minerva e Riflessoter. e Laserter., vol.I n.2 pp87:92

4.- Trelles M.A., Mayayo E., Smith V., Dalmases F. (1985) Observación experimental de los efectos de la irradiación láser de baja intensidad en las quemaduras y su aplicación clínica. Comunicación en el Congreso Láser España 85. Barcelona.

5.- Trelles M.A., Mayayo E., Miro L., Baudin G. (1986) Mast Cells and Low-Power Laser: Analysis of its components before and after Irradiation. Lasers in Medical Science, vol.I n.4 pp299

6.- Moore F.D., Saliba J. (1978) Remedio natural para las quemaduras. Tiempos Médicos, n.131 pp101:104

7.- Mayayo E. (1987) Low Power Laser Radiation Acts on Mast Cells Degranulation. Proceedings Optoelektronik, 87. En Prensa.

8.- Oraevskii A.N., Pleshanov P.G. (1978) Selective photochemical mechanisms of the biological action of laser radiation. Sov. J. Quantum Electron., 8(10) pp1263:1267

Effects of Laser Radiation over Zusanli Point on Egg of the Aged

Peng Yue. Gao-Hui He, Zhang Dong
Institute of Acupuncture and Moxibustion/Academy
of Traditional Chinese Medicine, Beijing. China
No.3 Haiyuncang, Dongzhimennei

For exploring the effects of laser radiation over ZuSanli point on the e EGG of the healthy aged, fourty-three subjects were selected for the study. The result as follows:

Fourty-three healthy ageds, aged above 45, free of disease and having not received medication for two weeks prior were selected for the study. 20 males and 23 females in the laser group, 2 males and 23 females in the control group. No drugs were administered during the course of this study.

Methods and Materials

The EGG was recorded with the apparatus of EGG-IA after and before radiation on ZuSanli point. The G2-1A of He-Ne laser fiber acupuncture apparatus was used for laser radiation on ZuSanli point. The wavelength was 6328A, output power 2-3mw and light spot diameter 2mm. At the beginning, the subject was kept lie still for 15'. In the meanwhile, EGG should be recorded. Then the ZuSanli point should be radia-ted by the laser for 15'. During the laser radiation and after radia-tion 15 minutes, the EGG should also be recorded. The control group was used the same method except no laser radiation on ZuSanli point.

Result and analysis:

This result showed that the frequency of EGG of body surface has not been changed by laser radiation on ZuSanli point. There was no signifi-cant difference in laser and control group($P > 0.05$). But the slow wave's amplitude could be regulated by laser radiation on ZuSanli point. After radiation on ZuSanli point, the lower wave's amplitude could be raised and the higher waves' amplitude reduced. Both of them indicated a statistically siginificant difference($P < 0.05$). There was no change in the normal waves' amplitude and control group after laser radiation($P > 0.05$).

Someone regarded as the slow waves' amplitude of EGG being raised during the increase of gastric motion or vice versa. So it should be considered that the effect of laser radiation over ZuSanli point on EGG is a normalizing action. The slow Waves' amplitude of EGG can be regulated according to the different condition of the gastric motion.

This result suggested that the effect of laser radiation over ZuSanl-li point on EGG is a biphasic regulating action. It is helpful to explain the mechanism of effect of health-care of ZuSanli point further.

Preliminary Study on the Biostimulation of Low Power Laser Therapy

K.Kamikawa
Meiji College of Oriental Medicine
Hiyoshicho, Funaigun, Kyoto 629-03, Japan

1. Introduction

Pain relief by low power laser is acknowledged as one of the biophysical laser applications. Generally He-Ne and diode lasers are used in pain clinics and YAG laser is used in some clinics. It is hard to find a standard for the practice of laser therapy of pain, becuase so many varieties of technical procedures and irradiation modalities have been reported. The thermographic findings during YAG and diode laser therapy of pain revealed more or less thermal effect on the lased region. The local circulatory increment produced by laser stimulation was influenced by the irradiation dose, however the therapeutic results were not always consistent with the irradiation dose and were not differentiated by continuous and pulsed irradiations. Absorption of these lasers in a milk showed similar patterns of energy distribution and the increased frequency of the pulsed laser resulted in an increment of average power in the pictures taken with infrared camera. It was interesting to find the interference fringe in the picture of the finger transilluminated with diode laser. These findings were reported in the Third International Nd:YAG Laser Symposium in 1986. The author hypothesized that coherency of laser beam may influence the structural water in the tissue and initiate a chemical process to produce the biostimulation. An experiment was designed to explore the influence of laser on water molecules in the living tissue.

2. Materials and Methods

A chemical shift of proton signal was recorded with FT-NMR apparatus (JNR FT-90Q, Japan Electron Optics Lavoratory) and figured with XY recorder. Materials were an albumen of a chicken egg, a slug and a silkworm. Material was put in the sample tube 5 mm in diameter and laser was irradiated through the glass wall of the tube. CW and pulsed diode lasers were used. The former was 830 nm of wavelength, 10 mW of exit power. The latter was 890 nm of wavelength, 10 W at peak power, 100 ns of pulse width, repetitive rate up to 10 kHz. Laser beam was focused

with lens in the spot of less than 1 mm in diameter. Proton sinnal was
recorded with RF of 89.55 MHz and the temperature in the box of the NMR
apparatus was set to keep the room temperature. As proton signals recorded from the animals were not stable, they were traced every 30 seconds on the same recording paper shifting from top to bottom. A slug
was chosen, as it was obtained through the year and was easy to be put
in the sample tube. A silkworm of proper size was fit with the tube to
minimize the movement of the body, but the available chance of it was
limitted. An albumen of a chicken egg was used as static material.
Following the recording of the proton signals, the material was irradiated with laser for 3 minutes. Immediately after the irradiation, the
sample tube was returned to the previous position and the recording was
continued for 10 minutes and was extended if necessary.

3.   Results

The experiment was carried out exclussively with a slug. Contorary to
expectation, the proton signals recorded from a slug were not always
stable even in the static state. Slight dislocation of the sample tube
caused significant influence on the proton signals. Needless to say,
the movement of the animal deformed the proton signals. The experiment
had little chance of success.

Fig.1 is one of available data. The upper five traces were recorded

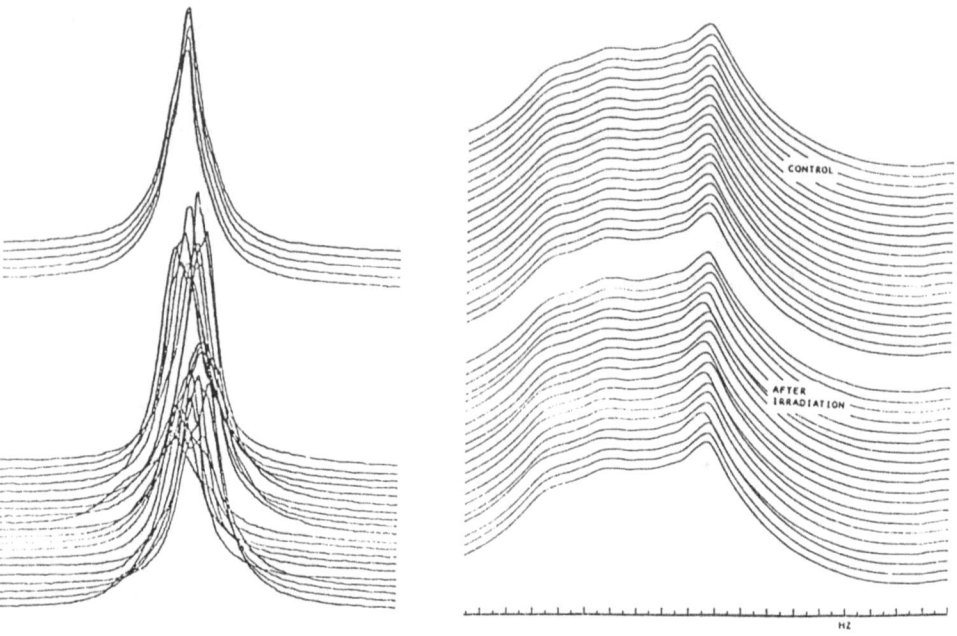

Fig. 1.   Fig. 2.

before irradiation. They looked stable at first glance, but the signals shifted to right and left spontaneously. The pulsed diode laser of 10 W at peak power, 1 kHz of repetitive rate was irradiated for 3 minutes. After irradiation the swing of the signals got remarkable and the signals were deformed a few minutes later. These changes suggested the movement of the animals. While the initial chemical shift seemed to be related the influence of laser on water mulecules in the living tissue. A dozen of the similar recordings were obtained, however there was no proof to confirm the speculation.

Concerning a silkworm, CW diode laser of 1 mW was irradiated to the rostral and caudal portion individually. The irradiation for 3 minutes resulted in moderate shift of the proton signals.

As illustrated in Fig.2, the proton signals of an albumen recorded with d6 acetone were stable. Irradiation of pulsed diode laser of 10 W at peak power, 10 kHz of repetitive rate, for 3 minutes caused moderate shift of the proton signals. They swung on both side for more than 10 minutes after irradiation and returned stable 30 minutes later.

4. Discussion

The animal showed spontaneous shift of the proton signals, which were deformed by the movement. It is hard to identify the chemical shift due to laser irradiation, because the proton signals were so susceptible to the environment. But the results recorded from an albumen indicated the influence of laser on the environment of water molecules. Lack of data during irradiation should be supplemented by the technical improvment. It is necessary to examine with lower dose of laser to avoid excessive stimulation. This experiment was designed based on the molecular theory proposed by L.Pauling.[1] He suggested the block of the ion transportation by the hydrate of the anesthetics. Influence of laser on the proton signals should be analyzed not only on free and structural water but also on OH radicals of high molecular compounds.

5. Summary

Based on a working hypothesis that an influence of laser beam on the structural water in the tissue may initiate a chemical process for biostimulation, NMR study was carried out with a slug, a silkworm and an albumen irradiated by diode lasers. The results suggested a possible influence of laser on water molecules in the tissue, but the hypothesis was not proved in the preliminary experiment.

6. Reference

1) Pauling L: A molecular theory of general anesthesia. Science 134; 15-21, 1961.

Histological Evaluation of Effect of Low Power Laser on the Synovial Membrane of Rheumatoid Arthritis

Jun Nishida[*], Takuya Iwasaki[*], Ryoichi Satodate[*],
Masataka Abe[*], Yoshinori Oyamada[**]

[*] Departments of Pathology and Orthopedic Surgery
School of Medicine, Iwate Medical University
Uchimaru 19-1, Morioka 020, Japan

[**] Division of Orthopedic Surgery, National Hospital
in Hanamaki, Hanamaki 025-03, Japan

Only a few studies have been carried out on the effects of low power laser irradiation on the joints affected by rheumatoid arthritis (RA). Goldman et al.[1] and Oyamada et al.[2,3] reported the improvement of symptoms and signs of RA by laser irradiation. We have histologically examined the effects of low power helium-neon laser irradiation on the synovial membrane of the RA-affected knee joints.

MATERIALS AND METHODS

Patients: We irradiated 20 knees in 18 patients who had suffered from RA for 4 to 16 years, 11 years on average. The patients were between 26 and 70 years old, 49 years on average. All patients had classical RA according to the criteria of the American Reumatism Association, and advanced RA according to the classification of rheumatoid progression and functional capacity.

Laser therapy: The laser used in this study: medium, helium-neon gas; out-put, 8.5mW; wavelength, 632.8nm; spot size, 0.2mm; laser assemblage, Model PDT, Senko Medical Instrument CO., Tokyo. The duration of irradiation was 15 minutes per day, and irradiation was performed every other day, for a total of 12 to 46 times, 26 times on average. The medial part of the knee was irradiated by the laser. The lateral part was not irradiated. The energy transmitted to the medial synovial membrane was $0.328\mu W$ on average. Transmittance of the laser to the synovial membrane was 0.00409% on average. The synovial membrane received the energy of $3.77 \times 10^{-4} J/cm^2$ on average during the 15-minute irradiation. The laser beam was not transmitted to the synovial membrane of the lateral part.

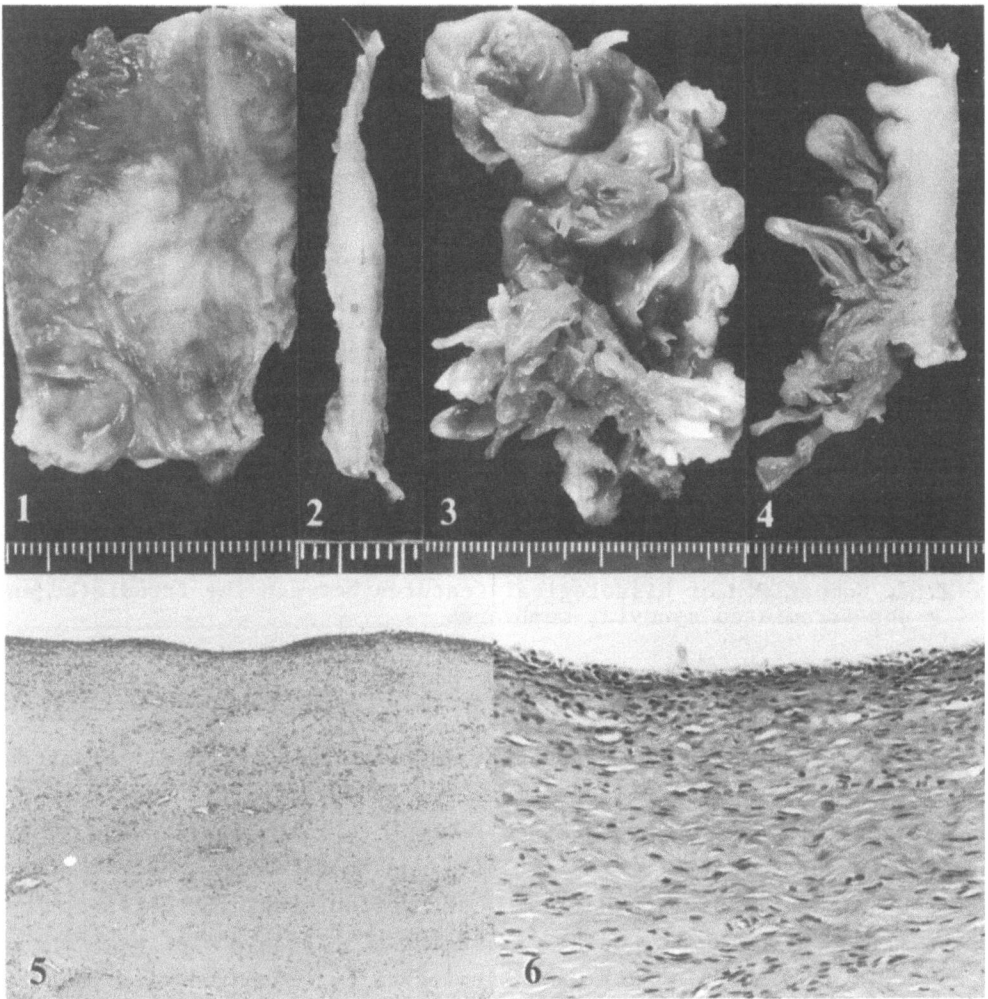

Figs. 1 and 2. Irradiated synovial membrane of the medial part of the knee. Villi disappear and the surface is flattened. The membrane becomes thin. Fig. 1, inner surface; and Fig. 2, cross section.

Figs. 3 and 4. Non-irradiated synovial membrane of the lateral part of the knee. Numerous villi proliferate on the synovial membrane. Fig. 3, inner surface; and Fig 4, cross section. Figs. 1-4 are the macroscopic views of the synovial membrane obtained from the same knee joint.

Figs. 5 and 6. Histological features of the irradiated synovial membrane. The surface of the synovial membrane becomes flattened. Cellular infiltration is slight. No proliferation of lining cells is seen. H.-E. stain. Fig. 6, 40 x; and Fig. 7, 110 x

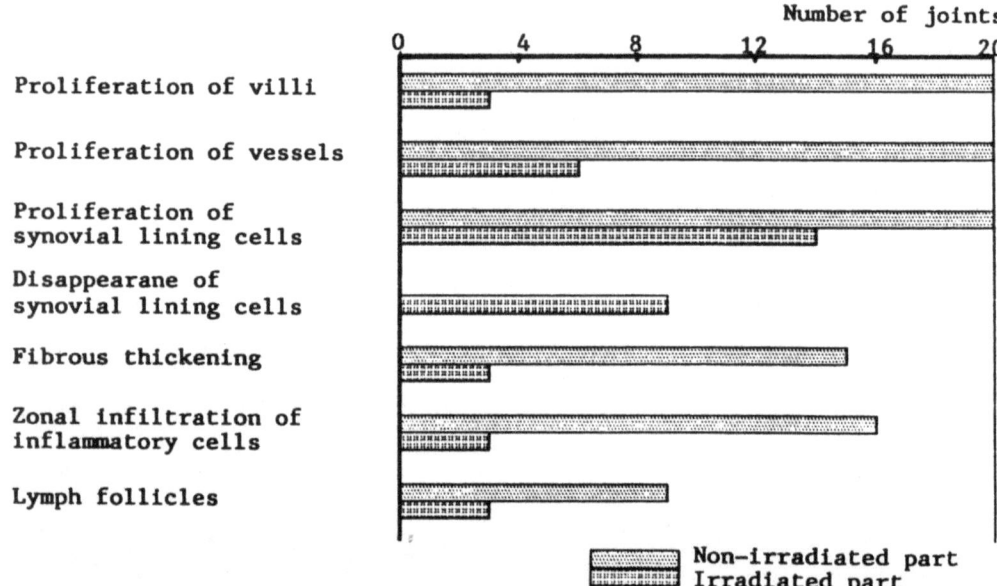

Fig. 7. Comparison of histological features between the irradiated and non-irradiated synovial membranes

Synovial membrane: The synovial membrane was obtained for microscopic examination at the operations for synovectomy or total knee replacement. The tissues were fixed in 15 % formalin for 4 days, dehydrated in an alcoholic series and embedded in paraffin. Sections were stained with hematoxylin and eosin, the periodic acid Schiff reaction, methylgreen pyronin and the Giemsa staining. The synovial membrane of the irradiated medial part was histologically compared with that of the non-irradiated lateral part.

RESULTS

The irradiated synovial membrane became smooth and thin (Figs. 1 and 2), but the non-irradiated synovial membrane was thick with numerous villi (Figs. 3 and 4). Figs. 5 and 6 show the histological features of the irradiated synovial membrane. The histological comparison of the irradiated and non-irradiated parts is summarized in Fig. 7.
In the irradiated synovial membrane, proliferation of villi was observed in 15% of the knees, proliferation of blood vessels in 30%, proliferation of lining cells in 70%, although those were observed in 100% in the non-irradiated synovial membrane. Partial disappearance

of lining cells was present in 45% in the irradiated synovial membrane. In addition, deposition of fibrin was decreased from 25% in the non-irradiated to 10% in the irradiated, fibrous thickening from 75% to 15%, zonal cellular infiltration from 80% to 15%, presence of lymph follicles from 45% to 15%, and germinal centers from 25% to 5%.

DISCUSSION

Biological effects of the laser have been classified into a thermal[4], photo-toxic[5], photo-chemical[6] and biostimulation effects[7,8]. In our study, the thermal effect on the synovial membrane could be excluded because we used a cold-type laser. The improvement of RA by low power laser irradiation may be the result of long-term and repeated biostimulation or a photo-toxic effect of the laser. In addition, the immunological effect of the laser may also be important because laser irradiation is thought to have an immunosuppressive effect[9,10].

Although the mechanism of the laser effect on the RA-affected joints could not be clarified in this study, the gross and histological appearances revealed that the low power laser irradiation was very effective for RA-affected joints.

REFERENCES
1. Goldman, J. A., Chiapella, J., Casey, H. et al.: Laser therapy of rheumatoid arthritis. Lasers Surg. Med. 1: 93-101, 1980.
2. Oyamada, Y. and Izu, S.: Application of low energy laser in chronic rheumatoid arthritis and related rheumatoid diseases. J. Japanese Soc. Laser Med. 6: 375-378, 1986. (In Japanese.)
3. Oyamada, Y., Tajima, Y., Yoshida, M. et al.: Therapeutic effect of low energy laser. Operation 40: 1905-1914, 1986. (In Japanese.)
4. Kleinkort, J. A., and Foley, R. A.: Laser acupuncture: Its use in physical therapy. Am. J. Acupuncture 12: 51-56, 1984.
5. Tomson, S. H.: Tumor destruction due to acridine orange photoactivation by argon laser. Ann. N. Y. Acad. Sci. 267: 191-200, 1976.
6. Schenk, P., Porteder, H. and Zetner, K.: Helium-Neon-Laser-Effekt auf Haut und orale Schleimhautgewebe. Laryng. Rhinol. Otol. 65: 146-150, 1986.
7. Fenyo, M.: Theoretical and experimental basis of biostimulation by laser irradiation. Optics and Laser Technology, 16: 209-215, 1984.
8. Kubasova, T., Kovács, L., Somosy, Z. et al.: Biological effect of He-Ne laser: Investigations on functional and micromorphological alterations of cell membranes, in vitro. Lasers Surg. Med. 4: 381-388, 1984.
9. Mester, E., Mester, A. F. and Mester, A.: The biomedical effects of laser application. Lasers Surg. Med. 5: 31-39, 1985.
10. Mester, E., Nagylucskay, S., Tisza, S. et al.: Neuere Untersuchungen über die Wirkung der Laserstrahlen auf die Wundheilung - Immunologische Effekte. Z. Exper. Chirurg. 10: 301-306, 1977.

Cont. Wave Infrared Low Power Application Significantly Accelerates Chronic Pain Relief Rehabilitation of Professional Athletes. A Double Blind Study

C. Diamantopoulos, O. Emmanouilidis
48 Woodland Gardens, GB-London N10-3UA

Unlike other patients, professional athletes demand from their therapists the quickest return into their games. The purpose of our study was to confirm that cont. wave infrared low power laser therapy accelerates their complete rehabilitation.

M&M: We used direct contact application on pain trigger points with a C.W. 820nm, 15mW I.R. laser diode incorporated into a Biotherapy 3 unit (Omega Univ. Tech. Ltd, London). Two groups of chronic cases were selected and matched according to pain and history/pathology and sport activities. The placebo group was given daily similar treatment with sham identical diode probes. Treatment was given daily for maximum 15 minutes irrespective of the number of pain trigger points. E ch selected pain trigger point was adminsitrered with 4J/cm². Contact thermography, VAP questionaire, point pressure and statistic tests were used to assess the results. Where applicable, swelling or other physiological changes were measured before and during the course of the treatments.

RESULTS

1) Out of the 31 athletes (9F/22M) in the placebo group, only 4 (3F/1M) showed significant pain relief after 10 placebo treatments.

2) In the laser group of 31 (9F/22M) athletes
   a) 18 were classified as healed by the 7,8,9,10th treatment. Irradiation continued to complete the relapse (excellent).
   b) 9 (3F/6M) showed complete pain relief by the 10th treatment (excellent) but 3M of this group returned for further treatment.
   A further treatment of 4 sessions produced again pain relief without relapse (good).

CONCLUSION

Since failure rates were very low we consider that the therapy with this I.R. low power laser diode in sport medicine is highly recommended.

Optoelektronik in der Medizin 1983
Optoelectronics in Medicine 1983

Vorträge des 6. Internationalen Kongresses
Proceedings of the 6th International Congress
Laser 83 Optoelektronik
Herausgeber/Editor: **W. Waidelich**
1984. 181 Abbildungen. XV, 273 Seiten
Broschiert DM 78,-. ISBN-13: 978-3-540-18130-9

Inhaltsübersicht: Highlights in der Lasermedizin. - Laser in der Neurochirurgie. - Laser in der Chirurgie. - Laser und Infrarot Koagulator in der Gastroenterologie. - Laser in der Urologie. - Laser in der Gynäkologie. - Laser in der Dermatolgie. - Laser Photomedizin. - Laser Photobiologie. - Laser Optoelektronische Diagnosesysteme. - Laser Sicherheit.

Optoelektronik in der Technik 1983
Optoelectronics in Engineering 1983

Vorträge des 6. Internationalen Kongresses
Proceedings of the 6th International Congress
Laser 83 Optoelektronik
Herausgeber/Editor: **W. Waidelich**
1984. 537 Abbildungen. XXII, 680 Seiten (320 Seiten in Englisch). Broschiert DM 118,-.
ISBN-13: 978-3-540-18130-9

Inhaltsübersicht: Laser-Systeme für Forschung. - Optoelektronische Komponenten und Sensoren. - Optronisches und lasertechnisches Messen und Prüfen. - Laser in der Materialbearbeitung. - Optoelektronische Signalübertragung. - Laser und Optoelektronik in der Weltraumtechnik. - Laser in der Umweltmeßtechnik. - Optoelektronische Displays. - Laser-Chemie. - Laser Sicherheit. - Photovoltaische Solartechnik. - VDI-Technologiezentrum: Industrielle Umsetzung der Lasertechnologie.

Springer-Verlag
Berlin Heidelberg New York
London Paris Tokyo

Optoelectronics in Medicine

Proceedings of the 5th International Congress
Laser 81
Editor: **W. Waidelich**
1982. 150 figures (11 figures in colour).
XI, 239 pages. Soft cover DM 62,-.
ISBN-13: 978-3-540-18130-9

Contents: Milestones in Laser Medicine. - Laser in Surgery. - Laser in Urology. - Laser in Dermatology. - Laser in Gynaecology. - Laser in Otorhinopharyncology. - Photobiology and Laser Photomedicine. - Laser and Optoelectronics in Medical Diagnosis. - Laser in Dental Technique.

Optoelektronik in der Technik
Optoelectronics in Engineering

Vorträge des 5. Internationalen Kongresses
Proceedings of the 5th International Congress
Laser 81
Herausgeber/Editor: **W. Waidelich**
1982. 504 Abbildungen. XXII, 580 Seiten (266 Seiten in Englisch). Broschiert DM 88,-.
ISBN-13: 978-3-540-18130-9

Contents: Laser Systeme/Laser Systems. - Laser-Spectroskopie und Laser-Chemie/Laser Spectroscopy and Laser-Chemistry. - Lasertechnisches Messen und Prüfen/Laser Measurement and Testing. - Laser in der Materialbearbeitung/Lasers in Material Processing. - Laser in der Umweltmesstechnik/Lasers in Environmental Measuring Techniques. - Laser und Optoelektronik in der Weltraumtechnik/Lasers and Optoelectronics in Space Techniques. - Optoelektronische Komponenten/Optoelectronic Components. - Optoelektronische Signalübertragung/Optoelectronic Signal Transmission. - Optoelektronische Bildaufnahme/Optoelectronic Image Pickup. - Optoelektronische Bild- und Datenaufzeichnungen/Optoelectronic Image and Data Recording. - Optoelektronische Bildverarbeitung/Optoelectronic Image Processing. - Optoelektronische Solartechnik/Optoelectronic Solar Technique.

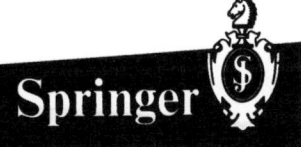

W. Waidelich
Laser/Optoelektronik in der Technik 1985
Laser/Optoelectronics in Engineering 1985
Vorträge des 7. Internationalen Kongresses
Proceedings of the 7th International Congress
Laser 1985 Optoelektronik

1986. 682 Abbildungen. XXVIII, 834 Seiten. (445 Seiten in Englisch). Broschiert DM 158,-. ISBN-13: 978-3-540-18130-9

Inhaltsübersicht: Sitzungsleiter. - Referenten. - Laser als Wirtschaftsfaktor. - Laser-Anwendung in der Chemie. - Laser-Komponenten. - Laser- und Optoelektronische Meßtechnik. - Laser-Systeme. - Laser in der Materialbearbeitung. - Holographische Interferometrie. - Optische Signalübertragung. - Laser und Optoelektronik in der Weltraumtechnik. - Laser und Optoelektronik in der Umweltmeßtechnik.

W. Waidelich, P. Kiefhaber
Laser/Optoelektronik in der Medizin 1985
Laser/Optoelectronics in Medicine 1985
Vorträge des 7. Internationalen Kongresses
Proceedings of the 7th International Congress
Laser 85 Optoelektronik

1986. 243 Abbildungen. XXVI, 531 Seiten. (334 Seiten in Englisch). Broschiert DM 118,-. ISBN-13: 978-3-540-18130-9

Inhaltsübersicht: Sitzungsleiter. - Referenten. - Laser-Dermatologie. - Laser-Chirurgie. - Laser-Gynäkologie. - Photodynamische Therapie. - Laser-Biostimulation. - Laser-Sicherheit. - Optoelektronische Meßverfahren und Laser für medizinische Anwendungen. - Laser-Photobiologie. 2nd International Nd: YAG Laser Conference (New Developments; Gastroenterology; Neurosurgery; Ophthalmology; Otolaryngology; Pulmonary Cardiology; Dermatology; Oral Surgery; Gynaecology; Urology).

Laser/Optoelektronik in der Technik 1987
Laser/Optoelectronics in Engineering 1987
Vorträge des 8. Internationalen Kongresses
Proceedings of the 8th International Congress
Laser 87 Optoelektronik

Herausgeber/Editor: W. Waidelich

1987. 575 Abbildungen. XXII, 710 Seiten. Broschiert DM 158,-. ISBN-13: 978-3-540-18130-9

Inhaltssübersicht: Lasersysteme/Laser Systems. - Optische Mess- und Prüftechnik/Optical Measuring and Testing. - Laser in der Materialbearbeitung/Laser in Material Processing. - Laser und Optische Informationstechnik/Laser and Optical Information Technique. - Laser und Optoelektronik in der Weltraumtechnik/Laser and Optoelectronics in Space Technology. - Workshop-VDI Technologiezentrum. - Industrie und Laser im Jahre 2000 - Einsatzbereiche und Anwendungen/Industry and Lasers in the year 2000 - Areas of Use and Applications.

Springer-Verlag
Berlin Heidelberg New York
London Paris Tokyo

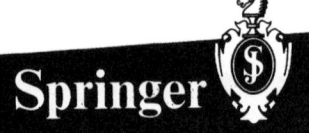

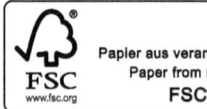

If you have any concerns about our products,
you can contact us on
ProductSafety@springernature.com

In case Publisher is established outside the EU,
the EU authorized representative is:
**Springer Nature Customer Service Center GmbH
Europaplatz 3, 69115 Heidelberg, Germany**

Printed by Libri Plureos GmbH
in Hamburg, Germany